Applied Basic Science for Basic Surgical Training

For Churchill Livingstone:

Commissioning editor: Laurence Hunter
Project development manager: Barbara Simmons
Project manager: Nancy Arnott
Designer: Erik Bigland
Artist: Peter Lamb

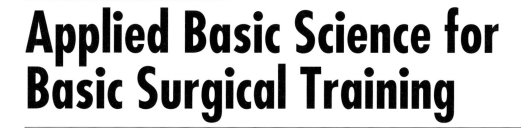

Applied Basic Science for Basic Surgical Training

Edited by

Andrew T. Raftery BSc MD CI Biol MI Biol FRCS

Consultant Surgeon, Sheffield Kidney Institute, Sheffield Teaching Hospitals NHS Trust, Northern General Hospital, Sheffield, UK;
Member (formerly Chairman) of the Court of Examiners, Royal College of Surgeons of England;
Examiner MRCS Royal College of Surgeons of Edinburgh;
Member of Panel of Examiners, Intercollegiate Speciality Board in General Surgery;
Honorary Senior Clinical Lecturer in Surgery, University of Sheffield

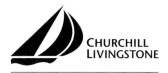

CHURCHILL
LIVINGSTONE

EDINBURGH LONDON NEW YORK OXFORD PHILADELPHIA ST LOUIS SYDNEY TORONTO 2000

CHURCHILL LIVINGSTONE
An imprint of Elsevier Limited

First published 2000

ISBN 0 443 06144 0
 Reprinted 2001, 2003, 2004 (twice), 2005

International Edition 0 443 06143 2
 Reprinted 2001, 2004 (twice), 2005

British Library Cataloguing in Publication Data
A catalogue record for this book is available from the British Library.

Library of Congress Cataloging in Publication Data
A catalog record for this book is available from the Library of Congress.

Medical knowledge is constantly changing. As new information becomes available, changes in treatment, procedures, equipment and the use of drugs become necessary. The author and the publishers have, as far as it is possible, taken care to ensure that the information given in this text is accurate and up to date. However, readers are strongly advised to confirm that the information, especially with regard to drug usage, complies with the latest legislation and standards of practice.

 ELSEVIER your source for books, journals and multimedia in the health sciences
www.elsevierhealth.com

Working together to grow
libraries in developing countries
www.elsevier.com | www.bookaid.org | www.sabre.org

ELSEVIER BOOK AID International Sabre Foundation

The
publisher's
policy is to use
**paper manufactured
from sustainable forests**

Printed in China
N/06

Preface

In recent years considerable changes have taken place in medical education at both undergraduate and post-graduate level. Formerly medical students would have had such a good grounding in basic medical sciences that when they subsequently took professional examinations as postgraduates it would merely have been a matter of revision and recall. With changes in the undergraduate medical curriculum the content of basic science is now greatly reduced and subsequently graduates who approach the basic professional examinations of the Surgical Colleges have a great deal more new information to learn. It is now not just a matter of revision and recall. Despite the fact that the content of basic science in the new Membership (MRCS) has been reduced, candidates still need to acquire a knowledge of basic science which will allow them to understand the principles behind the management of patients and the practical procedures that they will be expected to carry out as basic surgical trainees. The more detailed basic science will be learned as part of Higher Surgical Training in a chosen specialty.

This book has been written to encompass the basic anatomy, physiology and pathology required by the syllabuses of the Royal Colleges. The book is divided into two sections, the first covering the basic principles of pathology and microbiology and the second covering the anatomy, physiology and special pathology of the systems which a basic surgical trainee would be expected to know. An attempt has been made to indicate the clinical relevance of the facts and the reason for learning them. The authors are all experts in their field and many of them are experienced examiners at various Royal Colleges. There is some repetition and overlap between chapters which has been retained where it was considered necessary for the smooth continuity of reading a particular section, rather than cross-referring to other sections of the book. Although this book was written with basic surgical training in mind, it should provide a rapid revision for basic science for higher surgical training, and may even stimulate the motivated undergraduate who thirsts for more knowledge. I hope that this book will prove to be straightforward and readable and will provide the necessary knowledge in an integrated form that the basic surgical trainee requires for the MRCS examinations.

Acknowledgements

I am extremely grateful to the publishers Harcourt and in particular to Laurence Hunter, Commissioning Editor, and Barbara Simmons, Project Development Manager, for their support and help with this project. I am also grateful to my fellow authors for their time and effort in ensuring that their manuscripts were produced on time. Lastly, but by no means least, I would like to thank my secretaries, Miss Louise Griffiths and Mrs Maureen Woods for typing the manuscript and my wife Anne for collating, organising, and reorganising the whole manuscript on her word processor. I could not have completed the task without her.

Many of the illustrations have been reproduced from Textbook of Anatomy by A. W. Rogers, published by Churchill Livingstone in 1992, and General and Systematic Pathology edited by J. C. E. Underwood, 2nd edition, published by Churchill Livingstone in 1996.

Andrew T Raftery
Sheffield 2000

Contributors

Ken G. Callum MS FRCS
Consultant Vascular Surgeon, Derbyshire Royal
Infirmary, Derby, UK; Member of the Court of
Examiners, Royal College of Surgeons of England

Christopher R. Chapple BSc MD FRCS (Urol)
Consultant Urological Surgeon, Royal Hallamshire
Hospital, Central Sheffield University Hospitals,
Sheffield, UK; Director of the Postgraduate Office of the
European Association of Urology (The European School
of Urology)

Dennis W.K. Cotton BSc PhD BM MD FRCPath
Consultant Pathologist, Central Sheffield University
Hospitals, Sheffield; Reader in Pathology, University of
Sheffield School of Medicine, Sheffield, UK; Member of
the Court of Examiners, Royal College of Surgeons of
England; Examiner for the Royal College of
Pathologists; Examiner for the Royal Institute for Public
Health and Hygiene

Andrew Dyson MB ChB FRCA
Consultant Anaesthetist, Kings Mill Centre, Sutton in
Ashfield, Nottinghamshire, UK

William Egner PhD MB ChB MRCP MRCPath
Consultant Immunologist, Northern General NHS Trust
Sheffield, UK

David E. Hughes BMed Sci MB ChB PhD MRC Path
Consultant Histopathologist and Cytopathologist,
Department of Pathology, Chesterfield and North
Derbyshire Royal Hospital NHS Trust, Chesterfield;
Honorary Clinical Lecturer in Pathology, University of
Sheffield, UK

Samuel Jacob MB BS MS (Anatomy)
Senior Lecturer, Department of Biomedical Science,
University of Sheffield, Sheffield, UK; Member of the
Court of Examiners, Royal College of Surgeons of
England

Richard L. M. Newell BSc MB BS FRCS
Clinical Anatomist, School of Biosciences, University of
Wales, Cardiff, UK; Honorary Consultant Orthopaedic
Surgeon, Royal Devon and Exeter Health Trust, Exeter,
UK; Member of the Court of Examiners, Royal College
of Surgeons of England

M. Andrew Parsons MB ChB FRCPath
Senior Lecturer and Honorary Consultant in Ophthalmic
Pathology, Royal Hallamshire Hospital, Sheffield, UK;
Director, Ophthalmic Sciences Unit, University of
Sheffield; Examiner, Royal College of Ophthalmologists

George Proud MD BS BDS FRCS
Consultant Surgeon, Royal Victoria Infirmary,
Newcastle Upon Tyne, UK; Member of the Court of
Examiners and Chairman MRCS Clinical Examination
Group, Royal College of Surgeons of England; Regional
Adviser for Surgery, Northern Region and Regional
Specialty Adviser for General Surgery

Clive R.G. Quick MA MS FDS FRCS
Consultant Surgeon, Hinchingbrooke Hospital,
Huntingdon and Addenbrooke's Hospital, Cambridge,
UK; Member of the Court of Examiners, Royal College
of Surgeons of England; Associate Lecturer, University
of Cambridge, Cambridge, UK

Timothy J. Stephenson MA MD Dip HSM FRCPath
Consultant Histopathologist, Central Sheffield
University Hospitals, Sheffield, UK; Member of the
Histopathology Examiners Panel, Royal College of
Histopathologists

Jenny Walker ChM FRCS
Consultant Paediatric Surgeon, Sheffield Children's
Hospital, Sheffield, UK

Contents

General pathology and microbiology

1

Cellular injury

Dennis W K Cotton

The cell is a homeostatic mechanism which attempts to retain a stable state in the presence of environmental fluctuations. If the environmental fluctuations are sufficiently large, they will change the state of the cell, which will then attempt to return to its usual condition; if the changes in the cell are large enough to significantly disturb its function then we refer to these as cellular injury. In any particular case it may be difficult to tell whether a measured change is due to damage or is due to some meaningful response on the part of the cell.

By *cell injury* we mean that the cell has been exposed to some influence that has left it living, but functioning at less than optimum level. The end result of this may be:

(a) total recovery
(b) permanent impairment
(c) death.

On the whole, (b) is the least likely because cells are capable of significant reparative processes, and if they survive an insult, they generally repair it; if the damage is very severe but not lethal the cell may activate mechanisms that result in its own death.

Cell injury can be caused by a variety of mechanisms, including:

• physical
• chemical
• biological processes.

Cell death may result in replacement by:

• a cell of the same type
• a cell of another type
• non-cellular structures.

The cell is a highly structured complex of molecules and organelles that are arranged to fulfil routine metabolic housekeeping functions and the specialised functions that make one cell different from another. In order to carry out these functions the cell has energy needs and some transport mechanisms to facilitate import of metabolites and export of waste products. Injury to a cell results in relative disruption to one or more of theses structures or functions.

MORPHOLOGY OF CELL INJURY
LIGHT MICROSCOPY

The microscopic appearance of damaged cells is sometimes characteristic of a particular cell type but is seldom specific to the type of damage. When we refer to changes in appearance, we are talking about the appearances seen on histological preparations stained with various dyes; this is of course a long way from the biological processes that have caused the cell changes.

Hydropic change Cells that are damaged in some way that prevents control of fluid influx may swell and become pale as their contents are diluted. This is commonly the result of damage to membrane-bound ion pumps, the water following the ions passively.

Fatty change This is a characteristic change seen in liver cells as a response to cell injury from a variety of causes. Under the microscope the cells contain many small, or a single large vacuole. The vacuole(s) is empty because in life it contained fat but during histological processing this has dissolved out, leaving a hole. It is possible to identify the substance in such vacuoles by cutting a frozen section which does not involve exposure to fat solvents; the contents of the vacuoles can then be demonstrated using specific fat stains such as Sudan black or Oil red O. Fatty change in the liver occurs as a result of damage to energy-generating mechanisms and to protein synthesis since fat is transported out of the cell by energy-dependent protein carrier mechanisms and damage to these results in passive fat accumulation.

Eosinophilic change Haematoxylin stains acids such as DNA and RNA, and eosin stains proteins (proteins are amphoteric but contain many reactive bases). The cytoplasm contains proteins and RNA among other things. Cellular damage often results in a diminution of cytoplasmic RNA, and thus the colour of such cells becomes slightly less purple and more pink (eosinophilic). This is a characteristic of myocardiocytes in the early stages of ischaemia and may often be the only histologically visible change in postmortem tissue.

Nuclear changes These may be subtle, such as the disposition of chromatin around the periphery of the nucleus, often referred to as clumping, or more extreme alterations such as condensation of the nucleus (pyknosis), fragmentation (karyorhexis) and dilatation of the perinuclear cisternae of the endoplasmic reticulum (karyolysis). A small circular structure, the nucleolus, becomes more apparent as the nucleus is activated; this is the centre for the production of mRNA. The nucleolus can be demonstrated by silver stains (the resulting granules being termed AgNORs or 'silver-staining nucleolar organiser regions') although what is actually stained are specific regions of the chromosomes concerned with nucleolar function. AgNOR staining is particularly abnormal in malignant transformed cells. Severe clumping and fragmentation of chromatin together with nuclear shrinkage and break-up is suggestive of cell death and is characteristic of *apoptosis*.

ELECTRON MICROSCOPY

At higher magnification in the transmission electron microscope, fine indicators of cell damage can be seen earlier than those seen on ordinary light microscopy, but they are not much more specific. The general effects of loss of transmembrane ion and water control leads to swollen cells and swelling of mitochondria, both dependent upon the loss of ability to exclude calcium from the cell and from the mitochondrion. Smooth endoplasmic reticulum is dilated, and the ribosomes fall off the rough endoplasmic reticulum. Nuclear changes are similar to, but more pronounced than, those seen at light microscopy.

ACCUMULATIONS

If a late step in a non-branching metabolic pathway is defective, either genetically or because of some form of trauma, then intermediates earlier in the pathway will accumulate. In some cases where there is branching of the pathway the accumulating materials may be diverted off into alternative processes and the end effect of the insult will be a loss of the usual products occurring after the defective step. Accumulations may be relatively inert, such as lipids occurring in the liver as described above,

and their only significance may be as markers of damage. In other cases the accumulated materials may have deleterious effects resulting from direct metabolic influences, e.g. acidosis due to accumulated lactate, or by simple bulk effects such as those seen in various lysosomal storage diseases. Exogenous compounds may be metabolised or stored, but both of these processes may have deleterious consequences. Substances such as carbon tetrachloride are themselves not toxic, but the body has a limited and stereotyped series of responses to external agents and, whilst these responses are on the whole effective at detoxification, in some instances they can result in the production of molecular species more toxic than the original ingested material. In this manner carbon tetrachloride is metabolised in the liver with the production of free radicals which cause severe damage. This can be inferred histologically since the liver damage does not occur around the portal vein branches where the carbon tetrachloride enters the liver but only at some distance from this in zone II as it becomes metabolised. In the case of ingested asbestos particles, these are taken up into macrophages and cause the disruption of lysosomes, with the release of hydrolytic enzymes. There is consequent minute scarring from this single cell event, but the fibres are then taken up into another macrophage and the process is repeated. Some materials are totally inert, such as carbon, and serve only to show that the individual has a history of exposure to this substance and, more importantly, perhaps to other substances.

Amyloid This is an extracellular material that accumulates in many different conditions and causes problems by a simple bulk effect. It accumulates around vessels and in general causes problems by progressive vascular occlusion. The common feature of all the conditions underlying amyloidosis is the production of large amounts of active proteins. These proteins are inactivated by transformation of their physical form into beta-pleated sheets which are inert (silk is a beta-pleated sheet, which is why silk sutures are not metabolised in the human body). The human body has no enzymes for metabolising beta-pleated sheets, and amyloid therefore accumulates. The material is waxy in appearance and reacts with iodine to form a blue-black pigment similar to the product of reaction of starch and iodine (amyloid = starch-like). The disparate origins of the proteins constituting amyloid can be demonstrated, as the proteins often retain some of their immunohistochemical properties. The rationale of this process is that it removes excess metabolically active circulating proteins and stores them in an inert form, which is advantageous if the cause is short-lived but can be deleterious if the condition causing the protein production continues. The types of disease associated with amyloid production are: chronic inflammatory processes such as tuberculosis, rheumatoid disease and chronic osteomyelitis; tumours with a large production of protein, typically myeloma; and miscellaneous disease with protein production such as some inflammatory skin diseases, some tumours of endocrine glands and neurodegenerative diseases such as Alzheimer's.

Pigments Pigments of various sorts accumulate in cells and tissues. They may be endogenous or exogenous in origin and they represent a random collection of processes linked only by the fact that the materials happen to be coloured. When blood escapes from vessels into tissue the haemoglobin gives a dark grey-black colour to the bruise. As the haemoglobin is metabolised through bilirubin and biliverdin, it changes from green to yellow and is finally removed. Such haematomas generally have no significance unless they are very bulky or if they become infected. Other endogenous pigments include the bile pigments in obstructive jaundice. These can be seen in the skin and even more clearly in the sclera because they bind preferentially to elastin and this material occurs in greatest concentration in these tissues. Related pigments are found in the tissues in the porphyrias, but these absorb ultraviolet light and are not visibly coloured; however, they can transform this absorbed radiant energy into chemical energy, setting off free radical damage. Another pigment, beta-carotene, can be used in some porphyrias (erythropoetic protoporphyria) to quench free radical activity.

The commonest pigment in human skin is melanin, which is red, brown or black, but if it occurs in deep sites, as in blue naevi, can appear blue due to the Tindall effect. Melanin pigments do no harm, but they are often markers of pigmented tumour pathology. In widespread malignant melanoma the melanin production can be so great that melanin appears in the urine. Melanin production is under hormonal control, and ACTH, which is structurally related to MSH (melanocyte stimulating hormone), can cause pigmentation in situations in which it is produced in pathological amounts or iatrogenically. Melanosis coli is a heavy black pigmentation of the colon associated with anthracene laxative use and is unrelated to melanin and is itself inert.

Exogenous pigments are introduced in tattooing and some have been toxic in various ways. Another source for exogenous pigmentation is drugs and organic halogen compounds have often been implicated in abnormal pigmentation problems.

Crystal diseases These are another heterogeneous group of conditions, most of which affect joints, producing gout in the case of urate crystals and pseudogout in the case of pyrophosphate.

Lipofuscin This is a brown pigment that accumulates in ageing cells and is often called age pigment. It does not appear to cause any damage and is an incidental marker of ageing. It is mainly formed from old cellular membranes which have become cross linked as a result of free radical damage and which accumulate in residual bodies without being further metabolised. They are thought to be mainly of mitochondrial origin.

Calcification This occurs in two main pathological situations as well as physiologically in developing or healing bone: it occurs in normal tissues in the presence of high circulating levels of calcium ions (metastatic calcification) and in pathological tissue in the presence of normal serum levels of calcium (dystrophic calcification). Most calcium deposits are calcium phosphate in the form of hydroxyapatite and contain small amounts of iron and magnesium and other mineral salts.

Calcification occurs in two stages: *initiation* and *propagation*. Intracellular calcification begins in mitochondria, and in this context it is interesting to note that the earliest indicator of cell death is the influx of calcium into mitochondria. Extracellular initiation of calcification begins in small, membrane-bound matrix vesicles which seem to be derived from damaged or ageing cell membranes. They accumulate calcium and also appear to have phosphatases in them which release phosphate which binds the free calcium. Propagation is by subsequent crystal deposition which may be affected by a lowering of calcification inhibitors and the presence of free collagen.

CAUSATIVE AGENTS OF CELL DAMAGE
TRAUMA

This is a term that can be used to refer to the whole range of effects that can damage cells, tissues or organisms, but which is commonly restricted to mechanical damage. It is often lumped together with other non-chemical, non-biological forms of damage under the heading of *physical damage*, which includes extremes of temperature and the various forms of radiation.

Mechanical damage is seldom so specific that it acts only at the cellular level — such damage usually involves at least groups of adjacent cells — but the advent of laser techniques makes it possible to study individual cell damage at this level. If cells are damaged in this way they appear to be able to 'clot' small areas of cytoplasm and then to heal this by secreting new cell membrane.

Freezing cells slowly produces ice crystals which act as 'micro-knives' cutting macromolecules as they grow. Cryotechniques require very rapid freezing to prevent ice crystal formation, sometimes in conjunction with chemicals which inhibit crystal formation.

Heating cells introduces free energy and causes macromolecules to vibrate and break. Various intracellular mechanisms are present to repair these breaks, but there is a critical level at which cells are overwhelmed and death ensues. Enzymes have a temperature optimum at which their catalytic rate is maximum, and body temperature is carefully maintained in mammals and birds so that enzymes work close to this optimum. The optimum is not necessarily the maximum rate, and metabolism speeds up as temperature rises, so that fever states are catabolic. In some cases it seems that the body thermostat is deliberately reset at a higher level in an effort to deal with various infections, the causative organisms of which are even more temperature sensitive.

RADIATION

This may be in the form of electromagnetic waves or particles and also introduces free energy into cells. The longer the wavelength the lower the energy of the radiation, and at the very low wavelengths we are back in the realms of simple heat. In the case of radiation we have the added problem of iatrogenic damage since many medical activities involve exposing the patient to some form of radiation, including both diagnostic and therapeutic modalities. Most types of radiation used in medicine cause the formation of free ions; they are consequently lumped together as *ionising radiation*.

The problem of variation in energy level of radiation has led to considerable difficulty in establishing suitable measures of dose. The favoured unit currently is the *gray* (Gy) which is a unit of absorbed dose. One gray is equivalent to 100 rad (the older dose unit of *radiation absorbed dose*). However, since radiations are often mixed and since tissues have different sensitivities, a mathematically corrected dose called the effective dose equivalent is now used, and the unit of this is the *sievert* (Sv). The environment contains a number of sources of natural radiation and some degree of contaminant radiation. This varies from area to area and with occupations, but the average background exposure is in the area of 2.5 Sv/year in the UK. There is considerable debate as to what constitutes a safe level of background radiation or even if there is such a thing as a level of radiation below which no damage will occur. It seems reasonable to assume that no level of radiation can be considered safe

no matter how low it is since the safety is only a statistical statement of the likelihood of a mutational event and the probability can never be zero.

When radiation enters a cell it can be absorbed by macromolecules directly but more commonly it reacts with water to produce free radicals and these then interact with macromolecules such as proteins and DNA. Both enzyme and structural proteins depend on their three-dimensional structure for their function, and this three-dimensional structure is dependent upon various types of chemical bonds. These bonds are disrupted by radiation, mostly by the intermediation of free radicals, and the proteins are then incapable of performing their structural or enzymatic duties. Radiation-induced DNA damage includes

- strand breaks
- base alterations
- formation of new cross links.

DNA damage may have three possible consequences:

- cell death either immediately or at the next attempted mitosis
- repair and no further damage
- a permanent change in genotype.

Effects on tissues

Various tissues differ in their susceptibility to radiation, but in general the most rapidly dividing tissues are the most sensitive. Radiation damage to tissues is generally divided into acute and chronic effects, but the precise effects at any time are strongly dose related. Acute effects are related to cell death and are most marked in those cells that are generally dividing rapidly to replace physiological cell loss such as gut epithelium, bone marrow, gonads and skin. Damage is due to defective mitosis consequent upon DNA damage but also to vascular fragility as a result of endothelial damage. The chronic effects of radiation include atrophy which may be due to a reduction in cell replication combined with fibrosis. The initial insult may be vascular endothelial cell loss with exposure of the underlying collagen with subsequent platelet adherence and thrombosis. This is then incorporated into the vessel wall and is associated with intimal proliferation of endarteritis obliterans. With narrowing of the vessels due to endarteritis obliterans, there would be long term vascular insufficiency and consequent atrophy and fibrosis.

The effects of ionising radiation on specific tissues are indicated below.

Bone marrow

The effect of radiation is to suspend renewal of all cell

lines. Granulocytes are reduced before erythrocytes, which survive much longer. The ultimate outcome depends on the dose used and will vary from complete recovery to aplastic anaemia. In the long term survivor there is an increased incidence of leukaemia.

Skin

Irradiation of the epidermis results in cessation of mitosis with desquamation and hair loss. If enough stem cells survive, hair will regrow and any epidermal defects will regenerate. Damage to melanocytes will result in melanin deposition in the dermis, where it is ingested by phagocytic cells which remain in the skin and result in hyperpigmentation. Destruction of dermal fibroblasts will result in an inability to produce collagen and subsequently to thinning of the dermis. Damage to small vessels in the skin will result in thinning of their walls, with dilatation and tortuosity, and will result in telangiectasia. Larger vessels will undergo endarteritis obliterans with time.

Intestines

Irradiation of the surface epithelium of the small intestines will result in its loss with consequent diarrhoea and malabsorption. Damage to the full thickness of the wall will result in formation of strictures.

Gonads

Germ cells are very radiosensitive, and even with low doses sterility may be a consequence. Mutations may also occur in germ cells, which could result in a teratogenic effect.

Lung

The clinical effects of radiation toxicity to the lungs are dependent on the dose given, the volume of lung irradiated, and the duration of treatment. Progressive pulmonary fibrosis usually occurs.

Kidney

Irradiation of the kidney usually results in gradual loss of parenchyma, resulting in impaired renal function. Damage to renal vessels results in intrarenal artery stenosis with the development of hypertension.

Ionising radiation and tumours

This is further discussed in Chapter 5. There is a clear relationship between ionising radiation and tumours. This is firmly established for relatively high doses, but the carcinogenic affect of low levels of irradiation remains unclear. Tissues which appear to be particularly sensitive to the carcinogenic affects of ionising radiation include thyroid, breast, bone, and haemopoietic tissue.

Fractionation of irradiation

Because cells in mitosis are more susceptible to radiation, it is widely used to treat malignant tumours, which are characterised by high mitotic rates. The theory is that the radiation will kill cells in mitosis, leaving cells in interphase unaffected. Because of this, normal tissue, with a much lower mitotic rate, will lose a very small percentage of cells compared with the tumour. Similarly, normal tissue is better able to repair itself than is abnormal tumour tissue. Dividing the radiation into small doses timed to coincide with the next wave of tumour mitoses will further improve the kill rate in the abnormal tissue and will prevent the unwanted side effects of fibrosis and vascular damage. It has also been observed that tumours with low oxygen tensions are more resistant to radiation, so treatment is sometimes given together with raised concentrations or pressures of oxygen. The most probable explanation of this is that radiation damage is mediated by oxygen free radicals and that these are formed in greater numbers when the oxygen concentration is high.

POISONS

These are chemical agents which have a deleterious effect upon living tissue. They are usually distinguished from substances such as strong acids or alkalis which have a simple corrosive effect; poisons are viewed as interfering with some specific aspect of metabolism. Mechanisms of poisoning are varied but they all involve some degree of interaction between the poison and a cell constituent. A prime target for many poisons is the active site of an enzyme. By definition the active site is chemically reactive since it binds the substrate of that enzyme; the enzyme then undergoes a conformational change which alters the properties of the active site and this results in the catalytic change to the substrate that is the function of that enzyme. The product(s) of the reaction is then released and the enzyme returns to its normal conformation ready to bind another molecule of substrate. It is apparent from this description that the activities of enzymes can be modified by substances that bind inappropriately to the active site, but also by anything that alters the conformation of the enzyme molecule.

The three-dimensional shape of a protein is maintained by various types of crosslinks the stability of which is dependent upon pH and ionic concentration. Although the cell is buffered, changes in pH can occur if large numbers of acidic molecules are generated by some metabolic disturbance such as ketoacidosis resulting from a shift to anaerobic metabolism. This is quite a common event since many poisons affect the respiratory chain. Many of the classic poisons such as heavy metals and cyanide bind to the sulphydryl groups at the active site of respiratory enzymes. Such poisoning has a cascade effect in the cell as respiration is blocked, acidity rises, ATP levels fall, the energy-dependent detoxification processes begin to fail, and free radicals accumulate, resulting in membrane damage and loss of ionic control. Most pumps in the cell are energy dependent, and the stability of DNA as well as proteins requires a very narrow pH and ionic range. Carbon monoxide is a respiratory poison that binds strongly to haemoglobin, forming carboxyhaemoglobin and preventing the binding of oxygen. The complex is cherry pink, and people who have died of carbon monoxide poisoning have a paradoxically healthy pink colour. One of the most toxic natural elements is oxygen because of its very pronounced reactivity to almost everything. In evolutionary terms the respiratory mechanisms of the cell developed to protect it from free oxygen and only developed its respiratory function subsequently. Thus chemical blocking of respiratory mechanisms is effectively removing the cell's protection against oxygen, and the end results are typical oxygen toxicity. This can be seen very dramatically in the case of high levels of oxygen given to preterm infants with the development of respiratory distress syndrome.

There are many specific poisons such as animal venoms and plant toxins which specifically target one organ or cell type: for instance snake venoms are mostly neurotoxic or haemolytic in action.

INFECTIOUS ORGANISMS

These generally cause cell and tissue damage incidentally or indirectly by stimulating the host responses. In general there is no advantage to a parasitic organism in damaging the host, and most organisms that have parasitised man for a long historical period show reduced aggression and the hosts show some degree of tolerance. Organisms new to man or those which infrequently use man as a host tend to produce violent and life-threatening reactions. HIV is a new infection, and the infections that cause the deaths of most AIDs patients are infrequent parasites of man. Tuberculosis, leprosy and malaria cause considerable disability, but millions of people worldwide live out their lives and manage to reproduce in the presence of these infections which have been human companions for millennia. It is also notable that the most damaging effects of tuberculosis and leprosy are seen in those subjects who make the most brisk immunological response to the disease.

FREE RADICALS

The response to cell damage often involves the elaboration of new proteins and is therefore *energy dependent*. Such mechanisms require energy in the form of ATP, the synthesis of which is largely dependent upon available oxygen. Consequently it is often noticed that damaged tissue has a sudden requirement for increased amounts of oxygen: the so-called *respiratory burst*. The proteins secreted at this time may be responsible for clearing away a lot of cell debris and may appear to be destructive. This led to the identification of an apparently anomalous phenomenon called *reperfusion injury*. If myocardiocytes are damaged experimentally by ischaemia which is then maintained, the degree of damage is less than if they are damaged by ischaemia and then exposed to normal oxygen levels; the studies are performed by experimentally occluding coronary arteries in laboratory animals and releasing the occlusion at varying times. The animals are allowed to survive until the effects of ischaemia have had sufficient time to develop histologically and are then killed and the heart muscle examined microscopically. What is happening here is that energy-dependent processes are triggered by the initial ischaemia but they can only occur in the presence of adequate oxygen levels. Such reperfusion injury is the result of the experimental set-up, and the final long term result of the two experiments is roughly the same degree of injury except that the so-called *reperfusion injury* results in earlier and better scar formation. The mechanism of reperfusion injury is an example of another adaptive response to cell damage but this time mediated by *free radicals*. Free radicals are the final common pathway of many cellular processes, many, but not all, of which are involved in the response to cellular damage. A free radical is a molecule bearing an unpaired electron, in consequence of which it is highly reactive and short lived. Such molecules are used by the body to destroy bacteria and are found in lysosomes. Since they are highly reactive and are formed as a byproduct in many metabolic reactions, cells must be protected against them. Numerous substances, including vitamin D and glutathione act as free radical sinks, whilst enzymes such as superoxide dismutase actively metabolise free radicals; these are also oxygen/energy-dependent processes. Typical free radicals include superoxide, hydrogen peroxide, hydroxyl ions and nitric oxide.

MECHANISMS OF CELL DAMAGE

The basic mechanisms of cell injury have been briefly

mentioned above and will now be reiterated and discussed in further detail. They are:

- oxygen supply and oxygen free radicals
- disturbances in calcium homeostasis
- depletion of ATP
- membrane integrity.

Oxygen is a very reactive substance which combines with a vast range of molecules and is consequently handled with great caution by the cell. Free oxygen is very toxic, and oxidative processes in the cell are broken down into small, safe, metabolic steps such as the electron transport chain in the mitochondria. The small steps yield small discrete quanta of free energy which is coupled to energy storage mechanisms such as ATP. It is often said that the terminal phosphate bond in ATP is a *high energy* storage bond; this is not true. The significance of the terminal phosphate bond in ATP is that it is a *medium energy* bond and so can be formed by many oxidative reactions and can be used to fuel many other reactions; it stands at the centre of all energetic metabolic processes. ATP is the short term (minutes) energy storage molecule of most cells; longer term (hours) storage of sugars is in the form of glycogen. The virtue of glycogen is that one huge molecule containing many hundreds or thousands of sugar molecules exerts the osmotic pressure of only one molecule; the same number of free sugar molecules would rupture the cell. Longer term (days) storage of excess dietary calories is in the form of fats (ask any middle aged pathologist). When these stores are depleted the cell will begin to use structural proteins as a source of energy, but at this stage the individual is entering the pathological zone of starvation.

Some ATP can be produced by anaerobic processes (such as glycolysis), but these mechanisms cannot fully oxidise compounds such as sugars and result in the accumulation of only partially metabolised compounds that must subsequently be metabolised by aerobic processes. For example, in the case of sugars the anaerobic, glycolytic pathway results in the accumulation of lactic acid which must be further metabolised by aerobic pathways in the mitochondria. If this does not happen then lactic acidosis results. Most tissues can metabolise the resting levels of lactate that they produce, but at times of increased metabolic activity skeletal muscles and skin export their excess lactate into the blood stream where it is carried to the liver in which it is aerobically metabolised by the Krebs cycle of the liver mitochondria to carbon dioxide and water, yielding several more units of ATP. These two organs (skeletal muscle and skin) are very dependent upon good vascular supply not only for their own metabolic needs but also for the removal of lactate. A lack of oxygen (as a result of vascular disease, cardiac failure, respiratory disease, etc.) causes cells to switch from aerobic to anaerobic metabolism with consequent acidosis and lowered ATP levels because of the lower efficiency of anaerobic metabolism. Many cellular processes are ATP dependent, including the ionic membrane pumps and the integrity of membranes themselves. One of the earliest signs of irreversible cell damage is the failure to exclude calcium from cells and from mitochondria; while this may only be an incidental marker of cell damage it is also a very early event in apoptosis and may be an early cellular process actually leading to cell death. The various agents that cause cell injury (such as toxins, drugs, ultraviolet and other radiations, etc.) release free radicals, and in the presence of ATP depletion the enzyme processes and the scavenger mechanisms cannot operate, resulting in free radical damage to the phospholipids of various membranes such as cell membranes and organelle membranes (endoplasmic reticulum, mitochondria, lysosomes, etc.). Ischaemia and ATP depletion therefore results in the various morphological effects described above, together with destabilisation of lysosomal membranes and the leakage of hydrolytic enzymes into the cytoplasm with disorganisation of cytoskeletal structures and destruction of the enzymatic pathways on which the cells rely. Some of these enzymes of intermediary metabolism may leak from damaged cells into the blood and can be used as clinical markers of cell damage (lactic dehydrogenase from muscle; cardiac enzymes in myocardial infarction, etc.). When these changes become so severe that they cannot be reversed, cell death occurs. Curiously, leakage of these enzymes into the circulation rarely causes direct problems except in the case of pancreatic lipases in pancreatitis.

CELL DEATH

Cell death is the irreversible loss of the cell's ability to maintain independence of the environment. Living systems, including cells, are characterised by a relative stability of their internal milieu in the face of relatively wide environmental fluctuations in temperature, humidity and ionic concentration. Two major forms of cell death are recognised under pathological conditions: *necrosis* and *apoptosis*.

NECROSIS

This is characterised by death of large numbers of cells in groups and the presence of an inflammatory reaction.

This is the most familiar form of cell death and is associated with trauma, infection, ischaemia, toxic damage and immunological insults. Different patterns of necrosis are recognised and given specific names such as coagulative necrosis and liquefactive necrosis; in the former it is thought that autolytic processes dominate, and in the latter that heterolytic ones predominate. Certainly there are characteristic tissue differences: coagulative necrosis is the common event in most tissues, including myocardium, whilst liquefactive necrosis predominates in the brain. If there is no infection then the tissue can become mummified, and this is described as dry gangrene; if infection supervenes then anaerobic bacteria can cause wet gangrene. In tuberculous foci of infection a particular type of necrosis occurs with a mixture of cell membranes and bacterial debris with a 'cheesey' appearance known as caseous necrosis. This frequently undergoes subsequent calcification. The term fat necrosis does not really indicate a specific pattern of necrosis but is more a clinical term referring to a specific clinical entity around the pancreas when lipases have been released and autolysis occurs. In the breast, commonly following trauma, a rather specific and histologically startling form of fat necrosis occurs. This probably results from an inflammatory reaction to fat escaping from ruptured fat cells and can suggest carcinoma both clinically and mammographically although the diagnosis is usually obvious histologically.

APOPTOSIS

This is single cell death and may be associated with one or two lymphocytes (satellite cell necrosis) but not with a general inflammatory reaction. This type of cell death was first defined morphologically but its distinctive feature is that it is initiated by the cell itself. Apoptosis probably arose as a response to viral infection or mutation and represents a scorched earth policy where it is safer for the organism to sacrifice a cell rather than to allow the virus or the mutation to spread and threaten the whole individual. Apoptosis also occurs physiologically in hormonal involution.

The morphological hallmark of apoptosis is the apoptotic body which is eosinophilic and may contain some nuclear debris. It is a result of shrinkage of the cell cytoplasm and nuclear disruption. These apoptotic bodies are taken up by surrounding cells and digested; the cells are commonly, but not exclusively, the same cell type as the apoptotic cell. The early stages in apoptosis are characterised by surface blebbing and margination of chromatin followed by cell shrinkage and breakup into smaller apoptotic bodies. Epidermal apoptotic bodies are large

and pink because of their high content of cytoskeletal structures, while other cell types may be smaller and dominated by nuclear debris. Epithelial cells are often extruded from the epithelium into the underlying connective tissue stroma where they are taken up by macrophages. Since the process was seen for a long time before the mechanism was understood, apoptotic bodies in particular situations attracted specific names:

- Civatte or colloid bodies in lichen planus
- Kamino bodies in melanocytic lesions
- Councilman bodies in acute viral hepatitis.

The first recognised metabolic step is the production of endonucleases which cut the DNA into short double stranded fragments; this is an irreversible step. Calcium influx into the cell is an energy-dependent process in apoptosis in distinction to the passive entry in necrosis, but it is an early step and this indicates that it is an important mechanism in cell death generally. Inhibiting RNA and protein synthesis inhibits apoptosis, confirming the observation that it is a dynamic process and is energy dependent. Various factors concerned with apoptosis have been characterised and are listed in Table 1.1.

SENESCENCE

Senescence is certainly involved in cell death, but in many cases reduction in cell number is a function of normal cell loss together with a diminution in the ability to regenerate; thus the rate of cell death in the skin of the elderly is about the same as in youth or even less, but the ability of basal cells to divide is considerably reduced. Central nervous system cell loss may increase markedly in the elderly, but, after birth, neurons lose the ability to divide and all neuronal loss is permanent. If human fibroblasts are grown in cell culture they divide well for about fifty divisions but then they lose the ability to replicate further, this inbuilt limitation is known as the Hayflick limit. Cancer cells and most embryonic cells do not have this restriction. There are repetitive regions on some chromosomes that are shortened every time the cell divides, and in the adult human only gametes and tumour cells can resynthesise these regions since they possess the enzyme *telomerase*. There is a critical limit length to these telomeres, and when they reach this the cell can no longer divide.

CELL RENEWAL

Cells from different tissues differ in their ability to repli-

Table 1.1 Factors known to affect apoptosis	
Factors involved in apoptosis	Effects and modes of action
Bcl-2 (B-cell lymphoma / leukaemia-2 gene)	One of several 'survival genes' that prevent apoptosis until a 'trigger gene' is activated. Gene product is membrane located
p53	Tumour suppressor 'trigger' gene. Located on chromosome 17p, and mutation and heterozygosity are associated with many cancers. Associated with apoptosis in cells with damaged DNA. Suggested that p53 may stall cells in G1 to allow DNA repair and to trigger apoptosis if this fails
c-myc	Cellular oncogene which binds with protein *max* and binds to specific DNA sites in the vicinity of genes concerned with cellular growth such as PDGF
Glucocorticoids	Strongly stimulate apoptosis. They stimulate the production of calmodulin mRNA (a calcium-binding protein) and may influence calcium flux into the cell, which is an early step in apoptosis.
APO-1 or Fas	Membrane antigen member of the superfamily of tumour necrosis factor receptor/nerve growth factor receptor cell surface proteins; antibodies to this antigen strongly stimulate apoptosis.
T-cell antigen receptor in thymocytes	Stimulation of immature thymocytes results in apoptosis, stimulation of mature thymocytes results in cell activation. May protect against an immature and incomplete response.

From Cotton D W K 1997 Synopsis of general pathology for surgeons. Butterworth Heinemann, Oxford.

cate: some cells replicate freely (labile cells); some have a restricted ability to regenerate (stable cells); and some show no ability to replicate (permanent cells).

LABILE CELLS

These are typically epithelial cells that are readily shed under physiological conditions and are replaced from a population of *reserve* or *stem cells*. The skin, which is constantly growing from the base upwards, loses keratinocytes from the surface in the form of keratin flakes, and these are replaced by the division of cells in the basal layer. Not all cells in the basal layer divide; some are specialised for attachment of the epidermis to the dermis. Damage to this population of cells results in blister formation, but cell division is generally not affected and may even be increased. The lining of the gut is subject to constant insults due to the range of food and drink which passes over it, and surface cells are constantly being lost. Reserve cells in the gut are recognisable tiny cells with little cytoplasm which lie at the base of the various crypts and migrate upwards as they replicate. They are responsive to increased rates of loss from the surface, and trauma results in an adaptive burst of mitosis just as it does in the skin. Any failure to adapt the rate of cell division to the rate of cell loss results in a deficiency of the epithelium which is known as an ulcer. Other labile cell types include the glands which line the endometrial cavity. During the cyclical loss of this epithelium, the bases of the glands are retained, and in the proliferative phase of the menstrual cycle these become highly mitotic. The nuclei first move from their position at the base of the cell adjacent to the basement membrane, and then divide, closely followed by cytoplasmic division. Again, this division is closely associated with the rate of cell loss, but disturbances in hormonal balance can cause thickening of the cellular layers with resultant disturbances to the menstrual cycle. Histologically this type of hyperplasia can look very like neoplasia, and hyperplastic epithelia occurring as a response to trauma in general require careful distinction from well-differentiated neoplasia.

Both metaplasia and neoplasia are the result of changes to stem cells, but in the case of metaplasia the changes disappear when the stimulus is removed, while the changes of neoplasia are mutational events which are permanent. Consequently both metaplasia and neoplasia are commonest in epithelial tissues. Possibly because of the increased rate of mitosis and the consequent increase in opportunities for mutation in longstanding repair and the persistence of the injurious agents in metaplasia, both of these conditions have an increased risk of neoplasia. For instance, squamous cell carcinoma of the skin can arise in the margins of chronic skin ulcers (Marjolin's ulcer), and the majority of lung cancers are squamous although the lining of the lungs consists of mucus-secreting and ciliated columnar cells.

STABLE CELLS

These are capable of a limited mitotic response to trauma, but much less than is typical of labile cells. Hepatocytes can divide to replace cells lost to various types of metabolic trauma, as can renal tubular cells. However, the function of the organ depends very much on its three-dimensional structure in both cases, and this three-dimensional structure is maintained and formed by the collagen (reticulin) framework. The collagen framework is synthesised and repaired by fibroblasts and even under normal circumstances is in a state of constant, albeit very slow, flux. If it is damaged the rate of synthesis can increase considerably. But both normal turnover and repair depend upon the underlying orderly structure that was laid down during embryonic development, and if damage is severe enough to disrupt this pattern then synthesis results in a disorderly repair, the structure of which is so abnormal that function is impaired. The most striking example of this is diffuse toxic damage to the liver (alcohol, hepatitis, etc.) where masses of cells are destroyed, the reticulin framework disrupted and the regenerating hepatocytes grow in nodular masses resulting in disordered vascularisation and the condition known as cirrhosis. The reticular structure of the renal tubules is altogether simpler, and damage to the kidney tubules can be healed by regeneration, but the reticulin structure of the glomeruli is so complex that it can only be laid down in embryogenesis and cannot be regenerated in the adult. The fine surface patterning of the skin is determined by the orientation of collagen bundles in the dermis, and damage that is restricted to the epidermis is regenerated completely. Damage that involves the underlying dermis disrupts the normal orientation of collagen bundles and their cross links and results in a scar. Empirically this fact has been known to surgeons for many years, and the older books laid much stress upon the fact that scars could be minimised by cutting along Langer's lines rather than across them. These lines are the major orientation of the collagen bundles, and cutting across them results in damage to many fibres, which are subsequently repaired by random resynthesis of cut ends; incisions or splitting along Langer's lines means that disruption is more or less restricted to cross links and that there is minimal damage to the long axis of fibres.

PERMANENT CELLS

These have lost the ability to divide and have even lost the functional reserve of stem cells that would normally regenerate the tissue; typical examples are neurons and myocardiocytes. Damage to these tissues is therefore permanent. The various supporting cells still retain the ability to replicate: the response to damage in the central nervous system includes proliferation of glial cells, and in the heart there is fibrous scar formation by fibroblasts. On the face of it this would appear to be rather peculiar since not only are the heart and brain prone to a large number of traumatic events, their subsequent impaired function is often fatal. Presumably there is some overwhelming advantage to the loss of regenerative power that outweighs the disadvantages. Certainly the loss of regenerative ability means that tumours of adult neurons and cardiomyocytes do not occur, but this would hardly seem to compensate for the morbidity and mortality of strokes and heart attacks; the explanation probably lies in the fact that the spatial organisation of the cells of the brain and the heart are so specific that regeneration would result in functional chaos and even replacement of individual drop-out cells would be impossible to accomplish without considerable disorder.

Many cells lose the ability to divide as they mature and become specialised (they are often called 'postmitotic cells'). This is a different matter from *stable* cells in which no cell loss can be made good; postmitotic cells have functional reserve cells which can replace cell loss.

HEALING

Replication versus repair

Cell loss due to some form of trauma results in healing if the trauma has not been so severe as to endanger the continued existence of the individual. This healing can take two forms: the tissue can regenerate itself so that it is eventually much the same as it was before the trauma occurred, or it can form some sort of scar. With time, scars change because collagen is being actively metabolised and resynthesised, but the changes are slow. In some individuals scarring is very pronounced; in some cases it is so remarkable as to attract the term 'keloid'. The characteristics of keloid arise from disorganised masses of collagen that do not become more organised with time.

Primary versus secondary intention

This is a distinction that is made between wounds where the edges can be closely applied and those wounds in which there is a tissue deficiency that has to be filled in before healing can proceed. There is no fundamental difference between the two but there is a difference in emphasis between the various processes.

WOUND HEALING

Wound healing is the process by which a damaged tissue is restored, as closely as possible, to its normal state. The completeness or otherwise of wound healing depends upon the reparative abilities of the tissue, the type of damage, the extent of damage and the general state of health of the tissue and the organism in which the tissue exists. Wound healing has been most extensively studied in skin and bone, and many of the normal mechanisms have been elucidated in these tissues.

There have been significant advances in the understanding of cell and tissue growth in recent years, and a number of growth factors have been identified and characterised; these are generally referred to as *cytokines*, and some examples are listed in Table 1.2.

The steps in wound healing are generally listed in sequence, although in fact they all occur together, but at different stages of the process different mechanisms dominate:

- haemostasis
- inflammation
- regeneration
- repair.

Most wounds are accompanied by some degree of haemorrhage because blood vessels are damaged. Under these circumstances the free blood comes into contact with exposed collagen and with factors released from damaged cells, and clot formation occurs. A clot is a meshwork of fibrin with blood cells and platelets entrapped within it and which contracts due to cross linking and the transformation of fibroblasts into myofibroblasts. The clots thus form a framework for other cells to migrate over, and the entrapped cells, particularly macrophages and platelets, release various active agents that stimulate migration and replication of endothelial and epithelial cells. They also stimulate each other to grow and transform (see Table 1.2). This leads to a prolif-

Table 1.2 Some common cytokines and their actions	
Cytokine	Features
EGF (epidermal growth factor)	Binds to EGF transmembrane receptor on most mammalian cells (most numerous on epithelial cells) and causes relative dedifferentiation and proliferation
FGF (fibroblast growth factor)	Exists in two forms: acidic and basic (ten times more active); mitogenic for many mesenchymal cells and causes proliferation of capillaries
MDGF (macrophage-derived growth factor)	Secretion from macrophages stimulated by fibronectin and Gram negative endotoxins; stimulates proliferation of quiescent fibroblasts, endothelial cells and smooth muscle cells
PDGF (platelet-derived growth factor)	Stored in α-granules of platelets and released during platelet aggregation in haemostasis; chemotactic for monocyte/macrophages and neutrophils; mitogenic for mesodermal cells such as smooth muscle cells, microglia and fibroblasts; similar or identical factors produced by macrophages, endothelial cells, smooth muscle cells and transformed fibroblasts
TGFβ (transforming growth factor β)	Produced by transformed cells in culture; found in platelet α-granules, and the gene is induced in activated lymphocytes; induces granulation tissue
TNF (tumour necrosis factor or cachexin)	Produced mainly by monocyte/macrophages but also by T lymphocytes; induced by endotoxin and Gram positive cell wall products; mediator of general inflammation causing fever and production of IL-1, IL-6 and IL-8
Interleukins	IL-1 initiates granuloma formation in synergy with TNF; IL-2 increases size of granulomas; IL-6 induces acute phase proteins in hepatocytes and stimulates the final differentiation of B cells; IL-8 induces neutrophil chemotaxis, shape change and granule exocytosis as well as vascular leakage and increased expression of CD-11/CD-18; IL-1 receptor antagonist blocks the effects of IL-1, produced by monocyte/macrophages by the same stimuli that induce IL-1 and presumably limits the effects of IL-1
From Cotton D K W 1997 Synopsis of general pathology for surgeons. Butterworth Heinemann, Oxford	

eration of new vessels, mostly capillaries, which loop in and out of the healing wound and present a granular appearance on its surface (*granulation tissue*). Sometimes this granulation tissue may be so exuberant that the epithelium cannot close over it, resulting in an area of 'proud flesh' which is friable, bleeds easily and stops re-epithelialisation; this can be treated with a silver nitrate stick which reduces the granulation tissue to the extent that re-epithelialisation occurs.

At the same time as the formation of granulation tissue the process of inflammation is beginning with an influx of various plasma constituents leaking from damaged vessels and adjacent intact vessels which have dilated in response to the various local mediators of inflammation (Ch. 2) released by the trauma itself (Table 1.3). Any foreign material or infection stimulates the inflammatory reaction further and directs it down the most suitable pathways such as pus formation, foreign body giant cell reaction or granulomatous reactions to mycobacteria and fungi for example. Consequently, a reaction which begins as a stereotyped response to any trauma slowly evolves into a specific reaction tailored to the needs of the specific nature of the wound.

Fibroblasts crawl over the fibrin meshwork, removing it and laying down a loose network of collagen which is also constantly being broken down and reformed to produce a solid and mechanically tough meshwork for the support of the new epithelium. Factors released from a number of cell types, including epithelial cells themselves, and the absence of various inhibitors due to cell loss, result in increased epithelial division and migration over the wound surface. Any residual adnexal structures left in the supporting connective tissue layer can contribute to re-epithelialisation by stem cell dedifferentiation leading to a contribution to re-epithelialisation. The extent to which regeneration or repair figures in the healed tissue depends upon a variety of factors as discussed above and also to complicating factors both local and systemic.

Healing of specific tissues

Skin

The following is a description of the time course of events in the healing of skin:

- minutes: blood clot forms; surface dehydrates to form scab
- 24 hours: first phases of inflammation (neutrophils at the margins; edges of epidermis thicken and begin to migrate because of increased mitosis)
- 3 days: granulation tissue becoming covered by epidermis; vertical collagen fibres at edges; macrophages replace neutrophils
- 5 days: collagen fibrils begin to bridge wound; new vessels abundant; single-layered epidermis begins to become multilayered
- Week 2: collagen and vessels being remodelled; fibroblasts still active and proliferating; vessels reduced in number
- Week 4–5: wound strengthens; inflammatory infiltrate gone; collagen continues to remodel; adnexae do not regenerate.

The above account is typical for mucosal and skin healing, but other tissues have other specific features that modify this account. The most distinct difference is with bone.

Bone

Closed fractures of bone are generally sterile but may differ in the amount of bone fragments (comminuted fractures) that need to be removed by the processes of inflammation. Otherwise the wound healing processes are much the same as for incised skin wounds but modified to take account of the peculiar nature of bone and its functional modifications.

- Blood vessels within the bone and the periosteum are damaged and blood leaks out. This rapidly clots to form a haematoma.
- As in other tissues the haematoma forms a framework along which various cell types can migrate.
- The clot then organises over the next week, with inflammatory cells modifying the structure and fibroblasts secreting collagen.
- The inflammatory cells and the platelets release various growth factors: transforming growth factor α (TGFα); platelet-derived growth factor (PDGF); fibroblast growth factor (FGF).
- The osteoblasts normally resident in the periosteum become activated and begin to produce woven bone which is constantly being modified by mechanical forces exerted on it. These are translated into tiny electrical currents, and many experiments have been undertaken to study the effects of electrical current on fracture healing.
- The mesenchymal cells in the surrounding soft tissues also become activated and begin to secrete cartilage (fibrocartilage and hyaline cartilage) around the fracture site.
- By the second and third week the mass of healing tissue reaches its maximum girth but is still too weak for weight bearing.

Table 1.3 Chemical mediators of inflammation		
Mediators	Source	Release and actions
Cells Cationic proteins and neutral proteases	Lysosomes in neutrophils	Neutrophils release lysosomal contents in contact with bacteria and damaged tissues; they increase permeability and activate complement
Cytokines (including the lymphokines)	These were first described in lymphocytes (hence lymphokines) but are substances produced by many cells that influence other cells	See Ch. 2 for their relationships in inflammation
Histamine	Mast cells, basophils, eosinophils and platelets	Release is stimulated by C3a, C5a and neutrophil lysosomal proteins, resulting in vasodilatation and transiently increased vascular permeability
Leukotrienes	Neutrophils, mast cells, basophils and some macrophages contain the lipoxygenase pathway which converts arachidonic acid to various leukotrienes; a mixture of these forms slow-reacting substance of anaphylaxis (SRS)	The various cells are activated by interleukins and other products of inflammation to secrete leukotrienes, some of which (B4) are potent chemoattractants for neutrophils, monocytes and macrophages, while others (SRS) cause contraction of smooth muscle and enhance vascular permeability
Prostaglandins	Cells contain cyclo-oxygenase that makes prostaglandins from arachidonic acid; platelets produce thromboxane A2; endothelial cells produce prostacyclin; monocyte/macrophages produce any or all	
Nitric oxide	Also known as endothelium-derived relaxing factor, it is a short lived free radical produced by endothelium and macrophages	It is toxic to bacteria and appears to be a major factor in endotoxic shock
Plasma factors Coagulation proteins	Mostly synthesised in the liver in inactive form; when activated they release fibrin	Intermediates such as FXII are involved in activating other systems but the release of fibrin is an important part of inflammation
Complement	Series of 20 proteins synthesised in the liver and in macrophages; the liver produces most but macrophage complement is probably significant at sites of inflammation; the various components form an enzymatic cascade providing vast amplification of the initial effect	See Ch. 2
Fibrinolytic proteins	Mostly synthesised in the liver, they are the negative feedback arm that limits coagulation	Plasmin, which is released by the action of activated FXII, lyses fibrin clot to fibrin degradation products (FDP)
Kinins	Circulating clotting factor XII (Hageman factor), prekallikrein and plasminogen are synthesised in the liver and circulate as inactive plasma proteins	FXII is activated by negatively charged surfaces such as exposed basement membranes, proteolytic enzymes, bacterial LPS and foreign materials such as crystals; it converts plasminogen to plasmin and prekallikrein to kallikrein which in turn cleaves kininogen to release bradykinin; it also activates the alternative complement pathway

From Cotton D W K 1997 Synopsis of general pathology for surgeons. Butterworth Heinemann, Oxford

- As woven bone approaches the new cartilage this undergoes enchondral ossification and bridges the deficit with new bone.
- Remodelling may continue for many weeks, but eventually the repair may be indistinguishable from the original bone or it may be even stronger than previously.

Factors responsible for delayed wound healing

These include both local and systemic conditions (Box 1.1). Locally, wounds may be infected, which prolongs the inflammatory phase and delays the onset of regeneration and repair. In some situations the persistence of infection in a chronic form can prevent healing from ever taking place; chronic osteomyelitis following a compound fracture may persist for decades without resolution.

Persistence of an injurious agent such as a foreign body has much the same effect as infection in that it extends the period of inflammation and prevents the onset of healing. Foreign bodies induce a chronic granulomatous reaction (see Ch. 2) with typical foreign body giant cells.

Interruption of the nervous and vascular supply by trauma also slows healing, but injuries to an area in which vascular supply is poor also delay effective healing. Lacerations to the shins in the elderly can be very difficult to heal, particularly since poor vascularisation is often accompanied by venous stasis and oedema. Intact inner-

vation is important for wound healing, not only because of sensory warning about further trauma and the availability of normal muscle movement, but also because there seems to be a direct effect of intact nerve supply, although the nature of this remains obscure.

In fractures one of the major causes of delayed wound healing is instability of the fracture. If movement is not prevented, normal wound healing may be delayed and a fibrocartilage 'joint' may form which can even develop a synovial cavity mimicking a true joint.

Systemic diseases may have a large effect on wound healing. An obvious example that is of worldwide significance is poor nutrition. The gross effect of protein malnutrition is that there are not enough amino acids available for the high levels of protein synthesis required during healing. Vitamin and cofactor supplies are also deficient in malnutrition; substances such as vitamin C and zinc are essential in the molecular synthesis of collagen and many other components of connective tissue synthesis. An analogous situation arises in well-nourished individuals following trauma or surgery. The patients enter a severe catabolic state and may require parenteral nutrition even if they are capable of taking normal food. The elderly are often closer to the limits of nutrition and this, combined with the low regenerative capacity of old age generally, makes these individuals prone to delayed wound healing.

Concomitant diseases such as diabetes restrict the available nutritional supply to the wound, due to a mixture of the metabolic effects of the disease as well as a result of the vascular insufficiency common in longstanding diabetes. Diabetic patients are also prone to infection. Immunosuppression, both spontaneous and therapeutic, inhibits the inflammatory response, and steroids, either in natural diseases such as Cushing's or given therapeutically, have a similar effect. Advanced neoplasia results in immunosuppression directly, by cachexia and by bone marrow suppression, added to which the therapeutic modalities used to treat cancer are themselves immunosuppressive since they are aimed at rapidly replicating tumour cells and consequently also suppress bone marrow.

In general, wound healing aims at the restoration of the maximum similarity to the original tissue, although this is limited by the fact that the underlying structure of many tissues is laid down during development and cannot be recapitulated in the adult. However, equally complex structures can be developed in the adult of many species, particularly amphibians, so it may be possible in time to aim at complete wound healing, even in cases of traumatic or surgical amputation.

Box 1.1 Factors affecting wound healing

Local
- infection
- ischaemia
- foreign body
- haematoma
- malignancy
- denervation

Systemic
- poor nutrition
- deficiency of vitamins A and C
- protein deficiency
- zinc and manganese deficiency
- diabetes mellitus
- uraemia
- jaundice
- steroids
- immunosuppressive agents
- chemotherapeutic agents
- malignant disease
- irradiation
- age

2

Inflammation

Timothy J Stephenson

Inflammation is the local physiological response to tissue injury. It is not, in itself, a disease, but is usually a manifestation of disease. Inflammation may have beneficial effects, such as the destruction of invading microorganisms and the walling-off of an abscess cavity, thus preventing spread of infection. Equally, it may produce disease; for example, an abscess in the brain would act as a space-occupying lesion compressing vital surrounding structures, or fibrosis resulting from chronic inflammation may distort the tissues and permanently alter their function.

Inflammation is usually classified according to its time course as:

- *acute inflammation* — the initial and often transient series of tissue reactions to injury
- *chronic inflammation* — the subsequent and often prolonged tissue reactions following the initial response.

The two main types of inflammation are also characterised by differences in the cell types taking part in the inflammatory response.

ACUTE INFLAMMATION

The principal features of acute inflammation are as follows.

- An initial reaction of tissue to injury.
- In the vascular phase, dilatation and increased permeability occur.
- In the exudative phase, fluid and cells escape from permeable venules.
- Neutrophil polymorph is the predominant cell involved, but mast cells and macrophages are also important.
- Outcome may be resolution, suppuration (e.g. abscess), organisation, or progression to chronic inflammation.

Acute inflammation is the initial tissue reaction to a wide range of injurious agents; it may last from a few hours to a few days. The process is usually described by the suffix '-itis', preceded by the name of the organ or tissues involved. Thus, acute inflammation of the meninges is called meningitis. The acute inflammatory response is similar whatever the causative agent:

CAUSES OF ACUTE INFLAMMATION

The principal causes of acute inflammation are:

- microbial infections, e.g. pyogenic bacteria, viruses
- hypersensitivity reactions, e.g. parasites, tubercle bacilli
- physical agents, e.g. trauma, ionising irradiation, heat, cold
- chemicals, e.g. corrosives, acids, alkalis, reducing agents, bacterial toxins
- tissue necrosis, e.g. ischaemic infarction.

Microbial infections

One of the commonest causes of inflammation is microbial infection. Viruses lead to death of individual cells by intracellular multiplication. Bacteria release specific exotoxins — chemicals synthesised by them which specifically initiate inflammation — or endotoxins, which are associated with their cell walls. Additionally, some organisms cause immunologically-mediated inflammation through hypersensitivity reactions (Ch. 6). Parasite infections and tuberculous inflammation are instances where hypersensitivity is important.

Hypersensitivity reactions

A hypersensitivity reaction occurs when an altered state of immunological responsiveness causes an inappropriate or excessive immune reaction which damages the tissues. The types of reaction or classified in Chapter 6 but all have cellular or chemical mediators similar to those involved in inflammation.

Physical agents

Tissue damage leading to inflammation may occur

through physical trauma, ultraviolet or other ionising radiation, burns or excessive cooling ('frostbite').

Irritant and corrosive chemicals

Corrosive chemicals (acids, alkalis, oxidising agents) provoke inflammation through gross tissue damage. However, infecting agents may release specific chemical irritants which lead directly to inflammation.

Tissue necrosis

Death of tissues from lack of oxygen or nutrients resulting from inadequate blood flow (infarction, see Ch. 3) is a potent inflammatory stimulus. The edge of a recent infarct often shows an acute inflammatory response.

ESSENTIAL MACROSCOPIC APPEARANCES OF ACUTE INFLAMMATION

The essential physical characteristics of acute inflammation were formulated by Celsus (30 BC–AD 38) using the Latin words rubor, calor, tumor and dolor. Loss of function is also characteristic.

Redness (rubor)

An acutely inflamed tissue appears red: for example skin affected by sunburn, cellulitis due to bacterial infection or acute conjunctivitis. This is due to dilatation of small blood vessels within the damaged area.

Heat (calor)

Increase in temperature is seen only in peripheral parts of the body, such as the skin. It is due to increased blood flow (hyperaemia) through the region, resulting in vascular dilatation and the delivery of warm blood to the area. Systemic fever, which results from some of the chemical mediators of inflammation, also contributes to the local temperature.

Swelling (tumor)

Swelling results from oedema — the accumulation of fluid in the extravascular space as part of the fluid exudate — and, to a much lesser extent, from the physical mass of the inflammatory cells migrating into the area (Fig. 2.1).

Pain (dolor)

For the patient, pain is one of the best-known features of acute inflammation. It results partly from the stretching and distortion of tissues due to inflammatory oedema and, in particular, from pus under pressure in an abscess cavity. Some of the chemical mediators of acute inflammation, including bradykinin, the prostaglandins and serotonin, are known to induce pain.

Loss of function

Loss of function, a well-known consequence of inflammation, was added by Virchow (1821–1902) to the list of features drawn up by Celsus. Movement of an inflamed area is consciously and reflexly inhibited by pain, while severe swelling may physically immobilise the tissues.

EARLY STAGES OF ACUTE INFLAMMATION

In the early stages, oedema fluid, fibrin and neutrophil polymorphs accumulate in the extracellular spaces of the damaged tissue. The presence of the cellular component, the *neutrophil polymorph*, is essential for a histological diagnosis of acute inflammation. The acute inflammatory response involves three processes:

- changes in vessel calibre and, consequently, flow
- increased vascular permeability and formation of the fluid exudate
- formation of the cellular exudate — emigration of the neutrophil polymorphs into the extravascular space.

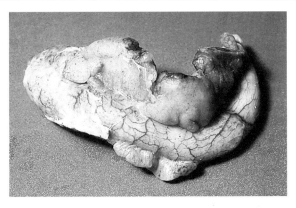

Fig. 2.1 Early acute appendicitis. The appendix is swollen by oedema, the surface is covered by fibrinous exudate, and there is vascular dilatation.

Changes in vessel calibre

The microcirculation consists of the network of small capillaries lying between arterioles, which have a thick muscular wall, and thin-walled venules. Capillaries have no smooth muscle in their walls to control their calibre, and are so narrow that red blood cells must pass through them in single file. The smooth muscle of arteriolar walls forms precapillary sphincters which regulate blood flow through the capillary bed. Flow through the capillaries is intermittent, and some form preferential channels for flow while others are usually shut down (Fig. 2.2).

In blood vessels larger than capillaries, blood cells flow mainly in the centre of the lumen (axial flow), while the area near the vessel wall carries only plasma (plasmatic zone). This feature of normal blood flow keeps blood cells away from the vessel wall.

Changes in the microcirculation occur as a physiological response: for example, there is hyperaemia in exercising muscle and active endocrine glands. The changes following injury which make up the vascular component of the acute inflammatory reaction were described by Lewis in 1927 as 'the triple response to injury': a flush, a flare and a wheal. If a blunt instrument is drawn firmly across the skin, the following sequential changes take place:

- A momentary white line follows the stroke. This is due to arteriolar vasoconstriction, the smooth muscle of arterioles contracting as a direct response to injury.
- The flush: a dull red line follows due to capillary dilatation.
- The flare: a red, irregular, surrounding zone then develops, due to arteriolar dilatation. Both nervous and chemical factors are involved in these vascular changes.
- The wheal: a zone of oedema develops due to fluid exudation into the extravascular space.

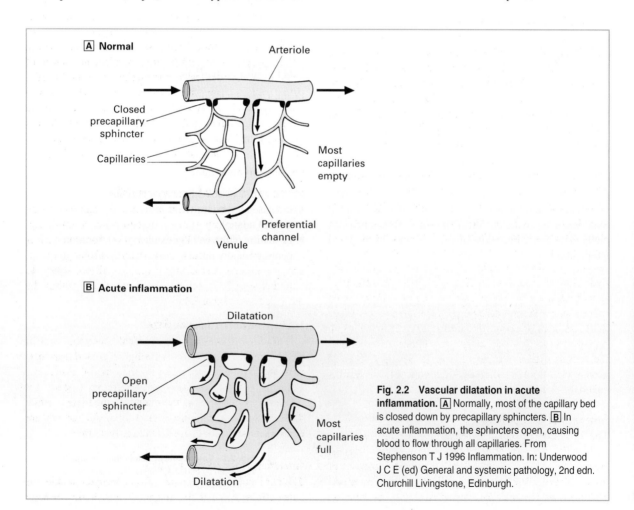

Fig. 2.2 **Vascular dilatation in acute inflammation.** [A] Normally, most of the capillary bed is closed down by precapillary sphincters. [B] In acute inflammation, the sphincters open, causing blood to flow through all capillaries. From Stephenson T J 1996 Inflammation. In: Underwood J C E (ed) General and systemic pathology, 2nd edn. Churchill Livingstone, Edinburgh.

The initial phase of arteriolar constriction is transient and probably of little importance in acute inflammation. The subsequent phase of vasodilatation (active hyperaemia) may last from 15 minutes to several hours, depending upon the severity of the injury. There is experimental evidence that blood flow to the injured area may increase up to ten-fold.

As blood flow begins to slow again, blood cells begin to flow nearer to the vessel wall, in the plasmatic zone rather than the axial stream. This allows 'pavementing' of leucocytes (their adhesion to the vascular epithelium) to occur, which is the first step in leucocyte emigration into the extravascular space.

The slowing of blood flow which follows the phase of hyperaemia is due to increased vascular permeability, allowing plasma to escape into the tissues while blood cells are retained within the vessels. The blood viscosity is therefore increased.

Increased vascular permeability

Small blood vessels are lined by a single layer of endothelial cells. In some tissues, these form a complete layer of uniform thickness around the vessel wall, while in other tissues there are areas of endothelial cell thinning, known as fenestrations. The walls of small blood vessels act as a microfilter, allowing the passage of water and solutes but blocking that of large molecules and cells. Oxygen, carbon dioxide and some nutrients transfer across the wall by diffusion, but the main transfer of fluid and solutes is by ultrafiltration, as described by Starling. The high colloid osmotic pressure inside the vessel, due to plasma proteins, favours fluid return to the vascular compartment. Under normal circumstances, high hydrostatic pressure at the arteriolar end of capillaries forces fluid out into the extravascular space, but this fluid returns into the capillaries at their venous end, where hydrostatic pressure is low (Fig. 2.3). In acute inflammation, however, not only is capillary hydrostatic pressure increased, but there is also escape of plasma proteins into the extravascular space, increasing the colloid osmotic pressure there. Consequently, much more fluid leaves the vessels than is returned to them. The net escape of protein-rich fluid is called *exudation*; hence, the fluid is called the *fluid exudate*.

Formation of the fluid exudate

The increased vascular permeability means that large molecules, such as proteins, can escape from vessels. Hence, the exudate fluid has a high protein content of up to 50 g/L. The proteins present include immunoglobulins, which may be important in the destruction of invading microorganisms, and coagulation factors, including fibrinogen, which result in fibrin deposition on contact with the extravascular tissues. Hence, acute inflamed organ surfaces are commonly covered by fibrin: the *fibrinous exudate*. There is a considerable turnover of the inflammatory exudate; it is constantly drained away by local lymphatic channels to be replaced by new exudate.

Ultrastructural basis of increased vascular permeability

The ultrastructural basis of increased vascular permeability was originally determined using an experimental model in which histamine, one of the chemical mediators of increased vascular permeability, was injected under the skin. This caused transient leakage of plasma proteins into the extravascular space. Electron microscopic examination of venules and small veins during this period showed that gaps of 0.1–0.4 μm diameter had appeared between endothelial cells. These gaps allowed the leakage of injected particles, such as carbon, into the tissues. The endothelial cells are not damaged during this process. They contain contractile proteins such as actin, which, when stimulated by the chemical mediators of acute inflammation, cause contraction of the endothelial cells, pulling open the transient pores. The leakage induced by chemical mediators, such as histamine, is confined to venules and small veins. Although fluid is lost by ultrafiltration from capillaries, there is no evidence that they too become more permeable in acute inflammation.

Other causes of increased vascular permeability

In addition to the transient vascular leakage caused by some inflammatory stimuli, certain other stimuli, e.g. heat, cold, ultraviolet light and x-rays, bacterial toxins and corrosive chemicals, cause delayed prolonged leakage. In these circumstances, there is direct injury to endothelial cells in several types of vessels within the damaged area (Table 2.1).

Tissue sensitivity to chemical mediators

The relative importance of chemical mediators and of direct vascular injury in causing increased vascular permeability varies according to the type of tissue. For example, vessels in the central nervous system are relatively insensitive to the chemical mediators, while those in the skin, conjunctiva and bronchial mucosa are exquisitely sensitive to agents such as histamine.

Formation of the cellular exudate

The accumulation of *neutrophil polymorphs* within the extracellular space is the diagnostic histological feature

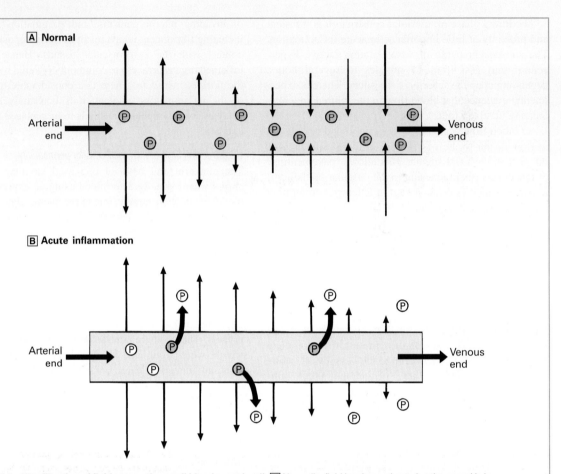

Fig. 2.3 Ultrafiltration of fluid across the small blood vessel wall. [A] Normally, fluid leaving and entering the vessel is in equilibrium. [B] In acute inflammation, there is a net loss of fluid together with plasma protein molecules (P) into the extracellular space, resulting in oedema. From Stephenson op. cit.

Table 2.1 Causes of increased vascular permeability	
Time course	Mechanisms
Immediate transient	Chemical mediators, e.g. histamine, bradykinin, nitric oxide, C5a, leukotriene B4, platelet activating factor
Immediate sustained	Severe direct vascular injury, e.g. trauma
Delayed prolonged	Endothelial cell injury, e.g. x-rays, bacterial toxins

of acute inflammation. The stages whereby leucocytes reach the tissues are shown in Figure 2.4.

Margination of neutrophils

In the normal circulation, cells are confined to the central (axial) stream in blood vessels, and do not flow in the peripheral (plasmatic) zone near to the endothelium. However, loss of intravascular fluid and increase in plasma viscosity with slowing of flow at the site of acute inflammation allow neutrophils to flow in this plasmatic zone.

Adhesion of neutrophils

The adhesion of neutrophils to the vascular endothelium which occurs at sites of acute inflammation is termed 'pavementing' of neutrophils. Neutrophils randomly contact the endothelium in normal tissues, but do not adhere to it. However, at sites of injury, pavementing occurs early in the acute inflammatory response and appears to be a specific process occurring independently of the eventual slowing of blood flow. The phenomenon is seen only in venules.

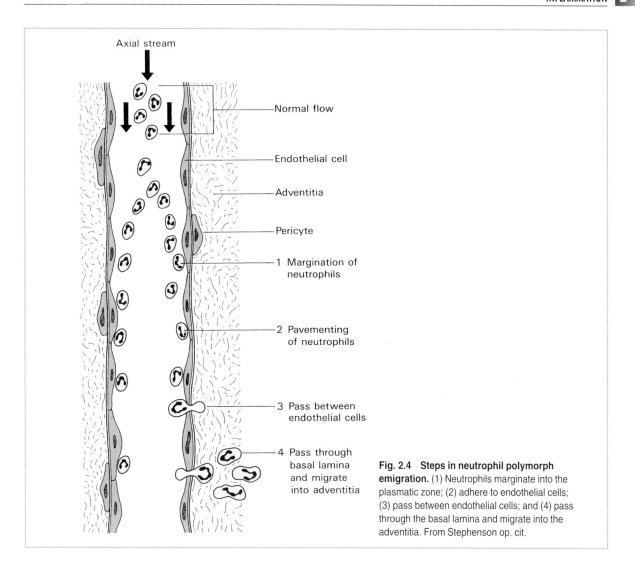

Fig. 2.4 Steps in neutrophil polymorph emigration. (1) Neutrophils marginate into the plasmatic zone; (2) adhere to endothelial cells; (3) pass between endothelial cells; and (4) pass through the basal lamina and migrate into the adventitia. From Stephenson op. cit.

Increased leucocyte adhesion results from interaction between paired *adhesion molecules* on leucocyte and endothelial surfaces. There are several classes of such adhesion molecules: some of them act as lectins which bind to carbohydrates on the partner cell. Leucocyte surface adhesion molecule expression is increased by:

- complement component C5a
- leukotriene B4
- tumour necrosis factor.

Endothelial cell expression of endothelial–leucocyte adhesion molecule-1 (ELAM-1) and intercellular adhesion molecule-1 (ICAM-1), to which the leucocytes' surface adhesion molecules bond, is increased by:

- interleukin-1
- endotoxins
- tumour necrosis factor.

In this way, a variety of chemical inflammatory mediators promote leucocyte–endothelial adhesion as a prelude to leucocyte emigration.

Neutrophil emigration

Leucocytes migrate by active amoeboid movement through the walls of venules and small veins, under the influence of C5a and leukotriene-B4, but do not commonly exit from capillaries. Electron microscopy shows that neutrophil and eosinophil polymorphs and macrophages can insert pseudopodia between endothelial cells, migrate through the gap so created between the endothelial cells, and then on through the basal lamina into the vessel wall. The defect appears to be self-sealing, and the endothelial cells are not damaged by this process.

Diapedesis

Red cells may also escape from vessels, but in this case the process is passive and depends on hydrostatic pressure forcing the red cells out. The process is called diapedesis, and the presence of large numbers of red cells in the extravascular space implies severe vascular injury, such as a tear in the vessel wall.

Chemotaxis of neutrophils

It has long been known from in-vitro experiments that neutrophil polymorphs are attracted towards certain chemical substances in solution — a process called chemotaxis. Video microscopy shows apparently purposeful migration of neutrophils along a concentration gradient. Compounds which appear chemotactic for neutrophils in vitro include certain complement components, cytokines and products produced by neutrophils themselves. It is not known whether chemotaxis is important in vivo. Neutrophils may possibly arrive at sites of injury by random movement, and then be trapped there by immobilising factors (a process analogous to the trapping of macrophages at sites of delayed type hypersensitivity by migration inhibitory factor; Ch. 6).

CHEMICAL MEDIATORS OF ACUTE INFLAMMATION

The spread of the acute inflammatory response following injury to a small area of tissue suggests that chemical substances are released from injured tissues, spreading outwards into uninjured areas. Early in the response, histamine and thrombin released by the original inflammatory stimulus cause upregulation of P-selectin and platelet activating factor (PAF) on the endothelial cells lining the venules. Adhesion molecules, stored in intracellular vesicles, appear rapidly on the cell surface. Neutrophil polymorphs begin to roll along the endothelial wall due to engagement of the lectin-like domain on the P-selectin molecule with sialyl Lewis^X carbohydrate ligands on the neutrophil polymorph surface mucins. This also helps platelet activating factor to dock with its corresponding receptor which, in turn, increases expression of the integrins lymphocyte function-associated molecule-1 (LFA-1) and membrane attack complex-1 (MAC-1). The overall effect of all these molecules is very firm neutrophil adhesion to the endothelial surface. These chemicals, called *endogenous chemical mediators*, cause:

- vasodilatation
- emigration of neutrophils
- chemotaxis
- increased vascular permeability.

Chemical mediators released from cells

Histamine. This is the best-known chemical mediator in acute inflammation. It causes vascular dilatation and the immediate transient phase of increased vascular permeability. It is stored in mast cells, basophil and eosinophil leucocytes, and platelets. Histamine release from these sites (for example, mast cell degranulation) is stimulated by complement components C3a and C5a, and by lysosomal proteins released from neutrophils.

Lysosomal compounds. These are released from neutrophils and include cationic proteins, which may increase vascular permeability, and neutral proteases, which may activate complement.

Prostaglandins. These are a group of long chain fatty acids derived from arachidonic acid and synthesised by many cell types. Some prostaglandins potentiate the increase in vascular permeability caused by other compounds. Others include platelet aggregation (prostaglandin I_2 is inhibitory while prostaglandin A_2 is stimulatory). Part of the anti-inflammatory activity of drugs such as aspirin and the non-steroidal anti-inflammatory drugs is attributable to inhibition of one of the enzymes involved in prostaglandin synthesis.

Leukotrienes. These are also synthesised from arachidonic acid, especially in neutrophils, and appear to have vasoactive properties. SRS-A (slow-reacting substance of anaphylaxis), involved in type I hypersensitivity (Ch. 6), is a mixture of leukotrienes.

5-hydroxytryptamine (serotonin). This is present in high concentration in mast cells and platelets. It is a potent vasoconstrictor.

Chemokines. This large family of 8–10 kDa proteins selectively attracts various types of leucocytes to the site of inflammation. Some chemokines such as IL-8 are mainly specific for neutrophil polymorphs and to a lesser extent lymphocytes, whereas other types of chemokines are chemotactic for monocytes, natural killer (NK) cells, basophils and eosinophils. The various chemokines bind to extracellular matrix components such as heparin and heparan sulphate glycosaminoglycans, setting up a gradient of chemotactic molecules fixed to the extracellular matrix.

Plasma factors

The plasma contains four enzymatic cascade systems — complement, the kinins, the coagulation factors and the fibrinolytic system — which are interrelated and produce various inflammatory mediators.

Complement system

The complement system is a cascade system of enzymatic proteins (Ch. 6). It can be activated during the acute inflammatory reaction in various ways:

- In tissue necrosis, enzymes capable of activating complement are released from dying cells.
- During infection, the formation of antigen–antibody complexes can activate complement via the *classical pathway*, while the endotoxins of Gram negative bacteria activate complement via the *alternative pathway* (Ch. 6).
- Products of the kinin, coagulation and fibrinolytic systems can activate complement.

The products of complement activation most important in acute inflammation include:

- C5a: chemotactic for neutrophils; increases vascular permeability; releases histamine from mast cells
- C3a: similar properties to those of C5a, but less active
- C567: chemotactic for neutrophils
- C56789: cytolytic activity
- C4b,2a,3b: opsonisation of bacteria (facilitates phagocytosis by macrophages).

Kinin system

The kinins are peptides of 9–11 amino acids; the most important vascular permeability factor is bradykinin. The kinin system is activated by coagulation factor XII (Fig. 2.5). Bradykinin is also a chemical mediator of the pain which is a cardinal feature of acute inflammation.

Coagulation system

The coagulation system (Ch. 10) is responsible for the conversion of soluble fibrinogen into fibrin, a major component of the acute inflammatory exudate.

Coagulation factor XII (the Hageman factor), once activated by contact with extracellular materials such as basal lamina, and various proteolytic enzymes of bacterial origin, can activate the coagulation, kinin and fibrinolytic systems. The interrelationships of these systems are shown in Figure 2.6.

Fibrinolytic system

Plasmin is responsible for the lysis of fibrin into fibrin degradation products, which may have local effects on vascular permeability.

Table 2.2 summarises the chemical mediators involved in the three main stages of acute inflammation.

ROLE OF TISSUE MACROPHAGES

These secrete numerous chemical mediators when stimulated by local infection or injury. Most important are the cytokines interleukin-1 (IL-1) and α-tumour necrosis factor (TNFα), whose stimulatory effect on endothelial cells occurs after that of histamine and thrombin. Other late products include E-selectin, an adhesion molecule which binds and activates neutrophils and the chemokines IL-8 and epithelial derived neutrophil attractant-78 which are potent chemotaxins for neutrophil polymorphs. Additionally, IL-1 and TNFα cause endothelial cells, fibroblasts and epithelial cells to secrete MCP-1, another powerful chemotactic protein for neutrophil polymorphs.

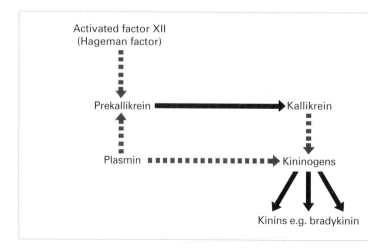

Fig. 2.5 The kinin system. Activated factor XII and plasmin activate the conversion of prekallikrein to kallikrein. This stimulates the conversion of kininogens to kinins, such as bradykinin. From Stephenson op. cit.

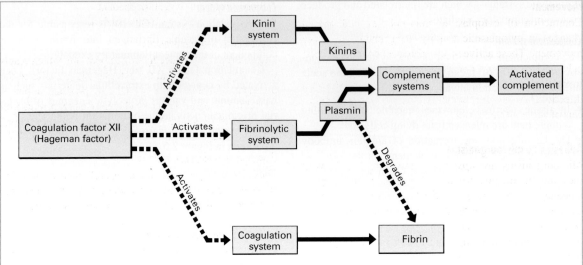

Fig. 2.6 Interactions between the systems of chemical mediators. Coagulation factor XII activates the kinin, fibrinolytic and coagulation systems. The complement system is in turn activated. From Stephenson op. cit.

Table 2.2 Endogenous chemical mediators of the acute inflammatory response	
Stages of acute inflammatory response	Chemical mediators
Vascular dilatation	Histamine, prostaglandins (PGE_2/I_2), VIP, nitric oxide, platelet-activating factor (PAF)
Increased vascular permeability	Transient phase — histamine Prolonged phase — mediators such as bradykinin, nitric oxide, C5a, leukotriene B4 and PAF potentiated by prostaglandins
Adhesion of leucocytes to endothelium	Upregulation of adhesion molecules on: • endothelium, principally by histamine, IL-1 and TNFα • neutrophil polymorphs, principally by IL-8, C5a, leukotriene B4, PAF, IL-1 and TNFα
Neutrophil polymorph chemotaxis	Leukotriene B4, IL-8 and others

ROLE OF THE LYMPHATICS

Terminal lymphatics are blind-ended, endothelium-lined tubes present in most tissues in similar numbers to capillaries. The terminal lymphatics drain into collecting lymphatics which have valves and so propel lymph passively, aided by contraction of neighbouring muscles, to the lymph nodes. The basal lamina of lymphatic endothelium is incomplete, and the junctions between the cells are simpler and less robust than those between capillary endothelial cells. Hence, gaps tend to open up passively between the lymphatic endothelial cells, allowing large protein molecules to enter.

In acute inflammation, the lymphatic channels become dilated as they drain away the oedema fluid of the inflammatory exudate. This drainage tends to limit the extent of oedema in the tissues. The ability of the lymphatics to carry large molecules and some particulate matter is important in the immune response to infecting agents; antigens are carried to the regional lymph nodes for recognition by lymphocytes (Ch. 6).

ROLE OF THE NEUTROPHIL POLYMORPH

The neutrophil polymorph is the characteristic cell of the acute inflammatory infiltrate. The actions of this cell will now be considered.

Movement

Contraction of cytoplasmic microtubules and gel/sol changes in cytoplasmic fluidity bring about amoeboid movement. These active mechanisms are dependent upon calcium ions and are controlled by intracellular concentrations of cyclic nucleotides. The movement shows a directional response (chemotaxis) to the various chemicals of acute inflammation.

Adhesion to microorganisms

Microorganisms are *opsonised* (from the Greek word meaning 'to prepare for the table'), or rendered more amenable to phagocytosis either by immunoglobulins or by complement components. Bacterial lipopolysaccharides activate complement via the alternative pathway (Ch. 6), generating component C3b, which has opsonising properties. In addition, if antibody binds to bacterial antigens, this can activate complement via the classical pathway, also generating C3b. In the immune individual, the binding of immunoglobulins to microorganisms by their Fab components leaves the Fc component (Ch. 6) exposed. Neutrophils have surface receptors for the Fc fragment of immunoglobulins, and consequently bind to the microorganisms prior to ingestion.

Phagocytosis

The process whereby cells (such as neutrophil polymorphs and macrophages) ingest solid particles is termed phagocytosis. The first step in phagocytosis is adhesion of the particle to be phagocytosed to the cell surface. This is facilitated by opsonisation, whereby the microorganism becomes coated with antibody, C3b and certain acute phase proteins, while phagocytic cells such as neutrophil polymorphs and macrophages have upregulated C3 and Ig receptors under the influence of inflammatory mediators, enhancing adhesion of the microorganism. The phagocyte then ingests the attached particle by sending out pseudopodia around it. These meet and fuse so that the particle lies in a phagocytic vacuole (also called a phagosome) bounded by cell membrane. Lysosomes, membrane-bound packets containing the toxic compounds described below, then fuse with phagosomes to form phagolysosomes. It is within these that intracellular killing of microorganisms occurs.

Intracellular killing of microorganisms

Neutrophil polymorphs are highly specialised cells, containing noxious microbicidal agents, some of which are similar to household bleach. The microbicidal agents may be classified as:

- those which are oxygen-dependent
- those which are oxygen-independent.

Oxygen-dependent mechanisms

The neutrophils produce hydrogen peroxide which reacts with myeloperoxidase in the cytoplasmic granules in the presence of halide, such as Cl^-, to produce a potent microbicidal agent. Other products of oxygen reduction also contribute to the killing, such as peroxide anions (O_2^-), hydroxyl radicals ($\cdot$OH) and singlet oxygen ($^1O_2$).

Oxygen-independent mechanisms

These include lysozyme (muramidase), lactoferrin which chelates iron required for bacterial growth, cationic proteins, and the low pH inside phagocytic vacuoles.

Release of lysosomal products

Release of lysosomal products from the cell damages local tissues by proteolysis by enzymes such as elastase and collagenase, activates coagulation factor XII, and attracts other leucocytes into the area. Some of the compounds released increase vascular permeability, while others are pyrogens, producing systemic fever by acting on the hypothalamus.

THE ROLE OF MAST CELLS

Mast cells have an important role in acute inflammation. On stimulation by the C3a/C5a complement components (Fig. 2.7) they release preformed inflammatory mediators present in their granules and metabolise arachidonic acid into newly synthesised inflammatory mediators (Table 2.3).

SPECIAL MACROSCOPIC APPEARANCES OF ACUTE INFLAMMATION

The cardinal signs of acute inflammation are modified according to the tissue involved and the type of agent provoking the inflammation. Several descriptive terms are used for the appearances.

Serous inflammation

In serous inflammation, there is abundant protein-rich fluid exudate with a relatively low cellular content. Examples include inflammation of the serous cavities, such as peritonitis, and inflammation of a synovial joint, acute synovitis. Vascular dilatation may be apparent to the naked eye, the serous surfaces appearing injected (Fig. 2.1), i.e. having dilated, blood-laden vessels on the surface (like the appearance of the conjunctiva in 'bloodshot eyes').

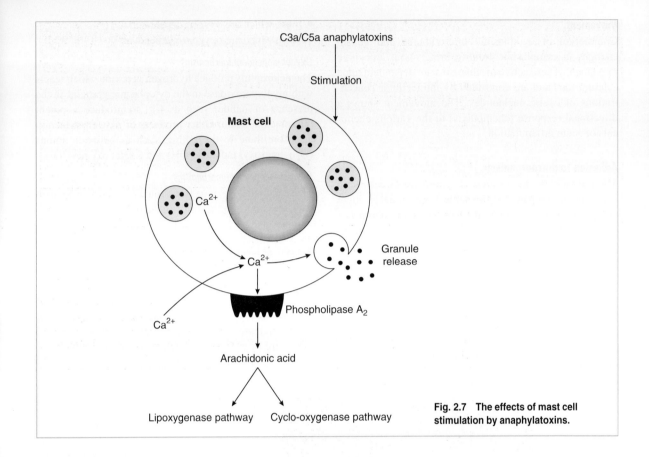

C3a/C5a anaphylatoxins

Stimulation

Mast cell

Ca^{2+}

Ca^{2+}

Ca^{2+}

Granule release

Phospholipase A_2

Arachidonic acid

Lipoxygenase pathway   Cyclo-oxygenase pathway

Fig. 2.7   The effects of mast cell stimulation by anaphylatoxins.

Catarrhal inflammation

When mucus hypersecretion accompanies acute inflammation of a mucous membrane, the appearance is described as catarrhal. The common cold is a good example.

Fibrinous inflammation

When the inflammatory exudate contains plentiful fibrinogen, this polymerises into a thick fibrin coating. This is often seen in acute pericarditis and gives the parietal and visceral pericardium a 'bread and butter' appearance.

Haemorrhagic inflammation

Haemorrhagic inflammation indicates severe vascular injury or depletion of coagulation factors. This occurs in acute pancreatitis, as a result of proteolytic destruction of vascular walls, and in meningococcal septicaemia, as a result of disseminated intravascular coagulation.

Suppurative (purulent) inflammation

The terms 'suppurative' and 'purulent' denote the production of pus, which consists of dying and degenerate neutrophils, infecting organisms and liquefied tissues. The pus may become walled-off by granulation tissue or fibrous tissue to produce an *abscess* (a localised collection of pus in a tissue). If a hollow viscus fills with pus, this is called an *empyema*: for example, empyema of the gallbladder (Fig. 2.8) or of the appendix (Fig. 2.9).

Membranous inflammation

In acute membranous inflammation, an epithelium becomes coated by fibrin, desquamated epithelial cells and inflammatory cells. An example is the grey membrane seen in pharyngitis or laryngitis due to *Corynebacterium diphtheriae*.

Pseudomembranous inflammation

The term 'pseudomembranous' describes superficial mucosal ulceration with an overlying slough of disrupted mucosa, fibrin, mucus and inflammatory cells. This is seen in pseudomembranous colitis due to *Clostridium difficile* colonisation of the bowel, usually following broad spectrum antibiotic treatment (Ch. 17).

Table 2.3	Two major pathways whereby mast cell stimulation leads to release of inflammatory mediators	
	Preformed	Effect
Granule release	Eosinophil chemotactic factor Neutrophil chemotactic factor	Eosinophil chemotaxis Neutrophil chemotaxis
	Histamine	Vasodilatation, increased capillary permeability, chemokinesis, bronchoconstriction
	Interleukins 3, 4, 5, 6 GM-CSF, TNF	Macrophage activation, triggering of acute phase proteins
	Neutral proteases β-glucosaminidase	Activates of C3 Cleaves glucosamine
	PAF	Mediator release
	Proteoglycan	Binds granule proteases
	Newly synthesised	Effect
Lipoxygenase pathway	Leukotrienes C_4, D_4 (SRS-A), and B_4	Bronchoconstriction, chemokinesis / chemotaxis, vasoactive
Cyclo-oxygenase	Prostaglandins Thromboxanes	Affect bronchial muscle, platelet aggregation and vasodilatation

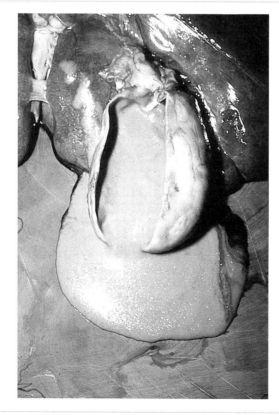

Fig. 2.8 Empyema of the gallbladder. The gallbladder lumen is filled with pus.

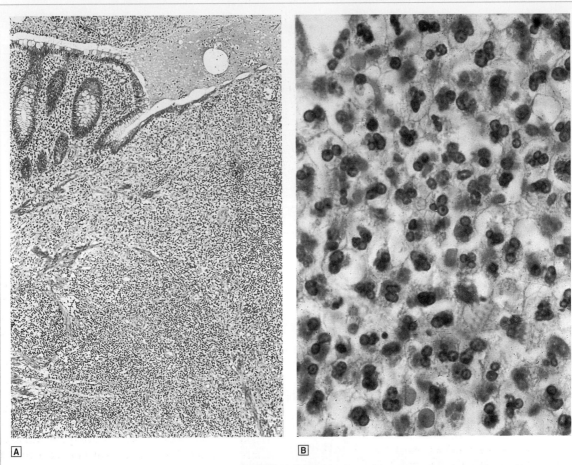

Fig. 2.9 Histology of acute appendicitis. [A] The appendix lumen is filled with pus, there is focal mucosal ulceration, and the appendicular wall and meso-appendix (bottom) are thickened because of an acute inflammatory exudate. [B] Pus in the lumen of the appendix. Pus consists of living and degenerate neutrophil polymorphs together with liquefied tissue debris.

Necrotising (gangrenous) inflammation

High tissue pressure due to oedema may lead to vascular occlusion and thrombosis, which may result in widespread septic necrosis of the organ. The combination of necrosis and bacterial putrefaction is *gangrene*. Gangrenous appendicitis is a good example (Fig 2.10).

EFFECTS OF ACUTE INFLAMMATION

Acute inflammation has local and systemic effects, both of which may be harmful or beneficial. The local effects are usually clearly beneficial — for example, the destruction of invading microorganisms — but at other times they appear to serve no obvious function, or may even be positively harmful.

Beneficial effects

Both the fluid and cellular exudates may have useful effects. Beneficial effects of the fluid exudate are as follows.

- *Dilution of toxins*, such as those produced by bacteria, allows them to be carried away in lymphatics.
- *Entry of antibodies* occurs due to increased vascular permeability into the extravascular space, where they may lead either to lysis of microorganisms, through the participation of complement, or to their phagocytosis by opsonisation. Antibodies are also important in neutralisation of toxins.
- *Transport of drugs*, such as antibiotics, to the site where bacteria are multiplying.

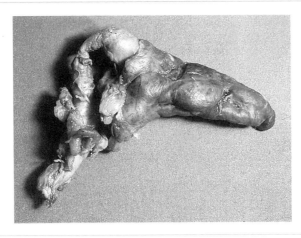

Fig. 2.10 Gangrenous appendix. The external surface is blackened as a result of acute inflammation with infarction.

- *Fibrin formation*, from exuded fibrinogen may impede the movement of microorganisms, trapping them and so facilitating phagocytosis.
- *Delivery of nutrients and oxygen*, essential for cells such as neutrophils which have high metabolic activity, is aided by increased fluid flow through the area.
- *Stimulation of immune response*, by drainage of this fluid exudate into the lymphatics, allows particulate and soluble antigens to reach the local lymph nodes, where they may stimulate the immune response.

The role of neutrophils in the cellular exudate has already been discussed. They have a lifespan of only 1–3 days and must be constantly replaced. Most die locally, but some leave the site via the lymphatics. Blood *monocytes* also arrive at the site and, on leaving the blood vessels, transform into *macrophages*, becoming more metabolically active, motile and phagocytic. Phagocytosis of microorganisms is enhanced by *opsonisation* by antibodies or by complement. In most acute inflammatory reactions, macrophages play a lesser role in phagocytosis than do neutrophil polymorphs. They appear late in the response and are usually responsible for clearing away tissue debris and damaged cells.

Both neutrophils and macrophages may discharge their lysosomal enzymes into the extracellular fluid by exocytosis, or the entire cell contents may be released when the cells die. Release of these enzymes assists in the *digestion of the inflammatory exudate*.

Harmful effects

The release of lysosomal enzymes by inflammatory cells may also have harmful effects, as follows.

- *Digestion of normal tissues*. Enzymes such as collagenases and proteases may digest normal tissues, resulting in their destruction. This may result particularly in vascular damage, for example in type III hypersensitivity reactions (Ch. 6).
- *Swelling*. The swelling of acutely inflamed tissues may be harmful: for example, in children the swelling of the epiglottis in acute epiglottitis due to *Haemophilus influenzae* infection may obstruct the airway, resulting in death. Inflammatory swelling is especially serious when it occurs in an enclosed space such as the cranial cavity. Thus, acute meningitis or a cerebral abscess may *raise intracranial pressure* to the point where blood flow into the brain is impaired, resulting in ischaemic damage, or may force the cerebral hemispheres against the tentorial orifice and the cerebellum into the foramen magnum (pressure coning; Ch. 8).
- *Inappropriate inflammatory response*. Sometimes, acute inflammatory responses appear inappropriate, such as those which occur in type I hypersensitivity reactions (e.g. hay fever; Ch. 6) where the provoking environmental antigen (e.g. pollen) otherwise poses no threat to the individual. Such allergic inflammatory responses may be life-threatening: for example, extrinsic asthma.

SEQUELAE OF ACUTE INFLAMMATION

The sequelae of acute inflammation depend upon the type of tissue involved and the amount of tissue destruction, which depend in turn upon the nature of the injurious agent. Both humoral and cellular mechanisms have evolved which regulate the inflammatory response. In the humoral control system there exist several complement regulatory proteins together with some acute phase proteins derived from the plasma transudate. At the cellular level, various prostaglandins, growth factors and glucocorticoids reduce cytokine production by T-lymphocytes and macrophages. The possible outcomes of acute inflammation are shown in Figure 2.11.

Resolution

The term resolution means the complete restoration of the tissues to normal after an episode of acute inflammation. The conditions which favour resolution are:

- minimal cell death and tissue damage
- occurrence in an organ or tissue which has regenerative capacity (e.g. the liver) rather than in one which cannot regenerate (e.g. the central nervous system)
- rapid destruction of the causal agent (e.g. phagocytosis of bacteria)
- rapid removal of fluid and debris by good local vascular drainage.

A good example of an acute inflammatory condition which usually resolves completely is acute lobar pneumonia (Ch. 11). The alveoli become filled with acute inflammatory exudate containing fibrin, bacteria and neutrophil polymorphs. The alveolar walls are thin and have many capillaries (for gas exchange) and lymphatic channels. The sequence of events leading to resolution is usually:

- phagocytosis of bacteria (e.g. pneumococci) by neutrophils and intracellular killing
- fibrinolysis
- phagocytosis of debris, especially by macrophages, and carriage through lymphatics to the hilar lymph nodes
- disappearance of vascular dilatation.

Following this, the lung parenchyma would appear histologically normal.

Suppuration

Suppuration is the formation of pus, a mixture of living, dying and dead neutrophils and bacteria, cellular debris and sometimes globules of lipid. The causative stumulus must be fairly persistent and is virtually always an infec-

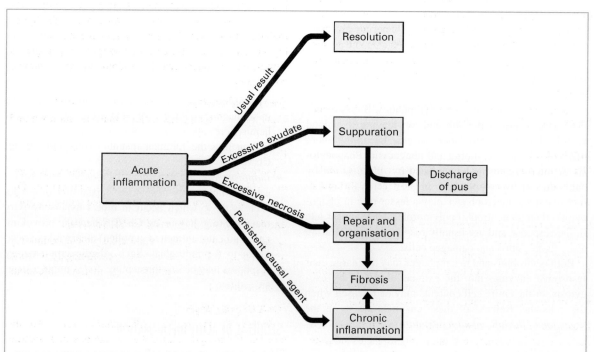

Fig. 2.11 The sequelae of acute inflammation. Resolution is the usual event, unless any of the adverse factors shown exist. From Stephenson op cit.

tive agent, usually pyogenic bacteria (e.g. *Staphylococcus aureus, Streptococcus pyogenes, Neisseria* species or coliform organisms). Once pus begins to accumulate in a tissue, it becomes surrounded by a 'pyogenic membrane' consisting of sprouting capillaries, neutrophils and occasional fibroblasts. Such a collection of pus is called an *abscess*, and bacteria within the abscess cavity are relatively inaccessible to antibodies and to antibiotic drugs (thus, for example, acute osteomyelitis, an abscess in the bone marrow cavity, is notoriously difficult to treat).

Abscess

An abscess (for example, a boil) usually 'points', then bursts; the abscess cavity collapses and is obliterated by organisation and fibrosis, leaving a small scar. Sometimes, surgical incision and drainage is necessary to eliminate the abscess.

If an abscess forms inside a hollow viscus (e.g. the gallbladder) the mucosal layers of the outflow tract of the viscus may become fused together by fibrin, resulting in an empyema (Fig. 2.8).

Such deep-seated abscesses sometimes discharge their pus along a *sinus tract* (an abnormal connection, lined by granulation tissue, between the abscess and the skin or a mucosal surface). If this results in an abnormal passage connecting two mucosal surfaces or one mucosal surface to the skin surface, it is referred to as a *fistula*. Sinuses occur particularly when foreign body materials are present, which are indigestible by macrophages and which favour continuing suppuration. The only treatment for this type of condition is surgical elimination of the foreign body material.

The fibrous walls of longstanding abscesses may become complicated by *dystrophic calcification*.

Organisation

Organisation of tissues is their replacement by granulation tissue. The circumstances favouring this outcome are when:

- large amounts of fibrin are formed, which cannot be removed completely by fibrinolytic enzymes from the plasma or from neutrophil polymorphs
- substantial volumes of tissue become necrotic or if the dead tissue (e.g. fibrous tissue) is not easily digested
- exudate and debris cannot be removed or discharged.

During organisation, new capillaries grow into the inert material (inflammatory exudate), macrophages migrate into the zone and fibroblasts proliferate under the influence of TGFβ, resulting in *fibrosis*. A good example of this is seen in the pleural space following acute lobar

pneumonia. Resolution usually occurs in the lung parenchyma, but very extensive fibrinous exudate fills the pleural cavity. The fibrin is not easily removed, and consequently capillaries grow into the fibrin, accompanied by macrophages and fibroblasts (the exudate becomes 'organised'). Eventually, fibrous adhesion occurs between the parietal and visceral pleura.

Progression to chronic inflammation

If the agent causing acute inflammation is not removed, the acute inflammation may progress to the chronic stage. In addition to organisation of the tissue just described, the character of the cellular exudate changes, with lymphocytes, plasma cells and macrophages (sometimes including multinucleate giant cells) replacing the neutrophil polymorphs. Often, however, chronic inflammation occurs as a primary event, there being no preceding period of acute inflammation.

SYSTEMIC EFFECTS OF INFLAMMATION

Apart from the local features of acute and chronic inflammation described above, an inflammatory focus produces systemic effects.

Pyrexia

Polymorphs and macrophages produce compounds known as *endogenous pyrogens* which act on the hypothalamus to set the thermoregulatory mechanisms at a higher temperature. Release of endogenous pyrogen is stimulated by phagocytosis, endotoxins and immune complexes.

Constitutional symptoms

Constitutional symptoms include malaise, anorexia and nausea.

Weight loss

Weight loss, due to negative nitrogen balance, is common when there is extensive chronic inflammation. For this reason, tuberculosis used to be called 'consumption'.

Reactive hyperplasia of the reticulo-endothelial system

Local or systemic lymph node enlargement commonly accompanies inflammation, while splenomegaly is found in certain specific infections (e.g. malaria, infectious mononucleosis).

Haematological changes

Increased erythrocyte sedimentation rate An increased erythrocyte sedimentation rate is a non-specific finding in many types of inflammation.

Leucocytosis Neutrophilia occurs in pyogenic infections and tissue destruction; eosinophilia in allergic disorders and parasitic infection; lymphocytosis in chronic infection (e.g. tuberculosis), many viral infections and in whooping cough; and monocytosis occurs in infectious mononucleosis and certain bacterial infections (e.g. tuberculosis, typhoid).

Anaemia This may result from blood loss in the inflammatory exudate (e.g. in ulcerative colitis), haemolysis (due to bacterial toxins), and 'the anaemia of chronic disorders' due to toxic depression of the bone marrow.

Amyloidosis

Longstanding chronic inflammation (for example, in rheumatoid arthritis, tuberculosis and bronchiectasis), by elevating serum amyloid A protein (SAA), may cause amyloid to be deposited in various tissues, resulting in *secondary (reactive) amyloidosis*.

CHRONIC INFLAMMATION

The principal features of chronic inflammation are as follows.

- Lymphocytes, plasma cells and macrophages predominate.
- Usually primary, but may follow recurrent acute inflammation.
- Granulomatous inflammation is a specific type of chronic inflammation.
- A granuloma is an aggregate of epithelioid histiocytes.
- May be complicated by secondary (reactive) amyloidosis.

The word 'chronic' applied to any process implies that the process has extended over a long period of time. This is usually the case in chronic inflammation, but here the term 'chronic' takes on a much more specific meaning, in that the type of cellular reaction differs from that seen in acute inflammation. Chronic inflammation may be defined as an inflammatory process in which lymphocytes, plasma cells and macrophages predominate, and which is usually accompanied by the formation of granulation tissue, resulting in fibrosis. Chronic inflammation is usually primary, sometimes called chronic inflammation ab initio, but does occasionally follow acute inflammation.

CAUSES OF CHRONIC INFLAMMATION

Primary chronic inflammation

In most cases of chronic inflammation, the inflammatory response has all the histological features of chronic inflammation from the onset, and there is no initial phase of acute inflammation. Some examples of primary chronic inflammation are listed in Table 2.4.

Transplant rejection

Cellular rejection of, for example, renal transplants involves chronic inflammatory cell infiltration.

Progression from acute inflammation

Most cases of acute inflammation do not develop into the chronic form, but resolve completely. The commonest variety of acute inflammation to progress to chronic inflammation is the suppurative type. If the pus forms an abscess cavity which is deep-seated, and drainage is delayed or inadequate, then by the time that drainage occurs the abscess will have developed thick walls composed of granulation and fibrous tissues. The rigid walls of the abscess cavity therefore fail to come together after

Table 2.4 Some examples of primary chronic inflammation	
Cause of inflammation	Example
Resistance of infective agent to phagocytosis and intracellular killing	Tuberculosis, leprosy, brucellosis, viral infections
Foreign body reactions	Endogenous materials, e.g. necrotic adipose tissue, bone, uric acid crystals Exogenous materials, e.g. silica, asbestos fibres, suture materials, implanted prostheses
Some autoimmune diseases	Organ-specific diseases, e.g. Hashimoto's thyroiditis, chronic gastritis of pernicious anaemia Non-organ-specific autoimmune disease, e.g. rheumatoid arthritis Contact hypersensitivity reactions, e.g. self-antigens altered by nickel
Specific diseases of unknown aetiology	Chronic inflammatory bowel disease, e.g. ulcerative colitis
Primary granulomatous diseases	Crohn's disease, sarcoidosis, reactions to beryllium

drainage, and the stagnating pus within the cavity becomes organised by the ingrowth of granulation tissue, eventually to be replaced by a fibrous scar.

Good examples of such chronic abscesses include: an abscess in bone marrow cavity (osteomyelitis), which is notoriously difficult to eradicate; and empyema thoracis which has been inadequately drained.

Some bacterial infections lead to chronic inflammation because the microbes have evolved defence mechanisms to phagocytosis. Some virulent organisms synthesise an outer capsule, which resists adhesion to phagocytes and covers carbohydrate molecules on the bacterial surface, preventing their recognition by phagocyte receptors. Some bacterial capsules physically block access of phagocytes to C3b deposited on the bacterial cell wall. Other organisms have positively antiphagocytic cell surface molecules or even secrete exotoxins which poison the leucocytes. Some bacteria bind to the surface of non-phagocytic cells to 'hide' from phagocytes. Poor activation of complement by some bacterial capsules, acceleration of complement breakdown by bacterial surface molecules such as sialic acid, and secretion of enzymes which degrade C5a are ways in which the complement system can be prevented from clearing infections. Evasion of immune responses by variation of surface antigens is encountered in viruses and parasites, but also to a lesser extent with some bacteria.

Another feature which favours progression to chronic inflammation is the presence of indigestible material. This may be keratin from a ruptured epidermal cyst, or fragments of necrotic bone as in the sequestrum of chronic osteomyelitis (Ch. 12). These materials are relatively inert, and are resistant to the action of lysosomal enzymes. The most indigestible forms of material are inert foreign body materials: for example, some types of surgical suture, wood, metal or glass implanted into a wound, or deliberately implanted prostheses such as artificial joints. It is not known why the presence of foreign body materials give rise to chronic suppuration, but it is a well-established fact that suppuration will not cease without surgical removal of the material.

Foreign bodies have in common the tendency to provoke a special type of chronic inflammation called 'granulomatous inflammation', and to cause macrophages to form multinucleate giant cells called 'foreign body giant cells'.

Recurrent episodes of acute inflammation

Recurring cycles of acute inflammation and healing eventually result in the clinicopathological entity of chronic inflammation. The best example of this is chronic cholecystitis, normally due to the presence of gallstones (Ch. 17): multiple recurrent episodes of acute inflammation lead to replacement of the gallbladder wall muscle by fibrous tissue, and the predominant cell type becomes the lymphocyte rather than the neutrophil polymorph.

MACROSCOPIC APPEARANCES OF CHRONIC INFLAMMATION

The commonest appearances of chronic inflammation are:

- *chronic ulcer*, such as a chronic peptic ulcer of the stomach with breach of the mucosa, a base lined by granulation tissue and with fibrous tissue extending through the muscle layers of the wall (Fig. 2.12).
- *chronic abscess cavity*: for example osteomyelitis, empyema thoracis
- *thickening of the wall of a hollow viscus* by fibrous tissue in the presence of a chronic inflammatory cell infiltrate: for example Crohn's disease, chronic cholecystitis (Fig. 2.13)
- *granulomatous inflammation* with caseous necrosis, as in chronic fibrocaseous tuberculosis of the lung
- *fibrosis*, which may become the most prominent feature of the chronic inflammatory reaction when most of the chronic inflammatory cell infiltrate has subsided. This is commonly seen in chronic cholecystitis, and peptic ulceration where fibrosis distorts the gastric wall and may even lead to acquired pyloric stenosis, and in the strictures which characterise Crohn's disease (Ch. 17).

MICROSCOPIC FEATURES OF CHRONIC INFLAMMATION

The cellular infiltrate consists characteristically of lymphocytes, plasma cells and macrophages. A few eosinophil polymorphs may be present, but neutrophil polymorphs are scarce. Some of the macrophages may form multinucleate giant cells. Exudation of fluid is not a prominent feature, but there may be production of new fibrous tissue from granulation tissue (Fig. 2.13). There may be evidence of continuing destruction of tissue at the same time as tissue regeneration and repair. Tissue necrosis may be a prominent feature, especially in granulomatous conditions such as tuberculosis. It is not usually possible to predict the causative factor from the histological appearances in chronic inflammation.

PARACRINE STIMULATION OF CONNECTIVE TISSUE PROLIFERATION

Healing involves regeneration and migration of specialised cells, while the predominant features in repair are

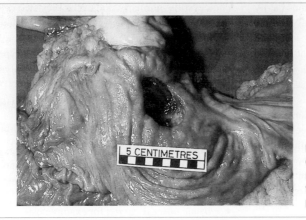

Fig. 2.12 Chronic peptic ulcer of the stomach. Continuing tissue destruction and repair cause replacement of the gastric wall muscle layers by fibrous tissue. As the fibrous tissue contracts, permanent distortion of the gastric shape may result.

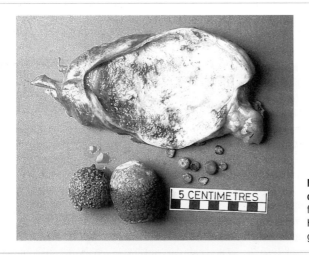

Fig. 2.13 Gallbladder showing chronic cholecystitis. The wall is greatly thickened by fibrous tissue. One of the gallstones was impacted in Hartmann's pouch, a saccular dilatation at the gallbladder neck.

angiogenesis followed by fibroblast proliferation and collagen synthesis. These processes are regulated by low molecular weight proteins called *growth factors* which bind to specific receptors on cell membranes and trigger a series of events culminating in cell proliferation (Table 2.5).

CELLULAR COOPERATION IN CHRONIC INFLAMMATION

The lymphocytic tissue infiltrate contains two main types of lymphocyte (described more fully in Ch. 6).

B-lymphocytes, on contact with antigen, become progressively transformed into plasma cells, which are cells specially adapted for the production of antibodies. The other main type of lymphocyte, the T lymphocyte, is responsible for cell-mediated immunity. On contact with

antigen, T lymphocytes produce a range of soluble factors called cytokines, which have a number of important activities.

- *Recruitment of macrophages into the area*. It is thought that macrophages are recruited into the area mainly via factors such as migration inhibition factor (MIF) which trap macrophages in the tissue. Macrophage activation factors (MAF) stimulate macrophage phagocytosis and killing of bacteria.
- *Production of inflammatory mediators*. T lymphocytes produce a number of inflammatory mediators, including cytokines, chemotactic factors for neutrophils, and factors which increase vascular permeability.
- *Recruitment of other lymphocytes*. Interleukins stimulate other lymphocytes to divide and confer on other lymphocytes the ability to mount cell-mediated immune

Table 2.5   Growth factors involved in healing and repair associated with inflammation

Growth factor	Abbreviation	Function
Epidermal growth factor	EGF	Regeneration of epithelial cells
Transforming growth factor α	TGFα	Regeneration of epithelial cells
Transforming growth factor β	TGFβ	Stimulates fibroblast proliferation and collagen synthesis, controls epithelial regeneration
Platelet-derived growth factor	PDGF	Mitogenic and chemotactic for fibroblasts and smooth muscle cells
Fibroblast growth factors	FGF	Stimulates fibroblast proliferation, angiogenesis and epithelial cell regeneration
Insulin-like growth factor-1	IGF-1	Synergistic effect with other growth factors
Tumour necrosis factor	TNF	Stimulates angiogenesis

responses to a variety of antigens. T lymphocytes also cooperate with B lymphocytes, assisting them in recognising antigens.

- *Destruction of target cells.* Factors, such as perforins, are produced which destroy other cells by damaging their cell membranes.
- *Interferon production.* Interferon γ, produced by activated T cells, has antiviral properties and, in turn, activates macrophages. Interferons α and β, produced by macrophages and fibroblasts, have antiviral properties and activate natural killer (NK) cells and macrophages.

These pathways of cellular cooperation are summarised in Figure 2.14.

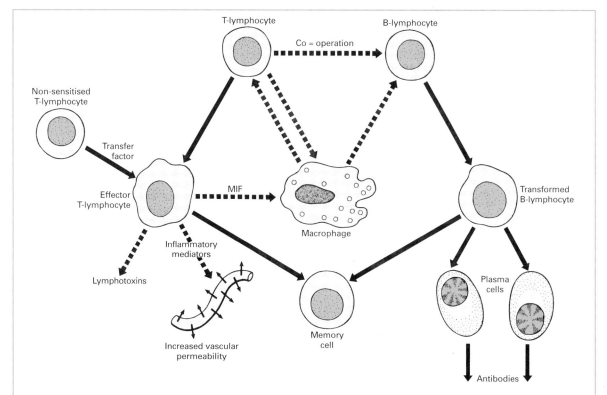

Fig. 2.14   Cellular cooperation in chronic inflammation. Solid arrows show pathways of cellular differentiation. Dotted arrows show intercellular communication. MIF = migration inhibition factor. From Stephenson op. cit.

MACROPHAGES IN CHRONIC INFLAMMATION

Macrophages are relatively large cells, up to 30 μm in diameter, which move by amoeboid motion through the tissues. They respond to certain chemotactic stimuli (possibly cytokines and antigen–antibody complexes) and have considerable phagocytic capabilities for the ingestion of microorganisms and cell debris. When neutrophil polymorphs ingest microorganisms, they usually bring about their own destruction and thus have a limited life-span of up to about 3 days. Macrophages can ingest a wider range of materials than can polymorphs and, being long-lived, they can harbour viable organisms if they are not able to kill them by their lysosomal enzymes. Examples of organisms which can survive inside macrophages include mycobacteria, such as *Mycobacterium tuberculosis* and *Mycobacterium leprae*, and organisms such as *Histoplasma capsulatum*. When macrophages participate in the delayed type hypersensitivity response (Ch. 6) to these types of organism, they often die in the process, contributing to the large areas of necrosis by release of their lysosomal enzymes.

Macrophages in inflamed tissues are derived from blood monocytes which have migrated out of vessels and have become transformed in the tissues. They are thus part of the *mononuclear phagocyte system* (Fig. 2.15). This system is in turn part of the *reticulo-endothelial system* which refers not only to the phagocytic cells, but also to interdigitating reticulum cells of lymph nodes and the endothelial cells in lymphoid organs.

The mononuclear phagocyte system, shown in Figure 2.15, is now known to include macrophages, fixed tissue histiocytes in many organs and, probably, the osteoclasts of bone. All are derived from monocytes which in turn are derived from a haemopoietic stem cell in the bone marrow.

The 'activation' of macrophages as they migrate into an area of inflammation involves an increase in size, protein synthesis, mobility, phagocytic activity and content of lysosomal enzymes. Electron microscopy reveals that the cells have a roughened cell membrane bearing filopodia, while the cytoplasm contains numerous dense bodies – phagolysosomes (formed by the fusion of lysosomes with phagocytic vacuoles).

Macrophages produce a range of important cytokines, including interferons α and β, interleukins 1, 6 and 8, and tumour necrosis factor (TNFα) (see Ch. 6).

Specialised forms of macrophages and granulomatous inflammation

A *granuloma* is an aggregate of epithelioid histiocytes.

Epithelioid histiocytes

Named for their vague histological resemblance to epithelial cells, epithelioid histiocytes have large vesicular nuclei, plentiful eosinophilic cytoplasm and are often

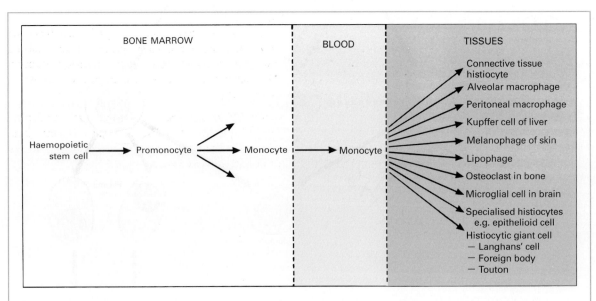

Fig. 2.15 The mononuclear phagocyte system. All of the differentiated cell types on the right are derived from blood monocytes. From Stephenson co. cit.

rather elongated. They tend to be arranged in clusters. They have little phagocytic activity, but appear to be adapted to a secretory function. The full range, or purpose, of their secretory products is not known, although one product is *angiotensin-converting enzyme*. Measurement of the activity of this enzyme in the blood can act as a marker for systemic granulomatous disease, such as sarcoidosis.

The appearance of granulomas may be augmented by the presence of caseous necrosis (as in tuberculosis) or by the conversion of some of the histiocytes into multinucleate giant cells. A common feature of many of the stimuli which induce granulomatous inflammation is indigestibility of particulate matter by macrophages. In other conditions, such as the systemic granulomatous condition *sarcoidosis*, there appear to be far-reaching derangements in immune responsiveness favouring granulomatous inflammation. In other instances, small traces of elements such as beryllium induce granuloma formation, but the way in which they induce the inflammation is unknown. Some of the commoner granulomatous conditions are shown in Table 2.6.

Histiocytic giant cells

Histiocytic giant cells tend to form where particulate matter which is indigestible by macrophages accumulates: for example, inert minerals such as silica, or bacteria such as tubercle bacilli which have cell walls containing mycolic acids and waxes which resist enzymatic digestion. The multinucleate giant cells, which may contain over 100 nuclei, are thought to develop 'by accident' when two or more macrophages attempt simultaneously to engulf the same particle; their cell membranes fuse and the cells unite. The multinucleate giant cells resulting have little phagocytic activity and no known function. They are given specific names according to their microscopic appearance.

Langhans' giant cells

Langhans' giant cells have a horseshoe arrangement of peripheral nuclei at one pole of the cell and are character-

Table 2.6	Causes of granulomatous disease
Cause	Example
Specific infections	Mycobacteria, e.g. tuberculosis, leprosy, atypical mycobacteria; many types of fungi, parasites, larvae, eggs and worms, syphilis
Foreign bodies	Endogenous, e.g. keratin, necrotic bone, cholesterol crystals, sodium urate Exogenous, e.g. talc, silica, suture materials, oils, silicone
Specific chemicals	Beryllium
Drugs	Hepatic granulomas due to allopurinol, phenylbutazone, sulphonamides
Unknown	Crohn's disease, sarcoidosis, Wegener's granulomatosis

istically seen in tuberculosis, although they may be seen in other granulomatous conditions. (They must not be confused with Langerhans' cells, the dendritic antigen-presenting cells of the epidermis.)

Foreign-body giant cells

So-called 'foreign-body giant cells' are large cells with nuclei randomly scattered throughout their cytoplasm. They are characteristically seen in relation to particulate foreign-body material.

Touton giant cells

Touton giant cells have a central ring of nuclei, while the peripheral cytoplasm is clear because of accumulated lipid. They are seen at sites of adipose tissue breakdown and in xanthomas (tumour-like aggregates of lipid-laden macrophages).

Although giant cells are commonly seen in granulomas, they do not constitute a defining feature. Solitary giant cells in the absence of epithelioid histiocytes do not constitute a granuloma.

3

Thrombosis, embolism and infarction

Dennis W K Cotton, Kenneth G Callum

Failure of the circulation to deliver blood to the tissues is termed vascular insufficiency. The main cause of this is thromboembolic disease, and when this is in the arterial circulation it is frequently associated with atherosclerosis. There are other causes (Box 3.1), which will be dealt with later in the chapter.

THROMBOEMBOLIC VASCULAR INSUFFICIENCY

Box 3.1   Causes of vascular insufficiency

- thromboembolism
  - venous — pulmonary embolism
  - arterial — systemic embolism
- non-thrombotic embolism
  - gas (air and nitrogen)
  - fat
  - tumour
  - amniotic fluid
  - foreign body, e.g. i.v. cannula, particulate matter with i.v. drug abusers
  - therapeutic, e.g. gelfoam, steel coils
- non-thromboembolic
  - atheroma
  - torsion
  - spontaneous vascular occlusion, e.g.spasm in Raynaud's
  - 'steal' syndrome
  - external compression, e.g. fractures, tourniquets, tumours

THROMBOSIS

A thrombus is defined as a solid mass formed in the living circulation from the components of the streaming blood. This serves to distinguish it from a clot which may form:

- outside the body

- in a dead body
- outside of the vasculature.

Thrombosis (the formation of thrombus) is a well-ordered series of events involving the blood platelets and the clotting cascade. Platelets adhere to areas of endothelial damage and if the stimulus is strong enough will go on to platelet activation with shape change and release of a number of substances which enhance the process of thrombosis at the same time as aggregating together.

Stages in the development of thrombosis

Thrombus may form in the heart, arteries, veins, or capillaries. The first stage involves platelets sticking to the damaged endothelium, and then a dense layer of fibrin and leucocytes adhere to the surface of the platelet. Blood clot (fibrin and red cells) develops on this layer of leucocytes and platelets, and then a secondary layer of platelets collects on the surface of the blood clot. The gradual extension of thrombosis leads to a propagated or consecutive thrombus. Organisation then begins with adherence to the wall of the vessel as mural thrombus. A second stage develops with a further batch of platelets laid down over the initial aggregate and then a further layer of blood clot. In this way alternate layers of platelets and blood clot form a laminar arrangement. This causes a differential contraction of platelets and fibrin and gives a rippled appearance reminiscent of rippling of the sand on a beach. This has also been described as having a coralline appearance. The ridges on the surface of the thrombi are known as the lines of Zahn after the pathologist who first described them. Further development depends on whether the endothelium is healthy and on the rate of blood flow. Thus in an artery with thrombosis secondary to atherosclerosis thrombosis may extend to the next branch after the endothelium becomes healthy again, assuming that there are collaterals with a reasonable blood flow. In veins, where the process tends to start in the pocket just above the valve, a number of things may happen: the process may end and the thrombus become covered with new endothelial cells; alternatively it may continue until a segment of vein is occluded. There is then a stagnant column of blood until the next tributary, and this stagnant column tends to coagulate, forming propagated thrombus. If the blood flow is reduced, the propagation may continue extensively. It may adhere to the sidewall of the veins in places or it may be largely free, simply attached to the site of origin. This latter type of thrombus can become dislodged relatively easily, forming a pulmonary embolism.

Causes of thrombosis

Several factors contribute to thrombus formation and these are usually grouped together under three headings (Virchow's triad). The factors in Virchow's triad are:

- damage to the vessel wall
- alterations in blood flow
- alterations in the constituents of the blood.

Not all these factors need to be present at the same time; some will be dominant in one clinical situation, whilst others will predominate in another. For example, venous thrombosis is commonly due to alterations in blood flow, while arterial thrombosis is more commonly due to vessel wall changes of atheroma, which does not occur in veins.

Damage to the vessel wall

- arteries — atherosclerotic plaques or synthetic grafts
- heart — congenital abnormalities or artificial valves
- veins — local injury caused by pressure on the calves from bed or operating table; or by insertion of intravenous cannulae; or distortion of the femoral vein during hip replacement.

Arterial thrombosis Atheroma of the arterial wall presents a good example of how vessel damage can lead to thrombosis and it is also a very common and important clinical situation. Atheroma is discussed in greater detail elsewhere (Ch. 9), but some points will be discussed here because they are relevant to the process of thrombosis. The first signs of atheroma appear in young adult life or even earlier and presents as fatty streaks. These are due to lipids accumulating within the vessel wall both intracellularly and in the connective tissue. This raises the intima into the vessel lumen and causes mild turbulence within the blood stream. Of themselves, fatty streaks are unlikely to cause significant disturbance to laminar blood flow but slowing of blood flow and increased viscosity acting together with larger fatty streaks could theoretically result in thrombi, but it would be expected that the thrombolytic system would deal with these.

Vascular endothelial cells have intrinsic fibrinolytic activity in which plasminogen, an inactive plasma protein synthesised in the liver, is converted to the active fibrinolytic enzyme plasmin. Whether thrombosis occurs or proceeds depends on the balance between the processes of thrombosis and fibrinolysis.

As fatty streaks progress they present more obstruction to normal flow, and endothelial cells may be lost. Fibrin and platelets may become deposited on the surface and protrude into the lumen, causing more turbulence, and a complicated atheromatous plaque develops. This plaque is also at risk from haemorrhage within it, and when it occurs it causes the plaque to protrude even further into the lumen. Several factors can increase the risk of atheroma and thus indirectly of thrombosis:

- smoking
- hypertension
- high blood cholesterol
- diabetes mellitus.

Smoking causes damage to endothelial linings and predisposes to atheroma formation. Hypertension increases atheroma formation, possibly because the increased pressure drives cholesterol through the intimal wall into the media, where it is taken up by macrophages and smooth muscle cells. Increased levels of cholesterol in the blood also directly contribute to atheroma formation even in the absence of hypertension, although the two commonly go together. Diabetes also contributes to atheroma formation through hyperlipidaemia, which is common in diabetes, but also as a result of direct metabolic processes, including collagen cross-linking, which traps cholesterol within the vessel wall, and increased 'stickiness' of platelets. Individuals with any one or combination of these factors are also at risk from thrombus formation on their atheromatous plaques.

Venous thrombosis Mechanical damage and vascular inflammation are the commonest causes of damage to venous walls, with subsequent thrombus formation. Inflammation of vessel walls, either arteries or veins, can cause thrombus formation, but the converse is also true. Thrombus initiates an inflammatory response, and in any given instance it can be difficult to say whether the process represents phlebothrombosis (thrombus due to inflammation) or thrombophlebitis (inflammation due to thrombosis). However, the commonest cause of venous thrombosis is alteration to blood flow.

Alterations in blood flow

The normal laminar flow may change to a turbulent pattern. This may happen with:

- prolonged inactivity following surgery, trauma, or a myocardial infarction

- heart failure
- proximal occlusion of the venous drainage.

Alterations in blood flow are critical in the venous system since pressure is much lower and the normal rate of flow is much slower than in the arteries. Because pressure is so much lower in the venous system and the vein walls are so much thinner than the walls of arteries of the same calibre, use is made of the pumping action of the surrounding muscle groups to aid return of blood to the heart. Consequently any decrease in muscle activity deprives venous blood of this added action and relative stasis occurs. Thus venous thrombosis becomes more likely in the veins of immobile subjects. The elderly are particularly at risk since they often have a degree of venous impairment or relative cardiac failure. One of the commonest deficiencies of the elderly venous system is impairment of the function of venous valves, and thrombosis is often seen to begin at the site of valves where, even under normal circumstances, some degree of turbulance is to be expected. For this reason it is particularly important to promote muscle contraction in the legs of the elderly in the postsurgical period. Another cause of relative immobility is long aeroplane journeys where immobility is combined with some degree of dehydration often due to alcohol consumption.

Alterations in the constituents of the blood
Alterations which may occur include:

- increased number of platelets following surgery or injury
- increased adhesiveness of young platelets produced at this time
- fluid loss, which may increase viscosity
- thrombophilia — abnormal balance of clotting factors and natural anticoagulants.

Alterations in the constituents of the blood may be due to relative water loss or to the presence of increased levels of blood constituents, resulting, in both cases, in an increase in blood viscosity. This not only slows flow but may also increase the tendency of blood to clot. Various constituents of the blood may increase in amount, generally as a consequence of other diseases such as myeloma. Some proteins show a tendency to slow circulation at lower temperatures, and thrombosis and infarction may therefore present rather dramatically in the cold-exposed peripheries.

Fate of thrombi
Thrombi may (Fig. 3.1):

- undergo complete resolution
- become organised as a scar

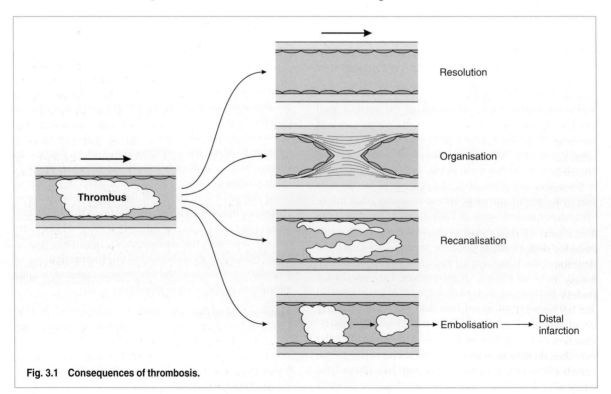

Fig. 3.1 Consequences of thrombosis.

- recanalise
- embolise in whole or in part.

It is not clear what factors determine which of these fates a thrombus will suffer, although size may be a factor. Small thrombi are being formed and resolved constantly, and some degree of disturbance of blood flow is probably required to tip the scales and cause a thrombus to organise. Certainly a larger thrombus will cause turbulence and/or inflammation and make it likely that further thrombosis will occur on its surface, causing the thrombus to lengthen, a process known as propagation. Resolution means that the clot is completely dissolved by processes of thrombolysis. In the clinical setting this is achieved by the use of thrombolytic enzymes, e.g. plasminogen activator or urokinase, but these have to be delivered onto the clot more or less directly, otherwise they diffuse through the blood stream and may become so dilute that they are ineffectual. Current therapies involve substances that act directly or indirectly on plasminogen activators. Compound such as aspirin and heparin help prevent further thrombus formation but do not help in lysis of an established thrombus. If the thrombus is not completely removed then the residue undergoes organisation.

Organisation is the process by which the thrombus is converted to a scar and eventually covered by endothelial cells. Intravascular scarring is essentially similar to those processes involved in the production of scars from thrombi in wound healing generally (Ch. 1). The main difference between intravascular granulation tissue and a thrombus is that with a thrombus the vascular phase of granulation tissue is prolonged and, if the thrombus does not resolve completely, the capillaries fuse together, resulting in one or several new vessels passing through the scar. This process is called recanalisation and in some cases may result in one or more functional vascular channels.

Thromboembolism is embolisation of a thrombus and should be distinguished from emboli of other materials since the clinical setting is different, as is the treatment. The effects of thromboemboli depend upon where the embolus settles, which in turn depends upon where the thrombus forms and what size the embolus is. Emboli arising from thrombi in veins will all go to the lungs (unless there is an abnormal connection between right and left heart). They will generally not arrest early in the circulation since the veins increase in diameter with the direction of blood flow as they approach the lungs, and only then do they start to turn into progressively smaller vessels of the lung bed. Arterial emboli will arrest in the artery with the smallest calibre which they can enter, and this will always be more peripheral than their origin because arterial size decreases in the direction of blood flow.

EMBOLISM

An embolus is an abnormal mass of undissolved material which passes in the blood stream from one part of the circulation to another, impacting in vessels too small to allow it to pass. The actual material which passes along the blood stream is termed an embolus. When it impacts and obstructs the flow of blood, this is known as an embolism. Thus when a thrombus in the leg breaks off, this is an embolus, and when it impacts in the pulmonary artery it is a pulmonary embolism. Emboli may consist of:

- thrombus
- gas (air and nitrogen)
- fat
- tumour
- amniotic fluid
- foreign body
- therapeutic emboli, e.g. gelfoam, muscle, steel coils.

Thromboembolism

Venous thromboembolism

The overwhelming majority of emboli arise from thrombus in the veins of the lower limbs. They then travel up through the inferior vena cava to the right side of the heart and finally impact in the pulmonary artery or one of its major branches, depending on the size of the embolus. The process of venous thrombosis and embolism is extremely common, and it has been estimated that approximately 30% of hospital inpatients have deep venous thrombosis and in approximately 10% of postmortem examinations there is evidence of pulmonary embolism.

The effect of an embolism depends on its size and the degree of arterial obstruction and also on whether there is any congestion in the pulmonary circulation. Pulmonary emboli may be small and clinically 'silent' and often multiple. These are frequently dissolved by endogenous thrombolysis or they may become incorporated into the vessel wall with an overlying new endothelium accompanied by proliferation of smooth muscle cells. If multiple small emboli occur over a period of time and become organised in this way, diffuse narrowing of small vessels can result in pulmonary hypertension.

If the embolus is large, as from an iliofemoral venous thrombosis, then a massive pulmonary embolism may occur. If both main pulmonary arteries are blocked then sudden death will ensue. If only one side is blocked, severe shortness of breath and circulatory collapse may occur. It is not known precisely why this happens, since ligation of the main pulmonary artery, as in pneumonectomy, does not cause this problem. A vagal reflex inducing spasm of the coronary and pulmonary arteries, perhaps associated with peripheral vasodilatation, has been suggested.

Peripheral arterial embolism

These arise most commonly (approximately 70%) from the left atrial appendage in atrial fibrillation. Mural thrombus following a myocardial infarction is another cause, or an arterial embolism may arise from an aneurysm, in particular those of the popliteal artery. Thrombi affecting heart valves are rare but may be associated with infective endocarditis, and in these circumstances the embolus may be infected (septic embolus). These may subsequently cause infection of the artery in which they impact, resulting in a mycotic aneurysm. Platelet emboli may occur arising from the surface of atheromatous plaques. Where these occur on a stenosis of the internal carotid artery, they are responsible for classical transient ischaemic attacks.

Gas embolism

These occur in two main situations: The introduction of gas accidentally during trauma or surgery, particularly to the neck, and in decompression sickness. The relative negative venous pressure in the neck can cause air to be sucked into the blood stream if these vessels are open, particularly with the patient in an erect or sitting position. The introduction of air via intravenous cannulae is possible with giving sets or syringes but is very uncommon, and volumes of air less than 100 mL very rarely cause serious problems. When air is introduced into the circulation it generally only causes a problem when it gets back to the heart and produces a frothy thrombus in the right ventricle and impedes output.

Nitrogen embolism may occur in decompression sickness when a diver ascends too rapidly. This results in nitrogen, which was in solution under high pressure, forming gas bubbles within the circulation as the pressure is rapidly reduced. Bubbles may also be formed in ligaments and joints, which can give severe pain, causing the patient to lie and bend himself up double in an attempt to relieve the pain — hence 'the bends'.

Fat embolism

Following fractures, most commonly of long bones, globules of fat may enter the circulation. This is actually relatively common but significant clinical consequences are rare. Pulmonary fat embolism is a frequent postmortem finding with fractures, although it is unlikely that this in itself was the cause of death, as the pulmonary vascular tree is so extensive. Sometimes the emboli may pass through the pulmonary vessels and into the systemic circulation, where they may become impacted in the capillaries of the brain, kidneys, skin, and other organs. This tends to be more serious with fever, respiratory distress and cerebral symptoms. Occasionally the brain damage is sufficiently severe for coma and death to result. A haemorrhagic skin eruption can occur, as may subconjunctival and retinal haemorrhages.

Tumour emboli

All malignant tumours tend to invade blood vessels at an early stage, and isolated malignant cells are commonly present in the circulation. A number of factors are responsible for survival of a metastatic tumour within the blood stream and for its ability to escape to surrounding tissue and to grow following impaction within a vessel bed of small enough calibre to impede its further progress. These factors seem to be related to a genetic event in the development of the cancer, and various factors have been identified as being related to the different metastatic capabilities (Ch. 5). It is likely that tumour emboli are coated by thrombus as a part of the defence mechanism of the body against tissue emboli, since they are rendered more attractive to phagocytic cells by this coating.

Amniotic fluid embolism

This occurs in labour when the placenta is detached from the uterine wall and amniotic fluid enters the maternal circulation. This eventually lodges in the lungs. The respiratory disturbance caused is often disproportionate to the volume of amniotic fluid, and the effects are likely to be chemical rather than simply mechanical. Consequently the condition is often referred to as amniotic fluid infusion to distinguish it from those conditions in which the major effects are simple blockage of vasculature. The condition is rare, occurring in only 1:50 000 deliveries, which is fortunate since the mortality is about 85% and treatment is largely ineffectual. Onset is indicated by severe respiratory difficulty with shock and fits followed by disseminated intravascular coagulation in many cases.

Foreign body embolism

This usually arises due to some intravenous instrumentation where pieces of cannulae are broken off and can move through the blood stream until they are arrested in a vessel too small to permit their further progress. Intravenous injections with undissolved drugs or contaminants can also result in foreign material moving into the blood stream. Such materials will become coated with thrombus and will eventually impact, with clinical effects dependent upon the significance of the occluded vessel. It is a rare phenomenon but may occur with recreational intravenous drug abuse.

Therapeutic embolism

Therapeutic emboli such as gelfoam, muscle, or steel coils may occasionally be used to stop haemorrhage, to thrombose aneurysms and small arteries, or to reduce the vascularity of a tumour prior to surgical removal.

NON-THROMBOEMBOLIC VASCULAR INSUFFICIENCY

This occurs when the blood supply is interrupted by mechanisms not involving primary thrombosis. Such conditions include:

- atheroma
- torsion
- spontaneous vascular occlusion, e.g. spasm
- 'steal' syndrome, i.e. redirected blood supply
- external pressure occlusion, e.g. tumours, tourniquets, fractures, tight plasters

ATHEROMA

Atheroma tends to occlude the lumen of the arteries progressively, causing relative ischaemia and an increased risk of thrombosis occurring on an atheromatous plaque. Thus a typical history might include atheroma of the lower part of the aorta, extending into the femoral arteries, causing intermittent claudication and mild skin atrophy progressively for some years. With thrombus formation, total occlusion may supervene, with gangrene due to infarction of the tissues distal to the occlusion if correction of the condition is not rapidly undertaken. The consequences of atheroma are further discussed in Chapter 9.

TORSION

Occlusion of vessels by external pressure causes the symptoms and signs of vascular insufficiency together with failure to drain the tissue via the veins. This is clearly seen in torsion of the testis. As the testis rotates on its pedicle (the spermatic cord or the mesorchium) the tension in the twisted region first affects the lowest pressure vasculature, which is the venous return. At first the arterial supply is unaffected and continues to pump blood into the testis, which becomes engorged, painful and swollen. Fluid leaks from the vessels (mainly veins) into the tissue spaces and causes further swelling which eventually reaches a pressure sufficient to cause arterial occlusion, adding to the anoxia of the tissues. The normal drainage system for tissue fluid is the lymphatic, but this is a low pressure system with no active pump mechanism and is therefore also occluded early in the process. If the situation is not resolved spontaneously or surgically infarction occurs. Torsion of the intestines, ovarian lesions (cysts and tumours) and strangulated hernias all demonstrate a similar sequence of vascular insufficiency.

SPONTANEOUS VASCULAR OCCLUSION

Vascular spasm is also capable of causing symptoms and signs of vascular insufficiency, and a large number of myocardial events (heart attacks) seem to be due to this rather than a thrombotic event. Such spasm is directly induced by cigarette smoke and is particularly common in vessels with some degree of intimal damage such as atheroma. Later, atheroma calcifies, and such vessels are protected from spasm to some extent by the calcification but are very prone to thrombus formation, usually secondary to plaque rupture (see Ch. 9). A milder degree of spasm is seen in Raynaud's disease, generally affecting the hand and in the similar condition seen in people who have worked with vibrating tools (vibration-induced white finger). The mechanism by which this spasm occurs is contraction of smooth muscle in the vascular wall. This is generally maintained in a relaxed state by nitric oxide (endothelium-derived relaxing factor) which is produced in response to vasoconstriction brought about by acetylcholine.

'STEAL' SYNDROME

'Steal' syndromes are rare but are another theoretical cause of relative vascular insufficiency. They occur when blood is redirected preferentially along one branch of a vessel to the detriment of the end territory of the other branch. This usually occurs when the branch from which the supply is stolen is already compromised by atheroma and the demands placed upon the shared supply could cause the flow in the defective branch to fall below a critical level. It can also occur where there is developmental disparity between branches and in extreme cases can result in congenital atrophy. It may also be seen with arteriovenous fistulae in the proximal part of a limb, especially when these are created between the brachial artery and cephalic vein at the elbow. The flow from the brachial artery goes preferentially through the cephalic vein if the anastomosis is large enough, very little blood going down the ulnar and radial arteries to supply the hand.

EXTERNAL PRESSURE OCCLUSION

This may be caused by tumours, tourniquets, or a tight plaster of paris cast. It may also be caused by fractures of long bones, the classical examples being a supracondylar fracture of the femur if the distal fragment is drawn backwards, compressing and damaging the popliteal artery. It may also occur in supracondylar fractures of the humerus in which the distal fragment is drawn forwards, impinging on the brachial artery.

ISCHAEMIA, INFARCTION AND GANGRENE

ISCHAEMIA

Ischaemia is the condition of an organ or tissue where the supply of oxygenated blood is inadequate for its metabolic needs.

Causes

General
Ischaemia may follow a sudden severe fall in cardiac output. Myocardial infarction occasionally results in symmetrical gangrene of the extremities. Different tissues may be affected with different degrees of severity, the brain being the most sensitive to ischaemia.

Local
Arterial obstruction This may be due to the following.

- Atherosclerosis. Where collateral supply has developed enough to provide an adequate blood supply at rest, symptoms of ischaemia (pain) only develop when the metabolic demands increase, as in angina pectoris and intermittent claudication. With increasing severity of ischaemia there may be symptoms at rest or tissue necrosis (infarction or gangrene).
- Intra-arterial thrombosis may occur and is most commonly secondary to atherosclerosis.

- Embolism may cause acute ischaemia, and, because there is no time for collaterals to develop, it is often more severe than with atherosclerosis and thrombosis.
- External pressure on an artery may cause ischaemia, as with twisting of an adhesive band in intraperitoneal adhesions, anterior tibial compartment syndrome, or a tight plaster cast.

Venous obstruction If this is extensive the tissues may become so engorged with blood that the arterial blood flow becomes blocked.

Examples include:

- strangulated hernias where initially it is the veins that are obstructed
- mesenteric venous thrombosis, which may subsequently lead to mesenteric infarction
- the rare condition of phlegmasia caerulea dolens, an iliofemoral thrombosis with venous engorgement so intense that the small distal arterioles may occlude, causing 'venous gangrene'.

Small vessel obstruction
This can be due to:

- vasculitis, when arterioles, capillaries, or venules may be occluded by inflammation
- frostbite, where spasm and cold can occlude the microcirculation
- microembolism, as in sickle-cell disease
- precipitated cryoglobulins
- thrombocythaemia, where the excess number of platelets blocks the microcirculation.

Severity of ischaemia
This depends on:

1. The speed of onset of arterial occlusion: where this is gradual there is time for collaterals to develop.
2. The extent of the obstruction: whether it is partial or complete and the length of the vessel occluded.
3. The extent and patency of the collateral circulation, which is a feature of both the speed of onset and the anatomical site of the obstruction. For example the central artery of the retina is an 'end artery', as are the smaller vessels to the cerebral cortex, so that occlusion of these vessels is likely to cause irreversible ischaemia. Although there is an extensive arcade of vessels arising from the superior mesenteric artery, the anastomoses between each branch are poor as compared with the collaterals joining with the branches of the inferior mesenteric artery. Infarction of the small bowel and proximal colon is much more common than

in the distal colon. On the other hand, the blood supply to the stomach is so rich that infarction of the stomach is extremely rare. The lungs and liver are unusual in having a double blood supply, so that they have a better chance of surviving the ravages of ischaemia. The patency of collaterals may be impaired if they are in spasm or themselves are affected by atherosclerosis.

4. The metabolic requirements of the ischaemic tissues: for example, the brain has a very high requirement for oxygenated blood and is the tissue which is most sensitive to ischaemia in the body, followed closely by the heart. It is particularly unfortunate that the collaterals to these organisms are poor and that the cells are unable to regenerate. Connective tissue tends to survive ischaemia better than the parenchymal cells specific to a particular organ.

INFARCTION

This can be defined as death of the tissue following acute ischaemia when irreparable damage has occurred. It usually forms a well-defined area of coagulative necrosis which, with the passage of time, frequently becomes organised into scar tissue.

Sequence of events

Shortly after death of the tissue blood continues to seep into the ischaemic area through the damaged capillary walls. Bleeding may increase partly from venous reflux and partly because the obstruction is often incomplete at the beginning of the episode. As a result the area may appear under the microscope to be 'stuffed' with blood (hence the name of the pathological process from the latin *infarcire* — to stuff). On cutting across an infarcted area in the initial stages, the blood may give a red appearance (hence the term 'red infarcts'). Over the next 24–36 hours swelling of the autolysing cells may squeeze out the blood and the area may become paler (hence the term 'pale infarcts'). However, the term infarction adds little to the understanding of the pathological process, and the colour depends largely on the tissue involved. For example, cerebral infarcts are usually pale, while the spongy lung tissue remains red right up to the stage of repair.

The dead tissue undergoes progressive autolysis of parenchymal cells and haemolysis of red cells. The living tissues surrounding the infarction undergo an acute inflammatory response. There is a rise in polymorph numbers and, after a few days, macrophage infiltration becomes prominent. This is known as the phase of demolition. Subsequently there is a gradual ingrowth of granulation tissue and the area is eventually organised into a fibrous scar (repair phase). Some dystrophic calcification may take place.

Systemic effects of infarction

These are fever, raised white cell count, and a raised ESR presumably as part of an acute phase response. There may be a rise in certain specific enzymes according to the tissue affected.

Effects of infarction in specific organs

The heart

(This is dealt with separately in Ch. 9.)

Central nervous system

Because of the high metabolic rate, nerve cells undergo functional changes within a few seconds of total ischaemia, and cell death occurs within a few minutes. The infarct is usually caused by a thrombosis secondary to atheroma or embolism, although 20% of strokes are haemorrhagic. The necrosis is typically liquefactive, which may subsequently result in formation of a cavity. After an initial neutrophil response there is intense phagocytic activity by microglial cells.

The lungs

Pulmonary infarction is very rare in healthy young people, even if a main pulmonary artery is occluded, because of the additional bronchial arterial supply. However, in heart failure and especially mitral stenosis, infarction is more likely. Pulmonary infarcts are caused by emboli of which 90% arise from the lower limb veins, and 10% from the right atrial appendage in patients with heart disease, especially mitral stenosis or atrial fibrillation from any cause. A pulmonary infarct tends to be wedge shaped with the base being on the pleural surface of the lung. It is the inflammation of this lung surface rubbing against the parietal pleura that gives the typical pleuritic pain. A transient pleural rub may be heard at the site of the pain, which disappears as a layer of fluid (effusion) develops over it and lubricates it. Patients may develop the symptoms and x-ray changes of a pulmonary infarction and yet recover, with return to normal x-ray appearances. This is because there is oedema and bleeding into the alveoli but no progression to necrosis, and thus subsequent resolution occurs. Strictly speaking this is not an infarct, as there is no necrosis.

Intestine

Small bowel infarction is usually due to a mechanical cause such as strangulated hernia or twisting round an adhesive band, although it can occur from superior mesenteric artery thrombosis or embolism. Occasionally it is due to mesenteric venous thrombosis. When the ischaemia is not severe enough to cause massive infarctions, sometimes the mucosa may undergo necrosis while the outer part of the bowel survives.

This is the mechanism of ischaemic colitis (see Ch. 17), which can closely mimic ulcerative colitis with toxic dilatation, in fact ischaemia is often the final common path in a variety of colitic diseases. Repair may lead to an ischaemic stricture. Transient ischaemic changes in the bowel can occur secondary to heart failure and shock. This has serious consequences, as the ischaemic bowel can allow bacterial translocation into the blood, causing a bacteraemia which may have a devasting effect in a patient who is already very ill.

Skeletal muscle

Ischaemic necrosis of skeletal muscle due to arterial occlusion alone results in a moderate degree of fibrous replacement. However, when there is additional venous obstruction there is a tendency to haemorrhage into the muscle, resulting in a much more intense fibrosis. This constitutes the basis of Volkmann's ischaemic contracture. This occurs most commonly in the forearm muscles following a supracondylar fracture of the humerus, but can occur at other sites.

GANGRENE

Gangrene is necrosis with putrefaction of the tissues, sometimes as a result of the action of certain bacteria notably clostridia. The affected tissues appear black because of the deposition of iron sulphide from degraded haemoglobin. True gangrene is particularly likely to occur in the gut, where putrefactive organisms abound.

In gradually progressive peripheral vascular disease, most commonly of the lower limb, the ischaemia may become severe enough to cause infarction of the toes and feet. The area becomes dry, shrivelled and black due to altered haemoglobins secondary to desiccation. An inflammatory zone develops at the junction of the living and dead tissue, which is known as the 'line of demarcation'. This version of necrosis is known an 'mummification' or 'dry gangrene'. Mummification occurs where the environmental humidity is low and the temperature high; dead tissue dries slowly, retaining its form. The description 'dry gangrene' is contradictory. If no infection supervenes, the dead tissue gradually separates and 'auto amputation' can occur. This is particularly likely to occur with a digit such as a toe.

If saprophytic infection and putrefaction occurs, the condition is known as 'wet gangrene'. Progressive infection of a site of necrosis accentuates the ischaemia, causing spreading gangrene and necessitating more proximal amputation where the blood supply is better.

Gas gangrene (see Ch. 7) is a dangerous form of spreading tissue necrosis which is likely to occur when the spores of clostridia gain access to a wound in which there is extensive soft tissue or muscle injury. The most common causal organism is *Clostridium perfringens*. Crepitus (a palpable crackling or bubbling) can often be detected under the skin due to the production of gas bubbles by the clostridia. Clostridia also produces powerful toxins which themselves cause tissue damage and thus enhance spread of the infection.

Other forms of infective gangrene due to particular organisms are the following.

- Meleney's gangrene. This may occur at the site of abdominal surgery or at the site of an accidental abrasion of the skin. Meleney attributed the condition to synergy between a micro-aerophilic, non-haemolytic streptococcus and *Staphylococcus auerus*. However, other bacteria were also isolated. It is probably best to look at the infection as being caused by a combination of anaerobic and aerobic bacteria which forms a cellulitis followed by gangrene.
- Fournier's gangrene. This is a spontaneous onset of rapidly progressive gangrene of the scrotum in otherwise healthy men. Elderly diabetics are particularly prone. It is caused by synergism between faecal bacteria and anaerobes. Fournier's gangrene and Meleney's gangrene probably have similar aetiological factors, and only the site of infection distinguishes the two.
- Necrotising fasciitis. This may follow minor abrasions or an otherwise simple and uncomplicated operation. The initial external appearance of the skin remains normal while the necrotising process spreads along fascial plains causing extensive necrosis. Later the overlying skin, deprived of its blood supply, becomes painful, red and finally necrotic. The patient is severely ill with fever and toxaemia. The infection is more likely to affect immunocompromised patients or diabetics. Small vessels are occluded by microthrombi, and the destruction of tissues occurs rapidly. The infection usually involves mixed microbial flora, often including micro-aerophilic streptococci, staphyloccci, Gram negative bacteria and anaerobes. The progression of this disease is dramatic, and extensive surgical procedures involving wide excision and occasionally amputation may be required, together with appropriate antibiotic therapy.

4

Disorders of growth, differentiation and morphogenesis

M. Andrew Parsons

Growth, differentiation and *morphogenesis* are the processes by which a single cell, the fertilised ovum, develops into a large, complex, multicellular organism with co-ordinated organ systems containing a variety of cell types, each with individual specialised functions. Growth and differentiation continue throughout adult life, as many cells of the body undergo a constant cycle of death, replacement and growth in response to normal (physiological) or abnormal (pathological) stimuli.

There are many stages in human embryological development at which anomalies of growth and/or differentiation may occur, leading to major or minor abnormalities of form or function, or even death of the fetus. In postnatal and adult life, some alterations in growth or differentiation may be beneficial, as in the development of increased muscle mass in the limbs of workers engaged in heavy manual tasks. Other changes may be detrimental to health, as in cancer, where the outcome may be fatal.

This chapter explores the wide range of abnormalities of growth, differentiation and morphogenesis which may be encountered in clinical practice, relating them where possible to specific deviations from normal cellular functions or control mechanisms.

DEFINITIONS
GROWTH

Growth is the process of increase in size, resulting from the synthesis of specific tissue components. The term may be applied to populations, individuals, organs, cells, or even subcellular organelles such as mitochondria.

Types of growth in a tissue (Fig. 4.1A) are:

- *multiplicative*, involving an increase in numbers of cells (or nuclei and associated cytoplasm in syncytia) by mitotic cell divisions; this type of growth is present in all tissues during embryogenesis

- *auxetic,* resulting from increased size of individual cells, as seen in growing skeletal muscle
- *accretionary,* an increase in intercellular tissue components, as in bone and cartilage
- *combined patterns* of multiplicative, auxetic and accretionary growth, as seen in embryological development, where there are differing directions and rates of growth at different sites of the developing embryo, in association with changing patterns of cellular differentiation.

DIFFERENTIATION

Differentiation is the process whereby a cell develops an overt specialised function or morphology which distinguishes it from its parent cell. Thus, differentiation is the process by which genes are expressed selectively and gene products act to produce a cell with a specialised function (Fig. 4.1B). After fertilisation of the human ovum, and up to the eight-cell stage of development, all of the embryonic cells are apparently identical. Thereafter, cells undergo several stages of differentiation in their passage to fully differentiated cells, such as, for example, the ciliated epithelial cells lining the respiratory passages of the nose and trachea. Although the changes at each stage of differentiation may be minor, differentiation can be said to have occurred only if there has been *overt* change in cell morphology (e.g. development of a skin epithelial cell from an ectodermal cell), or an alteration in the specialised function of a cell (e.g. the synthesis of a hormone).

MORPHOGENESIS

Morphogenesis is the highly complex process of development of structural shape and form of organs, limbs, facial features, etc. from primitive cell masses during embryogenesis. For morphogenesis to occur, primitive cell masses must undergo coordinated growth and differ-

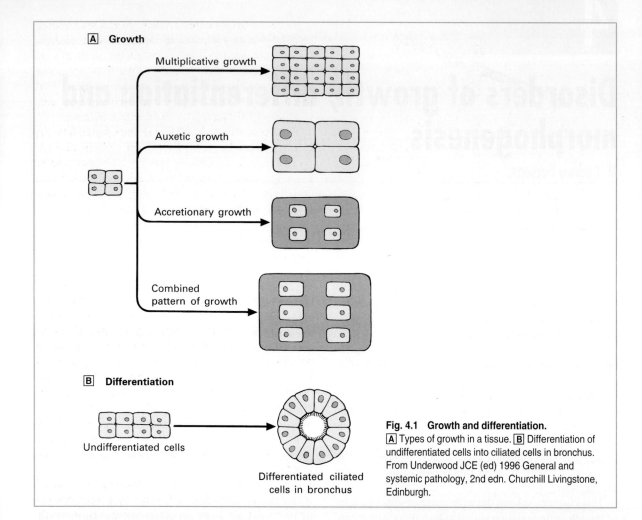

Fig. 4.1 Growth and differentiation.
A Types of growth in a tissue. B Differentiation of undifferentiated cells into ciliated cells in bronchus. From Underwood JCE (ed) 1996 General and systemic pathology, 2nd edn. Churchill Livingstone, Edinburgh.

entiation, with movement of some cell groups relative to others, and focal programmed cell death (apoptosis) to remove unwanted features.

CELL TURNOVER

In both fetal and adult life, tissue growth depends upon the balance between the increase in cell numbers, due to cell proliferation, and the decrease in cell numbers due to cell death (Fig. 4.2).

In fetal life, growth is rapid and all cell types proliferate, but even in the fetus there is constant cell death, some of which is an essential (and genetically programmed) component of morphogenesis. In postnatal and adult life, however, the cells of many tissues lose their capacity for proliferation at the high rate of the fetus, and cellular replication rates are variably reduced. Some cells con-

tinue to divide rapidly and continuously, some divide only when stimulated by the need to replace cells lost by injury or disease, and others are unable to divide whatever the stimulus.

REGENERATION

Regeneration enables cells or tissues destroyed by injury or disease to be replaced by functionally identical cells. The ability of cells to proliferate governs their regenerative potential. Mammalian cells fall into three classes according to their regenerative ability:

- labile
- stable
- permanent.

Labile cells proliferate continuously in postnatal life;

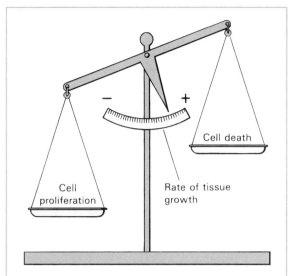

Fig. 4.2 Cell proliferation and death. Growth rate is determined by the balance between cell proliferation and cell death. From Underwood op. cit.

they have a short lifespan and a rapid 'turnover' time. Their high regenerative potential means that lost cells are rapidly replaced. However, the high cell turnover renders these cells highly susceptible to the toxic effects of radiation or drugs (such as anticancer drugs) which interfere with cell division. Examples of labile cells include:

- haemopoietic cells of the bone marrow, and lymphoid cells
- epithelial cells of the skin, mouth, pharynx, oesophagus, the gut, exocrine gland ducts, the cervix and vagina (squamous epithelium), endometrium, urinary tract (transitional epithelium), etc.

The high regenerative potential of the skin is exploited in the treatment of patients with skin loss due to severe burns. The surgeon removes a layer of the split skin which includes the dividing basal cells from the unburned donor site, and fixes it firmly to the burned graft site where the epithelium has been lost. Dividing basal cells in the graft, and dividing cells from residual basal and adnexal structures (such as the cells from the neck of pilosebaceous units) from the donor sites, ensure that squamous epithelium at both sites regenerates. This enables rapid healing to take place in a large burned area, when natural regeneration of new epithelium from the edge of the burn would otherwise be prolonged. Skin epithelium from a donor site can now be grown in the laboratory by tissue/organ culture for eventual grafting onto burned areas, and this is important for patients with extensive burns.

Stable cells (sometimes called 'conditional renewal cells') divide very infrequently under normal conditions, but are stimulated to divide rapidly when such cells are lost. This group includes cells of the liver, endocrine glands, bone, fibrous tissue and the renal tubules. Thus the liver is able to regenerate to its normal weight even after large partial resections for neoplastic disease.

Permanent cells normally divide only during fetal life and they cannot be replaced when lost. Cells in this category include neurons, retinal photoreceptors and neurons in the eye, cardiac muscle cells and skeletal muscle cells (although skeletal muscle cells do have a very limited capacity for regeneration).

CELL CYCLE

Successive phases of progression of a cell through its cycle of replication are defined with reference to DNA synthesis and cellular division. Unlike the synthesis of most cellular constituents, which occurs throughout the interphase period between cell divisions, DNA synthesis occurs only during a limited period of the interphase; this is the *S phase* of the cell cycle. A further distinct phase of the cycle is the cell-division stage or *M phase* (Fig. 4.3) comprising nuclear division (mitosis) and cytoplasmic division (cytokinesis). Following the M phase, the cell enters the *first gap (G_1) phase* and, via the S phase, the *second gap (G_2) phase* before entering the M phase again.

Some cells (e.g. some of the stable cells) may 'escape' from the G_1 phase of the cell cycle by temporarily entering a G_0 'resting' phase; others 'escape' permanently to G_0 by a process of *terminal differentiation,* with loss of potential for further division and death at the end of the lifetime of the cell; this occurs in permanent cells, such as neurons.

MOLECULAR EVENTS IN THE CELL CYCLE

At the molecular level, growth is stimulated initially by the receptor-mediated actions of *growth factors* — e.g. epidermal growth factor (EGF), platelet-derived growth factor (PDGF) and insulin-like growth factors (IGF-1 and IGF-2) — on cells in the quiescent G_0 phase of the cell cycle (Fig. 4.3) via intracellular second messengers. Stimuli are transmitted to the nucleus of the cell, where transcription factors are activated, leading to the initiation of DNA synthesis followed by cell division.

The process of cell cycling is modified by the actions of the *cyclin* family of proteins, which activate (by phos-

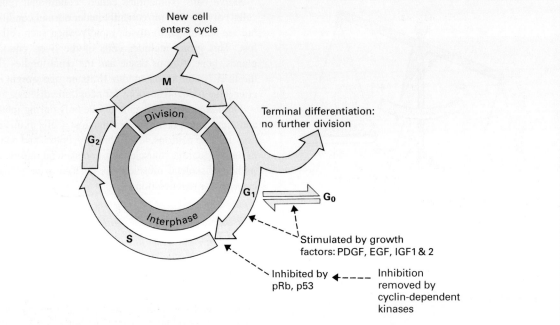

Fig. 4.3 The cell cycle. The four main stages of the cell cycle are the M phase (mitosis and cytokinesis, i.e. cell division) and the interphase stages G_1 (gap 1), S phase (DNA synthesis) and G_2 (gap 2). Cells may enter a resting phase (G_0), which may be of variable duration, followed by re-entry into the G_1 phase. Some cells may terminally differentiate from the G_1 phase, with no further cell division and death at the end of the normal lifetime of the cell. The sites at which growth factors and inhibitors act are shown. From Underwood op. cit.

phorylation) a number of proteins involved in DNA replication, mitotic spindle formation and other events in the cell cycle. Thus, for example, the inhibitory (antimitotic) action of the retinoblastoma gene product pRb is itself inhibited by the phosphorylating action of a cyclin-dependent kinase (Fig. 4.3); removal of this growth-inhibiting action of the retinoblastoma gene allows uncontrolled cellular proliferation to proceed, resulting in often rapid growth of this malignant eye neoplasm in children.

DURATION OF THE CELL CYCLE

In mammals, different cell types divide at very different rates, with observed cell cycle times (also called generation times) ranging from as little as 8 hours, in the case of gut epithelial cells, to 100 days or more, exemplified by hepatocytes in the normal adult liver. The principal difference between rapidly dividing cells and those which divide slowly is the time spent in the G_1 phase of the cell cycle; some cells remain in the G_1 phase for days or even years. In contrast, the duration of S, G_2 and M phases of the cell cycle is remarkably constant, and independent of the rate of cell division.

Therapeutic interruption of the cell cycle

Many of the drugs used in the treatment of cancer affect particular stages within the cell cycle (Fig. 4.4). These drugs inhibit the rapid division of cancer cells, although there is often inhibition of other rapidly dividing cells, such as the cells of the bone marrow and lymphoid tissues. Thus, anaemia, a bleeding tendency and suppression of immunity may be clinically important side effects of cancer chemotherapy.

CELL DEATH IN GROWTH AND MORPHOGENESIS

It seems illogical to think of cell death as a component of normal growth and morphogenesis, although we recognise that the loss of a tadpole's tail, which is mediated by genetically programmed cell death, is part of the metamorphosis of a frog. Cell death is a paradox of growth, and it is now clear that cell death has an important role in the development of an embryo, and in the regulation of tissue size throughout life. Alterations in the rate at which cell death occurs are important in situations such as hormonal growth regulation, immunity and neoplasia.

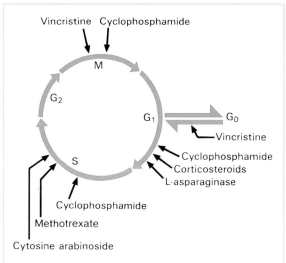

Fig. 4.4 Pharmacological interruption of the cell cycle.
The sites of action in the cell cycle of drugs that may be used
in the treatment of cancer. From Underwood op. cit.

APOPTOSIS

The term *apoptosis* is used to define the type of individual cell death which is related to growth and morphogenesis, but which appears to have an opposite function
in regulating the size of a cell population. Apoptosis is a
biochemically specific mode of cell death characterised
by activation of non-lysosomal endogenous endo-
nuclease which digests nuclear DNA into smaller DNA
fragments. Morphologically, apoptosis is recognised as
death of scattered single cells which form rounded, membrane-bound bodies; these are eventually phagocytosed
(ingested) and broken down by adjacent unaffected cells.

The coincidence of both mitosis and apoptosis within
a cell population ensures a continuous renewal of cells,
rendering a tissue more adaptable to environmental
demands than one in which the cell population is static.

Apoptosis can be triggered by factors outside the
cell or it can be an autonomous event ('programmed cell
death'). In embryological development, there are three
categories of autonomous apoptosis:

- morphogenetic
- histogenic
- phylogenetic.

Morphogenetic apoptosis This is involved in alteration of tissue form. Examples include:

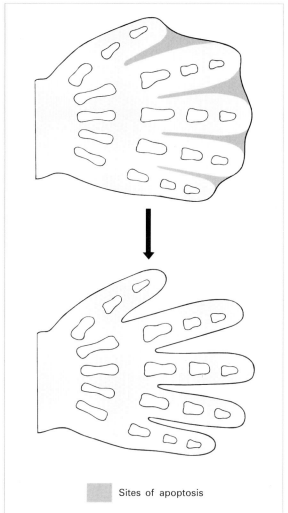

☐ Sites of apoptosis

Fig. 4.5 Morphogenesis by apoptosis. Genetically
programmed apoptosis (individual cell death) causing
separation of the fingers during embryogenesis. From
Underwood op. cit.

- interdigital cell death responsible for separating the
  fingers (Fig. 4.5)
- cell death leading to the removal of redundant
  epithelium following fusion of the palatine processes
  during development of the roof of the mouth
- cell death in the dorsal part of the neural tube during
  closure, required to achieve continuity of the
  epithelium, the two sides of the neural tube and the
  associated mesoderm
- cell death in the involuting urachus, required to
  remove redundant tissue between the bladder and
  umbilicus.

Failure of morphogenetic apoptosis in these four sites is a factor in the development of *syndactyly* (webbed fingers), *cleft palate* (see p. 73), *spina bifida* (see p. 72), and bladder diverticulum (pouch) or fistula (open connection) from the bladder to the umbilical skin.

Histogenic apoptosis This occurs in the differentiation of tissues and organs, as seen, for example, in the hormonally controlled differentiation of the accessory reproductive structures from the Müllerian and Wolffian ducts. In the male, for instance, anti-Müllerian hormone produced by the Sertoli cells of the fetal testis causes regression of the Müllerian ducts (which in females form the fallopian tubes, uterus and upper vagina) by the process of apoptosis.

Phylogenetic apoptosis This is involved in removing vestigial structures from the embryo; structures such as the pronephros, a remnant from a much lower evolutionary level, are removed by the process of apoptosis.

Regulation of apoptosis

When cells within tissues are stimulated to divide by mitogens the tissues enter a high turnover state, in which mitotic activity is accompanied by some degree of coincident apoptosis (Fig. 4.6). The ultimate fate of individ-

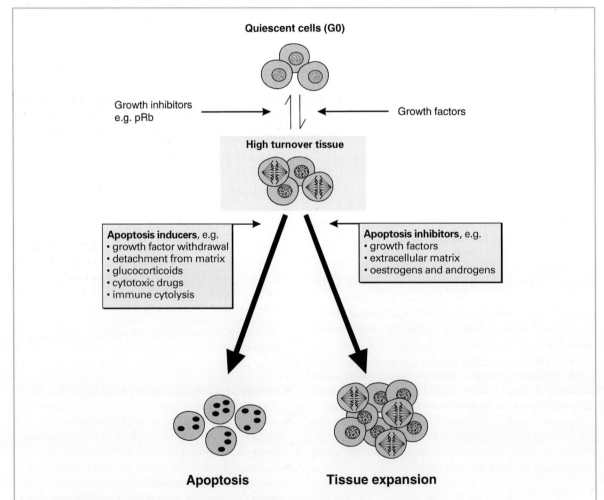

Fig. 4.6 Control of tissue growth by induction or inhibition of apoptosis. Quiescent (mitotically inactive) cells in G_0 are recruited into a high turnover (mitotically active) state by growth factors (see Fig. 4.3). Their subsequent fate depends on the presence or absence of apoptosis inducers or inhibitors. The inducers and inhibitors are mediated by the *bax* and *bcl-2* proteins, respectively, among others. From Underwood op. cit.

ual cells within the tissue — whether the cell will survive or undergo apoptosis — depends upon the balance between apoptosis inducers (survival inhibitors) and apoptosis inhibitors (survival factors). Although apoptosis can be induced by diverse signals in a variety of cell types, a few genes appear to regulate a final common pathway. The most important of these are the members of the *bcl-2* family (*bcl-2* was originally identified at the t (14;18) chromosomal breakpoint in follicular B-cell lymphoma, and it can inhibit many factors which induce apoptosis). The *bax* protein (also in the *bcl-2* family) forms *bax–bax* dimers which enhance apoptotic stimuli. The ratio of *bcl-2* to *bax* determines the cell's susceptibility to apoptotic stimuli, and constitutes a 'molecular switch' which determines whether a cell will survive, leading to tissue expansion, or undergo apoptosis.

The study of factors regulating apoptosis is of considerable importance in finding therapeutic agents to enhance cell death in malignant neoplasms. In retinoblastoma (a malignant neoplasm of the eye found in infants), the neoplasm has a very high mitotic rate, but also has extensive apoptosis. Occasionally the neoplasm undergoes spontaneous regression (possibly due to increased apoptosis), and agents which increase apoptosis might also induce this regression.

NORMAL AND ABNORMAL GROWTH IN SINGLE TISSUES

Within an individual organ or tissue, increased or decreased growth takes place in a range of physiological and pathological circumstances as part of the adaptive response of cells to changing requirements for growth.

INCREASED GROWTH: HYPERTROPHY AND HYPERPLASIA

The response of an individual cell to increased functional demand is to increase tissue or organ size (Fig. 4.7) by:

- increasing its size without cell replication (hypertrophy)
- increasing its numbers by cell division (hyperplasia)
- a combination of these.

The stimuli for hypertrophy and hyperplasia are very similar, and in many cases identical; indeed, hypertrophy and hyperplasia commonly coexist. In permanent cells (see pp. 11, 49) hypertrophy is the only adaptive option available under stimulatory conditions. In some circumstances, however, permanent cells may increase their DNA content (ploidy) in hypertrophy, although the cells arrest in the G_2 phase of the cell cycle without undergoing mitosis; such a circumstance is present in severely hypertrophied hearts, where a large proportion of cells may be polyploid.

An important component of hyperplasia, which is often overlooked, is a *decrease* in cell loss by apoptosis; the mechanisms of control of this decreased apoptosis are unclear, although they are related to the factors causing increased cell production (Fig. 4.6).

Physiological hypertrophy and hyperplasia

Examples of physiologically increased growth of tissues include:

- *muscle hypertrophy* in athletes, both in the skeletal muscle of the limbs (as a response to increased muscle activity) and in the left ventricle of the heart (as a response to sustained outflow resistance)

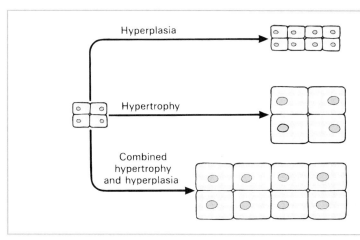

Fig. 4.7 Hyperplasia and hypertrophy. In hypertrophy, cell size is increased. In hyperplasia, cell number is increased. Hypertrophy and hyperplasia may coexist. From Underwood op. cit.

- *hyperplasia of bone marrow cells* producing red blood cells in individuals living at high altitude; this is stimulated by increased production of the growth factor, erythropoietin
- *hyperplasia of breast tissue* at puberty, and in pregnancy and lactation, under the influence of several hormones, including oestrogens, progesterone, prolactin, growth hormone and human placental lactogen.
- *hypertrophy and hyperplasia of uterine smooth muscle* at puberty and in pregnancy, stimulated by oestrogens.
- *thyroid hyperplasia* as a consequence of the increased metabolic demands of puberty and pregnancy.

In addition to such physiologically increased tissue growth, hypertrophy and hyperplasia are also seen in tissues in a wide range of *pathological* conditions.

REPAIR AND REGENERATION

The proliferation of vascular (capillary) endothelial cells and myofibroblasts in scar tissue, and the regeneration of specialised cells within a tissue, are the important components of the response to tissue damage.

Angiogenesis This is the process whereby new blood vessels grow into damaged, ischaemic or necrotic tissues in order to supply oxygen and nutrients for cells involved in regeneration and repair. Briefly, vascular endothelial cells within pre-existing capillaries are activated by angiogenic growth factors such as vascular endothelial growth factor (VEGF), released by hypoxic cells or macrophages. On activation, the endothelial cells secrete plasminogen activator and other enzymes, including the matrix metalloproteinases, which selectively degrade extracellular matrix proteins to allow endothelial cell migration to occur. Tissue inhibitors of metalloproteinases exist to prevent excessive matrix breakdown. Thus activated endothelial cells migrate (mediated by integrins, a family of cell-surface adhesion molecules) and proliferate towards the angiogenic stimulus to form a 'sprout'. Adjacent sprouts connect to form vascular loops, which canalise and establish a blood flow. Later, mesenchymal cells including pericytes and smooth muscle cells, are recruited to stabilise the vascular architecture, and the extracellular matrix is remodelled. Two other initiating mechanisms exist in addition to the above 'sprouting' form of angiogenesis: existing vascular channels may be bisected by an extracellular matrix 'pillar' (intussusception), and the two channels extend towards the angiogenic stimulus; and the third mechanism involves circulating primordial stem cells which are recruited at sites of hypoxia and differentiate into activated vascular endothelial cells. (Note that a similar process of angiogenesis occurs in response to tumour cells, as an essential component of the development of the blood supply of enlarging neoplasms. Such angiogenesis is an important new therapeutic target in the treatment of malignant neoplasms, although theoretically such drugs might impair angiogenesis and therefore delay healing of wounds.)

(Note that the term *'vasculogenesis'* should be reserved specifically for the blood vessel proliferation which occurs in the developing embryo and fetus.)

Myofibroblasts These often follow new blood vessels into damaged tissues, where they proliferate and produce matrix proteins such as fibronectin and collagen to strengthen the scar. Myofibroblasts eventually contract and differentiate into fibroblasts. The resulting contraction of the scar may cause important complications, such as:

- deformity and reduced movements of limbs affected by extensive scarring following skin burns around joints
- bowel stenosis and obstruction caused by annular scarring in Crohn's disease
- detachment of the retina due to traction caused by contraction of fibrovascular adhesions between the retina and the ciliary body, following intraocular inflammation.

Thus vascular endothelial cell and myofibroblast hyperplasia are important components of repair and regeneration at various sites in the body.

Skin

The healing of a skin wound is a complex process involving the removal of necrotic debris from the wound and repair of the defect by hyperplasia of capillaries, myofibroblasts and epithelial cells. Figure 4.8 illustrates some of these events, most of which are mediated by growth factors.

When tissue injury occurs, there is haemorrhage into the defect from damaged blood vessels; this is controlled by normal haemostatic mechanisms, during which platelets aggregate and thrombus forms to plug the defect in the vessel wall. Because of interactions between the coagulation and complement systems, inflammatory cells are attracted to the site of injury by chemotactic complement fractions. In addition, platelets release two potent growth factors — platelet-derived growth factor (PDGF) and transforming growth factor beta (TGFβ) — which are powerfully chemotactic for inflammatory cells, including macrophages; these migrate into the wound to remove necrotic tissue and fibrin.

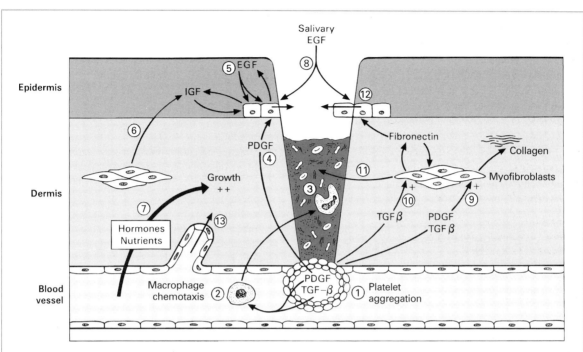

Fig. 4.8 Factors mediating skin wound healing. A wound is shown penetrating the skin, and entering a blood vessel. (1) Blood coagulation and platelet degranulation, releasing platelet-derived growth factor (PDGF) and transforming growth factor beta (TGFβ). (2) PDGF and TGFβ are chemotactic for macrophages, which migrate into the wound to phagocytose bacteria and necrotic debris (3). *In the epidermis:* (4) the released PDGF activates epidermal basal epithelial cells, which are also under autocrine and paracrine stimulation by epidermal growth factor (EGF) and insulin-like growth factors (IGF), (5), some derived from dermal myofibroblasts (6). Nutrients and oxygen (7) and circulating hormones and growth factors diffusing from blood vessels (including insulin, thyroxine, IGF-1 and IGF-2), and EGF (8) from saliva (if the wound is licked) all contribute to epidermal growth. *In the dermis:* (9) PDGF and TGFβ stimulate cell division in myofibroblasts, and (10) TGFβ stimulates these cells to produce collagen and fibronectin. Fibronectin stimulates migration of dermal myofibroblasts (11) and epidermal epithelial cells (12). Angiogenic growth factors (not shown) stimulate the proliferation and migration of new blood vessels into the area of the wound (13). From Underwood op. cit.

In the *epidermis,* PDGF acts synergistically with epidermal growth factor (EGF) and the somatomedins (IGF-1 and IGF-2) to promote the progression of basal epithelial cells through the cycle of cell proliferation (p. 49). PDGF acts as a 'competence factor' to move cells from their 'resting' phase in G_0 to G_1. EGF and IGFs then act sequentially in cell progression from the G_1 phase to that of DNA synthesis. Thereafter, the cell is independent of growth factors. In the epidermis, EGF is derived from epidermal cells (autocrine and paracrine mechanisms), and is also present in high concentrations in saliva when the wound is licked. IGF-1 and IGF-2 originate from the circulation (endocrine mechanisms) and from the proliferating cell and adjacent epidermal and dermal cells (autocrine and paracrine mechanisms).

(Note that, once a specialised adnexal structure such as a pilosebaceous unit has been destroyed, new units cannot regenerate from the basal layer of the epidermis.

Hairs will therefore not grow in areas where deep burns have destroyed adnexal tissues, even if split skin grafting is successful. Similarly, in 'scarring alopecia', hair loss is permanent once hair follicles have been destroyed.)

In the *dermis,* myofibroblasts proliferate in response to PDGF (and TGFβ); collagen and fibronectin secretion is stimulated by TGFβ, and fibronectin then aids migration of epithelial and dermal cells.

Capillary budding and proliferation are stimulated by angiogenic factors such as vascular endothelial growth factor (VEGF; see above). The capillaries ease the access of inflammatory cells and fibroblasts, particularly into large areas of necrotic tissue.

Hormones (e.g. insulin and thyroid hormones) and nutrients (e.g. glucose and amino acids) are also required. Lack of nutrients or vitamins, the presence of inhibitory factors such as corticosteroids or infection, or a locally poor circulation with low tissue oxygen concentrations, may all materially delay wound healing; these factors are very important in clinical practice.

Ulcers and erosions

An ulcer is a full-thickness defect in a surface epithelium or mucosa, which may also extend into subepithelial or submucosal tissue. An erosion is a partial-thickness defect in a surface epithelium or mucosa.

Both ulcers and erosions occur when adverse tissue circumstances ('ulcerating factors', such as hypoxia, factors such as gastric acid forming the local physico-chemical environment, or infection) cause local death of cells which cannot be replaced by regenerative cell pro-liferation, leading to net loss of epithelial or mucosal tissue. The presence of one or more of these 'ulcerating factors' therefore overpowers the local 'survival factors', such as the regenerative potential and oxygenation of the tissue, and an ulcer or erosion develops.

Once the 'ulcerating factor or factors' are removed, however, the residual 'survival and healing factors', or healing capacity of the tissue predominates, and cell pro-liferation exceeds cell loss, producing net tissue growth to fill the ulcer cavity. In deep ulcers (Fig. 4.9), angio-genic growth factors (produced by macrophages in the necrotic ulcer crater) stimulate growth and migration of capillaries into the base of the ulcer (producing vascular 'granulation tissue', seen as finely granular red tissue in the ulcer base). Myofibroblasts also migrate into the ulcer crater, where they proliferate and secrete collagen and matrix proteins, filling the ulcer crater. Once this has happened, the epithelial cells at the edge of the ulcer migrate over the new scar tissue; eventually the ulcer crater is filled, and the epithelium totally covers the former ulcer. Eventually, subepithelial scar tissue contracts (caused by myofibroblast contraction), and myofibroblasts differentiate into mature fibroblasts.

If 'ulcerating factors' persist, or if there are recurrent cycles of ulceration–healing–ulceration, an ulcer may be-come 'chronic', with a large deep crater and very exten-sive scar formation, perhaps leading to marked deformity of the tissue (such as, for example, an 'hour glass' defor-mity with possible stenosis in a stomach with a large chronic gastric ulcer).

At the epithelial edge of large chronic ulcers, persis-tent attempts to regenerate occasionally lead to the development of a malignant neoplasm (carcinoma).

If an ulcer fails to heal after 'ulcerating factors' have been removed, this may indicate that there is an under-lying neoplasm. Many malignant neoplasms, which arise in (or invade) epithelial or mucosal tissues, ulcerate as they outgrow their blood supply or invade local blood vessels. A classical example is basal cell carcinoma of the skin (a 'rodent' ulcer), but other examples include breast adenocarcinoma ulcerating overlying skin, and large ulcerated bowel adenocarcinomas.

Note that epithelial proliferation and regeneration alone are required to heal an erosion, once the causative factor has been removed.

Peritoneum

The practice of abdominal surgery requires an under-standing of the mechanisms of peritoneal healing and of the development of intra-abdominal fibrous adhesions (scars). In one large study, 31% of all cases of intestinal obstruction were due to adhesions, and of these patients 79% had undergone previous abdominal surgery, whilst 18% had inflammatory adhesions and 3% had congenital bands.

The process of healing and repair of a peritoneal defect is very different to that of an ulcerated epithelial surface, as the mesothelial surface cells do not grow over the defect from its edges. If even large peritoneal defects are left open (not sutured), macrophages migrate into the area to remove necrotic debris (Fig. 4.10). This is followed by a proliferation and migration of peritoneal perivascular connective tissue cells (which resemble pri-mitive mesenchymal cells) into the defect, which eventu-ally fills with these cells. The connective tissue cells on the 'new' surface then undergo metaplasia into mesothe-lial cells. As a result, peritoneal defects heal very rapidly, large defects heal as rapidly as small ones, and peritoneal healing occurs without formation of adhesions.

If, however, peritoneal defects are sutured, the suture compresses or tensions the mesothelium and underlying connective tissue, which tends to become relatively ischaemic as a result (Fig. 4.10). As a result, angio-genesis (new blood vessel formation) is stimulated, and capillaries (and later fibroblasts) migrate into the area. If fibrin and/or foreign material such as starch (used to lubricate the inside of surgical gloves) are on the peri-toneal surface, the capillaries and fibroblasts grow into the area, and are likely to cause adhesions to adjacent peritoneal surfaces, which may ultimately cause intesti-nal obstruction. In abdominal and pelvic surgery, there-fore, peritoneal surfaces which are left unsutured are less likely to cause adhesions, and both removal of fibrin and prevention of contamination by foreign body materials will reduce the chances of adhesion formation.

Peritoneal mesothelial cells have fibrinolytic activity, but damage to these cells at surgery reduces their ability to remove the peritoneal fibrin which promotes develop-ment of adhesions. In addition, growth factors such as

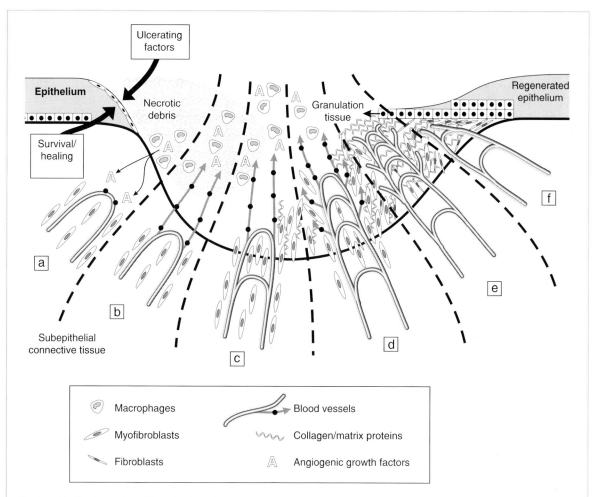

Fig. 4.9 Healing in an ulcer. These basic mechanisms apply to all ulcers, in different tissues of the body. In this ulcer the predominance of 'ulcerating factors' (factors such as anoxia, gastric acid, and infection) has caused loss of both the epithelium and subepithelial tissue (top left). Once these factors have been corrected, however, 'survival/healing factors' predominate, and healing, repair and regeneration can take place (sequence a–f). (a) Macrophages have migrated into the necrotic tissue of the ulcer, where they ingest necrotic debris. In addition, however, they secrete angiogenic growth factors (A), which diffuse into the tissue at the base of the ulcer. (b) Angiogenic growth factors stimulate vascular (capillary) endothelial cells to proliferate and migrate into the ulcer (forming 'sprouts'). (c) Adjacent endothelial cells sprouts join to form loops, and canalise (a lumen forms), allowing blood flow through the loop. New endothelial cell sprouts then develop. Myofibroblasts proliferate and migrate into the newly vascularised base of the ulcer. (d) More proliferation of capillaries occurs, producing granulation tissue (seen macroscopically as a red granular base to the ulcer). Myofibroblasts continue to proliferate, and produce collagen and other intracellular matrix proteins (to strengthen the developing scar). (e) Once the blood vessels and proliferating myofibroblasts fill the cavity of the ulcer, epithelial cells from the edge of the ulcer proliferate (stimulated by epithelial growth factors) and migrate over the regenerating subepithelial tissue (migration is aided by fibronectin secreted by myofibroblasts). (f) Eventually the myofibroblasts contract, with resulting contraction of the scar. The epithelium has now regenerated completely.

epidermal growth factor (EGF) and transforming growth factor beta (TGFβ) may directly influence cell growth in peritoneal healing. However, TGFβ (released in large quantities from platelets at sites of haemorrhage) and tumour necrosis factor (TNF) both probably increase plasminogen-activator inhibitor-1 (PAI-1) activity in peritoneal mesothelial cells, blocking fibrinolytic activity (and hence fibrin removal), and thereby promoting

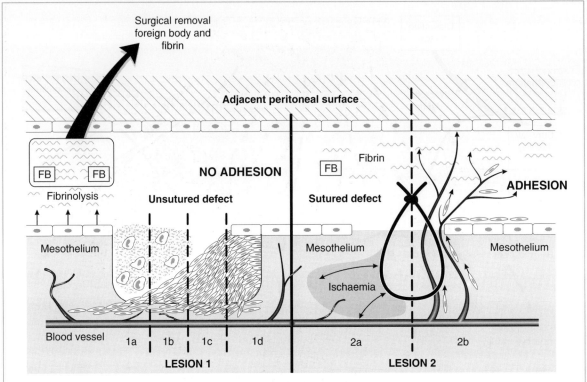

Fig. 4.10 Factors affecting peritoneal wound healing and adhesions. The figure represents two opposing peritoneal surfaces (top and bottom), with two surgically created wounds which have removed the mesothelium and some submesothelial connective tissue. In **lesion 1** (left) the surgeon has left the defect open, and has carefully removed foreign body (FB) material and fibrin from the surface. Under these circumstances: (1a) macrophages remove necrotic material from the wounded area, then (1b) subperitoneal perivascular connective tissue cells proliferate and migrate into the base of the defect, and (1c) fill the defect. Finally (1d) the surface layer of these cells undergoes metaplasia into mesothelial cells. As a result, healing takes place with *no* adhesions to adjacent peritoneal surfaces. In **lesion 2** (right), by contrast, foreign material and fibrin have not been removed by the surgeon. In addition, the peritoneal defect has been sutured, and as a result (2a) the tissue is relatively ischaemic as a result of the tension of the suture. Under these circumstances (2b) angiogenesis occurs, and proliferating blood vessels extend into the ischaemic tissue and into the fibrin on the surface of the wound, eventually accompanied by the proliferating myofibroblasts which grow over the adjacent mesothelium, and which eventually form the adhesions to the adjacent peritoneal surface (top). Contraction of these myofibroblasts, and accompanying scar contraction, may cause intestinal obstruction if the peritoneal adhesions are extensive.

adhesion formation. This is an important field in which further research may well influence the clinical management of patients undergoing abdominal surgery.

Bone

Cellular mechanisms involved in the healing of bone fractures are similar to those in healing in other tissues (Fig. 4.11 illustrates the events involved). Haemorrhage at the fracture site (inside and around the bone) produces a haematoma, in which there are fragments of necrotic bone, bone marrow, and soft tissues. As is the case in other sites, these necrotic tissues are removed by macrophages. Organisation of the haematoma in bone is

accomplished by ingrowth of capillaries and fibroblasts (as in other sites in the body), but is modified in bone by ingrowth of osteoblasts; the resulting proliferation of these cells produces an irregular mass of new irregularly woven bone, called 'callus'. Internal callus forms within the medullary cavity of the bone; external callus forms in relation to the periosteum, where it acts as a splint until it is finally removed by resorption and remodelling. Eventually, woven bone of the callus is remodelled into lamellar bone, with lamellae oriented according to the direction of mechanical stress on the bone.

Occasionally bone is lost at the time of fracture (for example, the fractured end of a bone may be removed by

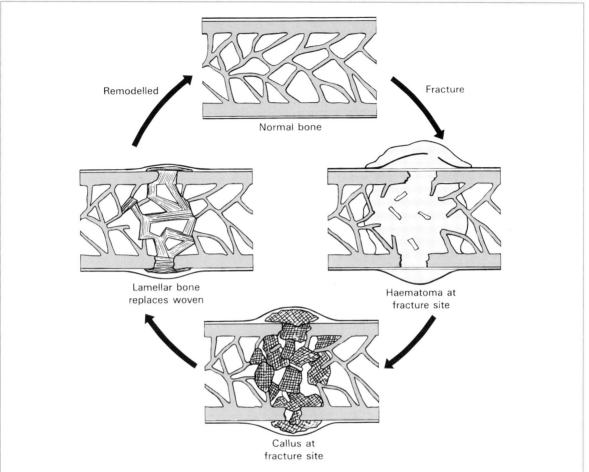

Fig. 4.11 Healing of a bone fracture. The haematoma at the fracture site gives a framework for healing. It is replaced by fracture callus, which is subsequently replaced by lamellar bone, which is then remodelled to restore the normal trabecular pattern of the bone. From Underwood op. cit.

the surgeon if heavy contamination has occurred when a compound fracture has penetrated the skin). Under such circumstances the two ends of the bone may be pinned and externally fixed and oriented on an external frame. After initial contact, the bone ends may be gradually separated by increasing traction over several weeks, allowing the bone to be drawn to its correct length whilst the healing process occurs.

Bone healing may be delayed or inhibited as a result of movement, gross misalignment, soft tissues interposed between the ends of the bone, infection, bone disease (such as osteoporosis or Paget's disease, or primary or secondary neoplasms), severe systemic illness or malnutrition. Excessive movement and soft tissue interposition may prevent bone fusion, and fibrous union of the bone may occur (perhaps producing a 'false joint').

Note that multiple fractures of different ages seen on x-ray may indicate an underlying bone disease such as severe osteoporosis or congenital osteogenesis imperfecta. In infants, children and weak dependants, however, such fractures may be the result of non-accidental injury (physical abuse).

Liver

In severe chronic hepatitis, extensive hepatocyte loss is followed by scarring, as is the case in the skin or other damaged tissues. Hepatocytes, like the skin epidermal cells, have massive regenerative potential, and surviving hepatocytes may proliferate to form nodules. Hyperplasia of hepatocytes and fibroblasts is presumably mediated by a combination of hormones and growth factors, although the mechanisms are far from clear. Regenerative nodules of hepatocytes and scar tissue are the components of cirrhosis of the liver.

Heart

Myocardial cells are permanent cells and so cannot divide in a regenerative response to tissue injury. In myocardial infarction, a segment of muscle dies and, if the patient survives, it is replaced by hyperplastic myofibroblast scar tissue. As the remainder of the myocardium must work harder for a given cardiac output, it undergoes compensatory hypertrophy (without cell division) (see Fig. 4.12). Occasionally, there may be right ventricular hypertrophy as a result of left ventricular failure and consequent pulmonary hypertension.

NON-REGENERATIVE HYPERTROPHY AND HYPERPLASIA

Many conditions are characterised by hypertrophy or hyperplasia of cells. In some instances, this is the principal feature of the condition from which the disease is named. The more common examples are summarised below.

Myocardium

The myocardium responds to an increased work load by increasing muscle mass by hypertrophy (myocardial cells cannot undergo mitosis). Right ventricular hypertrophy occurs in response to pulmonary valve stenosis, secondary to a ventricular septal defect, or in pulmonary hypertension. Left ventricular hypertrophy takes place in response to aortic valve stenosis or systemic hypertension.

Arteries

Hypertrophy of arterial smooth muscle arterial walls occurs in hypertension, in response to increased work load. Myointimal cell hyperplasia occurs as an important component of the development of atherosclerosis, when they proliferate in response to platelet-derived growth factors.

Capillary vessels

In the eye, capillaries grow from the retina into the vitreous gel, where they may cause reduced vision, especially if they bleed and stimulate scarring. Capillary hyperplasia is a response to retinal hypoxia, or (as proliferative retinopathy) as an important sight-threatening complication of diabetes mellitus.

Bone marrow

Erythrocyte precursor hyperplasia occurs in response to increased circulating erythropoietin concentrations,

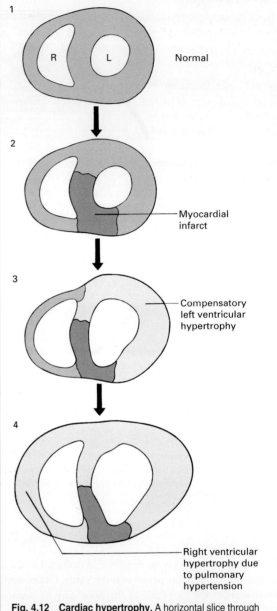

Fig. 4.12 Cardiac hypertrophy. A horizontal slice through the myocardium of the left (L) and right (R) ventricles. (1) Normal. (2) Area of anteroseptal left ventricular infarct. (3) Compensatory hypertrophy of the surviving left ventricle. (4) Right ventricular hypertrophy secondary to left ventricular failure and pulmonary hypertension. From Underwood op. cit.

due to increased secretion by the kidney resulting from decreased arterial oxygen tension (for example, as a result of living at high altitude, or due to anaemia).

Cytotoxic T lymphocytes

Hyperplastic expansion of T lymphocyte populations (Fig. 4.13) occurs in cell-mediated immune responses to, for example, organ transplants.

Breast

Juvenile hyperplasia of the breast may occur in females as an exaggerated response to female sex hormones at puberty. In males, breast hyperplasia (gynaecomastia) may occur at puberty, or be due to high oestrogen levels (e.g. in cirrhosis or oestrogen treatment of prostate cancer), or be secondary to drugs such as spironolactone, cimetidine or digoxin.

Prostate

With increasing age (particularly over 60 years), a relative excess of oestrogens stimulates oestrogen-induced hyperplasia of the epithelial and connective tissue of the prostate. This is most severe in the oestrogen-sensitive central zone of the prostate, where gland enlargement has maximum clinical effect by compression of the urethra.

Thyroid

Follicular epithelial hyperplasia is most commonly due to an IgG autoantibody to the thyroid-stimulating hormone (TSH) receptor; this has an inappropriate thyroid-stimulating effect (as a stimulatory hypersensitivity reaction), increasing thyroid activity and thyroxine secretion, and causing hyperthyroidism (Graves' disease). Hyperthyroidism may also result from increased TSH production by a pituitary adenoma.

Adrenal cortex

Adrenal cortical hyperplasia can result as a response to increased adrenocorticotrophic hormone (ACTH) production (e.g. from a pituitary tumour or, inappropriately, from a lung carcinoma).

APPARENTLY AUTONOMOUS HYPERPLASIAS

In some apparently hyperplastic conditions, cells appear autonomous, and continue to proliferate rapidly despite

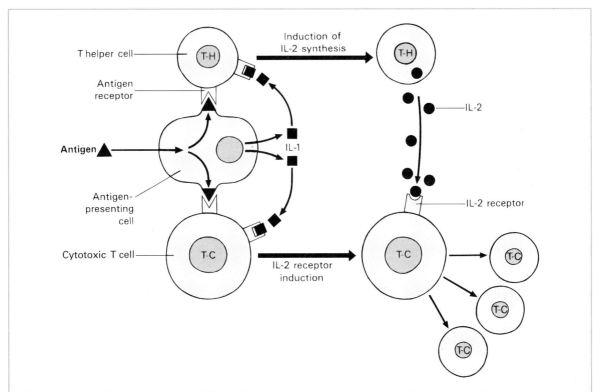

Fig. 4.13 Interleukins and cytotoxic T cell hyperplasia. Cytotoxic T cell hyperplasia is mediated by presentation of an antigen by an antigen-presenting cell (a macrophage) to T helper and T cytotoxic cells. Interleukin-1 (IL-1) acts on these cells via membrane receptors, stimulating the production of interleukin-2 (IL-2) by the T helper cell, and of IL-2-receptors by T cytotoxic cells. IL-2 from the T helper cells stimulates the now-receptive T cytotoxic cell to multiply. From Underwood op. cit.

the lack of a demonstrable stimulus or control mechanism. The question then arises as to whether these should be considered to be hyperplasias at all, or whether they are autonomous and hence neoplastic. If the cells can be demonstrated to be monoclonal (derived as a single clone from one cell) then this suggests that the lesion may indeed be neoplastic, but clonality is often difficult to establish.

Three examples are:

- *psoriasis,* characterised by marked epidermal hyperplasia
- *Paget's disease of bone,* in which there is hyperplasia of osteoblasts and osteoclasts resulting in thick but weak bone
- *fibromatoses,* which are apparently autonomous proliferations of myofibroblasts, occasionally forming tumour-like masses, exemplified by palmar fibromatosis (Dupuytren's contracture), desmoid tumour, retroperitoneal fibromatosis and Peyronie's disease of the penis.

DECREASED GROWTH — ATROPHY

Atrophy is the decrease in size of an organ or cell by reduction in cell size and/or reduction in cell numbers, often by a mechanism involving apoptosis (p. 51). Tissues or cells affected by atrophy are said to be atrophic or atrophied. Atrophy is an important adaptive response to a decreased requirement of the body for the function of a particular cell or organ. It is important to appreciate that, for atrophy to occur, there must be not only a cessation of growth but also an active reduction in cell size and/or a decrease in cell numbers, mediated by apoptosis.

Atrophy occurs in both physiological and pathological conditions.

Physiological atrophy

Physiological atrophy occurs at times from very early embryological life, as part of the process of morphogenesis, into late old age, where its results are regarded as the bane of existence (Box 4.1).

Pathological atrophy

There are several categories of pathological condition in which atrophy may occur.

Decreased function

As a result of decreased function as, for example, in a limb immobilised as a consequence of a fracture, there may be marked muscle atrophy (due to decrease in muscle fibre size). Extensive physiotherapy may be required

---

> **Box 4.1   Tissues involved in physiological atrophy**
>
> *Embryo and fetus*
> - branchial clefts
> - notochord
> - thyroglossal duct
> - Müllerian duct (males)
> - Wolffian duct (females)
>
> *Neonate*
> - umbilical vessels
> - ductus arteriosus
> - fetal layer adrenal cortex
>
> *Early adult*
> - thymus
>
> *Late adult and old age*
> - uterus, endometrium
> - testes
> - bone (particularly females)
> - gums
> - mandible (particularly edentulous)
> - cerebrum
> - lymphoid tissue
>
> From Underwood op. cit.

---

to restore the muscle to its former bulk, or to prevent the atrophy.

In extreme cases of 'disuse' atrophy of a limb, bone atrophy may lead to osteoporosis and bone weakening; this is also a feature of conditions of prolonged weightlessness, such as occurs in astronauts.

Loss of innervation

Loss of innervation of muscle causes muscle atrophy, as is seen in nerve transection or in poliomyelitis, where there is loss of anterior horn cells of the spinal cord. In paraplegics, loss of innervation to whole limbs may also precipitate 'disuse' atrophy of bone, which becomes osteoporotic.

Loss of blood supply

This may cause atrophy as a result of tissue hypoxia, which may also be a result of a sluggish circulation. Epidermal atrophy is seen, for example, in the skin of the lower legs in patients with circulatory stagnation related to varicose veins or with atheromatous narrowing of arteries.

'Pressure' atrophy

This occurs when tissues are compressed, either by exogenous agents (atrophy of skin and soft tissues overlying the sacrum in bedridden patients, producing 'bed sores') or endogenous factors (atrophy of a blood vessel wall compressed by a tumour). In both of these circumstances a major factor is actually local tissue hypoxia.

Lack of nutrition

Lack of nutrition may cause atrophy of adipose tissue, the gut and pancreas and, in extreme circumstances, muscle. An extreme form of systemic atrophy similar to that seen in severe starvation is termed 'cachexia'; this may be seen in patients in the late stages of severe illnesses such as cancer. In some wasting conditions, such as cancer, cytokines such as tumour necrosis factor (TNF) are postulated to influence the development of cachexia.

Loss of endocrine stimulation

Atrophy of the 'target' organ of a hormone may occur if endocrine stimulation is inadequate. For example, the adrenal gland atrophies as a consequence of decreased ACTH secretion by the anterior pituitary; this may be caused by destruction of the anterior pituitary (by a tumour or infarction), or as a result of the therapeutic use of high concentrations of corticosteroids (in, for example, the treatment of cancer), with consequent 'feedback' reduction of circulating ACTH levels.

Hormone-induced atrophy

This form of atrophy may be seen in the skin, as a result of the growth-inhibiting actions of corticosteroids. When corticosteroids are applied topically in high concentrations to the skin, they may cause dermal and epidermal atrophy which may be disfiguring. All steroids, when applied topically, may also be absorbed through the skin to produce systemic side effects, e.g. adrenal atrophy when corticosteroids are used.

DECREASED GROWTH — HYPOPLASIA

Although the terms 'hypoplasia' and 'atrophy' are often used interchangeably, the former is better reserved to denote the failure in attainment of the normal size or shape of an organ as a consequence of a developmental failure. Hypoplasia is, therefore, a failure in morphogenesis, although it is closely related to atrophy in terms of its pathogenesis. An example of hypoplasia is the failure in development of the legs in adult patients with severe spina bifida and neurological deficit in the lower limbs.

DIFFERENTIATION AND MORPHOGENESIS IN HUMAN DEVELOPMENT

Differentiation is the process whereby a cell develops an overt specialised function which was not present in the parent cell. It is an important component of morphogenesis; this is the means by which limbs or organs are formed from primitive groups of cells. Thus, abnormalities of differentiation often lead to abnormal morphogenesis and fetal abnormality. It must be remembered, however, that growth also plays an important role in morphogenesis; cells which vary in their differentiation may have very different growth characteristics. Variations in differentiation may also affect the ability of some cells to migrate with respect to others. Thus, normal

embryological development requires highly coordinated processes of differentiation, growth and cell migration which together comprise morphogenesis.

CONTROL OF NORMAL DIFFERENTIATION

A fertilised ovum may develop into a male or female, a human or a blue whale; the outcome depends on the structure of the genome. There are many similarities between the corresponding cell types in different species. Individual cell types are distinct only because, in addition to the many functional proteins required by all cell types for 'household' functions of respiration, repair, etc., each cell also produces a specific set of specialised proteins which are appropriate for only one cell type and one species.

Most differentiated cells contain the same genome as in the fertilised ovum. This has been demonstrated elegantly by injecting the nucleus of a differentiated tadpole gut epithelial cell into an unfertilised frog ovum, the nucleus of which was destroyed using ultraviolet light; the result was a normal frog with the normal variety of differentiated cell types (Fig. 4.14). In a more recent development, a mammal (sheep) has been cloned from a single ovarian cell.

There are very few exceptions to the rule that differentiated cells contain an identical genome to that of the fertilised ovum. In humans, for example, they include B- and T-lymphocytes which have antigen-receptor genes rearranged to endow them with a large repertoire of possible receptors.

TRANSCRIPTIONAL CONTROL

As most differentiated cells have an identical genome, differences between them cannot be due to amplification or deletion of genes. The cells of the body differ because they *express* different genes; genes are selectively switched on or off to control the synthesis of gene products.

The synthesis of a gene product can in theory be controlled at several levels:

- *transcription:* controlling the formation of mRNA
- *transport:* controlling the export of mRNA from the nucleus to the ribosomes in the cytoplasm
- *translation:* controlling the formation of gene product within the ribosomes.

In fact, many of the important 'decision' stages of differentiation in embryogenesis are under transcriptional control, and the manufacture of gene product is proportional to the activity of the gene.

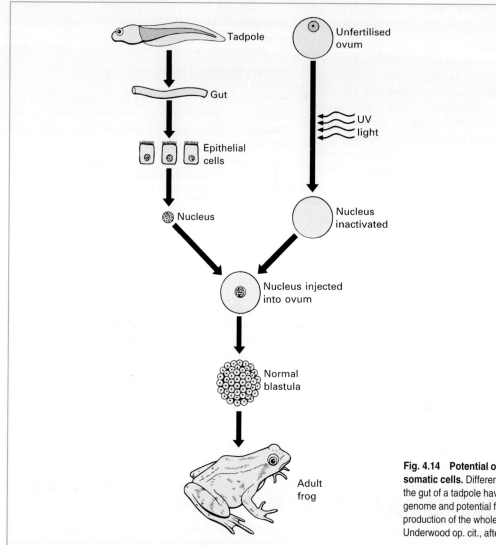

Fig. 4.14 Potential of the genome of somatic cells. Differentiated cells from the gut of a tadpole have the complete genome and potential for control of production of the whole frog. From Underwood op. cit., after JB Gurdon.

For a cell to differentiate in a particular way, given that it contains the potential of activation of the whole of the genome, some groups of genes must be switched on and other groups off. There is now ample evidence that the regulation of transcription of several (or many) individuals within a group of genes is mediated by the gene products of a small number of 'control' genes, which may themselves be regulated by the product of a single 'master' gene (Fig. 4.15).

CELL DETERMINATION

The homeobox-containing genes (single 'master' genes which control the development of major structures such as limbs in precise positions in the embryo), and other genes which regulate embryogenesis, act on the embryo at a very early stage, before structures such as limbs have begun to form. Nonetheless, by observing the effects of selective marking or obliteration of cells, a 'fate map' of the future development of cells in even primitive embryos can be constructed. Thus, some of the cells of somites become specialised at a very early stage as precursors of muscle cells, and migrate to their positions in primitive limbs. These muscle-cell precursors resemble many other cells of the limb rudiment, and it is only after several days that they differentiate and manufacture specialised muscle proteins. Thus, long before they differentiate, the developmental path of these cells is

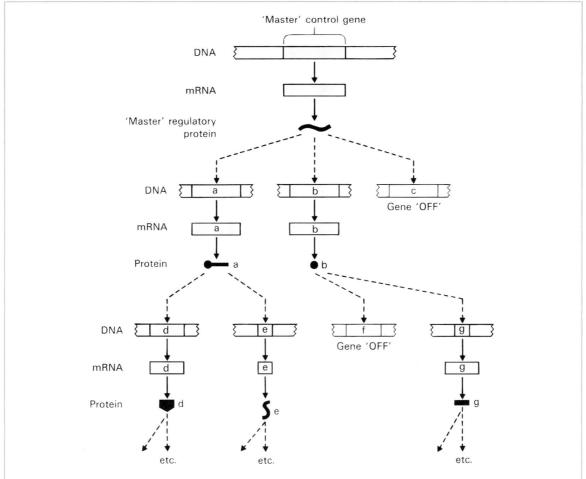

Fig. 4.15 Interaction of genes. A single master gene produces a regulatory protein which switches genes **a** and **b** on and gene **c** off; these in turn switch on or off a cascade of other genes. From Underwood op. cit.

planned; such a cell which has made a developmental choice before differentiating is said to be *determined*. A determined cell must:

- have differences which are heritable from one cell generation to another
- be committed and commit its progeny to specialised development
- change its internal character, not merely its environment.

Determination therefore differs from differentiation, in which there must be *demonstrable* tissue specialisation.

Some cells which are determined, but not differentiated, may remain so for adult life; good examples are the *stem cells*, such as bone marrow haemopoietic cells or

basal cells of the skin, which proliferate continuously and produce cells committed to a particular form of differentiation. Hypoplastic/aplastic anaemia, which result in anaemia, neutropenia, and thrombocytopenia, is thought to be due to a failure or suppression of bone marrow haemopoietic stem cells.

CELL POSITION AND INDUCTIVE PHENOMENA

Even before fertilisation, ova have cytoplasmic determinants of polarity; the manner in which major morphogenetic positional changes may occur under the influence of a small number of controlling genes has been discussed above. As the fields of cells over which spatial chemical signals act are generally small, large-scale changes to the whole individual occur early, and more specific minor features of differentiation within small areas of an organ or limb are specified later and depend on the position of the cell within the structure. Simple changes may occur in response to a diffusible substance (such as vitamin A in the developing limb bud), and serve to control local cell growth and/or differentiation according to the distance from the source. Additional differentiation changes may, however, occur as a result of more complex cellular interactions.

Many organs eventually contain multiple distinct populations of cells which originate separately but later interact. The pattern of differentiation in one cell type may be controlled by another, a phenomenon known as induction. Examples of *induction* include:

- the action of mesoderm on ectoderm at different sites to form the various parts of the neural tube
- the action of mesoderm on the skin at different sites to form epithelium of differing thickness and accessory gland content
- the action of mesoderm on developing epithelial cells to form branching tubular glands
- the action of the ureteric bud (from the mesonephric duct) to induce the metanephric blastema in kidney formation.

Inductive phenomena also occur in cell migrations, sometimes along pathways which are very long, controlled by generally uncertain mechanisms (although it is known, for example, that migrating cells from the neural crest migrate along pathways which are defined by the host connective tissue). Inductive phenomena control the differentiation of the migrating cell when it arrives at its destination — neural crest cells differentiate into a range of cell types, including sympathetic and parasympathetic ganglion cells, and some cells of the neuroendocrine (APUD) system.

MAINTENANCE AND MODULATION OF AN ATTAINED DIFFERENTIATED STATE

Once a differentiated state has been attained by a cell, it must be maintained. This is achieved by a combination of factors:

- 'cell memory' inherent in the genome, with inherited transcriptional changes
- interactions with adjacent cells, through secreted paracrine factors
- secreted factors (autocrine factors), including growth factors and extracellular matrix.

Even in the adult, minor changes to the differentiated state may occur if the local environment changes. These alterations to the differentiated state are rarely great, and most can be termed *modulations,* i.e. reversible interconversions between closely related cell phenotypes. An example of a modulation is the alteration in synthesis of certain liver enzymes in response to circulating corticosteroids.

In the neonatal stage of development, cell *maturation* may involve modulations of the differentiated state. Examples are:

- the production of surfactant by type II pneumonocytes under the influence of corticosteroids
- the synthesis of vitamin K-dependent blood-clotting factors by the hepatocyte
- gut maturation affected by epidermal growth factor (EGF) in milk.

DIFFERENTIATION AND MORPHOGENESIS IN HUMAN DEVELOPMENT

Control of normal differentiation

During development of an embryo, determination and differentiation occur in a cell by transcriptional modifications to the expression of the genome, without an increase or decrease in numbers of genes present. The factors involved are summarised in Figure 4.16. Expression of individual genes within the genome is *modified* during development by:

- positional information carried by a small number of 'control' gene products, causing local alterations in growth and differentiation
- migrations of cells and modifications mediated by adjacent cells (paracrine factors) or endocrine factors.

Maintenance and modulation of an attained differentiated state

Once attained, the differentiated state is *maintained* or *modulated* by:

- paracrine factors (interactions with adjacent cells)
- autocrine factors, such as growth factors and the extracellular matrix secreted by the cell.

External factors may cause alterations to the differentiated state of the cell, either during development or at any stage of adult life.

Normal differentiation and morphogenesis: summary

The main features of morphogenesis are summarised in Figure 4.17.

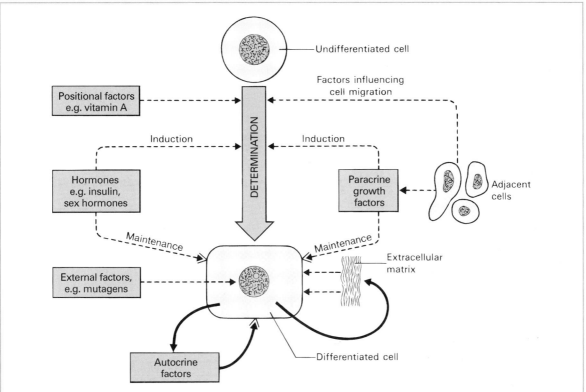

Fig. 4.16 Differentiation. Factors affecting determination, differentiation, maintenance and modulation of the differentiated state of a cell during embryogenesis include positional factors, hormones, paracrine growth factors and external factors such as teratogens. With the exception of positional factors, all of these are important in influencing the differentiated state of cells in postnatal and adult life. From Underwood op. cit.

CONGENITAL DISORDERS OF DIFFERENTIATION AND MORPHOGENESIS

The processes involved in human conception and development are so complex that it is perhaps remarkable that any normal fetuses are produced; the fact that they are produced is a result of the tight controls of growth and morphogenesis which are involved at all stages of development.

The usual outcome of human conception is abortion; 70–80% of all human conceptions are lost, largely as a consequence of chromosomal abnormalities (Fig. 4.18). The majority of these abortions occur spontaneously in the first 6–8 weeks of pregnancy, and in most cases the menstrual cycle might appear normal, or the slight delay in menstruation causes little concern. Chromosomal abnormalities are present in 3–5% of live-born infants, and a further 2% have serious malformations which are not associated with chromosomal aberrations. The most common conditions in these two categories are illustrated in Table 4.1.

Table 4.1 Incidence of some congenital abnormalities	
Chromosomal abnormality	Incidence per 1000 live births
Down's syndrome (47,+21)	1.4
Klinefelter's syndrome (47,XXY)	1.3
Double Y male (47,XYY)	<1
Multiple X female (47,XXX)	<1
Major malformations	Incidence per 1000 stillbirths + live births
Congenital heart defects	6
Pyloric stenosis	3
Spina bifida	2.5
Anencephaly	2
Cleft lip (± cleft palate)	1
Congenital dislocation of the hip	1
From Underwood op. cit.	

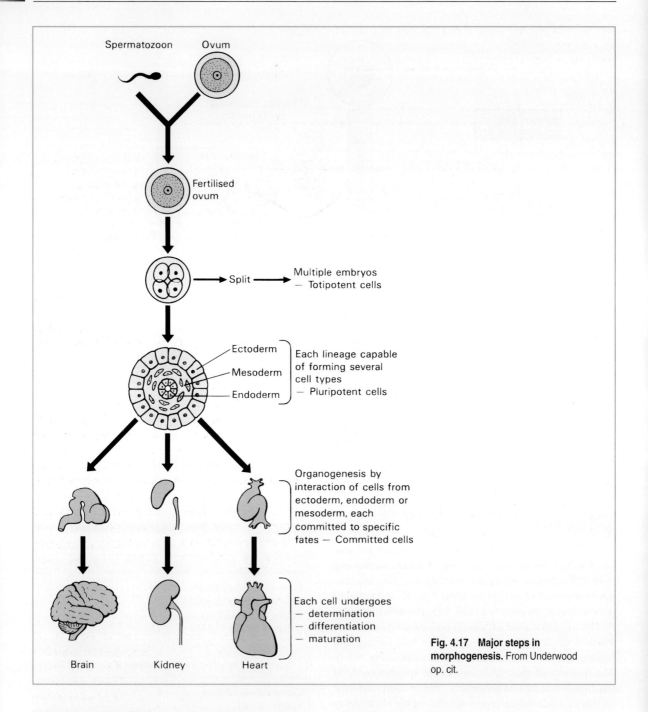

Fig. 4.17 Major steps in morphogenesis. From Underwood op. cit.

Chromosomal abnormalities affecting whole chromosomes

Autosomal chromosomes

The three most common autosomal chromosome defects involve the presence of additional whole chromosomes (trisomy). As the genome of every cell in the body has an increased number of genes, gene product expression is greatly altered and multiple abnormalities result during morphogenesis.

Trisomy 21 (Down's syndrome) affects approximately 1 in 1000 births; it is associated with mental retardation, a flattened facial profile, slanting eyes (producing a

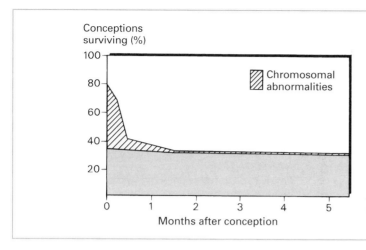

Fig. 4.18 Fate of human conceptions. Between 70% and 80% of human conceptions are lost by spontaneous abortion in the first 6–8 weeks of pregnancy, most as a consequence of chromosomal abnormality. Chromosomal abnormalities are present in 3–5% of live-born infants. From Underwood op. cit., after Witschi 1969.

'mongoloid' appearance) and prominent epicanthic folds. The hands are short, with a transverse 'simian' (i.e. monkey-like) palmar crease. There are also abnormalities of the ears, trunk, pelvis and phalanges. The incidence increases with maternal age.

Sex chromosomes

Chromosomal disorders affecting the sex chromosomes (X and Y) are relatively common, and usually induce abnormalities of sexual development and fertility. In general, variations in X chromosome numbers cause greater mental retardation.

Klinefelter's syndrome (47,XXY) affects 1 in 850 male births. There is testicular atrophy and absent spermatogenesis, eunuchoid bodily habitus, gynaecomastia, female distribution of body hair and mental retardation. Variants of Klinefelter's syndrome (48,XXXY, 49,XXXXY, 48,XXYY) are rare and have cryptorchidism and hypospadias in addition to more severe mental retardation and radio-ulnar synostosis.

Double Y males (47,XYY) form 1 in 1000 male births; they are phenotypically normal, although most are over 6 feet tall. Some are said to have increased aggressive or criminal behaviour.

Turner's syndrome (gonadal dysgenesis; 45,X) occurs in 1 in 3000 female births. About one-half are mosaics (45,X/46,XX) and some have 46 chromosomes and two X chromosomes, one of which is defective. Turner's syndrome females may have short stature, primary amenorrhoea and infertility, webbing of the neck, broad chest and widely spaced nipples, cubitus valgus, low posterior hairline and coarctation of the aorta.

Multiple X females (47,XXX, 48,XXXX) comprise 1 in 1200 female births. They may be mentally retarded,

and have menstrual disturbances, although many are normal and fertile.

True hermaphrodites (most 46,XX, some 46,XX/ 47,XXY mosaics) have both testicular and ovarian tissue, with varying genital tract abnormalities.

Parts of chromosomes

The loss (or addition) of even a small part of a chromosome may have severe effects, especially if 'controlling' or 'master' genes are involved, as these affect many other genes. An example of a congenital disease in this group is *cri-du-chat syndrome* (46,XX, 5p- or 46,XY, 5p-). This rare condition (1 in 50 000 births) is associated with deletion of the short arm of chromosome 5 (5p-), and was so named because infants have a characteristic cry like the miaow of a cat. There is microcephaly and severe mental retardation; the face is round, there is gross hyperteleorism (increased distance between the eyes) and epicanthic folds.

Single gene alterations

All of the inherited disorders of single genes are transmitted by autosomal dominant, autosomal recessive or X-linked modes of inheritance. There are more than 2700 known Mendelian disorders; 80–85% of these are familial, and the remainder are the result of new mutations. The alteration of expression of gene product constitutes at least a modulation of cell differentiation, and some have important effects on growth and morphogenesis.

Single gene disorders fall into four categories, discussed below.

Enzyme defects

An altered gene may result in decreased enzyme synthesis, or the synthesis of a defective enzyme. This may lead to accumulation of the enzyme substrate: for example,

- accumulation of galactose and consequent tissue damage in galactose-1-phosphate uridyl transferase deficiency
- accumulation of phenylalanine, causing mental abnormality, in phenylalanine hydroxylase deficiency
- accumulation of glycogen, mucopolysaccharides, etc. in lysosomes in the enzyme deficiency states of the lysosomal storage disorders.

A failure to synthesise the end products of a reaction catalysed by an enzyme may block normal cellular function. This occurs, for example, in albinism, caused by absent melanin production due to tyrosinase deficiency.

Defects in receptors or cellular transport

The lack of a specific cellular receptor causes insensitivity of a cell to substances such as hormones. In one form of male pseudohermaphroditism, for example, insensitivity of tissues to androgens, caused by lack of androgen receptor, prevents the development of male characteristics during fetal development.

Cellular transport deficiencies may lead to conditions such as cystic fibrosis, a condition in which there is a defective cell membrane transport system across exocrine secretory cells.

Non-enzyme protein defects

Failure of production of important proteins, or production of abnormalities in proteins, has widespread effects. Thus, sickle cell anaemia is caused by the production of abnormal haemoglobin, and Marfan's syndrome and Ehlers–Danlos syndrome are the result of defective collagen production.

Adverse reactions to drugs

The apparently innocuous condition of glucose-6-phosphate dehydrogenase (G6PD) deficiency does not result in disease until the antimalarial drug, primaquine, is administered; severe haemolytic anaemia then results. The prevalence of G6PD deficiency in the tropics may reflect evolutionary selective pressure, as the deficiency may confer a degree of protection against malarial parasitisation of red blood cells.

Functional aspects of developmental disorders

Abnormalities can occur at almost any stage of fetal development; the mechanisms by which the anomaly occurs are sometimes unknown. In most cases the genetic defect is unknown, although the majority are almost certainly the result of transcriptional alterations to an intact genome.

Embryo division abnormalities

Monozygotic twins (or multiple births) result from the separation of groups of cells in the early embryo, well before the formation of the primitive streak. On occasion, there is a defect of embryo division, resulting in, for example, *Siamese twins*; these are the result of incomplete separation of the embryo, with fusion of considerable portions of the body (or minor fusions which are easily separated).

Teratogen exposure

Physical, chemical or infective agents can interfere with growth and differentiation, resulting in fetal abnormalities; such agents are known as *teratogens*. The extent and severity of fetal abnormality depend on the nature of the teratogen and the developmental stage of the embryo when exposed to the teratogen. Thus, if exposure occurs at the stage of early organogenesis (4–5 weeks' gestation) then the effects on developing organs or limbs are severe.

Clinical examples of teratogenesis include the severe and extensive malformations associated with use of the drug thalidomide (absent/rudimentary limbs, defects of the heart, kidney, gastrointestinal tract, etc.), and the effects of rubella (German measles) on the fetus (cataracts, microcephaly, heart defects, etc.). Some other teratogens are listed in Table 4.2.

Failure of cell and organ migration

Failure of migration of cells may occur during embryogenesis.

Kartagener's syndrome   In this rare condition there is a defect in ciliary motility, due to absent or abnormal dynein arms, the structures on the outer doublets of cilia which are responsible for ciliary movement. This affects cell motility during embryogenesis, which often results in situs inversus (congenital lateral inversion of the position of body organs resulting in, for example, left-sided liver and right-sided spleen). Complications in later life include bronchiectasis and infertility due to sperm immobility.

Hirschsprung's disease   This is a condition leading to marked dilatation of the colon and failure of colonic motility in the neonatal period, due to absence of Meissner's and Auerbach's nerve plexuses. It results from a selective failure of craniocaudal migration of neuroblasts in weeks 5–12 of gestation. It is, interestingly, ten times more frequent in children with trisomy 21 (Down's syndrome), and is often associated with other congenital anomalies.

Undescended testis (cryptorchidism)   This is the result of failure of the testis to migrate to its normal position in the scrotum. Although this may be associated with severe forms of Klinefelter's syndrome (e.g. 48,XXXY), it is often

Table 4.2 Teratogens and their effects	
Teratogen	Teratogenic effect
Irradiation	Microcephaly
Drugs	
Thalidomide	Amelia/phocomelia (absent/rudimentary limbs), heart, kidney, gastrointestinal and facial abnormalities
Folic acid antagonists	Anencephaly, hydrocephalus, cleft lip/palate, skull defects
Anticonvulsants	Cleft lip/palate, heart defects, minor skeletal defects
Warfarin	Nasal/facial abnormalities
Testosterone and synthetic progestogens	Virilisation of female fetus, atypical genitalia
Alcohol	Microcephaly, abnormal facies, oblique palpebral fissures, growth disturbance
Infections	
Rubella	Cataracts, microphthalmia, microcephaly, heart defects
Cytomegalovirus	Microcephaly
Herpes simplex	Microcephaly, microphthalmia
Toxoplasmosis	Microcephaly
From Underwood op. cit.	

an isolated anomaly in an otherwise normal male. There is an increased risk of neoplasia in undescended testes.

Anomalies of organogenesis

Agenesis (aplasia)

The failure of development of an organ or structure is known as agenesis (aplasia). Obviously, agenesis of some structures (such as the heart) is incompatible with life, but agenesis of many individual organs is recorded. These include:

- *Renal agenesis.* This may be unilateral or bilateral (in which case the affected infant may survive only a few days after birth). It results from a failure of the mesonephric duct to give rise to the ureteric bud, and consequent failure of metanephric blastema induction.
- *Thymic agenesis* is seen in Di George syndrome, where there is failure of development of T lymphocytes, and consequent severe deficiency of cell-mediated immunity. Recent evidence suggests that there is failure of processing of stem cells to T cells as a result of a defect in the thymus anlage.
- *Anencephaly* is a severe neural tube defect in which the cerebrum, and often the cerebellum, are absent. The condition is lethal.

Atresia

Atresia is the failure of development of a lumen in a normally tubular epithelial structure. Examples include:

- *oesophageal atresia,* which may be seen in association with tracheo-oesophageal fistulae, as a result of anomalies of development of the two structures from the primitive foregut
- *biliary atresia,* which is an uncommon cause of obstructive jaundice in early childhood
- *urethral atresia,* a very rare anomaly, which may be associated with recto-urethral or urachal fistula, or congenital absence of the anterior abdominal wall muscles ('prune belly' syndrome).

Hypoplasia

A failure in development of the normal size of an organ is termed hypoplasia. It may affect only part of an organ, e.g. segmental hypoplasia of the kidney. A relatively common example of hypoplasia affects the osseous nuclei of the acetabulum, causing congenital dislocation of the hip, due to a flattened roof to the acetabulum.

Maldifferentiation (dysgenesis, dysplasia)

Maldifferentiation, as its name implies, is the failure of normal differentiation of an organ, which often retains primitive embryological structures. This disorder is often termed 'dysplasia', although this is a potential cause of confusion, as the more common usage of the term dysplasia implies the presence of a preneoplastic state (p. 76).

The best examples of maldifferentiation are seen in the kidney ('renal dysplasia') as a result of anomalous metanephric differentiation. Here, primitive tubular structures may be admixed with cellular mesenchyme and, occasionally, smooth muscle.

Ectopia, heterotopia and choristomas

Ectopic and heterotopic tissues are usually small areas of mature tissue from one organ which are present within another tissue (e.g. gastric mucosa in a Meckel's diverticulum) as a result of a developmental anomaly. Another clinically important example is endometriosis, in which endometrial tissue is found around the peritoneum in some women, causing abdominal pain at the time of menstruation.

A choristoma is a related form of heterotopia, where one or more mature differentiated tissues aggregate as a tumour-like mass at an inappropriate site. A good example of this is a complex choristoma of the conjunctiva (eye), which have varying proportions of cartilage, adipose tissue, smooth muscle, and lacrimal gland acini. A conjunctival choristoma consisting of lacrimal gland elements alone could also be considered to be an ectopic (heterotopic) lacrimal gland.

Complex disorders of growth and morphogenesis

Four examples of complex, multifactorial defects of growth and morphogenesis will be discussed: neural tube defects, congenital renal polycystic disease, disorders of sexual differentiation, and cleft palate and related disorders.

Neural tube defects

The development of the brain, spinal cord and spine from the primitive neural tube is highly complex and, not surprisingly, so too are the developmental disorders of the system (Fig. 4.19).

Neural tube malformations are relatively common in the United Kingdom and are found in about 1.3% of aborted fetuses and 0.1% of live births. There are regional differences in incidence, and social differences, the condition being more common in social class V than in classes I or II. The pathogenesis of these conditions —

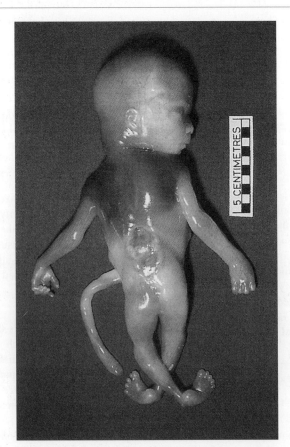

Fig. 4.19 Spina bifida. Dorsal view of a fetus from a pregnancy terminated after prenatal diagnosis of spina bifida. Extending from the lower thoracic to the sacral region there is an oval defect due to failure of spinal canal formation. Deformity and hypoplasia of the legs results from neurological deficit. From Underwood op. cit.

anencephaly, hydrocephalus and spina bifida — is uncertain and probably multifactorial.

Congenital renal polycystic disease

Cystic diseases of the kidneys are a heterogenous group of congenital and acquired conditions, some of which are important causes of renal failure. The congenital forms of renal polycystic disease are complex and involve not only the kidneys but other organs such as the liver. Although the diseases are familial, the precise mechanisms by which the cystic abnormalities develop are uncertain.

The two most important polycystic diseases affecting the kidneys are as follows.

Adult polycystic kidney disease (autosomal dominant polycystic kidney disease; ADPKD)   In this disease the Mendelian dominant trait has a high degree of penetrance (expression). At least one causative gene (ADPKD-1 gene) is known, located on the short arm of chromosome 6, but this gene is known not to be involved in some families, indicating that other gene defects may also be involved. Both kidneys are grossly enlarged (each commonly weighing more than 1000 g) and distorted by multiple cysts from a few millimetres to 100 mm in diameter, derived from all levels of the nephron. As they enlarge, the cysts compress adjacent functional tissue, which is eventually destroyed. Patients with this condition present at any age from late childhood, with symptomatology related to renal failure (around half have end-stage renal failure by 60 years of age) and/or hypertension. There is also an association of the disease with berry aneurysms of the vascular circle of Willis, which may rupture causing often fatal subarachnoid haemorrhage. Additional cysts may occur, especially in the liver, but also in the pancreas and lungs, but these do not affect organ function and are therefore clinically insignificant.

Childhood polycystic kidney disease (autosomal recessive polycystic kidney disease; ARPKD)   This is more rare than the adult form, and there are several subgroups, which may indicate that several gene defects may be involved. Around 10% of patients fall into the *perinatal subgroup,* with severe abnormalities at birth, and the baby is either stillborn or dies of renal failure and respiratory distress soon after birth. Their kidneys may be so enlarged as to be readily palpable, and renal enlargement may interfere with delivery. The multiple cysts (derived from collecting ducts) are characteristically elongated and arranged radially in the cortex and medulla. Children in the *neonatal, infantile* and *juvenile subgroups* have progressively less severe renal disease and survive proportionally longer.

Children with childhood polycystic disease all have additional liver abnormalities, which are probably due to developmental arrest of bile duct formation. These liver changes include cysts, secondary bile duct proliferation, and extensive fibrosis, often leading to hepatic failure and portal hypertension.

Disorders of sexual differentiation

Disorders of sexual differentiation are undoubtedly complex, and involve a range of individual chromosomal, enzyme and hormone receptor defects. The defects may be obvious and severe at birth, or they may be subtle, presenting with infertility in adult life.

Chromosomal abnormalities causing ambiguous or abnormal sexual differentiation have already been discussed (p. 69).

Female pseudohermaphroditism, in which the genetic sex is always female (XX), may be due to exposure of the developing fetus to the masculinising effects of excess testosterone or progestogens, causing abnormal differentiation of the external genitalia. The causes include:

- an enzyme defect in the fetal adrenal gland, leading to excessive androgen production at the expense of cortisol synthesis (with consequent adrenal hyperplasia due to feedback mechanisms which increases ACTH secretion)
- exogenous androgenic steroids from a maternal androgen-secreting tumour, or administration of androgens (or progestogens) during pregnancy.

Male pseudohermaphroditism, in which the genetic sex is male (XY), may be the result of several rare defects:

- testicular unresponsiveness to human chorionic gonadotrophin (hCG) or luteinising hormone (LH), by virtue of reduction in receptors to these hormones; this causes failure of testosterone secretion
- errors of testosterone biosynthesis in the fetus, due to enzyme defects (may be associated with cortisol deficiency and congenital adrenal hyperplasia)
- tissue insensitivity to androgens (androgen receptor deficiency)
- abnormality in testosterone metabolism by peripheral tissues, in 5a-reductase deficiency
- defects in synthesis, secretion and response to Müllerian duct inhibitory factor
- maternal ingestion of oestrogens and progestins.

These defects result in the presence of a testis which is small and atrophic, and a female phenotype.

Cleft palate and related disorders

Cleft palate, and the related cleft (or hare) lip, are relatively common (about 1 per 1000 births). Approximately

20% of children with these disorders have associated major malformations. The important stages of development of the lips, palate, nose and jaws occur in the first 9 weeks of embryonic life. From about 5 weeks' gestational age the maxillary processes grow anteriorly and medially, and fuse with the developing frontonasal process at two points just below the nostrils, forming the upper lip. Meanwhile, the palate develops from the palatal processes of the maxillary processes, which grow medially to fuse with the nasal septum in the midline at about 9 weeks.

Failure of these complicated processes may occur at any stage, producing small clefts or severe facial deficits (Fig. 4.20). A cleft lip is commonly unilateral but may be bilateral; it may involve the lip alone, or extend into the nostril or involve the bone of the maxilla and the teeth. The mildest palatal clefting may involve the uvula or soft palate alone, but can lead to absence of the roof of the mouth. Cleft lip and palate occur singly or in combination, and severe combined malformations of the lips, maxilla and palate can be very difficult to manage surgically.

Recently, lip and palate malformations have been extensively studied as a model of normal and abnormal states of morphogenesis in a complicated developmental system. It appears from the relatively high incidence of these malformations that the control of palatal morphogenesis is particularly sensitive to both genetic and environmental disturbances:

- genetic — e.g. Patau's syndrome (trisomy 13) is associated with severe clefting of the lip and palate
- environmental — e.g. the effects of specific teratogens such as folic acid antagonists or anticonvulsants, causing cleft lip and/or palate.

Recent experimental evidence has suggested that several cellular factors are involved in the fusion of the frontonasal and maxillary processes. The differentiation of epithelial cells of the palatal processes is of paramount importance in fusion of the processes. It is thought that the most important mechanism is mediated by mesenchymal cells of the palatal processes; these induce differentiation of the epithelial cells (p. 66), to form either ciliated nasal epithelial cells or squamous buccal epithelial cells, or to undergo programmed cell death by apoptosis (p. 51) to allow fusion of underlying mesenchymal cells. Positional information of genetic and chemical (paracrine) nature is important in this differentiation, and is mediated via mesenchymal cells (and possibly epithelial cells). In addition, the events may be modified by the actions of epidermal growth factor (EGF) and other growth factors through autocrine or paracrine mechanisms (p. 66), and by the endocrine actions of glucocorticoids and their intercellular receptors.

As yet, the precise way in which all of these factors interact in normal palatal development or cleft palate is unclear. In the mouse, it is known that physiological con-

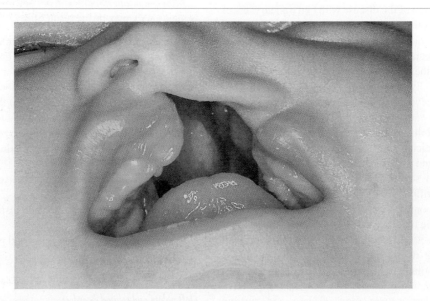

Fig. 4.20 Cleft palate. There is a large defect involving the upper lip, the upper jaw and the palate. From Underwood op. cit., courtesy of Mr D Willmott, Sheffield.

centrations of glucocorticoids, their receptors and EGF are required for normal development, but that altered concentrations may precipitate cleft palate.

ACQUIRED DISORDERS OF DIFFERENTIATION AND GROWTH

METAPLASIA

Metaplasia (transdifferentiation) is the reversible transformation of one type of terminally differentiated (epithelial or mesenchymal) cell into another fully differentiated cell type. Metaplasia often represents an adaptive response of a tissue to environmental stress, and is presumed to be due to the activation and/or repression of groups of genes involved in the maintenance of cellular differentiation. The metaplastic tissue is better able to withstand the adverse environmental changes.

Examples of metaplasia are listed in Table 4.3.

Epithelial tissues

Examples of metaplasia in epithelial tissues include the following.

Squamous metaplasia (a change to squamous epithelium)   This occurs in:

- transitional and ciliated respiratory epithelium of the *nasal cavity, sinuses, trachea* and bronchi in many tobacco smokers (note, dysplasia may also be present; see below)
- the epithelium of the *nose* and *sinuses* of nickel (hot metal) workers.
- *conjunctival* epithelium, and transitional and ciliated *nasal* epithelium, in vitamin A deficiency; note that conjunctival imprint cytology can be used (to detect loss of goblet cells) as a relatively inexpensive screening method for detecting vitamin A deficiency in famine victims
- duct epithelium of *salivary, pancreatic and bile ducts,* in the presence of stones

Table 4.3 Metaplasia and dysplasia in body tissues (refer to text for details)		
Organ	Metaplasia	Dysplasia (resulting malignancy)
Skin	Not applicable	Squamous cells in *actinic keratosis* (squamous carcinoma)
		Melanocyte dysplasia in *lentigo* and *dysplastic naevus* (malignant melanoma)
Eye	*Squamous metaplasia* of conjunctiva	Conjunctival/corneal *epithelial dysplasia* (squamous carcinoma)
	Osseous metaplasia of retinal pigment epithelial cells	Conjunctival melanocytes in *acquired atypical melanosis* (malignant melanoma)
Respiratory tract	*Squamous metaplasia* in nasal cavity, sinuses and bronchus	*Squamous dysplasia* in nasal cavity, sinuses and bronchus
	Osseous metaplasia of bronchial cartilage	
Oral oesophagus	Not applicable	Mouth and tongue *epithelial dysplasia*
	Glandular metaplasia of lower oesophagus (Barrett's oesophagus)	*Squamous dysplasia* (squamous carcinoma)
		Glandular dysplasia of lower oesophagus in Barrett's oesophagus (adenocarcinoma)
Stomach	*Intestinal metaplasia* of gastric epithelium	*De novo epithelial dysplasia,* and *dysplasia in adenomatous polyps* (adenocarcinoma)
Large bowel	Epithelial *metaplastic polyps*	*Epithelial dysplasia* in ulcerative colitis, and *dysplasia in adenomatous polyps* (adenocarcinoma)
Ducts (bile, salivary, pancreas)	*Squamous metaplasia*	Not applicable
Urinary tract	*Squamous metaplasia* of urothelium of kidney, ureters, bladder, prostate	*Transitional cell dysplasia* (transitional carcinoma); *squamous dysplasia* (squamous carcinoma)
Penis	Not applicable	*Squamous dysplasia* in *erythroplasia of Queyrat*
Female genital tract	Not applicable	*Squamous dysplasia* in *cervix uteri, vaginal* and *vulval intraepithelial neoplasia* (squamous carcinoma)
		Endometrial dysplasia/atypical hyperplasia (endometrial adenocarcinoma)
Breast	*Apocrine metaplasia*	*Breast duct endometrial dysplasia/atypical hyperplasia* (endometrial adenocarcinoma)

- *renal, ureteric and bladder epithelium* in the presence of ova of the trematode *Schistosoma haematobium* (note, dysplasia may also be present; see below)
- glands and ducts of the *prostate gland,* around areas of infarction in age-related prostatic hyperplasia.

Glandular metaplasia Glandular metaplasia of the lower oesophagus occurs when gastric acid reflux causes the normal squamous epithelium of the lower oesophagus to change to columnar epithelium, an appearance referred to as *Barrett's oesophagus.* Histologically the epithelium is of junctional (gastric cardiac), atrophic fundal (gastric secretory), intestinal or mixed type. Note that dysplasia may also be present, and that dysplasia (and not metaplasia) accounts for a 100-fold risk of malignancy when compared with the unaffected population.

Intestinal metaplasia This occurs in the stomach, as a consequence of chronic gastritis; under these circumstances the normal gastric mucosal neutral mucin-secreting cells are replaced by goblet cells containing acid glycoproteins typical of the intestine. Note that dysplasia may also be present in chronic gastritis (see below).

Metaplastic polyps Metaplastic polyps, with elongated crypts and hypermature 'serrated' surface cells, occur in the large bowel with increasing age, although their pathogenesis is unknown. These polyps have no malignant potential (see below).

Apocrine metaplasia This occurs in the breast as a frequent component of benign fibrocystic disease. Normal breast epithelial cells within small cysts are replaced by large columnar cells, with abundant eosinophilic cytoplasm. Apocrine metaplasia is not a risk factor for breast cancer development.

Mesenchymal tissues

Examples of metaplasia in mesenchymal tissues include bone formation (osseous metaplasia):

- following calcium deposition in atheromatous arterial walls
- in bronchial cartilage
- following longstanding disease of the uveal tract of the eye.

By definition, metaplasia does not itself progress to malignancy, although the environmental changes which initially caused the metaplasia may also induce dysplasia which, if persistent, may progress to tumour formation.

Metaplasia is sometimes said to occur in tumours as, for example, in squamous or glandular 'metaplasia'

which may occur in transitional carcinomas of the bladder. These examples of transdifferentiation certainly do occur in tumours, but the term 'metaplasia' is best reserved for changes in non-neoplastic tissues.

DYSPLASIA

Dysplasia is a *premalignant* condition characterised by increased cell growth, the presence of cellular atypia, and altered differentiation. Early mild forms of dysplasia may be reversible if the initial stimulus is removed, but severe dysplasia will progress to a malignant neoplasm unless it is adequately treated.

Dysplasia may be caused by longstanding irritation of a tissue, with chronic inflammation, or by exposure to carcinogenic substances.

In affected tissues (Fig. 4.21), dysplasia may be recognised by:

- evidence of increased growth, such as increased tissue bulk (e.g. increased epithelial thickness), and increased numbers of mitoses
- presence of cellular atypia, with pleomorphism (variation in the size and shape of cells and their nuclei), a high nuclear/cytoplasmic ratio, and increased nuclear DNA (recognised by hyperchromatism, i.e. more darkly stained nuclei)
- altered differentiation, as the cells often appear more primitive than normal. For example, dysplastic squamous epithelium may not show the normal differentiation from basal cells to flattened surface cells of the skin; this appearance is described as showing 'loss of epithelial polarity'.

Examples of dysplasia are listed in Table 4.3, and include the following.

Skin In the skin:

- In *squamous epithelial cells* of light-exposed areas, dysplasia produces *actinic keratosis,* where there are areas of thickened epithelium, hyperkeratosis (increased keratin production) and cellular atypia, often progressing to squamous carcinoma.
- In *melanocytes,* dysplasia may develop either in areas with increased numbers of confluent melanocytes (*lentigo*), or within pre-existing naevi (moles), particularly in *dysplastic naevus syndrome.* In this syndrome, some kindreds (families), termed 'BK mole' kindreds (the initials being those of the first patients described with this condition) have a high frequency of malignant melanomas developing from one or more naevi which are dysplastic histologically.

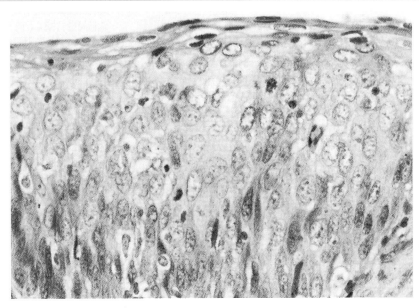

Fig. 4.21   Cervical intraepithelial neoplasia (CIN) grade 3. Note that in this severe dysplasia there is minimal surface differentiation (a few flattened epithelial cells). From Underwood op. cit.

Eye   In the *conjunctiva* of the eye:

- *Squamous epithelial dysplasia* may progress to squamous carcinoma.
- *Melanocyte dysplasia* (in *acquired atypical melanosis*) may affect wide areas of the conjunctiva, and gradually progress to malignant melanoma.

Respiratory tract   In the respiratory tract and especially in the *bronchus,* (but also in the *nasopharynx, sinuses* and *larynx*), dysplasia is most frequently caused by tobacco smoking (see above). The epithelium has often (but not always) already undergone squamous metaplasia, and superimposed dysplasia often progresses to malignancy (squamous carcinoma).

Mouth and tongue   In the mouth and tongue, dysplasia produces leukoplakia (a descriptive term only, meaning 'white patch', which can also be produced by other lesions, including carcinoma), and may progress to squamous carcinoma.

Oesophagus   In the oesophagus:

- *Dysplasia* of the *squamous oesophageal mucosa* may progress to squamous carcinoma.
- *Glandular dysplasia* of the lower oesophagus occurs in *Barrett's oesophagus* (see above), in areas of glandular metaplasia (when gastric acid reflux causes the normal squamous epithelium of the lower oesophagus to change to columnar epithelium). Under these circumstances, dysplasia accounts for 100-fold risk of malignancy (adenocarcinoma) when compared with the unaffected population.

Stomach   In the stomach:

- Dysplasia frequently develops in association with *Helicobacter pylori-associated chronic gastritis,* and often progresses over time to gastric adenocarcinoma. Given the good prognosis of early gastric adenocarcinoma confined to mucosa or submucosa (5 year survival of more than 90%), it is important to screen and monitor patients known to be at high risk (e.g. with chronic gastritis and dysplasia), as a means of preventing more advanced gastric cancer, which has a poor prognosis.
- Dysplasia frequently develops in existing *adenomatous polyps* (see below).

Large bowel   In the large bowel epithelium:

- Dysplasia and subsequent adenocarcinoma are frequent and important complications of longstanding *chronic inflammatory bowel disease* (and particularly in *ulcerative colitis*). The overall risk of colorectal cancer in ulcerative colitis is low (around 2%), but this increases to around 10% in patients affected for 25 years.

- Most *adenomas* (*adenomatous polyps;* see below) of the large bowel progress with time through increasing severity of dysplasia to malignancy (adenocarcinoma). In *familial adenomatous polyposis* (transmitted as a Mendelian dominant condition), adenomas (mainly of the large bowel, but also of the small bowel) develop during the second and third decades, become dysplastic, and undergo malignant change by the age of 35 years.

Kidney, ureters and bladder In the kidney, ureters and bladder:

- Dysplasia of the urothelium may arise *de novo* in transitional epithelium (progressing to transitional carcinoma), as described in rubber factory workers.
- It may be superimposed on squamous metaplasia (producing squamous carcinoma), as seen in epithelium in the presence of ova of the trematode *Schistosoma haematobium.*

Penis Dysplasia of the *glans penis* appears as a sharply defined, slightly raised erythematous (red) patch, with a moist keratinous surface (*erythroplasia of Queyrat*), which carries a high risk of progression to squamous carcinoma.

Female genital tract In the female genital tract:

- Dysplasia of the *cervix uteri* and, less commonly, of the *vagina* or *vulva,* carry a high risk of progression to invasive squamous carcinoma. These lesions (a spectrum of mild, moderate and severe dysplasia to in-situ squamous carcinoma) are classified as *cervical, vaginal and vulval intraepithelial neoplasia* (Fig. 4.21), and they can be recognised as microscopic changes in cells from exfoliative cytological and biopsy samples. Around 11% of cervical intraepithelial neoplasia stage 1(CIN 1) cases progress to CIN 3 within 3 years, and more than 12% of CIN 3 lesions would progress to invasive squamous carcinoma if untreated (although 30% of CIN 3 lesions would regress spontaneously).
- Dysplasia of the *endometrium* (known as '*atypical hyperplasia*') is recognised by microscopic architectural and cytological changes. There is a close correlation between the severity of atypia and subsequent development of adenocarcinoma; thus, in severe cytological atypia there is a 25% risk of malignancy in 3 years.

Breast In the female breast, dysplasia (again known as '*atypical hyperplasia*') is recognised within breast ducts, which are packed with disoriented epithelial cells, which have nuclear pleomorphism and mitotic figures.

The risk of developing breast adenocarcinoma is five times higher in women with atypical hyperplasia than in women with non-proliferative ductal lesions, and the risk increases further if the patient has a family history of breast cancer.

Note that the term 'dysplasia' is sometimes used misleadingly to denote the failure of differentiation of an organ which may retain primitive embryological structures. To avoid confusion, it is better to substitute the terms 'maldifferentiation' or 'dysgenesis' for this condition (see p. 71).

POLYPS

The term 'polyp' is used in medicine to describe the macroscopic ('naked eye') appearance of a smooth mass of tissue which projects outwards from the surface of an organ. This organ surface is usually an epithelium (such as the nasal mucosa, or the bowel epithelium), although lesions which could be described as 'polypoid' (polyp-like) might also occur on surfaces such as the peritoneum or synovium. Polyps are also described as 'sessile' when they are flat, and 'pedunculated' when they have a stalk (Fig. 4.22).

The term 'polyposis' is used to describe a condition or syndrome where there are multiple polyps in an organ (e.g. polyposis coli, affecting the colon) or an organ system (e.g. hamartomatous polyposis of the gastrointestinal tract in Peutz–Jeghers syndrome).

It is important to appreciate that the term 'polyp', when used alone and without further qualification, is purely descriptive of the shape of a lesion, and *does not signify any specific underlying pathological process* (such as hyperplasia, metaplasia, dysplasia or neoplasia). A polyp results from focal tissue expansion at a site at (or near) the organ surface, when the enlarging mass takes the line of least mechanical resistance as it expands outwards, rather than into the underlying tissue. The pathological process which causes both the focal tissue expansion and polyp formation may be either non-neoplastic (e.g. inflammation, hyperplasia, metaplasia, dysplasia) or neoplastic (e.g. neoplasms of epithelial, mesenchymal, lymphoid or other cellular origin). Non-neoplastic polyps and most neoplastic polyps are common and benign, but a small proportion of malignant neoplasms can have a polypoid appearance (e.g. lymphomatous polyposis of the gastrointestinal tract; polypoid adenocarcinoma of the large bowel). Note that some existing benign polyps (such as adenomatous polyps of the large bowel) can develop increasingly severe dysplasia over a period of time, and that eventually carcinoma-in-situ and

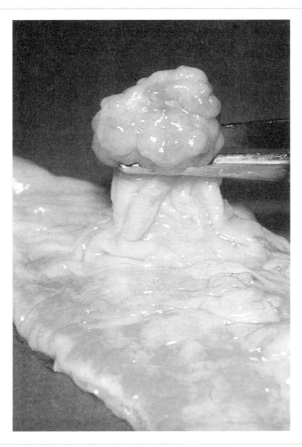

Fig. 4.22 Pedunculated adenomatous polyp of the colon. This common lesion has a clearly visible stalk enabling easy removal at endoscopy. Although benign, these lesions often progress through stages of dysplasia to adenocarcinoma of the large bowel. From Underwood op. cit.

invasive adenocarcinoma may threaten the life of the patient.

In medical and surgical practice, clinicians will encounter polyps in many organ systems. In each clinical situation, however, a diagnosis of 'polyp' is grossly inadequate, and further microscopic examination of the lesion must be made by a histopathologist to determine the precise pathological diagnosis. Figure 4.23 illustrates that there is great potential for misdiagnosis of sessile and pedunculated polyps of the large bowel, which may be non-neoplastic or neoplastic; of epithelial, mesenchymal, lymphoid or other cellular origin.

Systemic examples of polyps

Polyps of all types may be asymptomatic, or they may come to the attention of the patient and clinician because of their primary effects or complications; these include haemorrhage (associated with local trauma, torsion, inflammation, or ulceration), anaemia (due to chronic subclinical haemorrhage), and mechanical effects (obstruction or intussusception). Some of the common and important examples of polyps are described below.

Ear, nose and throat polyps

Aural polyps (non-neoplastic inflammatory) are a common complication of chronic inflammation in the middle ear, and consist of exuberant granulation tissue (capillary hyperplasia).

Nasal polyps (inflammatory) are very common and also result from chronic infective or allergic inflammation and consist of oedematous masses of connective tissue, with inflammatory cells and some incorporated glands.

Laryngeal polyps, also called laryngeal nodules (non-neoplastic; inflammatory/mechanical), also consist of oedematous connective tissue and deposits of fibrinoid (fibrin-like) material, beneath squamous epithelium — these are caused by vocal abuse, compounded by inflammation and, probably, by smoking).

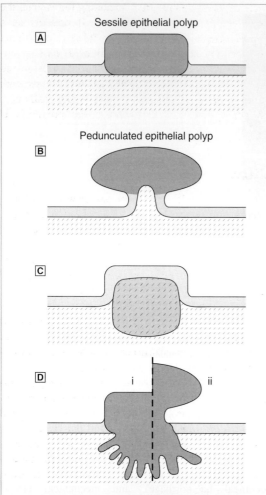

Sessile epithelial polyp

A

Pedunculated epithelial polyp

B

C

D   i   ii

Fig. 4.23   Types of polypoid lesions in the large bowel.
A A sessile epithelial polyp is flat, with no stalk. Examples: a metaplastic polyp, adenomatous polyp (adenoma). **B** A pedunculated epithelial polyp has a stalk (containing blood vessels and connective tissue; not shown). Example: adenomatous polyp (adenoma). **C** A sessile polyp due to a lesion arising in the mesenchymal subepithelial tissues. This could be a benign mesenchymal neoplasm such as a leiomyoma, derived from smooth muscle of bowel wall, or a malignant neoplasm such as lymphoma (lymphomatous polyp, derived from B lymphocytes). **D** A polypoid malignant epithelial neoplasm (adenocarcinoma) may look like (i) a sessile polyp (left), resembling **A** (above), or (ii) a pedunculated polyp (right), resembling **B** (above). The lesion may be only superficially invasive (e.g. invading the stalk of a pedunculated lesion) or deeply invasive (as shown).

Oral polyps

Oral polyps, arising from minor trauma to the oral (mouth, particularly gingival) mucosa, may cause an excessive repair reaction in some individuals. This produces an *epulis,* a fibrovascular polyp (non-neoplastic; regenerative/hyperplastic), with recognised 'congenital' and 'giant cell' variants. Similar vascular polyps are also associated with pregnancy.

Gastrointestinal polyps

The large bowel is by far the most common site of gastrointestinal polyps, followed by the stomach, whilst polyps of the small intestine are rare. The large bowel and stomach have a range of epithelial and non-epithelial, non-neoplastic and neoplastic polyps, involving a range of pathological processes. These include the following.

Inflammatory polyps (non-neoplastic) of the large bowel are seen in the context of inflammatory bowel disease, often with exuberant granulation or fibrovascular tissue. Note that 'pseudopolyps' are polypoid areas of surviving large bowel mucosa surrounded by deep ulcers, also seen in the context of inflammatory bowel disease.

Regenerative/hyperplastic/metaplastic polyps. (epithelial; non-neoplastic) are seen with *Helicobacter pylori*-associated gastritis in the stomach, although their pathogenesis is unknown elsewhere in the large bowel. These polyps are usually sessile, with elongated crypts, and no dysplasia. They have no malignant potential.

Hamartomatous polyps may be solitary as in *juvenile polyps,* or multiple (polyposis, as in *Peutz–Jeghers syndrome,* where they are associated with lip pigmentation), and may occur throughout the alimentary tract. These polyps are adenomyomas (consisting of epithelial and smooth muscle elements). They have no malignant potential.

Heterotopic polyps (epithelial non-neoplastic) are rare, and exemplified by a solitary stomach polyp containing heterotopic mature pancreatic tissue.

Adenoma/adenomatous polyps (epithelial; neoplastic, with varying degrees of dysplasia) are the most important of the polyps of the large bowel and stomach. Large bowel adenomas are very common (20% of 60 year olds have adenomas). They may be sessile or pedunculated; 75% are tubular, 10% are villous, and the remaining 15% have intermediate histology. Most adenomas of the large bowel and stomach progress with time through increasing severity of dysplasia to malignancy (adenocarcinoma), eventually with invasion and metastasis.

In *familial adenomatous polyposis* (transmitted as a Mendelian dominant condition), adenomas (mainly of the large bowel, but also of the small bowel) develop during the second and third decades, and undergo malignant change by the age of 35 years.

Polypoid malignant epithelial neoplasms are mostly adenocarcinomas of the stomach and large bowel which have developed from adenomatous polyps. Rarely, polypoid squamous carcinomas may occur in the oesophagus. Malignant neuroendocrine neoplasms (carcinoids) may also be polypoid.

Mesenchymal polyps (mesenchymal; neoplastic) are common; the benign forms include fibromas, haemangiomas, lipomas and lymphangiomas. Smooth muscle neoplasms are less likely to be polypoid, and they have an uncertain malignant potential.

Malignant non-epithelial polyps (neoplastic) are rare, and include sarcomas (equivalent to their benign mesenchymal counterparts) and malignant lymphomas (lymphomatous polyps).

Genitourinary polyps

Endometrial polyps (epithelial, non-neoplastic) are hyperplastic/metaplastic lesions occurring in the uterus of perimenopausal women, caused by an inappropriate response of the endometrium to oestrogenic stimuli. They consist of variably sized and often cystic glands (which may have metaplastic changes) within a cellular stroma containing thick-walled blood vessels. Malignant change is rare.

Cervical/endocervical polyps (epithelial, non-neoplastic) are common and consist of columnar mucus-secreting epithelium within oedematous stroma. They have no malignant potential.

Benign vaginal polyps (epithelial and mesenchymal, non-neoplastic) occur in adult women (around 40% are seen in pregnancy or hormone therapy) and consist of oedematous stromal tissue containing spindle-shaped (and often bizarre) cells covered by squamous epithelium. These benign hyperplastic lesions of adults may be mistaken histologically for the malignant botryoid rhabdomyosarcoma seen in infants (see below).

Botryoid rhabdomyosarcoma is an important (but rare) polypoid, highly malignant neoplasm of striated muscle of the urogenital tract, including the vagina, the uterine cervix and urinary bladder. It presents as a polypoid, grape-like (botryoid) in infants (occasional cases occur in adults), and consists of a mass of undifferentiated rounded or spindle-shaped cells mixed with larger, more differentiated rhabdomyoblasts with distinctive cross-striations. Although highly malignant, with appropriate modern treatment the prognosis is excellent.

NEOPLASIA

The word 'neoplasia' literally means 'new growth', and the lesion so produced is termed a *neoplasm*. A neoplasm is an abnormal tissue mass, the excessive growth of which is uncoordinated with that of normal tissues, and which persists after the removal of the neoplasm-inducing stimulus. The term *tumour* is often used to denote a neoplasm.

This chapter has so far only considered examples of alterations in growth and differentiation as a response to genetically programmed stimuli required in organ or embryonic development, or as a response to alterations in the environment or workload of a cell or tissue. Growth and differentiation, when appropriately controlled, are beneficial, allowing the body to respond flexibly to various environmental stimuli. In contrast, however, neoplasms result from uncontrolled growth and often disordered differentiation, which is excessive and purposeless. The growth of neoplasms continues in an autonomous manner, in the absence of normal physiological stimuli and without normal negative feedback mechanisms to arrest the cellular proliferation.

Numerous factors have been implicated in the development of human tumours, and these are discussed in detail in Chapter 5. It should be noted, however, that there are multiple steps in the development of neoplasms, and that many of these involve subversion of the normally controlled mechanisms of growth and cellular differentiation, e.g. hormones, growth factors and growth-factor-like proteins such as some of the oncoproteins.

5

Neoplasia

David E Hughes

A neoplasm ('new growth') is a lesion that results from abnormal growth of a tissue, which is partly or completely autonomous of normal growth controls and persists after the initiating stimulus has been removed.

Neoplasms usually manifest themselves as tumours (abnormal swellings). However, some neoplasms, most notably those derived from haemopoeitic cells do not form tumours, and clinically tumourous lesions can be caused by non-neoplastic disease (e.g. tuberculosis).

This chapter will describe how neoplasms form, how they are classified and how they behave.

CARCINOGENESIS

Carcinogenesis is the process by which normal cells are converted into cells capable of forming neoplasms. There is no single cause of neoplasia, and it is generally accepted that most neoplasms require several events to occur in a single cell (the multistep hypothesis) before a sustainable neoplasm can form. This accounts for the relative rarity of neoplasms when compared with the number of cells in the body, all of which, theoretically, have the potential to form neoplasms.

Another factor that protects most cells from neoplasia is that, in order to form a neoplasm, a cell must divide. Thus cells which are postmitotic, such as nerve cells and skeletal muscle cells, rarely form neoplasms, whereas cells such as the epithelium of the gut and the epidermis of the skin, which continually divide, form neoplasms more frequently.

This section will describe the factors that predispose to the formation of neoplasms. Some examples of carcinogens are given in Table 5.1.

CARCINOGENS

Carcinogens are agents which cause the formation of neoplasms from cells exposed to them. The nature of carcino-

Table 5.1 Examples of carcinogens

Carcinogen	Neoplasm caused
Chemical:	
3,4-benzpyrene (tobacco derivative)	Bronchogenic carcinoma
β-naphthylamine	Carcinoma of the bladder
Radiation:	
Ultraviolet light	Skin neoplasms
Ionising radiation	Leukaemia
Viruses:	
Human papilloma virus	Carcinoma of the cervix
Hepatitis B virus	Carcinoma of the liver
Others:	
Asbestos fibres	Mesothelioma
Aspergillus flavus aflatoxin	Carcinoma of the liver
Schistosoma	Carcinoma of the bladder

gens is diverse, but they all have the ability, directly or indirectly, to cause an inheritable change in the genes that control the growth and survival of the target cell.

Many carcinogens are now well known to the public as well as the medical profession: for example, tobacco smoke and asbestos. These have largely been identified by studies of the epidemiology of the neoplasms that they cause. Individual carcinogens can often cause neoplasms in more than one target tissue (e.g. tobacco derivatives can cause neoplasms of bronchial, laryngeal and bladder epithelium), and individual types of neoplasm can be caused by more than one carcinogen (e.g. bronchogenic carcinoma can be caused by tobacco derivatives, asbestos, nickel, or radon gas). However, for many types of neoplasm, the carcinogenic stimulus is not known.

Chemical

A variety of chemicals have been identified as carcinogens in man, and others are suspected to be on the basis of their carcinogenic effects in experimental animals.

There is no common structural link between the different types of chemical carcinogen, but they appear to have in common the ability to modify the structure of DNA: for example, by forming adducts or by adding alkyl groups.

Many chemical carcinogens are procarcinogens which require metabolic conversion to their active form by enzymes. If the enzyme required is present in all cell types, the carcinogenic effect is likely to occur at the site of exposure. However, some carcinogens require metabolism in another tissue, which influences where they exert their carcinogenic effects. This is well illustrated by the aromatic amine β-naphthylamine, which requires metabolism by the liver before being active, and as a result causes neoplasms of the bladder where it is concentrated during excretion.

The major classes of chemical carcinogens currently known are as follows.

Polycyclic aromatic hydrocarbons
The first example of an occupation-related neoplasm was the description by Percival Pott in 1777 of scrotal carcinomas in adults who had been employed as chimney sweeps during childhood. It has subsequently been shown that this was due to exposure to polycyclic aromatic hydrocarbons. This class of compounds was found to be the carcinogenic component of tar, which can cause skin neoplasms if applied experimentally to the skin of rabbits, and was probably responsible for the high incidence of skin cancers in oil shale miners in West Lothian in Scotland during the nineteenth century. Of greater importance today is the carcinogenic effect of polycyclic aromatic hydrocarbons present in tobacco smoke, most notably 3,4-benzpyrene. Polycyclic aromatic hydrocarbons are procarcinogens which require the action of hydroxylating enzymes such as aryl carbohydrate hydroxylase to become active carcinogens. These enzymes are ubiquitous, so polycyclic aromatic hydrocarbons can be carcinogenic at their site of contact, but as they can be absorbed into the blood stream, they are also carcinogenic at distant sites such as the kidney and bladder. This accounts for the fact that, although smoking tobacco is most strongly associated with carcinogenesis in tissues directly exposed such as the bronchus and larynx, smokers have a slightly increased risk of neoplasia in many other tissues.

Aromatic amines
Epidemiological studies have shown an increased risk of bladder neoplasms in workers in the rubber industry. This has been found to be due to the aromatic amine, β-naphthylamine, which is converted into the active carcinogen 1-hydroxy-2-naphthylamine in the liver. Glucu-

ronidation of this compound occurs in the liver, protecting the cells of the liver and other tissues from its carcinogenic effects. However, in the urinary tract, glucuronidase unconjugates the molecule, thus exposing the bladder urothelium to its carcinogenic effects.

Alkylating agents
The polycyclic aromatic hydrocarbons can act by alkylating DNA, so one would expect that the alkylating agents such as cyclophosphamide that are used as chemotherapeutic agents might also be carcinogenic. While this risk is not sufficiently strong to contraindicate their use, there is certainly evidence that patients treated with these compounds for conditions such as Hodgkin's disease have an increased risk of developing a different type of neoplasm later in life.

Azo dyes
These are an example of a class of compounds where recognition of their carcinogenic activity in laboratory studies has fortunately restricted their industrial use. For example, the dye dimethylaminoazobenzene causes liver cancer in rats.

Nitrosamines
This is another class of compounds that are strongly carcinogenic in laboratory animals. It is not known to what extent they are carcingenic in humans, but it is possible that generation of nitrosamines by fungi in poorly stored food could be responsible for some gastrointestinal neoplasms.

Radiation
Electromagnetic radiation of wavelengths shorter than the visible spectrum can cause damage to DNA that can result in neoplasia. Ultraviolet light is a signficant carcinogen because of the high levels of exposure that can occur during daily life, whereas ionising radiation (such as x-rays and gamma-rays) is significantly carcinogenic because of the ligh levels of energy it possesses.

Ultraviolet light
The relationship between exposure to ultraviolet light and skin neoplasms is now well established. Neoplasms of the epidermis (basal cell carcinoma and squamous cell carcinoma), and the related precancerous condition solar/ actinic keratosis, usually occur on sun-exposed sites and become more frequent with greater sun exposure. Similarly, malignant melanoma, a malignant neoplasm of melanocytes, is most common in fair-skinned individuals living in environments with high levels of sunlight exposure, such as white Australians. Malignant melanoma is uncommon in individuals of Afro-Carribean origin

because the greater density of melanin in their skin reduces the amount of ultraviolet light that reaches the melanocytes, which reside along the basal (deepest) layer of the epidermis.

Ionising radiation

The first indication of the carcinogenic potential of ionising radiation came from the frequency with which early x-ray workers developed skin cancers on their hands. Further evidence subsequently accumulated from the development of neoplasms, particularly leukaemia, in the survivors of the World War II atomic bombs. Ionising radiation can cause neoplasms in a wide variety of tissues: for example, therapeutic irradiation can result in the development of bone and soft tissue sarcomas, and the Chernobyl disaster has caused a large increase in thyroid cancers in the Ukraine because of the release of radioactive iodine which resulted; this element is of course concentrated and stored in the thyroid gland. One of the great dangers of radioactive substances is, depending on their half-life, the persistence of their effect within the body. A good example of this is the persistence of the thorium dioxide from the radiological agent thorotrast within the liver. This has caused the development of hepatic angiosarcomas in some patients many years after exposure.

Viruses

A growing number of viruses have been implicated in the developement of neoplasms. There are many examples of virally induced neoplasms in animals, study of which has done much to promote our understanding of the molecular genetics of neoplasia. Virally induced neoplasms in humans are (as far as we are aware) rather less common. The most ubiquitous oncogenic viruses are the human papilloma viruses; other viruses with well-established carcinogenic effects are the Epstein–Barr virus and the hepatitis B virus (see Table 5.2).

Table 5.2 Oncogenic viruses	
Virus	Neoplasm caused
Human papilloma virus	Common viral wart Carcinoma of the cervix
Epstein–Barr virus	Burkitt's lymphoma Nasopharyngeal carcinoma
Hepatitis B virus	Hepatocellular carcinoma
HTLV-1	T cell lymphoma/leukaemia

Mechanisms of viral carcinogenesis

DNA viruses can be carcinogenic either through integration into the host genome in such a way that interferes with the function of growth-controlling genes, or through their ability to produce proteins that interfere with growth-regulating factors. For example, human papilloma viruses produce proteins that inhibit the function of the p53 and Rb1 gene products (see section on genetics). The best-known examples of oncogenic DNA viruses are the Epstein–Barr virus, which is strongly associated with Burkitt's lymphoma and nasopharyngeal carcinoma, the hepatitis B virus, which is associated with hepatocellular (liver) carcinoma, and the human papilloma virus (HPV). HPV is associated with neoplasia of a number of different surface epithelia. It is responsible for the common viral wart of the skin and is also associated with carcinoma of the cervix, its precursor condition cervical intraepithelial neoplasia (CIN), and the analogous anal intraepithelial neoplasia (AIN). There are many different types of HPV. Individual types have preferred target tissues and have differing oncogenic potential. For example, many different HPV types infect the cervix, but only a small number of types (particularly types 16 and 18) are associated with the development of cervical carcinoma.

Oncogenic RNA viruses are retroviruses which integrate their genetic material into the host genome using the enzme reverse transcriptase. Although there are many examples of oncogenic retroviruses causing neoplasms in animals, this is rare in man. The best-known examples are Human T-Lymphotrophic Virus-1 (HTLV-1) which causes a form of lymphoma/leukaemia which is endemic in Japan and the Caribbean, and the Human Immunodeficiency Virus (HIV). However, HIV probably does not have a direct carcinogenic effect; the neoplasms that are associated with HIV infection probably arise as a consequence of immunosuppression and may actually be caused by other types of virus. Thus, HIV infection may act as a cofactor for oncogenesis by other viruses. There are other examples of this phenomenon, such as the Epstein–Barr virus requiring malaria infection as a cofactor in the development of Burkitt's lymphoma.

Other associations between viruses and neoplasms are being described — for example, herpesvirus 8 and myeloma — and it seems likely that further causative associations will be established in the future, particularly in neoplasms of the lymphoreticular system. The sequence of events by which viruses can cause neoplasia is outlined in Figure 5.1.

Other non-biological factors

Asbestos

The association between asbestos and malignant meso-

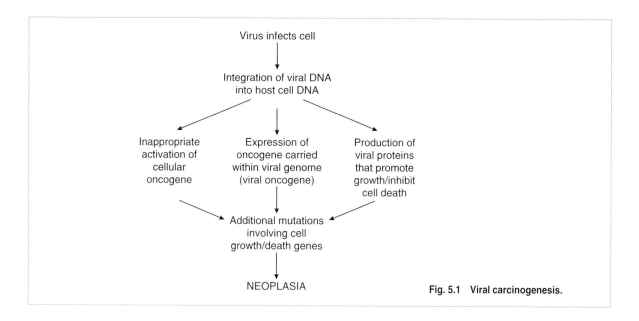

Fig. 5.1 Viral carcinogenesis.

thelioma (a neoplasm of the pleural, pericardial, or peritoneal mesothelial lining) is so strong that this disease is almost unknown in individuals who have not been exposed to asbestos. Asbestos was a widely used building material because of its fire resistance, before the health risks of asbestos exposure were known. As a result of this, the incidence of mesothelioma continues to rise despite the restrictions now placed on the use of asbestos. There is also a strong link between asbestos exposure and carcinoma of the bronchus. The mechanism responsible for the carcinogenic effect of asbestos is not known.

Metals
Industrial exposure to nickel is associated with an increased risk of nasal and bronchogenic carcinoma. In the setting of haemochromatosis, iron could be said to be an indirect carcinogen in the liver; however, the development of cirrhosis is required before the increased risk of hepatocellular carcinoma in this condition can be realised.

Betel nut
In some parts of Asia, betel nut chewing substitutes for tobacco smoking as the preferred local vice. It has similar hazards, as it is associated with an increased risk of the development of neoplasms of the oral cavity.

Other biological factors

Helicobacter pylori *infestation*
Helicobacter pylori infestation is a common cause of gastritis and peptic ulceration. Chronic *Helicobacter*

pylori gastritis sometimes leads to intestinal metaplasia of the gastric mucosa. This results in the normal secretory epithelium of the gastric antrum being replaced by an epithelium with intestinal characteristics. Sometimes this epithelium is well differentiated with a mixture of absorptive and goblet cells identical to those seen in the small intestine. In other cases the epithelium is less well differentiated, being identifiable as intestinal rather than gastric by the type of mucin that it produces. In the latter case, there is a small risk of the development of dysplasia (see below, under 'premalignant conditions') and ultimately gastric carcinoma. However, the association between *Helicobacter pylori* infestation and gastric carcinoma appears to be weak and presumably requires multiple cofactors. Nonetheless, this causative link has recently been confirmed in experimental animals infected with *H. pylori*.

There is a more direct link between Helicobacter infestation and a far less common neoplasm of the stomach, the so-called MALT (mucosa-associated lymphoid tissue) lymphoma. It has been shown that, despite having characteristics of a malignant neoplasm, such as clonality and invasiveness, MALT lymphomas sometimes regress when patients are treated with Helicobacter-eradicating antibiotics. However, it is more likely that Helicobacter infestation represents a growth-sustaining stimulus, rather than a conventional carcinogen. These observations have led to some debate about whether MALT lymphomas are true neoplasms or not.

Parasitic infestations

Schistosomiasis is associated with an increased risk of carcinoma of the bladder. Interestingly, Schistosomiasis-associated bladder carcinomas are squamous carcinomas, rather than transitional cell carcinomas which are the usual type of malignant neoplasm of the bladder. *Clonorchis sinensis,* the Chinese liver fluke, is also capable of inducing neoplasia of the bile ducts in which it dwells.

Hormones

Some neoplasms such as carcinomas of the breast and prostate may require the presence of hormones to maintain or promote their growth, as will be discussed below. There are also examples of abnormal exposure to some hormones being carcinogenic. For example, anabolic and androgenic steroids can cause the development of hepatocellular carcinoma, and oestrogens are associated with hepatocellular adenomas. Certain rare tumours of the female genital tract, such as clear cell carcinoma of the vagina, are very strongly associated with in-utero exposure to diethylstilboestrol, which was used therapeutically during pregnancy in the past.

Mycotoxins

It is likely that there are many toxins produced by fungi that are carcinogenic. To date the best-established carcinogenic effect is that of the aflatoxins produced by *Aspergillus flavus.* These toxins occur as dietary contaminants and are linked to the high incidence of hepatocellular carcinoma in some parts of central Africa.

HOST FACTORS

Age

Neoplastic disease is primarily a disease of old age. Although neoplasms can occur at any age, even in utero, neoplasms of almost all types become far more common after the age of 50. This reflects the cumulative effects of exposure to carcinogens over an individual's lifespan. A major reason for the continuing increase in the incidence of neoplastic disease is the increasing life expectancy of most populations.

Individual types of neoplasm have their own typical age distribution. For example, fibroadenoma of the breast usually occurs in women in their second, third and fourth decades, whereas carcinoma of the breast becomes more common after the menopause. Other types of neoplasm, for example neuroblastoma of the adrenal, are restricted to children and are almost unknown in adults.

It is a general rule that familial neoplasms — that is, those occurring in individuals who have a genetic predisposition to them (see below under genetic factors) — occur at a younger age than sporadic neoplasms.

Race

Different races are subject to different profiles of neoplastic disease. This is almost entirely due to differences in lifestyle. For example, the commonest fatal neoplasm in the United Kingdom and the United States of America is carcinoma of the bronchus, which is caused largely by tobacco smoking. The commonest fatal neoplasm worldwide is hepatocellular carcinoma, which in Africa and South-East Asia is related to exposure to dietary carcinogens and viral hepatitis. Immigrant groups tend to eventually assume the disease profile of their adopted countries. There are, however, occasional examples of genetically determined racial differences, such as a high frequency of familial breast cancer in Askanazy jews.

Endocrine status

Gender influences the risk of developing many types of neoplasm. This is generally related to differences in hormonal status, although lifestyle differences can play a part. For example, the far higher incidence of neoplasms of the breast in females than males is probably mainly due to endocrine influences, whereas, in the past, bronchogenic carcinoma was more common in men than women because of differences in the frequency of tobacco smoking between the sexes. There are, however, many examples where the influence of gender is not understood: for example, the higher frequency of osteosarcoma in males.

Diet

The risks of developing neoplasia as a result of dietary contaminants are well illustrated by the example of aflatoxin-induced hepatocellular carcinoma. Other dietary factors may also modify the risk of developing certain neoplasms: for example, a diet low in fibre is thought to increase the risk of colorectal carcinoma, and there is a link between high levels of dietary fat and breast carcinoma.

Genetic factors

Changes in the structure and function of a cell's genetic material are central to the development of neoplasia, and more than one such change is required in an individual cell before neoplasia can occur. If all of an individual's cells already have an abnormality in a relevant gene as a result of that individual's inherited genetic make-up (a germ-line mutation), then fewer subsequent changes are required for neoplasia to occur. This is well illustrated by the rare familial retinoblastoma syndrome (Fig. 5.2). If both alleles of the retinoblastoma (Rb1) gene in an indi-

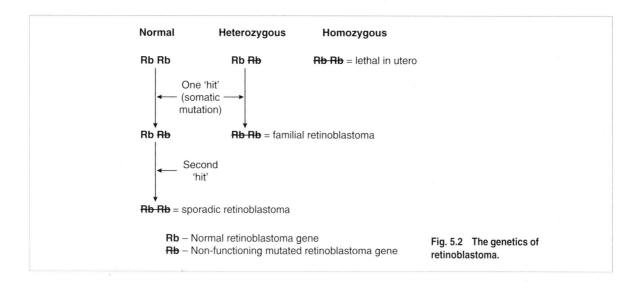

Normal   Heterozygous   Homozygous

Rb Rb   Rb R̶b̶   R̶b̶ R̶b̶ = lethal in utero

One 'hit'
(somatic
mutation)

Rb R̶b̶   R̶b̶ R̶b̶ = familial retinoblastoma

Second
'hit'

R̶b̶ R̶b̶ = sporadic retinoblastoma

Rb – Normal retinoblastoma gene
R̶b̶ – Non-functioning mutated retinoblastoma gene

Fig. 5.2 The genetics of retinoblastoma.

vidual retinal cell are non-functional, retinoblastoma can develop from that cell. Sporadic retinoblastoma is a rare tumour because it is unusual for both retinoblastoma alleles in an individual cell to acquire mutations that inhibit their function. However, if one allele is already non-functional because it was inherited in a defective form, then the chances of retinoblastoma developing as a result of a subsequent mutation of the other allele are very high. This also demonstrates that the 'retinoblastoma' gene is a tumour suppressor gene. This is a common property of the genes that are abnormal in the various familial cancer syndromes.

Another characteristic that the retinoblastoma syndrome shows what is common in familial cancer syndromes is that it affects more than one tissue. If individuals with the retinoblastoma syndrome survive the development of retinoblastomas (which are usually bilateral) early in childhood, they have a very high incidence of osteosarcoma during adolescence. The retinoblastoma syndrome is used here as an illustration because its genetics are simple and well characterised. However, there are a number of other familial cancer syndromes, many of which, such as familial polyposis coli, are more common. The best known examples are given in Table 5.3.

Immune response

Some neoplasms attract large numbers of inflammatory cells, usually lymphocytes, into their substance, and there is evidence that in some tumours this may convey a better prognosis. These observations have led to the development of the major research subspecialty of tumour immunology, but, at present, treating neoplasms by stimulating the host immune response is little more than a theoretical concept.

Table 5.3 Examples of familial cancer syndromes		
Syndrome	Gene affected	Resultant neoplasms
Li Fraumeni	p53	Breast, ovarian carcinomas, astrocytomas, sarcomas
Retinoblastoma	Rb1	Retinoblastoma, osteosarcoma
Familial polyposis coli	APC	GI tract carcinomas, mainly colon
von Hippel–Lindau	VHL	Renal carcinoma, phaeochromocytoma, haemangioblastoma
Multiple endocrine neoplasia syndromes (I–III)	RET, others	Tumours of pituitary parathyroids, thyroid, pancreas, adrenal (combination depends on which syndrome)
Familial breast cancer	BRCA 1, BRCA 2	Breast, ovarian syndrome prostatic carcinomas

However, evidence has been put forward that the immune system can detect and mount a response against neoplasms, principally via natural killer cells. The activity of these cells can be stimulated by lymphokines such as interleukin 2, and there is some evidence that factors like interleukin 2 could have therapeutic efficacy against some neoplasms. A more convincing example of an immunological treatment that can suppress the development of a neoplasm is the effect of BCG treatment on carcinoma-in-situ of the bladder.

The host immune response has another important indirect effect on the development of neoplasms. There is a strong positive link between immunodeficiency and the development of neoplasia. This is illustrated by the frequency of development of lymphomas and Kaposi's sarcoma in the Acquired Immune Deficiency Syndrome (AIDS), and cutaneous and anogenital squamous carcinomas in organ transplant recipients taking immunosuppressive therapy. In these settings the increased risk of neoplasia seems to be due to an inadequate immune response to oncogenic viruses.

PREMALIGNANT DISEASE

Given that malignant neoplasms usually develop as the result of multiple steps over a period of time, it is perhaps not surprising that many premalignant diseases have been described. Premalignant lesions are discrete identifiable lesions that may progress to become malignant neoplasms. These can be:

- benign neoplasms that can become malignant
- dysplasia/in-situ malignancy.

Premalignant conditions are non-neoplastic conditions that frequently lead to the development of neoplasms.

(The distinction between benign and malignant neoplasms will be defined below. The term dysplasia was defined in the previous chapter.)

Malignant change in benign neoplasms

The majority of benign neoplasms do not alter in any way, but some benign neoplasms have the ability to progress to become malignant neoplasms. Probably the best-characterised example of this phenomenon is the adenoma–carcinoma sequence in the colon. Adenomatous polyps of the colon are more numerous than colonic carcinomas, but all adenomatous polyps have the potential to develop into carcinomas, and many (but not all) carcinomas originate from adenomatous polyps. The polyps most likely to undergo malignant change show the greatest degree of histological dysplasia, and a sequence

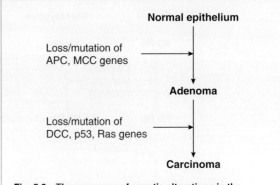

Fig. 5.3 The sequence of genetic alterations in the colorectal adenoma–carcinoma sequence. APC = adenomatous polyposis coli gene; MCC = mutated in colon cancer gene; DCC = deleted in colon cancer gene; Ras = a cellular oncogene involved in growth factors signal transduction; p53 = a tumour suppressor gene.

of genetic changes that leads to the development of colorectal carcinoma from normal epithelium via adenomatous polyps has now been described (Fig. 5.3).

Metaplasia–dysplasia sequence

Neoplastic transformation of cells occurs in cells undergoing proliferation, and is particularly likely to occur if the cells are also undergoing metaplasia (defined and described in the previous chapter). Neoplastic transformation of metaplastic epithelium usually follows a predictable and histologically identifiable sequence of low grade dysplasia progressing to high grade dysplasia / in-situ malignancy to invasive malignacy as additional genetic abnormalities are acquired in the neoplastic population. This progression is very well demonstrated in the cervix (Fig. 5.4). Other examples of the metaplasia–dysplasia sequence are shown in Table 5.4.

Premalignant conditions

These are usually conditions characterised by high cell turnover over a sustained period of time, usually resulting from a destructive form of chronic inflammation. Congenital abnormalities can also be premalignant conditions: for example, maldescent of the testis is associated with an increased risk of testicular neoplasia in later life. Some examples of premalignant conditions are given in Table 5.5.

CARCINOGENIC PROCESS

The carcinogenic process is the chain of events whereby

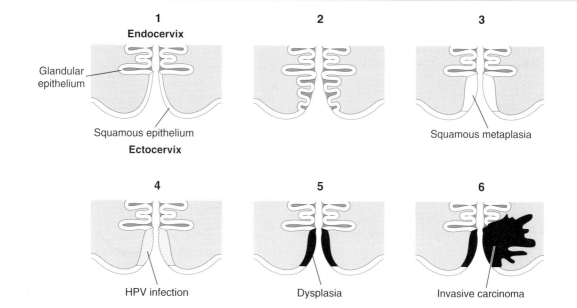

Fig. 5.4   The metaplasia–dysplasia–carcinoma sequence in cervical carcinoma. (1) In the prepubertal cervix there are stable squamous and glandular epithelia covering the ectocervix and the endocervical canal, respectively. (2) At puberty the rapid growth of the uterus causes the glandular epithelium to be drawn out onto the ectocervical surface. (3) The externalised glandular epithelium then undergoes squamous metaplasia. (4) This relatively unstable immature metaplastic epithelium is vulnerable to infection by human papilloma virus (HPV). (5) In some cases this leads to genetic changes that result in dysplasia within the squamous epithelium. (6) Ultimately, with additional genetic changes, this can lead to the development of invasive carcinoma.

Table 5.4 Examples of the metaplasia–dysplasia sequence		
Organ	Form of metaplasia undergoing dysplasia	Resulting malignancy
Oesophagus	Barrett's oesophagus (intestinal metaplasia)	Oesphageal adenocarcinoma
Stomach	Intestinal metaplasia (associated with achlorhydria)	Gastric adenocarcinoma
Bronchus	Squamous metaplasia	Brochogenic squamous carcinoma
Cervix	Squamous metaplasia	Cervical squamous carcinoma

Table 5.5 Examples of premalignant conditions	
Premalignant condition	Resulting neoplasm
Ulcerative colitis	Colorectal carcinoma
Chronic fistulae	Squamous carcinoma
Epithelial hyperplasia of the breast	Breast carcinoma
Paget's disease of bone	Osteosarcoma
Xeroderma pigmentosum	Skin malignancies

a carcinogenic stimulus leads to the formation of a neoplasm. The principal steps in this process are as follows:

1. exposure of cell/tissue to carcinogen (*initiation*)
2. alterations to genes controlling cell growth and/or survival (*promotion*)
3. irreversible change of growth control (*persistence*)
4. formation of neoplasm.

These four steps occur with decreasing frequency: exposure of cells to carcinogens is a very common event, and genetic alterations to growth-controlling genes probably occur quite frequently, but, because of inbuilt defence mechanisms, the latter two steps are relatively uncommon.

The division of the carcinogenic process into the stages of initation, promotion and persistence is based upon experimental evidence from models of tumour formation in which initiating and promoting stimuli are required. However, our increasing understanding of the molecular genetics of this process indicates that the stages described above simply reflect the requirements for more than one genetic change to occur before neoplasia becomes established.

The precise chains of molecular events in most tumour types have yet to be established.

GENETICS

Chromosomal abnormalities

Very crude DNA abnormalities may manifest themselves as visible changes in chromosomes isolated from neoplastic cells. These abnormalities can occur in a number of forms:

- translocations (part of one chromosome becomes attached to another chromosome)
- deletions (part of a chromosome is lost)
- extra chromosomes (usually trisomies – three copies of a chromosome rather than two)
- abnormal configurations such as ring chromosomes
- abnormalities associated with gene amplification, e.g. homogeneously staining regions.

The DNA of many neoplasms, particularly malignant ones, is inherently unstable, and random chromosomal abnormalities are common. However, there are a number of chromosomal abnormalities that are consistently found in certain tumour types, the best known being the 'Philadelphia chromosome' (a reciprocal, balanced translocation between chromosomes 9 and 22). At a purely descriptive level, these can be useful for diagnosis, particularly in groups of tumours in which the cells are morphologically similar, such as leukaemias and the 'small round cell tumours' of childhood such as neuroblastoma and alveolar rhabdomyosarcoma. Detailed molecular study of these chromosomal abnormalities has yielded some insight into the pathogenesis of some of the neoplasms with specific chromosomal abnormalities. A good example of this is the translocation between chromosomes 14 and 18 that occurs in follicular (low grade) B cell non-Hodgkin's lymphomas. This translocation results in the *bcl-2* gene coming under the control of the immunoglobulin heavy chain gene promoter. As B lymphocytes constitutively express their immunoglobin genes, this results in inappropriate overexpression of the *bcl-2* gene and thus overproduction of the bcl-2 protein. As bcl-2 is an anti-apoptotic protein, this results in the 'immortalisation' of the neoplastic B lymphocytes.

Oncogenes and tumour suppressor genes

Advances in molecular genetics have allowed more detailed study of the genes and genetic events associated with neoplasia than studies of chromosome structure allow. Research in this field has led to the discovery of genes which mediate the development of neoplasms. These genes are referred to as *oncogenes*. Another group of genes are negatively associated with neoplasia in that their inactivation promotes tumour formation. These are known as *tumour-suppressor genes* or *anti-oncogenes*.

The discovery of most oncogenes has resulted from study of retrovirally driven neoplasms in animals (such neoplasms are rare in humans). Study of oncogeneic retroviruses such as the Rous sarcoma virus revealed that they carried RNA templates for DNA sequences that caused transformation of normal cells. It was subsequently found that these viral oncogenes all had closely-related counterparts in the human genome (*proto-oncogenes*). It seems that retroviruses have the ability to 'hijack' these genes and incorporate them into their own genetic material. Study of the tumour-promoting genes in human neoplasms reveals that when they can be identified, they are usually proto-oncogenes with a known viral oncogene equivalent, although there are some proto-oncogenes that have not yet been found to be utilised by retroviruses.

Study of the nature of proto-oncogenes has revealed, perhaps not surprisingly, that they are all genes whose products are involved in the control of cell growth. The products of proto-oncogenes may be growth factors, growth factor receptors, proteins involved in transduction of signals through the cell membrane and cytoplasm following binding of growth factors to their receptors, or nuclear transcription factors. Examples of each class are given in Table 5.6.

Proto-oncogenes are therefore expressed in normal growing cells in a controlled manner. In neoplastic cells this control of their expression is lost. This can be due to activation by:

- mutation
- chromosomal translocation
- amplification.

Mutations affecting oncogenes are usually point mutations that occur at positions in the gene sequence that affect the regulation of production of the protein encoded by the gene, but not altering the structure of the active site of the protein. Chromosomal translocations can result in proto-oncogenes being realigned next to inappropriate promoter sequences. For example, in Burkitt's lymphoma, the *c-myc* proto-oncogene comes under the control of the immunoglobulin gene promoter, resulting in

Table 5.6	Examples of oncogenes
Oncogene	Type of protein produced
Growth factors and their receptors	
sis	Platelet-derived growth factor
erb-B	Epidermal growth factor receptor
fms	Macrophage colony-stimulating factor receptor
Signal transduction molecules (G-proteins, tyrosine kinases, etc.)	
ras	G-protein
src	Tyrosine kinase
abl	Tyrosine kinase
Transcription factors	
myc	Nuclear binding protein
fos	Transcription factor

uncontrolled growth of a population of B lymphocytes. When a gene is amplified, multiple copies of that gene are present within the genome, resulting in uncontrolled overproduction of the protein encoded by the gene.

Certain genes appear to have a 'protective' function, inhibiting or preventing the development of neoplasia. The best-known example of this class is *p53*. The product of this gene has the ability to direct cells with damaged DNA into apoptosis. If the *p53* gene is non-functional, DNA damage can accumulate within a cell, increasing the chances of the development of neoplasia. Mutations of *p53* are extremely common in malignant neoplasms, being detectable in up to half of all common epithelial malignancies.

TUMOURS — BENIGN AND MALIGNANT

CLASSIFICATION

Neoplastic disease can affect any organ or tissue, and each organ or tissue can give rise to a variety of neoplasms. This has led to a need to classify neoplastic disease in a way that is universally comprehensible. Broadly speaking, neoplasms are classified according to:

- their behaviour — benign or malignant
- their histogenesis — presumed cell type of origin.

Benign vs malignant

The most important factor that influences the behaviour and therefore the prognosis of a neoplasm is whether it is benign or malignant. Benign and malignant neoplasms tend to differ in a number of ways (Table 5.7 and Fig. 5.5), but the defining distinction is *invasiveness*. Malignant neoplasms invade surrounding tissue, whereas benign neoplasms do not. The invasiveness of malignant neoplasms also confers upon them the ability to *metastasise*. However, not all malignant neoplasms metastasise: for example, basal cell carcinomas of the skin very rarely metastasise, but are regarded as malignant because of their ability to invade the dermis and underlying tissues.

The distinction between benign and malignant is not always black and white, however. Some neoplasms are classified as being 'borderline' or 'of borderline malignancy'. Such neoplasms are usually either benign neoplasms with extensive dysplastic change or very low grade malignant tumours. A good example of this category is provided by borderline ovarian tumours. These tumours can be large and on histology show dysplastic features. However, follow-up studies show that these tumours have a good prognosis, rarely recurring or metastasising. This is perhaps not surprising when one considers that they are distinguished from ovarian carcinomas by the absence of invasiveness of the neoplastic epithelium — the defining feature of malignancy.

The rules of any classification are naturally subject to modification by their use in clinical practice, so not all terms commonly used to classify neoplasms correspond

Table 5.7	Characteristics of benign and malignant neoplasms	
Benign	Malignant
Non-invasive	Invade surrounding tissues
Do not metastasise	Capable of metastasis
Necrosis rare	Necrosis common
Ulceration rare	Ulceration common
Slowly growing	Rapidly growing
Histologically resemble tissue of origin	Variable resemblance to tissue of origin
Nuclear morphology usually normal	Nuclear morphology usually abnormal
Border usually circumscribed	Border usually irregular

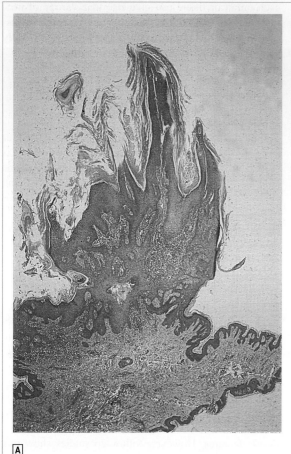

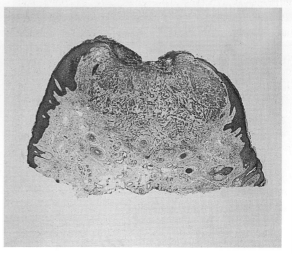

Fig. 5.5 Comparison of morphology of benign and malignant neoplasms. [A] shows a low power photomicrograph of a haematoxylin and eosin-stained histological section of a viral wart. [B] shows a similarly prepared histological section of a cutaneous invasive carcinoma at the same magnification. These therefore represent benign and malignant neoplasms arising in the same tissue and derived from the same cell type. The wart is exophytic, non-invasive and retains some elements of the normal organisation of the epidermis, for example formation of a distinct granular layer. In contrast, the squamous carcinoma has ulcerated the epidermis, invaded the dermis and lost most of its architectural resemblance to normal epidermis.

to the rules outlined above. For example, the term transitional cell carcinoma is often used to describe non-invasive papillary lesions of the urothelium. Theoretically, a more correct term would be 'transitional cell papilloma', which was indeed at one time the accepted term for these lesions. However, because of the tendency of these lesions to relentlessly recur and the lack of any histological hallmarks that distinguish those lesions that ultimately become invasive, they are now all regarded as carcinomas *ab initio*.

Nomenclature

The names given to neoplasms are a synthesis of their histogenesis and behaviour, incorporating the class of cell of origin (epithelial vs mesenchymal etc.), type of differentiation (glandular vs squamous etc.) and whether benign or malignant. All solid tumours have the suffix 'oma', meaning 'growth'. Circulating neoplasms of the haemopoietic and lymphoreticular system are referred to as leukaemias.

Epithelial neoplasms

Benign epithelial neoplasms are referred to as *adenomas* if they consist of glandular (exocrine or endocrine) cells, or *papillomas* if they have a papillary growth pattern — these are usually derived from a surface epithelium. Malignant epithelial neoplasms are referred to as *carcinomas*. This term usually has a prefix which refers to the pattern of growth or differentiation of the tumour, for example *adenocarcinoma* is the term used to describe a malignant epithelial neoplasm showing glandular differentiation. Often, a preceding adjective is used to describe the growth pattern or presumed cell of origin. In these situations the prefix 'adeno' may be dropped in common usage. Examples are papillary and follicular carcinomas of the thyroid (growth pattern) and ductal and lobular carcinomas of the breast (presumed cell of origin). The common macroscopic growth patterns of benign and malignant neoplasms are outlined in Figure 5.6.

Mesenchymal neoplasms

Benign mesenchymal neoplasms are named by combining a prefix describing their constituent cells with the suffix 'oma'. For example, a lipoma is a benign neoplasm of fat, and an angioma is a benign neoplasm of blood vessels. In malignant mesenchymal tumours the suffix becomes *sarcoma*; thus a liposarcoma is a malignant neoplasm of fat, and an angiosarcoma is a malignant neoplasm of blood vessels (or, more strictly speaking, endothelium). A list of terms used for mesenchymal and other neoplasms is given in Table 5.8.

Lymphoreticular neoplasms

All neoplasms derived from lymphocytes are referred to as lymphomas, with the exception of those that circulate, which are referred to as leukaemias (e.g. chronic lympho-

cytic leukaemia, hairy cell leukaemia), and neoplasms of plasma cells, which are termed plasmacytomas or myeloma depending on whether they affect single or multiple sites. The reason for the use of the blanket term 'lymphoma' is that the biology of these neoplasms is complex. Lymphomas are divided into Hodgkin's disease and non-Hodgkin's lymphomas. Hodgkin's lymphomas are defined by the presence of the Reed–Sternberg cell, a morphologically characteristic cell of uncertain origin. Non-Hodgkin's lymphomas exist in a bewildering diversity of forms which have spawned a number of different classifications. Broadly speaking, they can be subdivided into lymphomas of B lymphocytes or T lymphocytes and high grade or low grade lesions, the latter distinction being the most important for management and prognosis.

For practical purposes all lymphomas are regarded as malignant, but some, such as nodular lymphocyte-predominant Hodgkin's disease, have such a good prognosis that there is doubt as to whether they are true neoplasms.

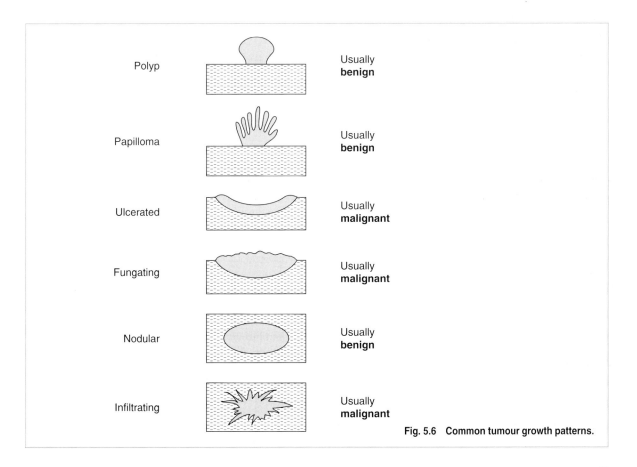

Fig. 5.6   Common tumour growth patterns.

Table 5.8 Common tumour names		
Tissue/cell type	Benign	Malignant
Epithelial		
Glandular	Adenoma	Adenocarcinoma
Squamous	Squamous papilloma	Squmous carcinoma
Mesenchymal		
Fibrous tissue	Fibroma	Fibrosarcoma
Smooth muscle	Leiomyoma	Leiomyosarcoma
Skeletal muscle	Rhabdomyoma	Rhabdomyosarcoma
Vascular	Angioma	Angiosarcoma
Nerve sheath	Neurofibroma	Neurogenic sarcoma
Fat	Lipoma	Liposarcoma
Bone	Osteoma	Osteosarcoma
Cartilage	Chondroma	Chondrosarcoma
Lymphoreticular		
Lymphocytes		Lymphoma
Lymphoid tissue		(Hodgkin's or non-Hodgkin's)
Primitive/embryonal		
Kidney		Nephroblastoma
Autonomic nerve		Neuroblastoma
Cerebellum		Medulloblastoma
Liver		Hepatoblastoma
Others		
Neuroendocrine	See Table 5.9	
Melanocytic	Naevi*	Malignant melanoma
Germ cells	Mature teratoma	Immature teratoma
		Seminoma

*Possibly hamartomas, rather than simple benign neoplasms

Neoplasms of nervous tissue

Mature nerve cells very rarely give rise to any type of neoplasm; however, their precursors can give rise to a variety of tumours such as neuroblastoma and medulloblastoma. These are examples of a variety of neoplasms bearing the suffix *blastoma* which are derived from embryonal cells and occur almost exclusively in children. Examples outside the nervous system include nephroblastoma (Wilm's tumour) of the kidney and hepatoblastoma of the liver. Neuroblastomas occasionally show a remarkable property by maturing from a primitive, poorly differentiated tumour into a benign ganglioneuroma.

The vast majority of tumours occurring in the nervous system are derived from support tissues. In the central nervous system these are most commonly astrocytomas; in the peripheral nervous system they are derived from Schwann cells or nerve sheath fibroblasts.

An important concept that is illustrated by tumours of the central nervous system is the distinction between histological and biological malignancy. A non-invasive cerebral neoplasm acts as a space-occupying lesion and therefore has the potential to kill the patient, although it may do this over a longer period of time than its histologically malignant counterparts.

Neuroendocrine neoplasms

This term referes to neoplasms that either form from cells of the APUD (amine and/or precursor uptake and decarboxylation) diffuse endocrine system which consists of cells such as the islet cells of the pancreas, the calcitonin-secreting C cells of the thyroid, and the endocrine cells of the gut epithelium, or epithelial neoplasms that show evidence of this form of differentiation through the presence of neurosecretory granules within their cytoplasm.

These neoplasms can be benign or malignant, and are characterised by their ability to secrete peptide hormones or vasoactive amines. They usually present with symptoms caused by the substance that they secrete rather than symptoms directly attributable to the tumour itself. The resultant syndromes will be discussed in more detail in the section below on clinical effects. The nomenclature of these neoplasms is variable and somewhat confused. However, it is common practice to refer to tumours secreting an identifiable product as causing a distinct syndrome according to their product, for example *insulinoma* or *gastrinoma*; others are referred to by the generic term *carcinoid*. These tumours are generally benign or of low to intermediate grade malignancy; their highly malignant counterpart is the so-called *small cell carcinoma*. The common examples of neuroendocrine tumours are shown in Table 5.9.

Melanocytic neoplasms

Benign proliferations of melanocytes are extremely common. These are known as melanocytic naevi and are often regarded as hamartomas rather than true neoplasms (this distinction will be explained below). Malignant melanocytic neoplasms are known as *melanomas.* Because this is a rather benign-sounding term, it is common practice to embellish this by referring to them as malignant melanomas (there is no such thing as a benign melanoma in humans, although they may occur in horses).

Germ cell neoplasms

Like other cell types, spermatogonia and oocytes are capable of forming neoplasms. Although germ cells themselves are haploid, the neoplasms that arise from them are generally diploid. In germ cell tumours arising in females, the sex chromosomes are invariably XX, whereas those arising in males can be XX or XY. The capacity of these cells to differentiate down the various embryonic lineages determines how germ cell neoplasms can manifest themselves. They may form neoplasms of essentially undifferentiated germs cells. In males these are referred to as *seminomas,* in females *dysgerminomas.*

Tumours that show differentiation beyond this stage are known as *teratomas* ('monster tumours'). The degree of differentiation of a teratoma is reflected in the maturity of the tissues it forms. The maturity of teratomas dictates their behaviour: mature teratomas are benign, whereas immature teratomas are malignant. In mature cystic teratomas, well-formed squamous epithelium, glandular epithelium, neural tissue and teeth are frequently seen and almost any other tissue can be present. The tissues present in immature teratomas resemble those of the early embryo. Other related tissues such as yolk sac and trophoblast may also be present in immature teratomas.

The majority of germ cell tumours arise in the gonads, but some arise in sites such as the mediastinum and retroperitoneum, reflecting the site of origin and path of migration of the primordial germ cells.

The majority of teratomas in females are mature, in males the majority are immature. Malignant germ cell tumours are far more sensitive to radiotherapy and chemotherapy than, for example, malignant epithelial neoplasms. This has resulted in an excellent prognosis for seminomas and a relatively good prognosis for teratomas, even when metastatic disease is present.

A related group of neoplasms are the gestational trophoblastic tumours which are derived, as their name indicates, from placental trophoblast following a pregnancy. They are very uncommon following normal pregnancies, but are relatively more common following (hydatidiform) molar pregnancies. Like normal trophoblast, the cells of these tumours are well equipped to invade and metastasise, but are fortunately highly sensitive to chemotherapy.

Mixed neoplasms

A number of neoplasms show more than one neoplastic component, most commonly both epithelial and mesenchymal, indicating origin from a cell capable of differentiating down both lineages. This is distinct from the recruitment of non-neoplastic stroma that occurs in

Table 5.9 Examples of neuroendocrine tumours			
Organ/tissue	Name	Product	Clinical manifestation
Pancreatic islet cells	Insulinoma	Insulin	Hypoglycaemia
	Glucagonoma	Glucagon	Hyperglycaemia
	Gastrinoma	Gastrin	Gastric ulceration (Zollinger–Ellison syndrome)
Gut and bronchial neuroendocrine cells	Carcinoid	Various, e.g. 5-HT	Flushing, palpitations (if liver metastases are present)
Thyroid C cells	Medullary carcinoma	Calcitonin	Silent

most epithelial neoplasms (see section on tumour dependency). Examples of benign mixed neoplasms are the fibroadenoma of the breast and the so-called pleomorphic salivary gland adenoma. Malignant neoplasms consisting of a mixture of epithelial and mesenchymal elements are generally referred to as carcinosarcomas; these occur most commonly in the female genital tract. There are some examples of mixed tumours which are distinctive clinicopathological entities such as synovial sarcoma (a misnomer because it is not derived from synovium) and the so-called pulmonary blastoma.

Poorly differentiated neoplasms

A proportion of malignant neoplasms do not show any evidence of differentiation, by conventional light microscopy. In the past these were assigned to the diagnostic dustbin of 'anaplastic tumours'. However, advances in electron microscopy and more particularly immunohistochemstry and cytogenetics now allow the majority of these neoplasms to be at least assigned to a broad category such as lymphoma or carcinomas, and sometimes to be diagnosed precisely. These distinctions can be of great importance to patient management: for example, an undifferentiated tumour that on further investigation proves to be a lymphoma may be highly responsive to appropriate chemotherapy.

Other lesions resembling neoplasms

Hamartomas are benign tumour-like lesions the growth of which are coordinated with that of the individual. They usually consist of one or more mature, well-differentiated tissue or cell types. Examples of such lesions are benign melanocytic naevi ('moles') and pulmonary hamartomas. It should be noted, however, that there is not a strictly defined distinction between hamartomas and other benign neoplasms.

Choristomas are tumour-like lesions which consist of a perfectly formed mature tissue in an ectopic site. These are sometimes referred to as 'rests'. Examples are ectopic adrenal tissue in the ovary, and ectopic pancreas in the wall of the gut. Like hamartomas, these are benign, non-neoplastic developmental abnormalities, the growth of which is coordinated with that of the individual in which they arise.

Eponymous neoplasms

As is the case in all areas of medicine, we delight in applauding our fellows, and inevitably, many tumours have gained eponymous names. Most eponymously-named tumours also have a histogenetic label: for example, the Grawitz tumour of the kidney is more commonly known as renal cell carcinoma. However, some tumours, usually of obscure histogenesis, are known only by their eponymous name. The best-known examples are Ewing's sarcoma of bone and Burkitt's lymphoma.

INVASION

As invasion is the *sine qua non* of the malignant neoplasms, the process of invasion might be expected to have been extensively studied and well understood. However, our knowledge of this subject is still at a very descriptive level.

Within tissue of origin

The invasiveness of epithelial neoplasms is easier to define and identify than that of other types of neoplasm. This is because there is a distinct anatomical barrier — the basement membrane — across which non-malignant epithelial cells do not cross. Thus it is possible to distinguish between carcinoma-in-situ and invasive carcinoma in tissues such as uterine cervix (Fig. 5.7), whereas in mesenchymal neoplasms, for example, diagnosis of malignancy tends to depend more upon the identification of surrogate features such as high mitotic activity or necrosis which are known to be associated with the ability to metastasise in that particular tumour type, unless there is clear evidence of invasion of structures such as neurovascular bundles.

As well as invading 'vertically' through the basement membrane into the underlying stroma, some neoplasms also invade 'horizontally' through the epithelium in which they arise. This form of invasion is termed *Pagetoid* because it characterises Paget's disease of the nipple in which ductal carcinoma-in-situ of the breast spreads along the lacteriferous ducts to the nipple epidermis. Pagetoid spread may precede or occur concurrently with invasion of the basement membrane and is also commonly seen in melanomas.

The ability to invade surrounding tissue presumably requires the acquisition of the ability to break down the physical barriers that normally prevent this happening. There is some evidence that this is due to the acquisition of the ability of neoplastic cells to secrete proteolytic enzymes such as metalloproteinases, and that this may be related to alterations in the interactions between the tumours cells and their basement membrane by alterations in their expression of adhesion molecules such as E-cadherin, the integrins (peptide cell adhesion molecules) and CD44 (a multifunctional cell surface proteoglycan). However, the precise significance of these events has yet to be fully defined.

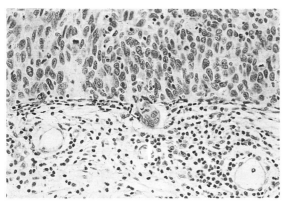

Fig. 5.7 Early invasion into squamous carcinoma. The upper part of this photomicrograph demonstrates squamous carcinoma-in-situ. The cells show no evidence of maturation, the nuclei are variable in size, show a course chromatin pattern, have no consistent orientation with respect to the basement membrane, and mitotic figures are present above the basal layer (where mitosis occurs in normal squamous epithelium). The arrow indicates a small group of cells that have penetrated the basement, membrane to invade the underlying stroma. This is the first step in the process that leads to the local establishment of a malignant neoplasm and, ultimately, to distant metastases.

Invasion of vessels

The ability of a neoplasm to metastasise depends upon its ability to invade vascular channels. In carcinomas, lymphatic vascular invasion usually precedes blood vessel invasion, so the first metastases to develop usually do so in the lymph nodes. Spread into the blood stream may then follow either from invasion of the efferent vessels in lymph nodes, or from blood vessel invasion at the site of the primary tumour. Non-epithelial tumours appear to play by slightly different rules: for example, lymph node metastases are uncommon in most sarcomas, haematogenous spread being the rule in these neoplasms.

The likelihood of vascular invasion in most tumours seems to correlate with their size or depth of invasion. This has been well established in colorectal carcinoma, cervical carcinoma and malignant melanoma. Thus it seems to relate more to the frequency with which the invading edge of the tumour encounters vessels, rather than requiring a phenotypic change in the same way as the transition between in-situ and invasive disease.

However, the story is not a simple one, and different tumours have individual patterns of behaviour. For example, papillary carcinomas of the thyroid have a high frequency of lymph node metastasis, but are rather reluctant to enter the blood stream, giving this tumour type a good prognosis, even when lymph node metastases are present. On the other hand, follicular carcinomas of the thyroid often invade blood vessels seemingly in preference to lymphatics, giving rise to skeletal and pulmonary metastases.

Local invasion of other tissues

Many of the most serious manifestations of malignant neoplasms are due to their ability to directly invade neighbouring tissues and structures. The pattern of local spread can vary from tumour to tumour: for example, adenoid cystic carcinomas of the salivary glands and some melanomas have a preference for perineural spread. Some structures are inherently resistant to invasion, but may nonetheless be affected by compression: for example, pelvic malignancies such as carcinomas of the cervix and ovaries can cause renal failure by constricting the ureters.

The extent to which a malignant neoplasm manifests itself through interfering with neighbouring structures depends, naturally, upon where the neoplasm arises. For example, a proximal bronchogenic carcinoma can cause morbidity and mortality in a number of ways without having to metastasise (Table 5.10).

METASTASIS

Along with invasiveness, the capacity to metastasise is a defining characteristic of malignant neoplasms. The term

Table 5.10 Consequences of local invasion of bronchogenic carcinoma	
Structure invaded/compromised	Consequence
Symphathetic chain	Horner's syndrome
Recurrent laryngeal nerve	Hoarseness
Brachial plexus	Pancoast syndrome
Phrenic nerve	Hemidiaphragmatic paralysis
Pericardium	Pericardial effusion
Superior vena cava	Facial swelling
Pulmonary vessels	Massive haemoptysis
Aorta	Massive haemoptysis
Oesophagus	Dysphagia

'metastasise' means 'to move house'. While this term may not recognise that the neoplasm also retains its original place of residence, it does infer that not only does the neoplasm have to find its way to a distant site, it also has to be able to establish itself there in order to be viable.

There are several possible routes by which a neoplasms can metastasise:

- via lymphatics
- via the blood stream
- transcoelomic spread (across cavities such as the peritoneum)
- via the cerebrospinal fluid
- 'seeding' during surgery.

The process of metastasis can be broken down into the following stages:

- invasion of vessel / body cavity
- homing to the 'recipient' organ or tissue
- establishment and growth of metastasis within the recipient tissue.

These stages are demonstrated in Figure 5.8. The first stage has been discussed above.

Tumour homing

In many cases, the site of a metastasis is determined by where the lymphatics or blood stream take it. This is demonstrated by the formation of lymph node metastases in carcinoma of the breast. It has been found that the first lymph node to which the lymph from a breast carcinoma drains can be identified by scintigraphy. This node is termed the *sentinel node*. If there is no metastasis in this node, the likelihood of metastases being present in other nodes draining that breast is low. The same principle probably applies to the formation of liver metastases in colorectal carcinoma, in that the blood vessels that are invaded in these neoplasms are tributaries of the portal vein.

A similar mechanism has been proposed for the localisation of bone metastases in prostate, breast and thyroid carcinomas. In prostatic carcinoma, bone metastases are far more common in the pelvis and lumbar spine than in other sites, in breast carcinoma the thoracic vertebrae are commonly involved, and in thyroid carcinoma the shoulder girdle and upper spine are common sites. In all three cases this is explained by retrograde spread through anastomosing venous plexi. However, this may not be the sole explanation, as these carcinomas are all capable of metastasising to sites in the skeleton distant from their anastomosing venous plexi, and often do so in preference

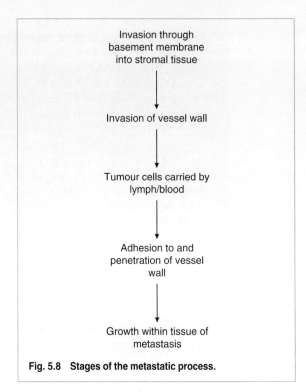

Fig. 5.8   Stages of the metastatic process.

to metastasising to other organs or tissues. This therefore infers a 'seed and soil' relationship in which a particular type of neoplasm has an affinity for a particular tissue. This may either be because of selective homing to that tissue, or because the recipient tissue provides a suitable environment in which the metastasis can grow, possibly through local growth factor production.

Our understanding of the balance between these two processes is far from complete. However, there are a few striking examples of where selective homing of neoplastic cells must occur. Neuroblastoma has the capacity to metastasise to bone, but for some reason commonly chooses the skull or orbit, despite the primary tumour arising in the adrenal medulla or sympathetic chain. Likewise, every medical student knows that the combination of a glass eye and hepatomegaly points to the diagnosis of liver metastases of ocular melanoma, a neoplasm that seems invariably to be able to find its way to the liver, apparently ignoring many other potential sites of metastasis on its way. The homing powers of haematological malignancies tend to be more obvious than those of other classes of neoplasm. An excellent example of this is given by gastric MALT (mucosa-associated lymphoid tissue) lymphomas. Although it is possible to demonstrate that neoplastic cells from gastric MALTomas circulate, if the tumour is removed surgically, the circulating cells generally fail to establish themselves elsewhere. This is because, like non-neoplastic MALT lymphocytes, the neoplastic lymphocytes home back to their tissue of origin. However, this does not apply to high grade gastric lymphomas in which the neoplastic cells appear to 'forget the rules' and are capable of dissemination.

The molecular basis of tumour homing is not yet understood. It presumably involves cell adhesion molecules such as the addressins, selectins and molecules like CD44 and certain integrins which are known to mediate homing of non-neoplastic lymphocytes.

Process of metastasis formation

In order for a metastasis to establish itself in a recipient tissue, it has to:

- interact with the vascular endothelium in order to come out of the circulation
- enter the tissue
- survive and grow within the tissue
- establish its own blood supply.

The interaction between the neoplastic cells and the vascular endothelium may be direct, mediated by cell adhesion molecules, or in many cases it may depend upon the neoplastic cells being contained within fibrin or thrombus material which then binds to the vascular endothelium or is simply 'filtered out' in capillaries.

Most neoplasms are dependent to some extent on the presence of suitable growth factors to promote cell division and prevent apoptosis (programmed cell death — many neoplastic cells have a surprisingly tenuous hold on life). The requirement for growth factors may simply be for ubiquitous ones such as platelet-derived growth factor (PDGF) or the insulin-like growth factors (IGFs/somatomedins). Alternatively, the requirement may be more specific. For example, the high affinity of myeloma cells for bone appears to be due to their requirement for interleukin-6, a factor produced in large quantities by bone cells. Alternatively, the neoplasm itself may produce a factor that suitably modifies its environment. For example, bone metastases of breast carcinoma commonly produce parathyroid hormone-related peptide which stimulates resident osteoclasts to resorb bone and thus make way for growth of the metastasis.

The subject of establishment of a blood supply is essentially the same for metastases as it is for primary tumours. This is dealt with below under 'tumour dependency'.

BIOLOGY OF NEOPLASTIC CELLS

Neoplastic cells, even undifferentiated ones, retain most of the characteristics of normal cells in terms of their structure and metabolism. There is no truly definitive abnormality shared by all neoplastic cells, although it is probably true to say that they all have alterations in their DNA and do not resemble their normal counterparts completely in their metabolism and function.

DNA abnormalities

The qualitative genetic abnormalities occurring in neoplastic cells have been discussed in the section on genetics, above. These qualitiative changes do not tell the whole story, however. Neoplastic cells, particularly those of malignant tumours, have inherently unstable DNA. Not only do they retain the genetic abnormalities that resulted from the initial carcinogenic process, they continue to acquire additional ones. This results in heterogeneity within the tumour with generation of genotypically and phenotypically different clones. The importance of this is that these clones often have differing susceptibilities to chemotherapy. Thus, chemotherapy tends to select out resistant clones. This explains why combination chemotherapy is generally more effective than single agents, and why post-chemotherapy recurrences tend to be resistant to the regime originally used.

Within the neoplastic cells, the accumulation of genetic abnormalities often manifests iself in quantitative DNA abnormalities. While the cells of benign or well-differentiated malignant neoplasms may have a *diploid* chromosomal configuration (i.e. identical to normal somatic cells), many malignant neoplastic cells are either:

- *polyploid* (contain multiples of the normal number of chromosomes) or
- *aneuploid* (contain a number of chromosomes that is other than the normal number or a multiple thereof).

Such abnormalities are not stable and tend to become more extreme as the neoplasm progresses. In general, aneuploid neoplasms tend be behave more aggressively than their diploid or polyploid counterparts.

These DNA abnormalities manifest themselves histologically as abnormalities of nuclear morphology, such as hyperchromatism, abnormalities of chromatin distribution, multiple or enlarged nucleoli and increased and variable nuclear size. These features can be vital for the pathological diagnosis of malignancy, particularly in cytological specimens.

Mitosis and apoptosis

An increased frequency of mitosis is a common feature of malignant neoplasms, but is less usual in benign neoplasms. Characterisitcally, this mitotic activity is independent of any regulatory stimulus, in contrast to the increases in mitotic activity ocurring in physiological situations such as wound healing. Frequent cell division accounts for why most malignant neoplasms grow in size. However, they generally only increase in size at a small fraction of the rate that would be expected if all of the cells produced survived. The reason for this is that the majority of cells produced perish rapidly through apoptosis. Apoptosis is a natural suicide mechanism that is programmed into almost all cells and is controlled by many of the same genes that control proliferation. Thus, highly proliferative cells are usually also highly vulnerable to apoptosis. However, in some neoplastic cells, the mechanism leading to apoptosis is defective, resulting in 'immortal cells'. This is the case in some low grade B cell lymphomas where an anti-apoptotic gene, *Bcl-2*, is inappropriately switched on by being linked to the immunoglobulin heavy chain gene promoter by a chromosomal translocation. The frequency of mitosis in these neoplasms is very low, so they grow by a gradual accumulation of cells. This is reflected in their slow but relentless clinical course. Melanomas, on the other hand, often have the particularly deadly combination of increased proliferation and decreased apoptosis.

Other metabolic abnormalities

Despite the high metabolic demands of rapid proliferation, neoplastic cells are often surprisingly resistant to hypoxia. This may be due to their tendency to generate energy by anaerobic glycolysis. Neoplastic cells also often have quantitative and qualitative abnormalities of protein synthesis. Thus they may either overproduce a normal product in an unregulated way or they may produce a protein which is abnormal for their tissue of origin. An example of the former is insulin production by insulinomas; an example of the latter is ectopic ACTH production by bronchogenic carcinomas. Protein production by some tumours has the clinical utility of giving rise to tumour markers which can be used for diagnosis or for monitoring response to therapy. Examples of such markers are given in Table 5.11.

CLINICAL EFFECTS — LOCAL AND SYSTEMIC

The clinical effects of neoplasms are many and varied, being influenced by the site, size and type of neoplasm, its pattern of spread and the actions of its products.

Table 5.11 Examples of tumour markers	
Tumour type	Marker
Prostatic adenocarcinoma	Prostate-specific antigen
Hepatocellular carcinoma	Alpha-fetoprotein
Seminoma	Placental alkaline phosphatase
Choriocarcinoma	Beta-human chorionic gonadotrophin
Ovarian carcinoma	CA 125
Colorectal carcinoma	Carcinoembryonic antigen
Myeloma	Monoclonal immunoglobulin
Phaeochromocytoma	Catecholamines and their breakdown products

Local effects

The commonest clinical manifestations of the primary neoplasm are:

- a mass (palpable or visible)
- bleeding (due to ulceration)
- symptoms of irritation of the tissue of origin (e.g. cough due to carcinoma of the bronchus)
- pain
- obstruction of a hollow viscus
- compression of or damage to adjacent structures, e.g. nerves.

Mass

This applies particularly to superficial lesions of tissues such as the skin and breast, although neoplasms arising in deeper structures such as the stomach and colon may be palpable on clinical examination. Increasingly the presence of a mass manifests itself radiologically, rather than as a presenting complaint or on clinical examination.

Bleeding

This is a common presenting complaint for tumours arising in a large hollow viscus such as the colon or bronchus and reflects the tendency of these neoplasms to ulcerate. Bleeding may be overt or occult, manifesting itself as iron-deficiency anaemia.

Symptoms of irritation

This depends upon the site of the neoplasm. For example, laryngeal neoplasms usually present with hoarseness, bronchogenic carcinoma often causes a cough, and colorectal carcinoma commonly causes alterations in bowel habit.

Pain

Although the public perception of cancer is that it is a painful disease, a large proportion of primary neoplasms are painless. Where pain does occur, it is often related to perineural invasion or is caused indirectly by damage to neighbouring structures or obstruction of a hollow viscus.

Obstruction of a hollow viscus

This depends upon the relative size of the tumour and the viscus in which it arises. For example, a colonic carcinoma can present with symptoms of obstruction, but this is not the most typical manifestation, whereas dysphagia is the rule in carcinoma of the oesophagus.

Compression or damage to adjacent structures

The classical example of this phenomenon is obstructive jaundice caused by carcinoma of the head of pancreas, which is the usual clinical presentation of this neoplasm. Nerves are probably the most eloquent structures when it comes to indicating the presence of a neigbouring tumour. A good example of this is bitemporal hemianopia resulting from compression of the optic chiasma by a pituitary tumour.

Effects of metastases

Once they have metastasised, the vast majority of malignant neoplasms are incurable, and disseminated malignancy is generally accepted to be the cause of death in most patients dying of malignant disease. However, the precise mechanism by which metastatic disease brings about death is often obscure.

Metastases often cause clinical effects that differ from those attributable to the primary tumour. For example, lung metastases may cause breathlessness, cerebral metastases may cause convulsions or focal neurological signs, bone metastases may cause pathological fractures, and peritoneal deposits may cause ascites. Much of the pain caused by malignant disease is due to secondary deposits in sites such as bone and liver. Extensive metastatic deposits may also worsen effects caused by tumour products (for example, hypercalcaemia due to parathyroid hormone-related peptide) by increasing the total tumour volume.

Ultimately, replacement of a large proportion of the volume of an organ by metastases can cause impairment or failure of the function of that organ. For example, liver metastases commonly declare their presence by causing jaundice, and extensive bone marrow deposits can cause anaemia or pancytopenia.

Paraneoplastic effects

Paraneoplastic effects are those which occur in the presence of a neoplasm but which are not directly caused by the tumour itself or its metastases. These can be divided into the following categories:

- humoral (i.e. mediated by a secreted tumour product)
- immunological (usually tumour-associated autoimmune phenomena)
- uncertain cause.

Examples of paraneoplastic syndromes are given in Table 5.12.

Humoral

Syndromes caused by the secretion of an 'appropriate' product, such as insulin by insulinomas or catecholamines by phaeochromocytomas, have been described above. Many other neoplasms secrete 'inappropriate' products such as ACTH or antidiuretic hormone by bronchogenic carcinomas. The commonest of these syndromes is humoral hypercalcaemia of malignancy, which is caused by secretion of parathyroid hormone-related peptide (PTHrP). The normal function of this peptide, which is produced by many epithelial tissues, is not known. It causes hypercalcaemia by binding to the parathyroid

Table 5.12 Examples of paraneoplastic syndromes		
Syndrome	Associated tumour	Cause
Paraneoplastic Cushing's syndrome	Bronchogenic carcinoma	ACTH
Syndrome of inappropriate ADH	Bronchogenic carcinoma	ADH
Humoral hypercalcaemia of malignancy	Various	PTHrP
Carcinoid syndrome	Carcinoid (liver metastases)	5-HT, others
Dermatomyositis	Various	Autoantibody induction
Eaton–Lambert syndrome	Bronchogenic carcinoma	Anti-neurotransmitter receptor autoantibodies
Acanthosis nigricans	Pancreatic carcinoma	? epidermal growth factor
Hypertrophic pulmonary osteoarthropathy	Bronchogenic carcinoma	Unknown

hormone receptor in kidney and bone. It is possible that, to some extent, the weight loss and cachexia associated with many malignant neoplasms is due to secretion of catabolic factors, but it is more likely that in most cases it is multifactorial.

Immunological

Autoimmune disease can be triggered by malignant neoplasms. A significant proportion of patients with dermatomyositis, particularly those developing it for the first time later in life, have an underlying malignancy. Also, membraneous glomerulonephritis, a cause of neph-rotic syndrome, which results from immunological damage to the glomerular basement membrane, can be initiated by an underlying neoplasm. A variety of neuro-logical syndromes can be associated with malignant neoplasms, most commonly small cell carcinoma of the bronchus. Examples of this are the myasthenia-gravis-like Eaton–Lambert syndrome, cerebellar ataxia and dementia. The majority, if not all, of these syndromes seem to be caused by the production of autoantibodies against nerve cell components such as neurotransmitter receptors, possibly due to an immune response to anti-gens shared by tumour cells and neurons.

Syndromes of uncertain cause

The cause of some paraneoplastic syndromes has not been fully established, but in the majority of cases the syndrome is probably caused by an unidentified product secreted by the tumour. Examples of this category are finger clubbing and hypertrophic pulmonary osteoarthro-pathy associated with carcinoma of the bronchus.

TUMOUR DEPENDENCY

In many senses, neoplasms have a parasitic relationship with the individuals in which they arise. In order to grow they need to be supplied with the nutritional requirements of any tissue, and although their growth is autonomous, for most neoplasms this term is relative and they retain some requirement for growth factor / endocrine support. This relationship with the host has more than a purely academic significance; in some tumours it proves to be their therapeutic Achilles heel.

Angiogenesis

No solid tumour of normal cellularity can grow beyond a couple of millimetres in diameter without recruiting its own blood supply. The ability to do this is one of the few characteristics that most neoplasms have in common. However, precisely how they do so is not clearly estab-lished and may vary from neoplasm to neoplasm. It is

likely that most neoplasms can produce cytokines or growth factors that stimulate the proliferation and dif-ferentiation of endothelial cells, although there is also evidence to suggest that these factors may be produced by non-neoplastic accessory cells that are present within the tumour, most notably macrophages. It is likely that tissue hypoxia is an important stimulus for angiogenesis.

Apart from being biologically important in tumour development, inhibiting angiogenesis may also be signifi-cant in future treatment strategies for malignant neoplasms. Indeed, inhibition of angiogenesis may contribute to the efficacy of some existing chemotherapeutic regimes.

Growth factor/hormone dependency

Although autonomy of growth is a feature of neoplasia, in many cases this is relative; a neoplasm requires less stimulation by growth factors than its parent tissue, but still requires some stimulation, at least for optimal growth. Thus many neoplasms require, or benefit from, the common growth factors such as platelet-derived growth factor (PDGF) or the insulin-like growth factors (IGFs/somatomedins), but other neoplasms are more specific in their requirements. Three good examples of the latter class are carcinomas of the breast, prostate and thyroid (Table 5.13).

Breast carcinoma

A large proportion of carcinomas of the breast express oestrogen receptors. The degree of oestrogen receptor expression in a carcinoma correlates well (but not perfectly) with the therapeutic response of that tumour to oestrogen blockade using agents such as the selective oestrogen receptor-modulating drug tamoxifen. Overall, oestrogen receptor-positive carcinomas tend to be of lower grade and have a better prognosis than their oestrogen receptor-negative counterparts.

Prostate carcinoma

Prostatic epithelium is dependent upon androgenic stimulation for its growth and survival; castration of male

Table 5.13 Neoplasms dependent on growth factors/hormones	
Neoplasm	Growth factor/hormone
Breast carcinoma	Oestrogens
Prostate carcinoma	Androgens
Thyroid carcinomas	TSH
Endometrial carcinoma	Oestrogens
Myeloma	Interleukin 6

rats results in apoptosis of prostate epithelial cells and partial involution of the gland. This characteristic is retained by most prostatic carcinomas, allowing their growth to be inhibited by androgen blockade. This can be achieved by orchidectomy (removal of the main source of androgens) or by interfering with the hypothalamo-pituitary-testicular axis. Luteinising hormone (LH) released from the pituitary stimulates androgen production by Leydig cells in the testis. LH production can be inhibited either by treatment with oestrogens or luteinising hormone releasing hormone (LHRH) agonists which, after a transient stimulation, cause a long term depression of LH release.

Unfortunately, after a period of time, prostatic carcinomas usually lose their androgen senstivity, so the treatments described above are not curative.

Thyroid carcinoma

Papillary and follicular carcinomas of the thyroid respond in the same way as normal thyroid follicular epithelium to the growth-promoting effects of thyroid stimulating hormone (TSH). TSH suppression is used in combination with surgery and radio-iodine therapy to treat these neoplasms. It can be achieved by the negative feedback effect of replacement doses of thyroxine.

PROGNOSIS

How a neoplasm behaves clinically is determined by more than simply being benign or malignant. Some benign tumours are life-threatening, particularly those of the central nervous system, and the prognosis of malignant tumours varies from that of the cutaneous basal cell carcinoma, which can be reliably cured by adequate local excision, to incurable neoplasms such as malignant mesothelioma. Predicting the 'typical' or 'average' prognosis of a group of comparable neoplasms can be done quite accurately, but predicting the future course of an individual neoplasm can be less certain.

The prognosis of benign tumours can generally be stated to be that they are cured by adequate excision. Some benign tumours have a tendency to recur locally. This can be due to:

- difficulty in identifying the margins of the tumour at the primary excision
- tendency to be multiple at one site.

The exceptional benign tumours that have a poor prognosis are those which impinge upon vital structures and are difficult or impossible to remove surgically: for example, gliomas affecting the mid- or hind-brain.

Significance of grade and stage

The most important prognostic factors within most individual malignant tumour types are stage and grade, usually in that order.

The *stage* of a malignancy describes how far advanced that tumour is in terms of its *extent of growth*. The principle of staging was first established by Cuthbert Dukes, who found that the prognosis of carcinoma of the rectum after resection could be predicted by examining the extent of growth of the tumour within the resection specimen. Dukes' staging remains in widespread use today and is described in Chapter 17.

It is usual to describe four stages, in which stage I represents disease localised to the tissue of origin, stage IV respresents disseminated disease, and stages II and III are steps in between which are therapeutically or prognostically significant for that tumour type. An alternative commonly used method of staging is the TNM classification, which includes separate scores for the local extent of the tumour (T), the extent of its lymph node metastases (N) and its visceral metastases (M). The TNM classification is useful for carcinomas (it is generally not relevant to non-epithelial neoplasms) as it contains more information than stage alone. Staging can be defined according to anatomical boundaries, or be judged by direct measurements. For example, Clark staging of melanomas relies on the former, the different stages being defined by invasion of different anatomical layers of the skin, whereas Breslow staging of melanomas is done by measuring the greatest depth of invasion of the lesion.

The *grade* of a tumour is a measure of its *inherent potential for growth*. Stage for stage, high grade tumours progress more rapidly, are usually less easily controlled by treatment and therefore have a worse prognosis than their low grade counterparts. The grade of a neoplasm is judged according to its histological appearance, with the degree of differentiation (i.e. resemblance to the tissue or cell type of origin), proliferative activity and extent of necrosis (in effect a surrogate for rate of growth) being taken into account.

Generally speaking, stage is more prognostically significant than grade, but increasingly the value of combining both in judging prognosis and planning treatment is being recognised. For example, the Nottingham Prognostic Index for breast carcinoma (based on a large retrospective series of cases) is calculated by adding scores for tumour size, grade and lymph node status (perhaps surprisingly, grade and lymph node status have equal weight in this system).

Significance of histogenesis

Within a particular tumour type, stage and grade are usually the most important prognostic factors. However, neoplasms derived from different cell types behave inherently in different ways. For example, lymphomas and sarcomas usually differ from carcinomas in their patterns of spread and which organs or tissues they preferentially involve. Comparison of basal cell carcinoma and melanoma provides a good example of how strongly histogenesis can influence behaviour of a neoplasm within one tissue, in that basal cell carcinomas are indolent and locally invasive, rarely metastasising, whereas melanomas develop more rapidly and metastasise as a rule if not locally excised at an early stage of their development.

Other factors of prognostic significance

Numerous other factors have been shown to influence the prognosis of individual types of neoplasms, although these are often linked to grade or stage and do not influence the outcome of individual cases. For example, aneuploidy (see above) is usually associated with a worse prognosis, but also correlates with high grade. Increasingly, specific genetic characteristics are being shown to influence prognosis. For example, amplification of the *N-myc* gene conveys an unfavourable prognosis in neuroblastoma.

Of greatest practical utility is a prognostic factor that predicts or detects a response (or lack thereof) to a particular form of therapy. The best-established examples of this are oestrogen receptor status of breast carcinomas (response prediction) and serum tumour markers such as alpha-fetoprotein (response detection).

SCREENING

Despite great advances in our understanding of the pathology and pathogenesis of malignant tumours in recent years, the improvements in the prognosis of the common epithelial malignancies such as lung, prostate, colon and breast carcinomas has been rather disappointing. One of the reasons behind this is the tendency of many malignant neoplasms to present clinically at an advanced stage when local spread is too extensive for curative surgery or when metastases are already present. Theoretically, prognosis of these tumours should be improved if they could be detected at an earlier stage, before they became symptomatic. This has led to the development of screening programmes, the best established of which are those for carcinomas of the cervix and carcinoma of the breast.

Principles of population screening

It is possible to screen individuals for a variety of neoplastic diseases on an ad hoc basis by simple 'fishing' with appropriate diagnostic tests. However, to have an impact on a disease within a population, a coordinated screening programme is required. Population screening programmes are aimed at reducing morbidity and mortality from a particular disease within the entire population. In order to be able to establish a screening programme, it is necessary to fulfil the following criteria.

- There must be a diagnostic test available that can practically be applied to large numbers of people and can be repeated on different occasions in the same individual.
- The test must have high levels of sensitivity (the proportion of tests carried out in individuals who have the disease that detect the disease) and specificity (the proportion of positive tests that are due to the disease, rather than other diseases or artefacts).
- The test must give comparable results between different centres.
- It must be possible to apply the test to a high proportion of the target population.
- There must be established and effective treatments for the disease.
- There must be evidence that screening for the disease in question can reduce levels of morbidity and mortality from that disease.

In practice, however, issues of funding and political pressures are also strongly influential in decisions regarding population screening.

Existing screening programmes

Cervical carcinoma screening

Squamous carcinoma of the cervix and its precursor lesion, cervical intraepithelial neoplasia (CIN), can be detected by exfoliative cytology. Given that these diseases affect a relatively accessible site in a relatively young age group, and that by the time cervical carcinomas become symptomatic, they are often locally advanced, screening for cervical carcinoma has been widely practised for many years. However, only recently has a co-ordinated national screening programme been developed in the United Kingdom.

The test employed, microscopic examination of exfoliative cytology samples stained by the Papanicolaou technique, is highly sensitive and specific. It has the considerable advantage of allowing detection of the precursor condition, CIN, and thus allowing simple local curative treatment to be carried out before invasive carcinoma develops. The major disadvantage is that it is labour-intensive and therefore expensive and prone to subjective error. However, despite this, the UK cervical carcinoma screening programme appears to be successful, because prevalence and death rates from cervical carcinoma in the UK are declining. It is probable that this is attributable to the screening programme, but this cannot be stated with absolute certainty as the screening programme represents (for obvious ethical reasons) an uncontrolled experiment.

Breast carcinoma screening

After carcinoma of the bronchus, carcinoma of the breast is the commonest cause of death from neoplastic disease for women in the UK. There has been some improvement in the prognosis of this disease in recent years, probably mainly due to the introduction of oestrogen receptor antagonists such as tamoxifen, but approximately half of women developing this disease will die of it. Prognosis in carcinoma of the breast is most strongly related to stage. It therefore should follow that detecting lesions at an earlier stage should improve the overall prognosis. It is often possible to detect carcinomas of the breast, or their precursor lesion, ductal carcinoma-in-situ, by mammography before they become palpable. This has led to mammography being used for screening purposes. In the UK this occurs in the setting of a coordinated national screening programme.

Breast carcinoma screening programmes have been shown to be associated with an improved prognosis. However, this improvement is probably at least partially due to *lead time artefact*. This means that screening detects some lesions earlier than they would have presented, but earlier treatment does not affect their natural history. Thus some screening-detected patients simply have their diagnosis for longer rather than surviving for longer. This artefact is less of a problem in interpreting survival data in populations that have been screened for longer, but even in these populations, the improvements in outcome are disappointingly small.

Future of screening

There is much debate about screening for two other common carcinomas, namely those of the prostate and large bowel. Prostatic carcinoma can be screened for by measuring serum prostate-specific antigen. This is a relatively inexpensive and simple test which has a high degree of sensitivity and fairly good specificity. However, because the value of radical prostatectomy (the only potentially curative treatment) is still uncertain, the value of screening is also unproven. Colorectal carcinoma can be detected by testing for faecal occult blood. This is a simple and inexpensive investigation that has been shown to be effective in pilot screening programmes and may in future be used in a coordinated screening programme. Individuals with a strong family history of colorectal carcinoma are currently screened, but usually using the far more sensitive (but more expensive and invasive) modality of colonoscopy.

6

Immunology

William Egner

THE IMMUNE RESPONSE

Immunity is defined as resistance to disease. At its most basic level this consists of a physical barrier (the mucosal surfaces and skin) and the antibacterial actions of certain components of secretions such as lactoferrin and enzymes. Much more effective defences are accomplished by two systems which amplify and focus inflammatory responses onto invading foreign substances (or damaged self components). Basic immune responses can be divided into innate (non-adaptive) and specific (adaptive) effector mechanisms (Fig. 6.1).

INNATE IMMUNITY

Innate immune defences consist of:

- physical barriers such as mucosal epithelium
- secretions with antibacterial activity, including lactoferrin
- phagocytic cells: monocytes, macrophages and neutrophils
- natural killer (NK) cells (lymphocytes capable of non-MHC-restricted killing);
- soluble mediators which can enhance the activity of innate and specific responses: C-reactive protein (CRP), mannose-binding lectin (MBL), cytokines

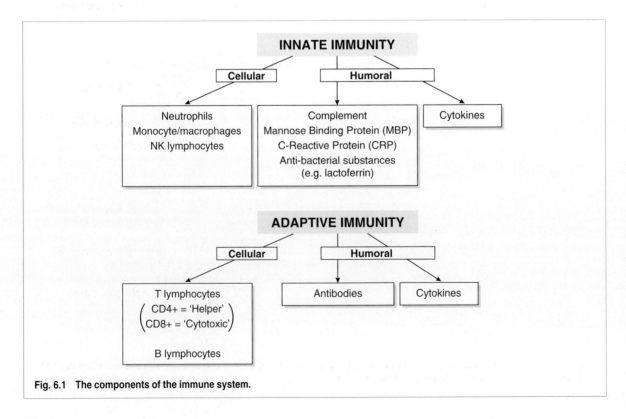

Fig. 6.1 The components of the immune system.

- soluble enzymic cascades such as the complement system, which is activated directly by exposure to pathogens and serves to directly lyse the pathogen, or to enhance and target the activity of innate and specific effector cells by opsonisation and activation via cell surface receptors for complement components.

The innate immune system cannot adapt to recognise an organism which has evolved to evade it, it does not develop memory (enhanced responses on subsequent encounters with the same antigen), and it does not possess antigen specificity.

SPECIFIC IMMUNE RESPONSES

Specific (adaptive) immune responses are more effective than innate ones and are mediated by lymphocytes and antibodies which amplify and focus non-specific responses and provide additional effector functions. These cells are organised into lymphoid tissues (Fig. 6.2). Humoral immunity often refers to the antibody arm of the specific immune response. Cellular (cell-mediated) immunity refers to lymphocyte-mediated effector responses (T helper (Th) and cytotoxic cells) of the specific immune response. These two arms of the specific im-

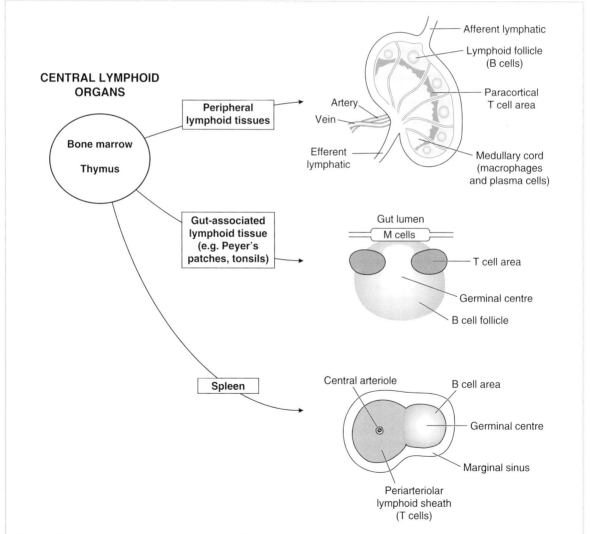

Fig. 6.2 The organisation of the lymphoid system. The lymphoid system is organised to ensure efficient recirculation and interaction of T lymphocytes, B lymphocytes and antigen-presenting cells.

mune response are not really separable, since antibodies are usually not produced without some cell-mediated response to the same antigen and vice-versa. T and B lymphocytes possess infinitely variable antigen receptors which can clonally expand. Antigen receptors which can be secreted into interstitial fluid and onto mucosal surfaces are called antibodies. Antibodies can activate complement and also enhance opsonisation of antigen via phagocyte surface receptors for the Fc region of immunoglobulins (FcR). Both innate and adaptive mechanisms exponentially amplify the immune response, since clonal expansion of lymphocytes increases the number of cells reactive with an antigen. Cytokines and complement components recruit other immune effector mechanisms and antibodies activate complement and phagocytes.

T helper cell responses which help antibody production by B cells are called Th2 type reponses, and those which promote the inflammatory activity of phagocytes such as macrophages are called Th1 type. The effectiveness of each type of response in the prevention of individual infections or in the pathogenesis of autoimmune diseases differs. Antibodies, complement and phagocytes are important in protecting against extracellular bacteria such as the pneumococcus and meningococcus; antibodies and phagocytes against intracellular bacteria such as salmonella; activated macrophages against intracellular mycobacterial infections; IgA antibodies in preventing mucosal penetration (immune adherence) by viruses (e.g. poliovirus, influenza); and T cell responses (CD8 cytotoxic) and NK cells are important to eliminate established intracellular viral infections. The specific adaptive immune response is thus flexible, capable of responding to antigens which have not been previously encountered, including those generated in organisms by the selection pressures of an effective adaptive immune response. Many pathogens have specific adaptations/mutations to evade previous immunological memory responses (e.g. influenza antigen variability) or to suppress the normal mechanisms of immune destruction.

COMPLEMENT

The complement system is a soluble enzymic cascade which focuses and amplifies the activity of the specific and innate immune systems as well as having lytic activity against bacteria (Fig. 6.3). It is part of the innate defences since it has no intrinsic antigen specificity.

The complement cascade has a final common pathway which leads to the insertion of a multimeric pore-forming structure (membrane associated complex (MAC) consisting of complement components C5–9) into bacterial cell membranes, leading to osmotic lysis. The production of this lytic complex is achieved via two mechanisms called the classical and alternative pathways.

Classical pathway

The classical pathway is triggered by antigen–antibody immune complexes which bind circulating complement factor C1q to the Fc region of the antibody tail, which has undergone conformational changes as a result of antibody binding. The resultant sequential activation of complement proteins results in the formation of a C3 convertase (C4b2b) which cleaves C3, thus forming a C5-convertase (C4b2b3b) which catalyses the production of the C5–9 pore-forming complex. In the process, C2, C3 and C4 are split into fragments, the smaller of which (C2a, C3a, C4a) are chemotactic and the larger of which (C3b, C4b) bind to immune complexes to opsonise or solubilise them, or to a pathogen surface to opsonise it. Thus multiple effects ensue on other effector mechanisms as a result of complement activation. CRP and MBL can directly activate the classical pathway of complement without the intervention of immune complexes.

Alternative pathway

The alternative pathway is phylogenetically older than the classical pathway and is triggered by contact with exposed bacterial capsules without the need for prior antibody production. Factors B and D (analogous to the classical pathway C4 and C2) again lead to the production of a C3 convertase (C3bBb) and a C5 convertase (C3bBb3b), leading to opsonisation, chemotaxis and the final common pathway in a similar way to the classical pathway.

ANTIGENS

An antigen is any substance which can elicit a specific immune response. An antigen consists of many epitopes. An epitope is a specific sequence of a protein or carbohydrate recognised by the receptor molecules of the immune system (antibody or T cell receptor). Antigens can be divided into foreign (non-self, allogeneic, xenogeneic, etc.) and self-antigens (autoantigens). Although an antigen usually elicits an immune response, if the antigen is encountered in appropriate circumstances the specific immune response may be switched off by a variety of mechanisms which will be important to consider when discussing the immunology of transplantation and autoimmune diseases.

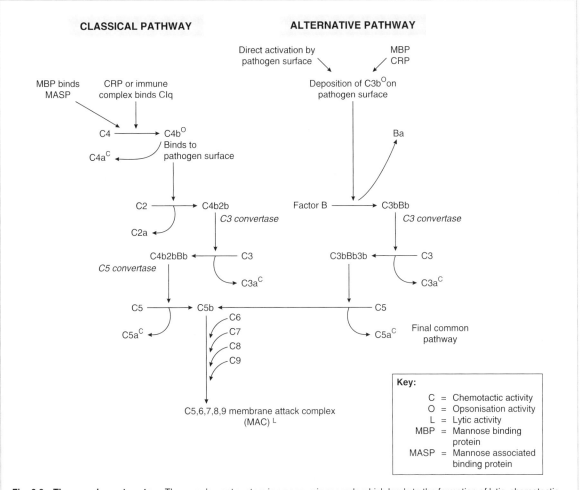

Fig. 6.3 The complement system. The complement system is an enzymic cascade which leads to the formation of lytic, chemotactic and opsonising factors. 'Classical' activation by antibody or 'alternative' activation by other means result in similar pro-inflammatory effector function. c = chemotactic activity; o = opsonisation activity; L = lytic activity.

ANTIBODIES

An antibody is a soluble protein immune receptor produced by B lymphocytes, consisting of two identical antigen-binding sites. Each binding site is formed by the N terminal ends of a heavy chain (coded by V(ariable), D(iversity) & J(oining) genes) and light chain (coded by V & J genes) joined to a common Fc tail (coded by two or three C(onstant) region genes) (Fig. 6.4). The antigen specificity of the antibody resides in the antigen-binding variable regions (the fragment antigen-binding, Fab, portion). Antibodies are divided into different isotypes (classes) which have different functional attributes (ability to bind cells via Fc receptors and activate com-plement) due to the Fc (fragment constant) tails coded by the constant region genes of the heavy chain, thus different constant region genes produce different antibody classes. Antibodies which bind to antigen or cells and activate complement via the Fc region thus activate, amplify and target non-specific defence mechanisms.

Multiple different copies of V, D and J region genes are inherited to provide variability. The antigen-binding variable regions are further (infinitely) diversified by a combination of programmed and random mutations to the V genes in the hypervariable regions (mutation hotspots) and to the joins between V, D and J genes, enabling anti-bodies to be produced which can bind to virtually any natural or synthetic antigen encountered. Up to 10^{10}

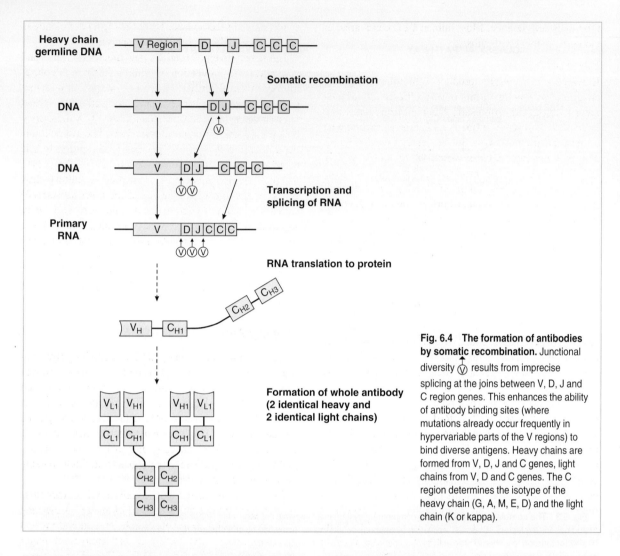

Fig. 6.4 The formation of antibodies by somatic recombination. Junctional diversity Ⓥ results from imprecise splicing at the joins between V, D, J and C region genes. This enhances the ability of antibody binding sites (where mutations already occur frequently in hypervariable parts of the V regions) to bind diverse antigens. Heavy chains are formed from V, D, J and C genes, light chains from V, D and C genes. The C region determines the isotype of the heavy chain (G, A, M, E, D) and the light chain (K or kappa).

different antibody specificities may be produced in any individual. Each cell producing antibody which binds an epitope of an antigen is stimulated to clonally reproduce, and thus further amplification of the immune response occurs with the progeny of each cell producing exactly the same antibody but many different clones expanding.

Most antibody immune responses are polyclonal (many cell clones expand, each recognising different, sometimes overlapping, epitopes on the antigen); oligoclonal responses occur when a limited number of clones expand for some reason (e.g. prolonged inflammation); monoclonal proliferations are usually representative of malignant transformation of a single clone of a B cell at some point in its differentiation (early or late B cells = lymphoma, and often produce IgM; terminally differentiated plasma cells = myeloma and usually produce IgG/A isotypes).

The antigens recognised by antibodies are often conformational (that is, require a folded 3D structure for recognition), often bringing widely separated areas of a larger molecule together to form the epitope (which is therefore discontinuous in linear sequence, unlike the epitopes recognised by T cells). Antibodies thus tend to recognise native folded 3D structures.

Most antibody production is 'T cell dependent' (i.e. very inefficient in the absence of T cells, which recognise linear epitopes on the same antigen as that recognised by the antibody, but not necessarily the same epitope). A small number of relatively 'T-independent' B lymphocytes exist which bear the CD5 surface antigen. They tend to recognise conserved carbohydrate epitopes on pathogens (including human ABO blood groups), produce IgM and may represent a phylogenetically older type of B cell defence. Most human CLL cases arise as clones from this B cell subset.

Isotypes and subclasses

B lymphocytes initially produce IgM upon a primary encounter with antigen; this is very efficient at complement fixation and opsonisation, but IgM circulates as a large pentameric (five antibody molecules) structure with a short half-life (~5 days). Subsequently an individual B cell will undergo a class-switch to IgG (~3 weeks), IgA (~1 week), or IgE production, but class-switching depends on effective T cell help following T cell recognition of an epitope on the same antigen. Memory develops in parallel with the class switch. Both these processes are dependent on surface CD40–CD40L interactions between B cells, APC and T cells. IgG diffuses well into extracellular spaces and can neutralise circulating viruses and bacteria (prevent binding by blocking receptors), opsonise via complement or Fc receptors or lyse via complement activation. IgG is divided into four subclasses (IgG1, IgG2, IgG3, IgG4) which have different Fc regions (and thus is coded by different heavy chain constant region gene segments). These classes and subclasses have different half lives and abilities to fix complement, or bind Fc receptors (Table 6.1).

There are several different types of Fc receptors (FcRI or CD64, FcRII or CD32, FcRIII or CD16) which bind some IgG subclasses better than others and are distributed differently on each effector cell type. IgG1 constitutes 60–70% of the circulating IgG in man; IgG2 constitutes 20–40%. IgG3 constitutes 15–20%. IgG4 circulates in trace amounts and its functional significance is unknown, although it may be important in IgE-mediated antiparasite and allergic responses. IgG1 and IgG3 tend to be produced in response to protein antigens; IgG2 in response to polysaccharide antigens (such as those of bacterial capsules), thus IgG2 deficiency may predispose to bacterial infections. While several subclass deficiency syndromes are recognised, IgG2 (+/– IgA) deficiency is probably the only one of clinical importance.

IgA is secreted preferentially onto mucosal surfaces and is important in prevention of initial adherence to epithelium or mucosal penetration (blocks interaction with cell surface receptors) of bacterial and viral pathogens spread via respiratory or gastrointestinal routes. IgA deficiency thus predisposes to mucosal infections. The gut contains peptidases which degrade IgG and IgM rapidly. IgA is protected from destruction by a remnant of the polyIg receptor (which selectively transports secretory IgA across epithelium to the outside of the mucosal surface) called the secretory component, and IgA is usually secreted as a dimer joined by a j(oining)-piece. Most secretory IgA is of the IgA2 subclass; most circulating in serum is IgA1. The significance of this is uncertain. Unlike most IgG subclasses or IgM, IgA does not efficiently fix complement via the classical pathway of complement activation.

T LYMPHOCYTES

T cell responses are clonal, and are normally polyclonal (multiple clones capable of recognising many different epitopes). Oligoclonal (limited number of clones) and monoclonal (single clone) T cell proliferations occur as for B cells. Monoclonal proliferations can be recognised by looking for a single clonal rearrangement of the T cell receptor (TCR) genes (a member of the immunoglobulin gene superfamily analogous to antibodies) using molecular biology techniques.

In contrast to antibodies, T cells tend to recognise short linear peptides on the surface of antigen-presenting cells (APC) which digest the whole antigen and present the fragments on the surface in the grooves of major histocompatibility complex (MHC) Class I or II molecules. The T cell receptor requires various coreceptor molecules (LFA-1, CTLA-4, CD28, CD40L) associated

Function	Class/subclass						
	IgG1	IgG2	IgG3	IgG4	IgM	IgA	IgE
Classical complement	++	+	+++	–	–	–	–
Alternative complement	–	–	–	–	–	?	–
FcR binding phagocytes	+	+/–	+	–	–	–	–
Mast cell binding	–	–	–	–	–	–	+++
Mean plasma level (g/L)	9	3	1	6.5	1.5	3	0.00005

Table 6.1 The functional attributes of different immunoglobulin molecules

Table 6.2 T cell subtypes			
	Th1	Th2	Cytotoxic
Surface marker	CD4	CD4	CD8
Function	Pro-inflammatory Macrophage activation	B cell help	Cytotoxic for intracellular pathogens
Cytokines	IL-2 IFNγ TNFα IL-12 GM-CSF	IL-2 IL-4 IL-5 IL-10 IL-13 TGFβ	IL-2 (IFNγ) (TNFβ) (TNFα)
Infections if compromised	Mycobacteria Leishmania Pneumocystis	Tetanus Pneumococcus Poliovirus	Influenza Listeria Toxoplasma

with it on the cell surface to enable efficient antigen recognition and signalling via antigen-presenting cells (CD3, CD4, CD8). Thus all T cells have CD3 on the surface. CD4-bearing T cells generally have 'helper' functions; those which aid B cell antibody production are called Th2 and those which activate mononuclear phagocytes and thus promote cellular inflammatory activity are called Th1 (Table 6.2). These T cells types tend to produce different cytokine profiles when activated by antigen; Th1 produce pro-inflammatory IFNγ, IL-1, IL-12, TNFα; Th2 produce IL-4, IL-5, IL-13, TNFα and others which promote antibody production. In immune responses one type of T helper activity will often dominate. This is important both in defence against infection and in pathogenesis of immunologically mediated diseases. CD8 positive T cells in contrast often have cytotoxic effector properties and are important in certain viral infections.

T cells recognise antigen fragments only on the surface of APC which express MHC Class I and II molecules on the surface. MHC molecules have an antigen-binding groove on the surface which can bind antigen fragments of 9–11 amino acids (MHC Class I) or 14–20 amino acids (MHC Class II). They thus act as display platforms on which the TCR can recognise antigen, but because they bind antigen fragments themselves the MHC molecules also influence the immune responses in any individual. The TCR binds to a portion of the lips of the groove as well as the antigen fragment. Thus the TCR is also self-restricted, since it binds only to the combination of self antigen (MHC) + foreign antigen. A T cell will not operate effectively with non-self APC bearing different MHC molecules. They can however cooperate with non-self cells provided they express the same MHC molecules (as in allogeneic bone marrow transplantation). MHC Class I is recognised by CD8, and MHC Class II by CD4 on the T cell surface (Fig. 6.5). Virtually every nucleated cell expresses MHC Class I on the surface, but MHC Class II expression is restricted to certain cell types, usually when activated. APC express MHC Class II in high density and thus are the major activators of CD4 positive lymphocytes. MHC Class I restricted CD8 positive T cells are also stimulated by APC, but these cells often have effector cytotoxic function against intracellular pathogens, particularily viruses. They recognise an infected target cell by seeing viral antigen in the surface groove of self-MHC Class I, and are activated to deliver a lethal attack on the cell. Not surprisingly, viruses adapted to reduce MHC Class I surface expression (e.g. adenovirus) can partially evade their attentions. Degraded intracellular antigens in the cell's cytosol tend to get access to the MHC Class I groove in the process of MHC assembly in the endoplasmic reticulum, and thus responses to intracellular antigens tend to occur via the MHC Class I pathway (Fig. 6.6). Extracellular antigens from bacteria phagocytosed and digested in the lysosomes of APC tend to gain access to MHC Class II most readily since the assembly pathway of MHC Class II intersects with the lysosomal pathway and degraded extracellular antigen gains access to 'empty' MHC Class II molecules after the invariant chain (which occupies the MHC groove prior to antigen binding) is displaced by alterations in the intralysosomal pH.

Memory

T and B lymphocyte memory probably involves both

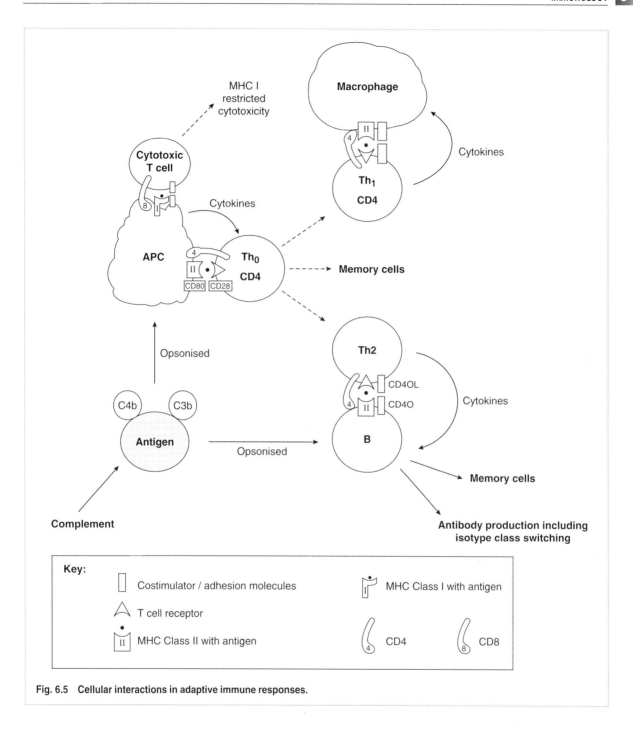

MHC I
restricted
cytotoxicity

Macrophage

Cytokines

**Cytotoxic
T cell**

Th₁

CD4

Cytokines

APC

Th₀

CD4

CD80 CD28

- - - > **Memory cells**

Opsonised

Th2

CD4OL

CD4O

Cytokines

B

C4b   C3b

Antigen

Opsonised

Memory cells

Complement

**Antibody production including
isotype class switching**

Key:

☐ Costimulator / adhesion molecules

⌐• MHC Class I with antigen

△ T cell receptor

(CD4 (4)

) CD8 (8)

•
⊓ MHC Class II with antigen
II

Fig. 6.5 **Cellular interactions in adaptive immune responses.**

long-lived and constantly restimulated cells (B cells use long-lived reservoirs of antigen on the follicular dendritic cells (FDC) in lymph nodes). A secondary (memory) response thus involves the activation of an expanded panel of antigen-reactive clones, which have differen- tiated to produce IgG or IgA rather than IgM (which dominates primary responses), giving a response magni- fied in both quantity and quality. Previously activated cells have been 'primed' and thus are more readily acti- vated by small amounts of antigen on APC. During an

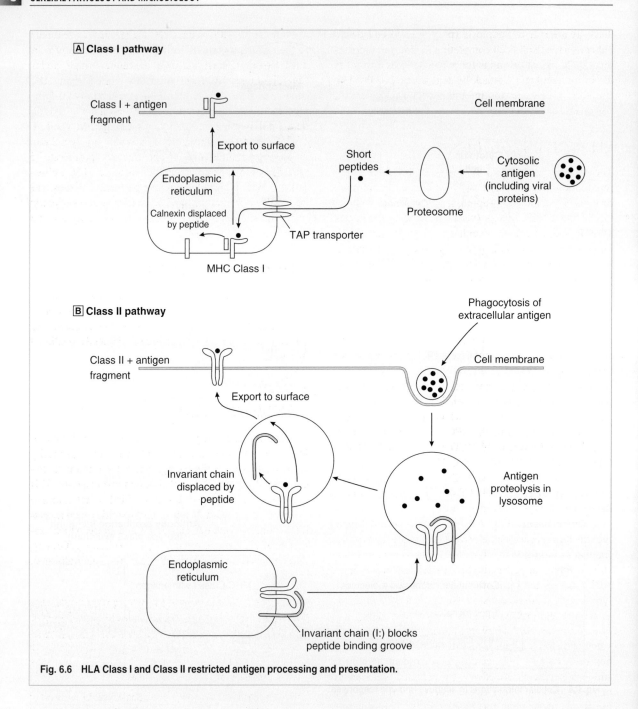

Fig. 6.6 HLA Class I and Class II restricted antigen processing and presentation.

immune response, B cells are selected by competition for antigen on FDC in the lymph nodes; those binding strongly survive, others die through inability to compete for antigen and loss of a survival signal. Thus the antibody response undergoes a process of affinity maturation (each generation of antibodies produced binds better to antigen).

Apoptosis

In order to prevent an escalating cycle of destruction leading to inevitable death there are cellular and humoral mechanisms which downregulate the response of both innate and adaptive responses. This may involve cellular death as a result of apoptosis (programmed cell death) either as a result of a cell completing its lifespan (approximately 20 clonal divisions for a T cell) or as a result of direct immunological attack by regulatory T cells. This apoptotic process is non-inflammatory, unlike necrotic cell death.

ANTIGEN-PRESENTING CELLS (APC)

The initial interaction of lymphocytes with antigen is important in determining whether a specific immune response is promoted or suppressed. The default pathway in unprimed 'naïve' cells (which have not encountered specific antigen before) is either to become specifically unresponsive to the antigen (anergy) or to die (apoptosis) if the antigen is encountered in an insufficiently stimulating context. Naïve lymphocytes are relatively refractory to stimulation, and require potent signals to activate them to clonally proliferate and/or become effector cells. This usually occurs centrally in the lymph nodes, bone marrow or spleen, but can occur elsewhere. These extra signals are complex and multifactorial but act in addition to the recognition of antigen and MHC by the TCR/CD3/ (CD4 or CD8) complex and include adhesion molecules which stabilise contact between lymphocyte and APC, and costimulator molecules which provide activation signals to the T cell from the APC. Important interactions include those between: B7.1(CD80) or 7.2 and CD28 or CTLA-4; LFA-3 (CD58) and CD2; ICAM-1(CD54) or ICAM-2(CD102) or ICAM-3 (CD50) and LFA-1(CD18/ CD11a), CD40 and CD40L. CD40–CD40L is essential to the formation of long-lived memory B cells and immunoglobulin class-switching. APC of several different types provide these second signals while presenting a processed fragment of antigen to a lymphocyte (Fig. 6.5). Primary stimulation of naïve T cells requires a potent professional APC (such as the Dendritic cell (DC) or an activated B lymphocyte) with potent stimulatory capacity and ability to acquire and process (digest) antigen by phagocytosis or endocytosis. Secondary restimulation of recently activated or memory T cells is less stringent and can occur on non-professional APC which are not potent enough to stimulate naïve cells effectively, e.g. activated endothelium or monocytes and other cells expressing MHC Class II molecules. Activated monocytes appear to present antigen to primed T cells in secondary responses, unless specifically differentiated by cytokine combinations to develop potent DC-like function for naïve T cells. It is not yet clear whether the superior stimulatory ability of professional APC relates to the quantity or the quality of stimulatory molecules displayed.

Professional APC such as DC are resident as sentinels in the skin (Langerhans' cells) or in the interstitium of most tissues (interstitial DC) including lymph nodes (interdigitating DC). On encounter with antigen, DC become activated (mature) and migrate centrally via lymphatics to become resident in the T cell areas of lymph nodes (paracortical area) as interdigitating cells. There, T cells recirculating through lymph nodes via lymphatic drainage encounter antigen and clonally proliferate if they carry the appropriate antigen-specific TCR. Subsequently they migrate back to the peripheral tissues and elicit a local immune response. Similar processes occur in the spleen and Peyer's patches. B cells may also be stimulated directly by DC.

CLASSIFICATION OF IMMUNE RESPONSES

Gell and Coombs classified immune responses in the 1930s (Table 6.3). This is of limited clinical usefulness since mixed patterns are always seen but is useful for the general understanding of immunologically mediated diseases.

AUTOIMMUNE DISEASES

An autoimmune disease is one in which an immunological attack directed against self-antigens is primarily responsible for the clinical picture. All autoimmune diseases are disorders of the specific immune response. This definition encompasses diseases which affect multiple systems (also known as non-organ-specific) such as systemic lupus erythematosis (SLE) and those which primarily affect a single organ (organ-specific, e.g. Graves' disease, myaesthenia gravis (MG), autoimmune Addison's).

Table 6.3 Classification of specific immune (hypersensitivity) responses

Type	Mechanism	Clinical example
I	IgE-mediated	Allergy
II	Antibody against cell surface antigens	Some penicillin reactions Haemolytic anaemias
III	Immune complex deposition	Extrinsic allergic alveolitis Serum sickness
IV	Cell-mediated immunity	Delayed type hypersensitivity skin test Contact dermatitis

The immunological effector mechanisms may include direct cellular or humoral responses to an autoantigen, immune complex deposition or interference with normal function of the target antigen (e.g. anti-acetylcholine receptor antibodies in MG, anti-TSH receptor antibodies in autoimmune thyroid disease). Autoimmune diseases are usually more common in women (probably related to oestrogen), may be associated with infections (ankylosing spondylitis, Reiter's, insulin-dependent diabetes), and are associated with certain MHC haplotypes (A1, B8, DR3) or antigens (e.g. B27, DR3, DR4, DQ2). In many diseases there is dysregulation of immune responses to multiple autoantigens, with an increased incidence of autoantibodies and other autoimmune diseases.

SELF-TOLERANCE

T cells recognise antigen together with self-MHC epitopes in the antigen-binding groove of MHC molecules. Strongly self-reactive cells are eliminated (deleted) by encounter with self-antigen on thymic APC (thymic epithelium and DC) in early fetal life. Some self-antigens are probably not expressed in the thymus and remain hidden from the immune system (cryptic epitopes, e.g. intraocular antigens), and tolerance is not established. These antigens tend to reside in immunopriviledged sites, and an immune response does not occur unless released by trauma (e.g. sympathetic ophthalmitis). In adults any cells capable of some degree of self-reactivity which escape deletion in the thymus are probably actively sup-

pressed or made unresponsive (anergised) by mechanisms not yet understood but which involve CD4 (and CD8) positive T cells. Allograft tolerance can be transferred by these cells ('infectious tolerance'). The potential for self-reactivity thus exists in all individuals but is usually prevented from becoming a pathogenic mature immune response. Some anti-self immune responses are involved in 'housekeeping' activities such as the removal of effete RBC. Low titres of non-pathogenic autoantibodies (often IgM isotype) are therefore commonly found in the unwell elderly without any immunological disease.

Autoimmune disease may occur either by reactivation of anergised cells by encounter with potent APCs in certain circumstances which override their programmed unresponsiveness (e.g. where a strong immune response to another antigen results in bystander help sufficient to activate self-reactive T cells in the vicinity), by cross-reactivity between self- and foreign antigens, or as a result of inherited or acquired defects in molecules important in the control of immune responses and maintainance of anergy (e.g. Fas/FasL). The clinical phenotypes of the autoimmunity probably reflect the predominant effector mechanisms and the organ specificity of the antigen(s) and may result in direct damage or interference with normal function. The identity of many autoantigens is now known (Table 6.4). Some are receptors, some enzymes.

Organ-specific autoimmunity manifests itself by damage or malfunction of a single organ as a result of a specific immune response, usually to multiple antigens or to multiple organs on the basis of shared antigens

Table 6.4	Autoantigen specificities and disease	
Disease	Autoantigen	Function
Pemphigus	Desmoglein 1 & 3	Intracellular adhesion (desmosomal cadherin)
Pemphigoid	BPAg 1 & 2	Basement membrane adhesion (hemidesmosome)
Graves' disease	TSHR (stimulator	Hormone receptor
Hypothyroidism	TSHR (blocking)	Hormone receptor
Myasthenia gravis	AcHR	Receptor for neuromuscular transmitter
Goodpasture's	NC domain collagen IV	Basement membrane constituent
Addison's disease	21 hydroxylase 17 hydroxylase Cytochrome p450 side chain cleavage enzyme	Enzymes involved in steroid hormone metabolism (p450SCC shared with ovary/testis)
Autoimmune CAH	p450IID6, p450IIC9, p450IA2	Liver microsomal enzymes
PBC	E2 subunit of pyruvate dehydrogenase	2-oxoacid dehydrogenase pathway in mitochondria

(e.g. steroid cell antibodies linking Addison's disease and premature ovarian failure, or the lung and kidney damage of Goodpasture's syndrome). In some conditions (e.g. myasthenia gravis) humoral responses are responsible for many of the disease manifestations, but are unlikely to occur without cellular responses which may also be important. In other diseases, cellular mechanisms may be the predominant pathogenic responses: e.g. extrinsic allergic encephalomyelitis (EAE, a model for multiple sclerosis) to myelin basic protein (MBP) and other intra-cerebral autoantigens. In systemic autoimmunity such as SLE, pathogenesis is multifactorial and involves multiple unrelated antigens. Humoral and cellular responses to multiple nuclear (nucleosome) and cytoplasmic compo-nents are seen, particularly anti-double-stranded DNA antibodies (dsDNA) which can cause an immune com-plex nephritis, although the precise mechanism is unclear. Sometimes titres of antibodies or complement levels (reduced by immune complex deposition) reflect disease activity in an individual, but in others they do not. In some diseases, the autoantibodies or lymphocytes are patho-genic in models of disease (e.g. anti-dsDNA antibodies in SLE; anti-GBM antibodies in Goodpasture's). In other diseases they are not, and may be secondary markers of damage (e.g. many antinuclear antibodies (ANA) in SLE, antithyroid peroxidase antibodies in thyroid malignancy).

MHC ANTIGENS AND AUTOIMMUNITY

MHC antigens are inherited (along with a package of minor antigens) as a haplotype consisting of an HLA-A, -B, -C (Class I); -DR, -DP, -DQ (Class II) allele from each parent (Fig. 6.7). Allogeneic immune responses (against a foreign MHC antigen from the same species) can be generated after transplantation.

Table 6.5 MHC associations with disease		
Disease	HLA allele	Relative risk
Ankylosing spondylitis	B27	90
Goodpasture's syndrome	DR2	16
Pemphigus vulgaris	DR4	14
Anterior uveitis	B27	10
SLE	DR3	6
Multiple sclerosis	DR2	5
Graves' disease	DR3	4
Rheumatoid arthritis	DR4	4
IDDM	DR3 & 4	3
Myasthenia gravis	DR3	2.5

The MHC may provide predisposition, protection or modify disease expression, and certain alleles or haplo-types are associated with particular diseases (Table 6.5). Both organ-specific and non-organ-specific autoimmune diseases are associated with similar MHC haplotypes in some cases, suggesting an inherited predisposition. This susceptibility may be based on differences in antigen-presentation since the MHC molecules inherited by an individual will alter the strength of immune responses to certain antigens or susceptibility may result from linked genes (such as those for complement proteins C2, C4 and factor B and TNF inherited in the MHC Class III region) (Fig. 6.7). Other genes in the MHC Class III region code the proteasome components LMP2 and LMP7 and the TAP transporter involved in processing and transporting antigens onto the MHC antigens. The closer two genes are in the genome the less likely that they will be sepa-rated by recombination, a phenomenon called linkage disequilibrium. Few MHC associations with diseases are very strong (most strongly B27 and ankylosing spondyli-tis), most conditions are probably the result of a combina-

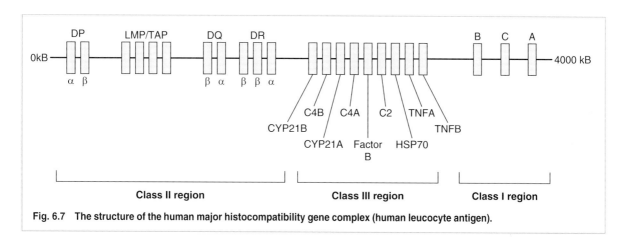

Fig. 6.7 The structure of the human major histocompatibility gene complex (human leucocyte antigen).

tion of genes and additional environmental influences, perhaps including infection. The apparent association of MHC Class I alleles (e.g. HLA-B27) and MHC Class II (e.g. DQB1) may also be due to molecular mimickry between pathogen and MHC, resulting in autoimmune attack. (Heat shock protein (HSP) 60 is widely conserved and generates immune responses in bacterial infection and some autoimmune diseases.)

TRANSPLANTATION

Transplantation is the process of surgically implanting an organ from one individual (donor) into another (recipient). Unfortunately the adaptive immune system treats the new graft like any foreign antigen and mounts a specific immune response to it, resulting in graft rejection. In order to obtain long term acceptance one has to either suppress the recipient immune response or induce a state of tolerance.

The ideal immunosuppressive regime would be donor-specific (no impairment of defence mechanisms against pathogens, no increase in malignancy, and no impairment of responses to a third party allograft). As yet this is only achieved in animal models. Some degree of toler-ance is implied by long term microchimaerism in human recipients of solid organ and bone marrow grafts, where recipient macrophages/DC replace donor ones in the solid organ graft and donor APC may migrate into the lymphoid tissues of the new host. This observation gave rise to the hypothesis that microchimaerism is important in maintaining long term graft acceptence by maintaining tolerance. However it is equally possible that this long term persistance of donor cells results from immuno-suppression or tolerance rather than being its cause.

Graft alloantigens may be displayed to T cells by direct presentation (donor HLA antigen is recognised directly on the surface of donor APC, either as an antigen fragment in donor HLA molecules or by direct stimula-tion of the TCR by the allogeneic HLA molecule) or indirect presentation (processed antigen fragments of donor HLA are phagocytosed, digested and presented on recipient APC, in the antigen-binding grooves of recipient HLA molecules, as is the case with any other antigen, and this process is dependent on surface co-stimulatory molecules on the APC). The direct pathway predominates in graft rejection, at least initially.

TRANSPLANTATION BARRIER

The means to provide a more widely available transplant programme between unrelated donors began with ABO

and HLA matching, immunosuppressive drugs, and may continue with xenograft technology. Non-self antigens are subject to immune-mediated attack by adaptive humoral and cellular mechanisms. The most important antigens are those most widely expressed on the graft, e.g. ABO blood group antigens, and those eliciting strong responses, e.g. disparate MHC antigens (allogeneic response). Any other polymorphic cell surface molecule on the graft which is not expressed by the recipient will also elicit an immune response. In the case of cross-species grafting (xenogeneic transplantation), rejection response is even stronger as a result of increased disparity between the MHC molecules and the presence of broadly reactive anticarbohydrate antibodies which bind to the graft and cause hyperacute rejection.

The aim of immunosuppression is to depress the effec-tor immune response to prevent graft rejection (at least initially). The hope is that subsequently either tolerance or graft acceptance will result from downregulation of the antigraft response and enable withdrawal of immuno-suppression. The aim of ABO-matching and HLA-matching (tissue typing) is to reduce the antigenic disparity between the graft and the recipient. Since at least four important HLA antigens are inherited from each parent (HLA-A, HLA-B, HLA-C, HLA-DR) as a haplotype, an ideal match (such as that from an identical twin) will be matched for all eight alleles. Other antigens clearly exist, but matching for these is not currently prac-ticable; however, genetic linkage of genes means that related donors with a haplotype match are likely to share the same non-MHC genes. The same is not true of appar-ently HLA-matched unrelated donors, who may have differences in other genes. The technique for determining the HLA-type is important. The serological techniques for HLA Class-I matching may be unable to distinguish between certain alleles, and apparent identity may miss minor differences in sequence which can be recognised by the immune system. In general, molecular techniques such as oligonucleotide probes are more specific.

Cyclosporin A (CsA), a fungal metabolite, prolonged survival of renal transplants in man in the late 1970s. By this time, however, graft survival from living related donors had reached a plateau, suggesting that early graft survival results from ABO matching and immunosup-pressive drugs, with some contribution from HLA-DR matching (which is more effective than HLA-B or HLA-A matching). Some have therefore argued that the benefit of HLA matching is insignificant with modern immuno-suppressive drug regimes; however, it appears that long term graft survival appears more dependent on HLA-A and -B matching (Fig. 6.8).

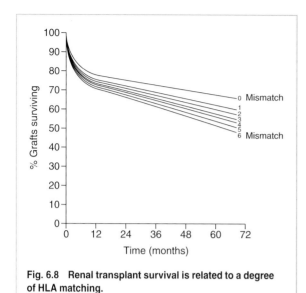

Fig. 6.8 Renal transplant survival is related to a degree of HLA matching.

Solid organ grafts contain passenger leucocytes, including lymphocytes and APC. The most important passenger leucocytes in the graft are dendritic cells expressing high levels of MHC Class II. Experimental depletion of these APC pretransplant improves graft survival, but this strategy is not in routine use in human transplantation.

MATCHING

Currently, renal transplants are matched for ABO blood group, direct cross-match for anti-HLA alloantibodies and HLA matching (Table 6.6). Cross-matching is usually performed using lymphocytotoxicity assays for HLA Class I reactive IgG and IgM lytic antibodies (predictive of antibody-mediated hyperacute rejection). Recipient sera are stored at intervals while awaiting a donor for retrospective analysis. Flow cytometric cross-match may be better in previously sensitised patients and is non-lytic. The accuracy of HLA typing depends on technology employed. HLA-DR matching confers better protection against graft loss in the first year than HLA-A or -B in the presence of cyclosporin. HLA-DR mismatch increases graft loss by five-fold, HLA-B mismatch by three-fold and HLA-A mismatch by two-fold. However this translates to only a minor (3–5%) increment in graft survival when immuosuppression with cyclosporin A is used, and it is often better to use a fresh but mismatched kidney locally rather than endure prolonged ischaemic time in search of a better match elsewhere.

REJECTION

A renal transplant is most likely to be lost in the first 3 months, but rejection is only one possible cause of graft loss. Most patients have at least one episode of acute rejection. Major immunologically mediated antitransplant responses can be directed against several antigens, including A, B, O blood group antigens, MHC Class I and II molecules and cell-surface carbohydrates (e.g. alpha-gal in xenogeneic transplantation) (Fig. 6.9). Antitransplant responses can also occur against other cell-surface antigens which are poorly defined and for which matching is currently not performed except serendipitously in transplants from identical twins or close relatives. The presence of a non-self MHC on a cell surface will generate a strong allogeneic cellular and humoral immune response. 50% of renal grafts have at least one episode of acute rejection. Paradoxically, this response is even stronger if the source is the MHC of another species (xenogeneic response). This recognition of allogeneic MHC/antigen combinations is difficult to explain since T cells are self-restricted (i.e. designed only to recognise antigen and self-MHC combinations) and a T cell restricted to one HLA-A allele (an allele is one version of a gene) will not usually recognise the same antigen on a different HLA-A allele. The fact that each HLA allelic variant will bind a different set of self-peptides increases the likelihood of a strong response provided the recipient's T cells can interact with the allogeneic MHC. In practice, between 1 in 10 to 1 in 1000 T cells can recognise allogeneic MHC molecules, possibly due to cross-reactivity of different antigen/MHC combinations.

Hyperacute rejection

Hyperacute rejection is caused by pre-existing, complement-fixing antibodies. Rapid allograft rejection (coagulopathy, infarction and neutrophil infiltrate mediated by antibody and complement) occurs within minutes or hours and is caused by IgG anti-HLA Class I (not IgM), or ABO antibodies (hence utility of cross-matching and ABO matching pretransplant). There is no effective therapy except prevention by screening allograft recipients and rapid graft excision once established.

Pre-existing 'natural antibodies' in xenogeneic transplants are usually IgM and IgG anti-α-gal which is expressed by the graft but not on human cells. These xenogeneic antibodies are probably formed by exposure to bacterial capsular polysaccharides. Neutralising complement effector function by producing transgenic animals which express cell-surface human complement regulatory genes (CD46, CD55, CD59), which prevent lysis by the terminal attack complex, is a potential solution.

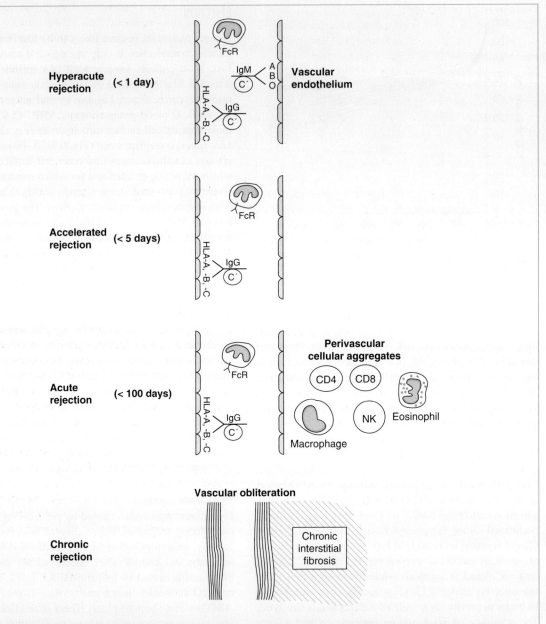

Fig. 6.9 Mechanisms of graft rejection. Hyperacute and accelerated rejection appear to be predominantly mediated by antibodies and complement. Acute rejection appears to be mediated by humoral and cellular mechanisms. The vasculopathy of chronic rejection is of unknown aetiology.

Accelerated rejection (< 5 days)

Accelerated rejection is usually mediated by pre-existing non-complement-fixing anti-HLA antibodies in sensitised patients. Flow cytometry may pick up positive cross-matches missed by standard lymphocytotoxicity testing. Early biopsy reveals interstitial cellular or vascular rejection. Some centres biopsy high risk grafts early to pick this up. Antilymphocyte agents such as OKT3 may be effective but less so than for acute rejection.

Acute rejection (< 100 days)

Acute rejection probably represents a combination of T cell effector function (cellular rejection) and antibody-mediated endothelial damage (acute vascular rejection). The antibodies involved include IgM isohaemagglutinins in ABO mismatch and IgG anti-HLA Class I antibodies in multiparous or previously transfused/transplanted patients. IgM anti-Class I antibodies do not appear to adversely affect graft survival, even if they can lyse in vitro. Thus ABO cross-matching and pretransplant recipient screening for anti-donor-HLA Class I is essential for renal and heart/lung recipients. Some centres also screen for anti-HLA Class II, but the significance of these antibodies is controversial. Peak antibody titres may wane with time while awaiting renal transplantation, but in view of the possibility of recrudescent immunological memory, screening is often performed against this peak serum as well as the current serum. Anti-HLA antibodies are not looked for in all transplant types. Liver transplants are relatively insensitive to HLA Class I mismatches, and cross-matching is not practical in others because of constraints of time and limited donor availability. Hepatocytes may be protected by low level surface HLA expression or the secretion of soluble blocking Class I molecules. Acute rejection reflects major antigenic disparity between graft and recipient. In renal cellular rejection, most T cells are usually CD8 positive, yet the process is thought to be primarily driven by CD4 positive Th1 cells which recruit and activate effectors such as monocyte/macrophages, eosinophils, NK cells and cytotoxic T cells, and CD8 positive T cells are not essential for experimental graft rejection. There is usually tubulitis (invasion of tubules) with interstitial oedema and infiltration.

In antibody-mediated vascular rejection there is endothelial damage (fibrinoid necrosis, fibrin and platelet thrombi if severe) with lymphocytic vascular invasion and perivenous aggregates. Initially rejection may be focal and be missed by a biopsy needle.

Early treatment with high dose corticosteroids (pulsed doses of methyl prednisolone) is effective within 2–4 days in most cases. In steroid-resistant rejection ALG, ATG, or OKT3 may be effective.

Chronic rejection (> 100 days)

Chronic rejection may reflect antibody responses to antigen mismatches which are not effectively suppressed by immunosuppressive agents, unlike acute rejection. The greater the mismatch (especially for HLA-DR) the more severe the chronic rejection, and number of acute rejection episodes correlates with the likelihood of chronic rejection (50% of renal recipients with one or more rejection episodes show some chronic rejection within 5 years). Reduction of immunosuppression accelerates rejection, suggesting an immunological mechanism. 3–5% of allogeneic renal grafts are lost annually after the first year. Chronic renal rejection is a poorly understood vasculopathy of medium and small arterioles, to which hypertension, hyperlipidaemia and infection may contribute. Similar vascular changes occur in heart and lung transplantation. Vessels are thickened with elastic reduplication and intimal proliferation, medial necrosis and fibrin deposition. Cellular infiltrates are infrequent, but interstitial fibrosis occurs. There is no effective therapy.

Recurrence of original disease

Recurrence is infrequent in immunologically mediated disease, since graft recipients are heavily immunosuppressed. Latent infections may recrudesce however.

Donor-specific tolerance

A form of tolerance (antigen-specific immunological unresponsiveness) occurs in a few long term human renal transplant recipients who can discontinue immunosuppressive drugs without graft loss. Although induction of tolerance would be a long term goal for transplantation, there is as yet no reliable method to induce this.

Until 25 years ago blood transfusion was avoided if possible because of the risk of allosensitisation (in 20–30%) of the potential renal graft recipient which would restrict the number of suitable donors. However, transfusion paradoxically gave a survival benefit to the graft, perhaps as a result of specific induction of tolerance. Early work suggested that transfusion can induce alloantigen-specific tolerance, improving graft survival in heart and renal transplantation (if there was a single DR match). However, the benefit is modest, and it has rarely been used since the introduction of cyclosporin (CsA), because a similar improvement in graft survival is achieved by the drug without the risk of allosensitisation, and there is no evidence that transfusion brings additional benefit to most patients. Tolerance in T cells has been induced in rodents by blocking APC/T cell interaction using CsA or monoclonal antibodies (mAbs) directed against T cell markers (CD4/8 or adhesion/costimulator molecules CD18/11a/CD54/CTLA-4/CD80); this may turn stimulatory antigen presentation into anergy-inducing non-professional presentation, which is later maintained by the graft. An alternative hypothesis is that persisting donor APC (microchimaerism) are essential to the survival of the graft and maintainance of tolerance, and augmenting these with simultaneous BMT (containing DC precursors) has been tried, with minimal success.

RENAL TRANSPLANTATION

Renal transplantation is used for end stage renal failure with > 90% loss of nephrons and severe uraemia. Glomerulonephritis, pyelonephritis, interstitial nephritis, adult polycystic disease and diabetes are the most common causes in all age ranges. Usually an ABO-matched HLA Class I and Class II compatible cadaveric donor (maintained on life support and clinically brain dead) is used, occasionally a live first-degree relative is the donor. HLA-matching is not the only factor important for successful grafting (Tables 6.6 and 6.7, Fig. 6.8); adequate cold preservation, with minimal cold ischaemic time (up to 48 h) and minimal warm ischaemia during reperfusion, is also important. Heart, liver and two kidneys may be retrieved, flushed with cold storage solution and stored on ice. Lymph node and spleen are taken from the donor for tissue typing (because they are rich in lymphocytes). The extraperitoneal right iliac fossa pouch is now the most common site for renal transplantation, and immuno-suppression is started 4–12 h before transplantation. Twin–twin transplants were known to work in skin grafting, and 29 such renal transplants were performed in Boston up to 1976 with a 20 year survival rate of 50% for both patients and grafts. Cadaver grafts or those from living but unrelated donors all failed by 12 years, and only 40% were still functioning at 1 year. Transplants from living and related donors, however, had a 40% chance of functioning at 17 years.

Table 6.6 Matching criteria for transplantation

Organ	ABO	XMI	A	B	C	DR	DQ	XMII
Kidney	y	y	y	y	y	y	n	n
BM	n	n	y	y	y	y	y	n
Heart	y	n	n	n	n	n[a]	n	n
Lung	y	n	n[a]	n[a]	n[a]	n[a]	n	?
Heart/lung	y	n	n[a]	n[a]	n[a]	n[a]	n	?
Liver	y	n[a]	n[a]	n[a]	n[a]	n[a]	n	n
Small bowel	y	y	n[a]	n[a]	n[a]	n[a]	n	?
Pancreas	y	y	n	n	n	n	n	n
Cornea	n	n	n[b]	n[b]	n	n	n	n

HLA XM in heart transplantation if highly sensitised recipient only (10–20% panel reactive).
n[a] not routine but may retrospectively determine need for immunosuppression / risk of rejection.
n[b] only for vascularised high risk grafts.

Table 6.7 Landmarks in human renal transplantation

Date	Procedure
1902	First successful autologous kidney transplant (lasted 5 days), Ullman
1908	Functional canine renal homografts excised and replaced, Carrel
1936	First human to human kidney transplant (failed), Voronoy
1942	Immunological rejection of skin grafts demonstrated by Medawar & Gibson
1951	Plastic-encased renal allograft transplantation into the thigh, some with prednisolone cover (one graft functioned for 5½ months), USA
1951	Eight iliac fossa grafts anastomosing renal to iliac vessels (failed), France
1950s	Six mercaptopurine and steroids used
1954	Human twin–twin transplant (functioned for 8 years), Murray, USA
1958	Mercaptopurine (MP) postpones canine renal allograft rejection
1958	Total body irradiation, results poor
1960	Azathioprine (6-MP derivative) developed
1963	Prednisolone and azathioprine (6-MP derivative) in canine renal allografts
1978	Cyclosporin prolongs renal graft survival, Calne

BONE MARROW TRANSPLANTATION

The ideal is to obtain complete HLA-A, -B, -DR, -DQ matching by serological and PCR techniques for the best possible match using first degree relatives or volunteer donor panels. There is a much higher risk of graft-versus-host disease than in solid organ grafts, because of the transplantation of immunocompetent donor T cells. Best results are seen with haplotype-matched first degree relatives. Unrelated donors, who inevitably include other antigen mismatches even if HLA match appears good, have a worse prognosis. Therefore if the donor is un-related, only a single minor mismatch is allowed, whereas if the donor is related a single antigen major mismatch may be accepted.

HEART TRANSPLANTATION

Cardiac transplantation for end-stage cardiac disease began in 1967 and now has a 75% 5-year survival. HLA matching is usually impractical due to limited organ preservation times (4–6 h) and low organ availablility, but a known positive anti-HLA antibody cross-match contraindicates transplantation.

HLA-DR matching may reduce early cardiac rejection, but it is uncertain whether this improves survival or reduces the accelerated atherosclerosis seen in 40% of recipients at 5 years (also seen in chronic rejection of kidneys and liver). It is hypothesised that accelerated atherosclerosis may be immune-mediated and secondary to endothelial damage, since it is worse in MHC Class I mismatches and allosensitised individuals. Antiplatelet drugs may slow progression, but retransplantation is the main therapeutic option. Immunosuppressive requirements are stricter than for renal transplants, with CsA, steroids, azathioprine, and ATG (antithymocyte globulin) or Campath (a lytic monoclonal antibody directed against surface CD52 on all leucocytes) being used. 85% of recipients get one or more rejection episodes. Weekly endomyocardial biopsies may be performed to monitor rejection. Focal and perivascular interstitial lymphocyte infiltrates (neutrophils if severe) are seen in rejection, similar to renal rejection. Rejection may be aborted with steroids, ATG or OKT3. Infections are the most common cause of death within 3 months of transplantation.

LUNG TRANSPLANTATION

Single lung tranplantation is used in some interstitial lung diseases. Matching criteria are the same as for heart–lung transplantation, with a 2 year survival of 60%. No hyperacute rejection has been documented, but there is no time to cross-match anyway due to time constraints on organ preservation (< 6 h). Acute cellular rejection produces perivascular lymphocytic infiltrates and bronchiolitis. Chronic rejection produces bronchiolitis obliterans.

LIVER TRANSPLANTATION

This is used for end-stage liver failure. Cross-matching is not routinely done for anti-HLA antibodies although a positive cross-match for anti-HLA Class I antibodies may predispose to chronic rejection. The degree of HLA-A, -B, -DR, -DQ mismatch may determine the need for immunosuppression retrospectively. Re-infection of the graft is a particular problem with liver transplantation for end-stage hepatitis B or C infection in the immunosuppressed recipient. Autoimmune diseases such as primary biliary cirrhosis (PBC) or autoimmune chronic active hepatitis (AICAH) rarely recur in the graft. CsA, corticosteroids, azathioprine, tacrolimus and OKT3 are used for immunosuppression and treatment of acute rejection. Chronic rejection produces intraluminal biliary fibrosis analogous to the vasculopathy in other types of organ transplantation.

SMALL BOWEL TRANSPLANTATION

This is a potential solution for intestinal failure. The small bowel contains large amount of lymphoid tissue as Peyer's patches and mesenteric lymph nodes, thus rejection and graft-versus-host disease are a greater problem than with other organs, and the bowel is very intolerant of ischaemia. In addition the infection risk is high because the bacteria in the gut translocate easily across damaged mucosa, causing sepsis. A combined small bowel and liver graft may be performed. Graft survival is improved by CsA, prednisolone, azathioprine, OKT3, and tacrolimus. Prostaglandin (PGE1) infusion may be beneficial. Graft survival of up to 75% has been reported at 1 year. Cadaveric donors with minimal graft cold ischaemia (< 6 h) are used. Acute and chronic rejection occurs.

PANCREATIC ISLET TRANSPLANTATION

ABO and anti-HLA Class I cross-matching are essential for this tissue. No other matching is practicable for vascularised gland or isolated islet cells. The latter approach excludes passenger leucocytes and reduces rejection potential. The islets themselves do not express costimulator molecules and thus do not invoke rejection (and may even tolerise the host). Loss of APC is accelerated experimentally by in-vitro culture in 95% oxygen or UV irradiation before transplantation. There has been little clinical success in humans as yet, perhaps because the transplant becomes susceptible to the same autoimmune assault endured by the original pancreas.

CORNEAL TRANSPLANTATION

No matching is required, because this non-vascular graft is made to a relatively immunoprivileged site. The graft can be stored for 28 days. HLA-A and -B matching is used only for high risk grafts with previous rejection or a vascularised corneal bed, but the effectiveness is disputed. Topical corticosteroids are the main means of preventing rejection, but oral cyclosporin may be used in high risk patients. Rejection is treated with increased topical treatment or intravenous methylprednisolone, but success rates of 98% at 5 years are achieved.

HEART–LUNG TRANSPLANTATION

The main advantage of this approach (for lung disease, cystic fibrosis and pulmonary hypertension) over lung transplantation is not immunological but preservation of tracheal blood supply. 2 year survival for heart–lung transplants approaches 50%. HLA matching is impracticable due to the cold ischaemia time limit of 6 h. HLA-A, -B, -DR, -DQ matching may determine the level of immunosuppression required subsequently. Immunosuppressive regimes are similar to those of heart transplantation. The lungs are very vascular and susceptible to immunological attack, showing the first signs of rejection. Monitoring of graft function (FEV1, PO_2, CXR), bronchiolar lavage and transbronchial biopsy for the interstitial perivascular mononuclear infiltrates of rejection are used. Obliterative bronchiolitis occurs in 50% of recipients at 8–12 months as result of chronic rejection with intimal vasculopathy. Obliterative bronchiolitis is treated with steroids and ATG, but the prognosis is poor.

IMMUNOSUPPRESSION IN TRANSPLANTATION

In the absence of mechanisms for producing donor-specific tolerance, we are left to fall back on general impairment of the host immune responses in order to prevent immune-mediated graft rejection. These drugs, however, predispose the patient to infections and neoplasia (Table 6.8). Post-transplantation EBV positive lymphoproliferative disorders are increased with prolonged immunosuppression (particularly with ATG, ALG, OKT3, CsA) and in those with primary EBV infections post-transplantation.

The mode of action of immunosuppressive drugs is described later. Azathioprine was first used in renal trans-

plantation in the 1960s. Corticosteroids are still used for their multiple anti-inflammatory and immunomodulatory effects. CsA and, more recently, FK506 (tacrolimus) have markedly improved the outlook in clinical solid organ transplantation. Antilymphocyte immunoglobulins (ALG, ATG) and anti-T cell monoclonal antibodies (ATG, Campath, OKT3) are effective in T cell depleting bone marrow and treating cellular rejection. Newer drugs such as mycophenolic acid, rapamycin, Brequinar, 15-deoxyspergualin, and anticostimulatory or adhesion molecules on T cell and APC surfaces are promising new alternatives, the latter holding out the possibility of specific tolerance induction.

GRAFT-VERSUS-HOST DISEASE (GVHD)

The transfer of immunologically competent T cells (and their precursors) may result in an attack on the host by donor lymphocytes. These cells clonally proliferate in the new host. This is a major problem in bone marrow transplantation but is also occasionally seen in solid organ transplantation (particularly small bowel) depending on the number of lymphoid cells in the graft. Acute GVHD (onset < 100 days post-transplant) may resolve with treatment. Chronic GVHD (> 100 days) is an aggressive disease with autoimmune-like features and multiple organ involvement with fibrosis. Preventative drug strategies, including methotrexate and CsA, are mandatory for allogeneic bone marrow transplantation, and some

Table 6.8	Infections in immunosuppressed transplant recipients			
Transplant	Infection / site	Bacterial	Fungal	Viral
Renal	Pyelonephritis Pneumonia Bacteraemia	Gram negative enteric Enterococci Staphylococci Streptococci	Candida Aspergillus Cryptococcus	CMV HSV-1/2 EBV
Heart–lung	Pneumonia Mediatinitis Bacteraemia	Staphylococci Streptococci Gram negative enteric Pseudomonas (lung)	Aspergillus Candida Cryptococcus (lung)	CMV HSV-1/2 EBV Adenovirus
Liver	Hepatic/abdo abscess Cholangitis Bacteraemia	Gram negative enteric Enterococci Staphylococci	Candida Aspergillus	CMV HSV 1/2 EBV Adenovirus Hep B & C
Bone marrow	Bacteraemia Pneumonia Multiple sites	Gram negative enteric Staphylococci Streptococci Mycoplasma	Candida Aspergillus Cryptococci	CMV HSV 1/2 EBV Parvovirus

estimation of risk can be made from specialised quantitation of precursors of cytotoxic recipient-reactive T cells in the donor (CTLPp). The mechanisms regulating the balance between long term chimaerism, where donor lymphoid cells persist in the new host without damage, and GVHD are unknown.

TUMOUR IMMUNOBIOLOGY

It has been assumed for many years that the immune system is important in the suppression of neoplastic growth. Immunodeficient or immunosuppressed individuals (particularly those with T cell dysfunction and renal recipients treated with OKT3) have a clearly increased incidence of certain tumours (viral(EBV)-induced B cell lymphomas and non-viral lymphoid tumours). Some primary antibody-deficient patients (CVID) also have an increased incidence of neoplasia (particularly stomach and B cell non-Hodgkin's lymphoma (NHL)). HIV infection has increased knowledge of the role of intact immunity in tumour suppression and refocused attention in the potential role of oncogenic viruses such as HPV 16/18 (cervical cancer), EBV (Burkitt's lymphoma), HTLV-1 (T cell leukaemia) and HSV-8 (Kaposi's sarcoma) in producing tumours in man.

Virally or chemically induced tumours are most immunogenic; but tumours are very heterogeneous, with many eliciting little or no specific immunity. Melanoma, renal cell carcinoma and lymphomas appear most susceptible to immune surveillance, which is predominantly mediated by CD8 positive cytotoxic T lymphocytes and NK cells. Many tumours evade immune responses by low expression of immunogenic molecules such as HLA, by the secretion of immunomodulatory cytokines or the direct induction of anergy in reactive lymphocytes. Many tumours continue to grow despite the activities of tumour-infiltrating lymphocytes (TIL). A unique tumour antigen for cellular immune responses is necessary in order to enhance specific immune responses against a tumour. A variety of tumour antigens and approaches have been used for immunologically mediated therapy in recent years. Suitable antigens for immunotherapy are either uniquely expressed in a neoplastic cell or heavily overexpressed in the tumour.

IMMUNE SURVEILLANCE

In immune surveillance, the immune system is able to recognise variants from normal antigen expression and focus an immunologically mediated attack on them. The

Table 6.9 Immune avoidance by tumours

Strategy	Mechanism
Reduced HLA Class I expression	Allelic loss under selection pressure Virus mediated (adenovirus) Oncogene mediated Reduction of TAP transporters
Induction of anergy	Tumour acting as non-professional APC
Immunosuppressive factors	Endogenous TGFβ, IL-10 Viral IL-10 (EBV) Endogenous prostaglandin E2
Immunoprivileged sites	CNS, testis, ovary
Immunocompromised host	Old age, HIV infection, drugs, pregnancy

antigens recognised include overexpressed tissue-specific antigens, mutated self-antigens, or normally repressed antigens to which tolerance has not been established (e.g. BCR/ABL, p53, C-myc, p21Ras, MAGE-1, MART-1, gp100). Since tumours are clonal populations, often with a high mutation rate, it is possible for immunological election pressure to favour the evolution of less immunogenic variants (immunological escape). Many tumours evade effective immune responses by a variety of mechanisms (Table 6.9)

TUMOUR MARKERS

Any soluble circulating antigen in serum or plasma measurable by biochemical or immunoassay can be used as a tumour marker. Most are proteins secreted in excess, and thus are not absolutely specific for any given tumour, interpretation depending on the absolute level. They are thus often more suited to monitoring response to treatment rather than diagnostic screening. Some are cytokines or hormones secreted by the tumour (e.g. β human chorionic gonadotrophin, alpha-fetoprotein) others are cell surface antigens shed into the circulation (e.g. cell surface mucins in adenocarcinomas, CA125, CA159). Levels generally reflect tumour mass. Many also have non-neoplastic sources and can be affected by non-specific inflammation, liver disease, etc.

TUMOUR IMMUNOTHERAPY

Attempts to use the immune system to treat tumours have utilised several approaches: (1) use of specific antibodies or cells to attack tumour cells, (2) induction of antitumour immune responses, or (3) enhancement of pre-existing antitumour responses, both innate and specific (Table 6.10).

Passive antibody immunotherapy

The detection of tumour-specific surface antigens may enable the use of targeted therapies where a monoclonal antibody is the carrier molecule which specifically directs and concentrates a therapeutic drug, prodrug, toxin, or isotope to the neoplasm. In practice the specificity of the toxin or isotope on the conjugate molecule is not absolute and there is some collateral damage to normal tissue. This technique has been used with some success in B cell lymphomas, with conjugates targeted to B cell specific surface molecules such as CD22. In addition, the antibodies may attach to Fc receptors of effector cells and recruit additional cellular effectors. This technique is also of use in radioimaging of tumours.

Vaccination

Attempts to vaccinate with crude cell extracts and tumour specific antigens have been made with some success but depend on the existence and isolation of a relatively tumour specific antigen. Virally induced tumours can be reduced by preventing primary infection by vaccination (e.g. hepatitis B).

Cellular immunotherapy

Certain tumours are susceptible to the action of activated CD8 positive cytotoxic T lymphocytes and NK cells, both in animal models and humans. Adoptive transfer or cellular immunotherapy is an attempt to activate or clonally expand pre-existing tumour specific T and NK cells in vitro. One form is called lymphokine-activated killer cells (LAK) because IL-2 is used in their generation in vitro. Unfortunately this form of therapy requires isolation and sterile in-vitro expansion of PBMC or T cells using IL-2 before re-infusion into the patient. It is a

cumbersome, individualised, tumour specific therapy, and impractical for general usage.

Gene therapy

Animal models suggest that the direct conversion of poorly immunogenic tumours into potent APC may enhance effective tumour specific immunity. This can be accomplished by transfection of cytokine genes such as TNFα, IL-2, IL-4, IFNγ, GM-CSF or costimulatory molecules such as B-7 (CD80). This has yet to be shown to be of use in humans.

Another strategy to enhance the induction of anti-tumour responses is to transfect skeletal muscle with the DNA sequence of a tumour specific antigen. The skeletal muscle cell transiently expresses the antigen and acts as an APC. A costimulatory molecule may be transfected simultaneously. This approach is currently undergoing phase I studies in man and can induce immune responses against B cell lymphomas using transfected sequences of the patient's own immunoglobulin idiotype (i.e. using the antigen-binding region of the immunoglobulin of the B cell clone as the immunogen). This is a cumbersome, individualised therapy for each patient.

APC enhancement

Another approach is to attempt to boost the immune repsonse of the host by the use of potent autologous professional APC which have been pulsed with tumour antigen. This works well in animal models and is being developed for use in man. There is also the possibility of enhancing APC activity by using cytokines, or targeting gene transfection to APC using lineage-specific promotors.

Cytokine immunotherapy

This is used in an attempt to boost cellular (T and NK) immune responses in the tumour host or to alter the

Table 6.10 Strategies for immunomodulation	
Strategy	Action
Specific cancer vaccine	Vaccinate with tumour/virus specific antigens
Targeted immunotherapy	Use antibodies to target drug or radiation therapy to specific tumour or tissue
Viral vaccine	Prevent primary infection and thus viral induced tumours
Enhance tumour immunogenicity	Gene transfection with costimulator or cytokine genes to enhance local imune responses
Cellular adoptive immunotherapy	IL-2, PHA or CD3 activated LAK, PBMC, CD8+ T cells, TIL
Boost general cellular immunity	Cytokine, infusions, e.g. IL-2 to activate NK cells and other cellular effectors

immunogenicity of the tumour cells. IL-2 therapy has been used in melanoma and renal carcinoma with very limited success, and significant side effects. IL-12 and IL-7 are currently being assessed. The local release of IFNγ as a result of cytokine exposure may enhance the susceptibility of some tumour cells to lysis.

IMMUNODEFICIENCY

An immunodeficiency is an impaired ability to mount effective immune responses to infectious agents. These may be global (affecting T cells, B cells and phagocytes) or may affect one or more components of specific (severe combined immunodeficiency (SCID), primary antibody deficiencies (PAD)) or non-specific (chronic granulomatous disease, CGD) defences. Impaired immunity may be primary (e.g. primary antibody deficiencies) or secondary (to disease, drugs, infection). The majority are secondary to other conditions. Immunodeficiency results in differing types of infections (bacterial, viral, fungal) depending on the defence mechanisms affected (Table 6.11).

SECONDARY IMMUNODEFICIENCY

There are multiple causes of secondary immunodeficiency (Fig. 6.10). It is well recognised that lymphopro-

liferative disease, including chronic lymphatic leukaemia (CLL) and myeloma, result in impairment of specific adaptive immunity in later stages of disease progression, and increased susceptibility to bacterial infection. Non-neoplastic diseases such as systemic lupus erythematosis (SLE) or rheumatoid arthritis (RA) show an inherently increased susceptibility to infections, although the direct cause of the impairment is unknown. Drug therapy is an important cause of immunosuppression affecting both specific and innate mechanisms. Infections can cause immunosuppression either directly (e.g. HIV-induced T cell destruction) or indirectly (EBV, CMV).

Inflammation can cause transient impairment of responses — e.g. after surgery, trauma, burns (where there is also loss of serum proteins) — and increased susceptibility to infection, although abnormalities of functional assays are usually more pronounced than clinical problems (depressed CMI skin tests, depressed in-vitro lymphocyte proliferations, alterations in granulocyte and NK functions), reflecting the plasticity of the immune response as a whole. Postoperative infections in patients given perioperative blood transfusions appear to be increased due to an ill-defined immunosuppressive effect of some component of the blood given (RBC or WBC).

Secondary immunodeficiency as a result of surgery

The most common way a surgical procedure predisposes to infection is by breaching a mucosal barrier. In addi-

Table 6.11 Immunodeficiency and infection				
	Infections	Primary defect	Secondary defect
Neutrophils (neutropenia)	Endogenous bacteria, including *Pseudomonas*	Autoimmune neutropenia, cyclical neutropenia	Drug-induced neutropenia
Neutrophils (functional defect)	Catalase positive *Staphylococcus*, *Salmonella*, *Aspergillus*	CGD, LAD	
Complement	Bacteria (*Neisseria meningitidis*)	Specific complement component deficiency	
Macrophages	Atypical mycobacteria		HIV
T cells (generalised defect)	Viruses, fungi, mycobacteria, *Pneumocystis*, *Listeria*, etc.	SCID, Di George	HIV, immunosuppressive drugs
T cells (specific defect)	*Candida*	CMC	
B and T cells (combined)	Encapsulated bacteria + opportunists (variable)	HIV (children), some SCID, some CVI, HIGM	Drug induced immunosuppression
B cells (generalised)	Encapsulated bacteria (also loss of protection against viruses)	XLA, CVI,	CLL, myeloma
B cells (specific defect)	Encapsulated bacteria	Specific antibody deficiency to polysaccharide antigens	

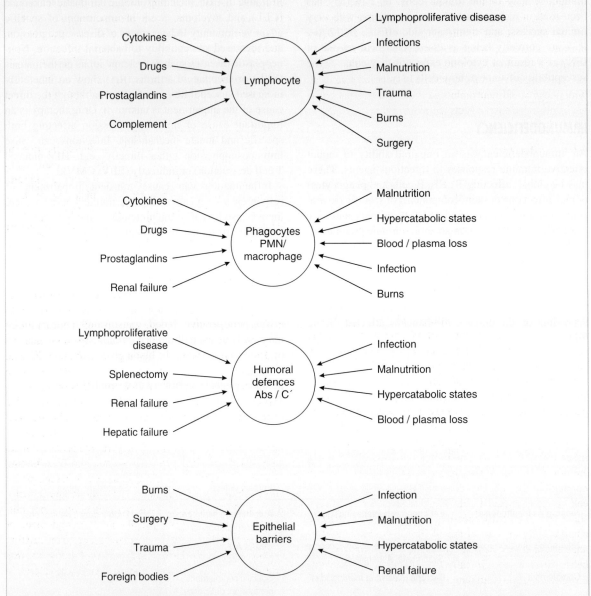

Fig. 6.10 The causes of secondary immunodeficiency. Many causes of secondary immunodeficiency act on several different components of the immune response.

tion, barriers may be compromised by haemorrhagic shock or jaundice, gut immobility, ischaemia, burns or malnutrition resulting in defective killing of organisms by phagocytes, with subsequent penetration across mucosa (translocation), perhaps inside macrophages or neutrophils. The presence of drains or other foreign bodies also provides both routes of entry and niduses of infection. Surgery results in severe metabolic alterations

with an initial hypometabolic phase followed by a hyper-metabolic phase. 6–7% of body weight may be lost in the first 3 days after major gut surgery. There is a potential for infection from endogenous or exogenous sources. A similar impairment of specific and innate defence mechanisms operates in trauma and generalised inflammatory responses due to disease or infection, but in elective surgery careful attempts to maintain homeostasis during the period of anaesthesia may reduce this impairment. The precise causes of immunosuppression are unknown but may involve circulating cytokines, loss of blood or plasma (depleting immunoglobulins or complement), hypercatabolic states, or renal and hepatic failure. These effects make it important to perform functional studies on lymphocytes and neutrophils at times when a patient is well. These multiple effects are sometimes referred to as surgical stress

Cellular effects of surgical stress

In vivo there is delayed-type hypersensitivity (DTH) skin test anergy in postsurgical patients, and impairment is more frequent in those with a worse outcome, although it is not clear if this is cause or effect. Patients with burns, viral infections and sarcoidosis all have variable and transient depression of DTH to unrelated antigens, but have other reasons to be susceptible to infections. Likewise, in-vitro T cell IL-2 production and antigen specific proliferation are inversely related to the severity of injury. T cells are activated (increased CD25 (IL-2R) expression), but proliferation (specific antigen, allogeneic cells and mitogens) is generally impaired, perhaps due to soluble factors (complement fragments or cytokines), which can suppress neutrophil chemotaxis and NK cell activity.

Lymphocyte numbers are not consistently altered by surgical stress. CD4 T cell numbers only fall in major trauma (by day 2–4). This may be reflected in the total lymphocyte count. This phenomenon may result from redistribution of cells to peripheral organs or lymphoid tissue rather than a decline in numbers. CD4/CD8 ratios are not useful, since they reflect a dynamic ratio of two populations and take no account of absolute numbers. NK cell numbers appear stable. B cell numbers may remain stable or transiently decline. Some of the observed changes may be due to the pharmacological effects of anaesthetic drugs, which can reduce proliferation of B cells. There is no clinically useful correlation between these observations and outcome of surgery.

Cytokine effects of surgical stress

Failure to produce cytokines such as IL-1 and IL-2 is associated with fatal outcomes. There also appears to be decreased production of IFNγ in trauma, which may impair phagocyte activation and B cell proliferation and increase immunosuppressive PGE2 production. Many other cytokines are produced, including PAF and TNFα which induces production of IL-1, IL-6 and PGE2.

Complement activation by surgical stress

Both classical and alternative pathways are affected by trauma, the alternative pathway (AP) in burns. This is primarily complement consumption in the early stages, with the production of complement fragments which affect phagocyte function. Complement can also be directly activated by drugs, methylmethacrylate resins in orthopaedic surgery and dialysis or cardiopulmonary bypass pump membranes but the effect is often subclinical or results in an adverse reaction rather than immunosuppression.

Antibody production in surgical stress

Any fall in total immunoglobulin levels is due to haemodilution by i.v. fluid replacement or exudative loss of plasma (in severe burns). Defects in specific antibody production to vaccination following major injury have been demonstrated. Thermal injury and trauma reduces vaccine responses to tetanus but not to polysaccharide antigens, suggesting that some of these defects may reflect T cell dysfunction.

Phagocyte dysfunction in surgical stress

A neutrophil leucocytosis is usual and proportional to the degree of inflammation/trauma. This may be due to mobilisation of marginalised neutrophils from pulmonary vasculature or new emigrants from the bone marrow under cytokine control. Neutrophil activation is seen with transiently decreased adhesiveness followed by an increase which parallels changes of adhesion molecule expression on damaged vascular endothelium. This enables homing of neutrophils, activation and extravasation at the site of injury. However, neutrophil chemiluminescence, NBT reduction, and superoxide production are suppressed and antibacterial lysosyme and B12 binding protein are reduced. In-vitro chemotaxis is decreased for up to 9 days even after minor trauma, and longer in major trauma. Reduced chemotaxis correlates with poor outcome in burns patients. Depletion of complement or immunoglobulins due to hypercatabolism, consumption and loss may secondarily impair neutrophil opsonisation and chemotaxis. In severe trauma, acute phase protein production may be depressed.

APC function in surgical stress

Although there is often an initial monocytosis after surgery, with a transient increase in phagocytosis, enzyme content and cytochrome oxidase activity, this is transient and often becomes impaired subsequently. MHC Class II expression may be reduced after surgery or haemorrhage. Impairment of APC function has not been formally demonstrated in man.

Endothelial effects of surgical stress

Endothelial injury with subsequent coagulation, platelet activation, increased vascular permeability, endothelial cell and platelet production of cytokines or prostaglandins/ leukotrienes and upregulation of adhesion molecules are central events in surgical and traumatic injury. Subsequent cytokine-mediated effects on distant organs produce the classical systemic signs of fever (IL-1 and IL-6 are the 'endogenous pyrogen' acting on the hypothalamic axis; IL-1 produces leukocytosis and activates phagocytes, IL-6 upregulates production of complement and other acute phase proteins from mononuclear phagocytes and the liver).

Neuroendocrine effects of surgical stress

The role of the neuroendocrine system is of increasing interest but poorly understood. There are increases in circulating hormones and cytokines, including colony-stimulating factors, corticosteroids and catecholamines, which result in increased neutrophil emigration and production in the marrow as well as pro-inflammatory cytokines such as IL-1, IL-2 and IFNγ. Beta-endorphins can increase T cell cytotoxicity in vitro, but the clinical relevance of these changes is unknown.

IMMUNOLOGICAL IMPAIRMENT AFTER SPLENECTOMY

Severe immunological impairment is caused by splenectomy. Splenic preservation should be attempted whenever possible. Splenectomy removes both secondary lymphoid tissue in the white pulp and a major phagocytic site for the removal of senescent erythrocytes, opsonised bacteria and intracellular parasites. The spleen is a major site of antibody production, particularily IgM, and is a reservoir of lymphocytes. Splenectomy therefore results in a T cell lymphocytosis and an impaired antibody response to the polysaccharide antigens of bacterial capsules. The result is an increased susceptibility to overwhelming bacterial sepsis, especially in children. Estimates of risk vary, but the risk is especially high in children less than 4 years old, and in the first few years after splenectomy. It is likely that the underlying disease influences prognosis, because the risk is greater after splenectomy for pathology, e.g. thalassaemia, than for trauma.

Infections may present insidiously, then rapidly deteriorate. Encapsulated bacteria such as *Streptococcus pneumoniae*, *Haemophilus influenzae* and *Neisseria meningitidis* predominate, because antibodies to bacterial polysaccharide capsules are important in defence. Mortality is up to 50–70%. Most children receive prophylactic penicillin for 5 years postsplenectomy, but practice varies in adults, and compliance with long term therapy may be a problem. Many patients carry prophylactic

antibiotics for self-medication, and all need education on the risks and importance of rapid presentation of symptoms to a doctor. All splenectomised individuals should be immunised with polysaccharide vaccines against *Pneumococcus*, *Neisseria meningitidis* (A & C) and *Haemophilus influenzae* B. These are best given 10 days before splenectomy (when a functional spleen is present) or, if pre-immunisation is not possible, 2 weeks after surgery. If possible, patients lacking a spleen should not travel to malaria or babesia endemic areas, because of increased susceptibility.

CONTROLLING IMMUNOSUPPRESSION IN THE SURGICAL PATIENT

Attempts can be made to reduce immunosuppression after surgery. Homeostasis and pain control reduces any potential neuroendocrine effects. Avoiding ischaemia improves entry and function of immune effector cells and reduces the likelihood of bacterial infection. Early wound closure and removal of drains reduces potential portals of bacterial entry. Blood transfusion should be minimised where possible (to reduce possibility of blood-borne transmission of infection and the putative immunosuppressive effects of transfusion). It is also helpful, wherever possible, to avoid use of broad spectrum antibiotics which alter normal flora in the gut and increase translocation of pathogens. Nutritional support may be important in some procedures.

NUTRITIONAL SUPPORT IN SURGERY

Nutritional support (calories and protein) to meet the increased metabolic needs following surgery may reduce immunosuppression, particularly in gastrointestinal procedures. Parenteral nutrition does not appear to have any clinical benefit despite correction of nitrogen balance, perhaps due to mucosal atrophy in the gut, and the invasive procedure itself increases the risk of iatrogenic sepsis. Enteral arginine supplements produce improvements of in-vitro tests of lymphocyte function in burns patients which may be of clinical benefit, as may omega-3 fatty acids. Enteral feeding does not produce the mucosal atrophy associated with parenteral nutrition and thereby may reduce the translocation of pathogens across the gut mucosa and maintain local mucosal IgA secretion. Enteral, but not parenteral, glutamine supplementation may improve mucosal integrity and aid macrophage and lymphocyte function. These interventions have yet to be subjected to double-blind clinical trials of efficacy.

Various experimental therapies, including cyclooxygenase inhibitors (which decrease immunosuppressive PGE2 production), ATP-MgCl$_2$ (to improve the ATP-depleted post-trauma state), and calcium channel blockers (to reduce intracelluar calcium levels which impair mitochondrial function), are effective in experimental animals but do not yet have a proven clinical role.

Immunodeficiency in uraemia

Both uraemia and haemodialysis lead to an immunocompromised state. Infections are a major cause of mortality in renal failure. Vascular access and cutaneous staphylococcal carriage result in increased risk of infection. Haemodialysis membranes may activate the alternative pathway of complement, leading to C5a generation which affects neutrophil function and causes transient peripheral pooling in the lungs. Metabolic derangement impairs cellular function, and dryness and ulceration of mucosal barriers increases translocation of bacteria. T cell lymphopaenia occurs with impaired proliferation, depressed DTH skin test responses, and some impairment of antibody responses to vaccination.

Immunodeficiency in nephrotic syndrome

Nephrotic patients have a peculiar susceptibility to pneumococcal sepsis. Loss of IgG (180 kD) may be relevant in some patients. IgM is generally retained due to its larger size. Complement factor B may also be lost in the urine. Raised complement C3 and C4 levels are usually seen in the nephrotic syndrome due to compensatory hepatic and mononuclear phagocyte production. There is no such feedback regulation of IgG, and low IgG levels persist. There is a demonstrable defect of opsonisation and phagocytosis in vitro, reflecting impairment of antibody, complement and neutrophil function.

Immunodeficiency in connective tissue diseases

Primary immunodeficiencies predispose to autoimmunity, but patients with autoimmune diseases are often immunocompromised as a consequence of the disease itself, as well as immunosuppressive drug therapies. Patients with SLE have acquired abnormalities of complement due to consumption by immune complexes and may have dysregulated polyclonal antibody production. Patients with rheumatoid arthritis may have secondary abnormalities of neutrophil function which may predispose to staphylococcal infection, possibly by immune complex formation altering neutrophil function. Despite these observations, the use of potent immuosuppressive drugs dominate the clinical immunosuppression in patients with CTD.

Immunodeficiency in malnutrition

Malnutrition is the most common cause of immunodeficiency worldwide, increasing childhood and perinatal mortality from infectious diseases, such as measles. The metabolic demands of established infection (negative nitrogen balance) further compromise the infected host. Impaired DTH, decreased cytokine production, reduced T cell numbers and proliferation to antigen or mitogens is seen. Vaccine responses and total IgG levels are often normal in mild malnutrition, but impaired in severe cases; however, IgA levels often fall. C3 levels fall due to reduced hepatic synthesis and consumption. Neutrophil chemotaxis and opsonisation may be normal but bacterial killing is impaired.

Immunodeficiency as a result of infection

Some impairment of immune responses is common after viral infections where transiently reduced T cell function and DTH anergy are often found (measles, Hep B, EBV, CMV, rubella). The clinical relevance of these functional alterations is not clear, although clearly some viruses gain a survival advantage by suppressing host antiviral responses. Herpes viruses (EBV, CMV) appear to directly suppress T cell cytokine production (IFNγ) and proliferation. Specific antibody production is unimpaired, yet autoantibody production may be increased.

HIV infection is a special case which causes T cell depletion (and thus causes secondary B cell malfunction) by a combination of direct cytopathicity and immune-mediated CD8 positive cytotoxic attack on infected T cells and APC. This may eventually lead to clonal exhaustion of T cell precursors (possibly by direct infection of T cell progenitor cells) and eventual loss of antigen specific T cells, leading to total immunoparesis. Full discussion of the possible pathogenesis of immunodeficiency in HIV infection is beyond the scope of this chapter. Some bacterial infections (TB, leprosy) and fungal infections (*Aspergillus*) can also cause reduced T cell and macrophage function.

Immunodeficiency as a result of malignancy

An immunocompromised state is often found in disseminated lymphoid and non-lymphoid malignancy. Leukaemias and lymphomas cause reduced DTH and mitogen T cell responses, sometimes with impairment of antibody production. CLL can cause hypogammaglobulinaemia and infections, and may require intravenous immunoglobulin (IVIG) replacement. The host is immunocompromised by radiotherapy, chemotherapy or splenectomy. Hodgkin's disease suppresses T cell function and specific antibody responses to carbohydrate antigens by an unknown mechanism, but IgG levels are normal. Myeloma impairs T and B cell function by an unknown mechanism, thus despite normal or elevated IgG levels (which may be predominantly monoclonal paraprotein) specific antibody responses to pathogens and vaccines are impaired. Bacterial pneumonia is common.

Immunosuppression in sarcoidosis

Sarcoidosis classically produces DTH skin anergy to other antigens; the mechanism is unknown, but this appears to have little clinical significance, as patients with sarcoidosis are not unduly susceptible to infection unless treated with corticosteroids.

Age-related immunodeficiency

Premature children have insufficient maternal IgG transfer (predominantly occurs in the last few weeks of pregnancy) and may have transient hypogammaglobulinaemia until endogenous production of immunoglobulins restores normal IgG levels at 6–9 months of age. Phagocytosis, T and B cell function, chemotaxis and complement levels are also impaired in comparison with normal neonates. IgA production may not reach adult levels until 5 years of age in many otherwise normal children. Responses to polysaccharide antigens are generally poor in normal children before 2 years of age.

In old age some impairment of immunity is suggested by the increased incidence of infections, monoclonal paraproteins, autoantibodies, DTH anergy, and reduced antibody responses to vaccines and lymphoproliferative disorders. This is reflected in decreased T cell numbers, increased CD45RO expression, and decreased T cell proliferation and cytokine production. Macrophages are also impaired, with decreased cytokine production or responsiveness. B cell numbers tend to increase with age, while IgE production reduces and many allergies remit.

Immunodeficiency as a result of metabolic disturbances

Diabetes (susceptible to staphylococci) and cirrhosis (*Escherichia coli* peritonitis) result in ill-defined defects in cell-mediated and humoral immunity. The suceptibility is probably multifactorial, with both tissue ischaemia and increased glucose levels contributing.

Drug-induced immunosuppression

This is probably the most common iatrogenic immuno-compromised state. Some drugs have immunosuppressive properties which are secondary to their primary usage (e.g. hydroxychloroquine, dapsone, some antibiotics and phenytoin).

Table 6.12 Frequency of UK primary antibody deficiency 1996 (in 1921 patients)	
Deficiency	Percentage
Common variable immunodeficiency	44
IgG subclass deficiency	11
X-linked agammaglobulinaemia	9
SCID	5
IgA deficiency	5
Chronic granulomatous disease	3
Combined T/B disorders (including HIGM)	2.5
Neutropaenia	2
Specific antibody deficiency	2
Complement deficiency (including MBL)	2

PRIMARY IMMUNODEFICIENCY

Some immunodeficient states are inherited, although the expression of the immunodeficiency may in some cases be triggered by environmental triggers at a later stage in life such as EBV in X-linked lymphoproliferative disorder (XLP). These immunodeficiencies may present with unduly prolonged, recurrent or severe infections in childhood or adulthood (Table 6.12). The genetic bases of many are now known (Fig. 6.11).

INNATE IMMUNODEFICIENCIES

Phagocyte immunodeficiencies

Defects in neutrophil function include chronic granulomatous disease (CGD), where there is a genetic abnormality in a subunit of the cytochrome b558 enzyme complex (NADPH oxidase). This complex produces oxygen free-radicals in neutrophil and monocyte cytoplasmic phagosomes which kill pathogens in conjunction with hydrogen peroxidase. Some bacteria or fungi produce the enzyme catalase which neutralises hydrogen peroxidase, thus CGD patients get recurrent, deep-seated and severe infections with catalase positive *Staphylococcus*, *Salmonella* and *Aspergillus*.

Since the most common missing component is p91phox (*ph*agocyte *ox*idase located on the X chromosome), CGD is usually X-linked and manifest in males, with female carriers, although an autosomal form exists due to deficiency of p47phox and p67phox. Patients have problems in early childhood and often require surgical drainage of deep abscesses. Prophylactic antibiotics to cover *Staphylococcus* and *Aspergillus* are necessary, sometimes augmented with subcutaneous injections of the neutrophil-activating cytokine IFNγ.

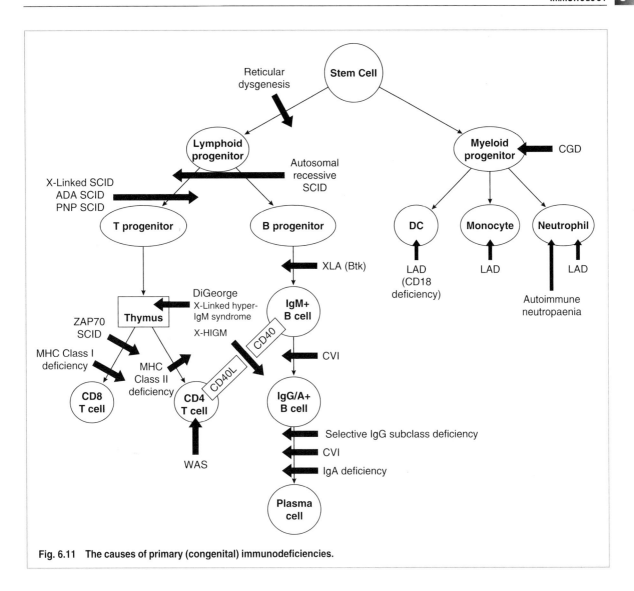

Fig. 6.11   The causes of primary (congenital) immunodeficiencies.

Leucocyte adhesion deficiency (LAD)

LAD-1 results from the deficiency of the CD18 chain integrin component of the adhesion molecules LFA-1 (CD18/CD11a), CR3 (CD18/CD11b) and CR4 (CD18/CD11c). Deficiency results in abnormal neutrophil adhesion and complement receptors, and failure to form pus at the sites of infection because of impaired migration across inflamed endothelium (diapedesis).

Myeloperoxidase (MPO) deficiency

MPO enables hydrogen peroxidase to form toxic halides which enhance bacterial killing in the phagosome. MPO deficiency may predispose to infection in conjunction with other immunological defects (e.g. mannose-binding

lectin, MBL) but probably not in isolation, since deficiency is quite common.

Primary antibody deficiency (PAD)

Patients with the severe combined T and B cell immunodeficiencies (SCID) will not survive into adulthood without bone marrow transplantation (BMT), which may well restore a functional immune system. SCID will not be mentioned further here. The most common clinical problem resulting from primary antibody deficiency encountered by surgeons is excision of bronchiectatic lung tissue, or ENT sinus drainage procedures for persistent sinus disease. Most primary antibody deficiencies are disorders of B cell development or function with impaired or absent antibody production. Some have minor abnormalities of T cell function and have an increased incidence of autoimmunity and malignancy. The most common type, common variable immunodeficiency (CVI), has a prevalence of 12–20 per million.

PAD presents with pneumonia, sinus and gastrointestinal infections due to the absence of IgG and IgA. Lack of IgA leads to susceptibility to mucosal pathogens entering by the respiratory and gastrointestinal tract. Patients get: respiratory infections with encapsulated bacteria (*Haemophilus influenzae* (usually untypable) and *Streptococcus pneumoniae*) and *mycoplasma*; gastrointestinal infections with *Giardia*, *Campylobacter* and *Salmonella*; *Mycoplasma* arthritis; and rarely *Neisseria meningitidis* meningitis (more usual in complement deficiency).

Antibody deficient patients usually clear viral infections normally, although they never develop antibody-mediated resistance against re-infection. They do not get infections with opportunists or unusual organisms, except in hyper-IgM syndrome (HIGM) due to a T cell defect, where pneumocystis pneumonia and cryptosporidial gastroenteritis occur. X-linked agammaglobulinaemia (XLA) patients occasionally get fatal enteroviral meningoencephalitis and myositis. Since XLA is a B cell disorder, this suggests that antibodies mediate important enterovirus protection.

Treatment consists of intravenous immunoglobulin (IVIG, predominantly IgG) replacement prepared from a large pool of healthy donors screened for infectious disease. We cannot replace IgA yet, and a major problem with monomeric IgG infusions is poor penetration onto mucosa and the rapid enzymic destruction once there (normal dimeric IgA is specifically secreted and protected by the secretory component). Adjunctive surgery or prophylactic antibiotics may be necessary, especially if end-organ damage such as bronchiectasis or chronic sinusitis becomes established because of delayed diagnosis.

Patients with CVI have an increased risk of malignancy and autoimmunity. Gastric carcinoma, associated with achlorhydria, gastric atrophy and pernicious anaemia, is increased 40 fold, and extranodal B cell lymphomas are increased 100 fold. Occasionally, T cell lymphomas occur. PAD patients may also have autoimmune thrombocytopaenias (which must be mediated by non-antibody mechanisms) and may require splenectomy if unresponsive to treatment. Diagnosis of autoimmune disease or infections may be difficult because serological tests are useless, since patients do not make antibodies. Vaccinations are equally useless, and live vaccines are avoided because a concurrent deficit of cell-mediated immunity

in some antibody deficient patients may lead to fatal dissemination.

PAD patients with low IgG levels (pre- or post-treatment) are susceptible to mycoplasma arthritis. This can result in joint destruction and chronic pain requiring operative intervention under cover of tetracyclines.

Sinus disease remains problematic in many patients. Drainage procedures such as Caldwell–Luc procedures were generally unsuccessful in the past, perhaps because of inadequate therapy. The role of new endoscopic procedures such as FESS (functional endoscopic sinus surgery) remains to be defined.

Regional lymphadenopathy and splenomegaly can occur, particularly in CVI and HIGM. In each case there may be a requirement for excision biopsy of lymph nodes to exclude a lymphoma or other neoplasm. Approximately 1 in 5 CVI patients have a granulomatous variant (GAD), with splenomegaly, reduced CD4 positive T cells, raised CD8 positive T cells, low B cell numbers and sarcoid-like non-caseating granulomata in multiple organs. These may cause diagnostic confusion with mycobacteria (antibody deficient patients are not unduly susceptible to tuberculosis) and other granulomatous disorders (Whipple's, syphilis, toxoplasmosis). Benign reactive nodular hyperplasia of the gut lymphoid tissue is present in many antibody deficient patients, and may mimic other intra-abdominal pathology. HIGM may present with a lymphoproliferative picture with enlarged and dysplastic secondary lymphoid tissue with abnormal follicular development. This results from the genetic abnormality of the CD40 ligand (CD40L) on activated T cells, which impairs the T and B cell interaction which is critical for the formation of normal lymphoid follicular architecture as well as the proper function of T cells, B cell class switching from IgM to IgA and IgG, and memory cell generation. B cells thus get stuck in an immature IgM-producing stage.

IMMUNOSUPPRESSION

Immunosuppression by disruption of the immune response to a specific antigen is the ultimate goal of immunologists and surgeons and may result from improved understanding of the role of clonal anergy and deletion in the maintainance of self-tolerance and tolerance to foreign antigens (including MHC). Meantime, patients have to live with the inadequacies and potentially fatal side effects of pharmacological immunosuppression. The various drugs used may be subdivided according to their principal mode of action (Table 6.13, Fig. 6.12)

Table 6.13 The principal mechanisms of action of immunosuppressive drugs

Drug	Anti-inflammatory	Proliferation	Cytokines	Adhesion/Costimulator	Phagocyte	T cell	B cell	APC
Corticosteroids	y	y	y	y	y	y	y	y
CsA		y	y		?	y	?	?
FK506		y	y			y		
Rapamycin		y				y		
Cyclophosphamide	y			y	y	y	y	
Methotrexate		y			y	y	y	y
Mycophenolate	y	y		y		y	y	
Leflunamide		y				y	y	
Brequinar	y				y	y		
15 Deoxyspergulain	y					y	y	
Azothiaprine		y			y	y	y	
TBI		y			y	y	y	y
T cell mAb		y		y		y		
Anticytokine mAb	y		y					
Antiadhesion	y	y		y	y	y	y	y

CORTICOSTEROIDS

Corticosteroids cross the cell membrane to bind to cytosolic glucocorticoid receptors, which translocate to the nucleus to bind to glucocorticoid responsive elements which activate gene transcription over 6–12 h. They also have multiple anti-inflammatory effects on neutrophils, vascular adhesion, cytokine production, wound repair, 5-lipo-oxygenase and cytokine production such as IL-1. Corticosteroids also affect B cells (reduce antibody secretion, promote apoptosis), T cells (reduce cytokine secretion and proliferation). Their big disadvantage comes from side effects including adrenal suppression, cataracts, osteoporosis, diabetes, increased susceptibility to infections, and the masking of systemic signs of infection.

ANTICYTOKINES

IL-1RA is anti-inflammatory in RA but is not helpful in transplantation.

ANTI-APC

15-Deoxyspergualin (15DS) binds to heat shock proteins (HSP) and interferes with their ability to act in loading of antigenic peptides onto HLA molecules. 15DS only has a modest effect in transplantation. Cytokines and costimulatory molecule expression are unaffected, but multiple toxicities including leucopenia limit its utility. 15DS also suppresses B cell proliferation, inhibiting antibody formation.

NUCLEOSIDE SYNTHESIS INHIBITORS

Azathioprine

Azathioprine is a cytotoxic drug used in transplantation, autoimmune diseases and vasculitis. Azathioprine is a precurser of 6 mercaptopurine which undergoes intracellular conversion to the purine analogue thiosinic acid which inhibits DNA/RNA synthesis. It kills lymphocytes, phagocytes, megakaryocytes and erythroblasts and any other proliferating cell indiscriminately. In transplantation (and autoimmunity), antigen specific, clonally proliferating cells are killed more rapidly than resting cells.

The main side effects are thus infections, bone marrow suppression, hepatotoxicity, hair loss and late malignancy.

Brequinar sodium

Brequinar sodium inhibits pyrimidine synthesis and may complement CsA in renal transplantation. Thrombocytopenia occurs as a side effect.

Mycophenolic acid

Mycophenolic acid blocks purine synthesis and is an alternative to azathioprine. It is relatively lymphocyte specific and also inhibits glycosylation of adhesion molecules, interfering with immune responses on many levels. Mycophenolic acid also inhibits smooth muscle proliferation and may be useful in preventing chronic vascular rejection.

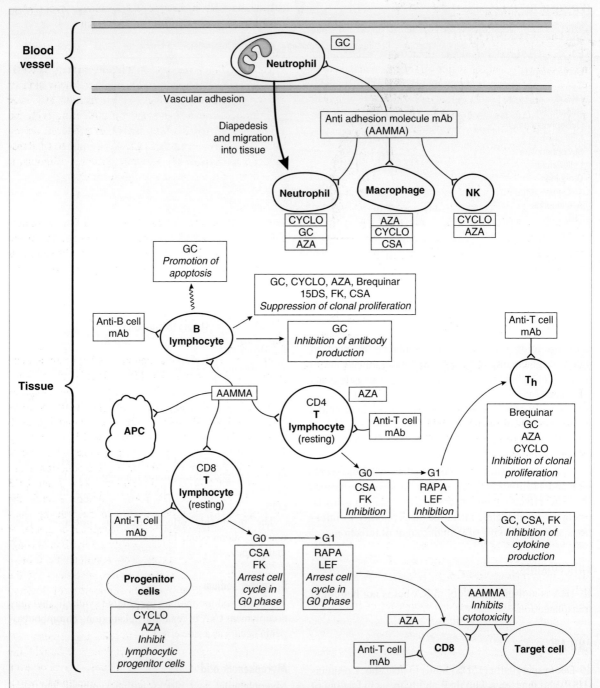

Fig. 6.12   Sites of action of immunosuppressant drugs. GC = glucocorticoid (steroid); RAPA = rapamycin; CYCLO = cyclophosphamide; LEF = leflunamide; AZA = azathioprine; 15-DS = 15-deoxyspergualin; CSA = cyclosporin A; FK = FK506 (tacrolimus)

CYTOTOXIC THERAPIES

Total body irradiation (TBI)

TBI was used briefly in human renal transplantation, can induce tolerance, but has major side effects and may need rescue progenitor cell transplantation. TBI kills lymphocytes indiscriminately in the secondary lymphoid tissues, and the lymphopenia blunts graft rejection reponses. Occasionally, Y-mantle irradiation is used for highly sensitised recipients.

Cyclophosphamide

Cyclophosphamide is used in autoimmune diseases, vasculitis and in higher doses in ablation of recipient marrow pre-BMT (conditioning). It is an alkylating agent which chemically modifies the bases of DNA to prevent normal replication by cross-linking. Thus it is both mutagenic and cytotoxic. Cyclophosphamide's main side effects include mucositis, infertility, infection, bone marrow suppression, hair loss and malignancy (bladder and other late tumours). In high doses the drug Mesna is used to neutralise the bladder toxicity of the acrolein metabolite.

ANTI-T CELL-PROLIFERATION/ACTIVATION DRUGS

Cyclosporin

CsA is a lipid-soluble fungal derivative, and was the first T cell specific drug which inhibits cytokine synthesis and clonal proliferation in T cells. It is indiscriminate, because it inhibits all T cells in the early calcium-dependent G0 phase of activation, not just antigen specific cells. CsA binds to the cell surface receptor cyclophylin, becomes internalised to bind to calcineurin (a calcium/calmodulin-dependent phosphatase) leading to transcription factor inhibition (preventing NFAT dephosphorylation and nuclear translocation). It thus suppresses cytokine and cytokine receptor production (e.g. IL-2/IL-2R, IL-3, IL-4, IFNγ, TNFα, GM-CSF). Because CsA inhibits T cell proliferation and cytokine production it impairs B cell and macrophage T helper-dependent functions. CsA also inhibits B cells and macrophages directly and acts synergistically with corticosteroids. The main side effects include nephrotoxicity, hepatotoxicity, hypertrichosis, gingival hyperplasia, tremor and infection. There is also an increased incidence of neoplasia, especially lymphomas.

FK506

FK506 (tacrolimus) is similar to CsA, acting on the G0 phase of proliferation, but binds to a separate FK506-binding protein (FKBP) which then interacts with calcineurin. FK506 has apparent advantages over CsA in liver transplantation but has similar toxicity.

Rapamycin

Rapamycin binds the FK506 binding protein (FKPB) but does not inhibit calcineurin or T cell activation or cytokines. It probably blocks cell activation at a later calcium-independent G1 stage by interfering with the cellular events triggered by cytokines produced during early T cell activation (including IL-1, IL-4 and IL-6). Rapamycin can reverse early allograft rejection. Although it antagonises FK506, it may complement CsA.

Leflunamide

Leflunamide inhibits B and T cell signalling by inhibiting the lck and fyn tyrosine kinases important in the calcium-independent G1 phase of cell proliferation. It prolongs renal allograft survival in dogs and rodents but is toxic.

MONOCLONAL ANTIBODIES

Anti-T cell mAb

Humanised monoclonal antibodies (mAb) promise to be more specific than polyclonal heterologous antisera such as antilymphocyte (ALG) or antithymocyte globulins (ATG). New technologies for rapid production such as phage display will probably improve availability. mAb can be divided into those which deplete cell numbers (by lysis or inducing redistribution) and those which block important cell surface costimulatory and adhesion molecules, or a combination of these effects (as with anti-CD3 (e.g. OKT3) or anti-CD4 mAb). Problems include the development of 'resistance' due to neutralising antibodies against the foreign protein sequences of species of origin of the mAb. This can be reduced by 'humanising' the antibody (i.e. replacing with a human Fc protein sequence but retaining the binding specificity of the original mouse/rabbit mAb). The properties of the final molecule can be adjusted since the Fc portions of each human immunoglobulin isotype have different abilities to activate complement or bind to cellular receptors.

Side effects of mAb include cytokine release with the first dose (pyrexia, flu-like symptoms, rigors or even hypotension and pulmonary oedema), infections, including opportunistic infections (CMV, fungi), HSV reactivation, and late onset EBV lymphoproliferation and B cell lymphomas (especially with OKT3).

Antibodies can be directly conjugated to toxins for immunotherapy of tumours, but anti-IL-2R-toxin conjugate has been used experimentally for immunosuppression. In the future, combinations of antibodies are likely to be used.

Cytoreductive antibodies include Campath (CDw52, pan-leucocyte), anti-CD3 (OKT3, anti-T cell murine IgG2a mAb against the CD3ε chain of the TCR complex), anti-CD2 and anti-CD45 (used to deplete passenger APC in experimental grafts). Only OKT3 is used routinely as yet, the rest are experimental.

Anti-costimulatory/adhesion ligand mAb

These antibodies interfere with antigen presentation, T cell proliferation and T/B cooperation at an early stage of T cell activation. They include anti-CD80 (B7.1), anti-CD4, anti-CD25 (IL-2 receptor), anti-LFA-1(CD18/CD11a), anti-ICAM-1(CD54), and anti-CD28. In addition to mAb, chimaeric molecules can be produced using molecular techniques consisting of a receptor or its ligand attached to a human Fc immunoglobulin tail. These agents block the physical interaction between a receptor/ligand pair. One example is CTLA-4-Ig (which binds to B7.1 and blocks interaction with CD28 or CTLA-4 on T cells). Anti-CD4 produces infectious tolerance which can be adoptively transferred by T cells from one animal to another. Anti-CD8 have not been tried, since CD8 cells are not essential for experimental transplant rejection and have had minimal effects in animal models. CTLA4-Ig prolongs allograft survival in animals and can induce tolerance to xenogeneic human pancreatic islet grafts.

Anti-LFA-1/ICAM-1 combination therapies interfere with antigen presentation/costimulation and cell adhesion in lymphocytes and phagocytes, and can produce experimental tolerance in primates. ICAM-1 mAb are currently being trialled for treatment of rejection and graft-versus-host disease in humans. Anti-IL-2R mAb are effective in prevention of renal allograft rejection. Anti-IL-4 and anti-IL-4R may prolong experimental allograft survival, suggesting that other such combinations may be useful. However, prolongation is not the establishment of long

term tolerance, and the redundancy of the cytokine network complicates matters.

MALIGNANCY IN IMMUNOSUPPRESSION

Organ transplant recipients

There is a three-fold increase in neoplasia in transplant recipients, usually in young adults about 60 months after transplantation, which is related to the degree of pharmacological immunosuppression, especially with agents such as OKT3. Kaposi's sarcoma is 500 times more common in renal recipients than age-matched controls. Kaposi's sarcoma tend to occur earlier (mean 23 months), lymphomas at 37 months, and squamous carcinomas of vulva or perineum after 100 months. Carcinoma of the cervix is increased 14 fold and is human papilloma virus associated (HPV16 and 18). Immunosuppressed solid organ recipients also tend to get ultraviolet and virus-induced squamous tumours of skin and lip (human papilloma virus type 5) which are more aggressive than in immunocompetent hosts, but in contrast do not have an increased incidence of basal cell carcinoma. Non-Hodgkin's lymphoma (NHL) is increased 28–49 fold, and these are mostly of B cell origin and EBV positive. These statistics demonstrate the importance of a functional immune system in the surveillance of virally induced tumours. Thus some lymphomas regress on reduction of immunosuppression (or acyclovir), but as a result the graft may be lost.

Others

The incidence of tumours is also increased in anyone on long term immunosuppressive treatment for autoimmunity, after chemotherapy for a primary malignancy, and SLE and Sjögrens have an intrinsically increased risk of B cell NHL which is enhanced by immunosuppressive treatment. In addition, cyclophosphamide therapy increases the incidence of bladder carcinoma, because of renal excretion of toxic metabolites.

7

Basic microbiology

Andrew T Raftery

SURGICALLY IMPORTANT MICROORGANISMS

This section will concentrate only on those microorganisms which cause surgical problems. Microbes may be divided into:

- conventional pathogens, i.e. those which may cause infection in the previously healthy person
- conditional pathogens, i.e. those which cause infection in those who have a predisposition to infection
- opportunistic pathogens, i.e. those that are usually of low virulence but which will cause infection in the immunocompromised patient.

Examples of the above are shown in Box 7.1.

Microorganisms which are of the greatest significance in surgery are usually bacteria. Bacteria may be classified as follows:

- shape
  bacilli — rod shaped
  cocci — spherical
- Gram staining
  Gram positive — blue
  Gram negative — pink

Box 7.1 Microbial infections

- Conventional
  Staphylococcus aureus — wound infection
  Haemophilus influenzae — chest infection
  Neisseria gonorrhoea — gonorrhoea

- Conditional
  Pseudomonas aeruginosa — wound infection
  Klebsiella — urinary tract infection

- Opportunistic
  Pneumocystis carinii — chest infection
  Candida albicans — oesophagitis
  Aspergillus fumigatus — aspergillosis

- growth requirements
  aerobic
  anaerobic
  facultatively anaerobic.

GRAM POSITIVE COCCI

The important ones are staphylococci and streptococci.

Staphylococci

These tend to be arranged in grape-like clusters. They may be divided into coagulase positive and coagulase negative. Coagulase positive staphylococci are called *Staph. aureus*. They are responsible for the following:

1. superficial infections, e.g. boils, abscesses, styes, conjunctivitis, wound infections.
2. deep infection, e.g. septicaemia, endocarditis, osteomyelitis, pneumonia
3. food poisoning
4. toxic shock syndrome.

Coagulase negative staphylococci, e.g. *Staph. epidermidis* are of lower pathogenicity and rarely cause infection in healthy people. They form part of the normal skin flora. However, they may be responsible for infection in association with foreign bodies, e.g. prosthetic cardiac valves, intravenous lines, continuous ambulatory peritoneal dialysis, and vascular grafts. These infections may lead to septicaemia and endocarditis and become life threatening. Their treatment with antibiotic alone is often inadequate, and the prosthesis may require removal.

Staph. saprophyticus, a commensal, may cause urinary tract infections in sexually active women.

Antibiotic sensitivity

Staph. aureus appears in multiple resistant forms, especially in hospital practice. Recently there has been an increase in MRSA (methicillin-resistant *Staph.*

aureus) which presents a major threat to surgical patients. Antibiotics active against *Staph. aureus* include:

- penicillin (80% of hospital strains are resistant)
- flucloxacillin (active against beta-lactamase-producing organisms)
- erythromcyin
- clindamycin
- fusidic acid
- cephalosporins
- vancomycin.

Streptococci

These are spherical or oval cocci occurring in chains. They are classified by their ability to lyse red blood cells present in blood containing culture medium. They are further subdivided by serology, on the basis of polysaccharide antigens present on their surface, into Lancefield groups. The species responsible for sepsis are the beta-haemolytic strains where colonies completely lyse the blood cells on a culture plate, causing a colourless, clear, sharply defined zone. They include Lancefield groups A, B, C and G.

Lancefield Group A

Strep. pyogenes causes:

- tonsillitis and pharyngitis
- peritonsillar abscess (quinsy)
- otitis media
- mastoiditis
- wound infection with cellulitis and lymphangitis
- erysipelas
- necrotising fascititis.

Antibiotic sensitivity   Penicillin is the drug of choice. All strains are sensitive. In patients sensitive to penicillin, erythromycin is the drug of choice, but some strains are resistant.

Lancefield Group D

This group includes the enterococci. *Strep. faecalis* is the most important surgically in this group. It may cause urinary tract infections and abdominal wound infections and may be isolated from the bile in acute cholecystitis. Enterococci are sensitive to ampicillin, moderately resistant to penicillin, and resistant to cephalosporins.

'Viridans' streptococci: These show alpha haemolysis on blood containing culture plates with a green (hence the term viridans) discoloration around the colonies. Most human strains are commensals of the upper respiratory tract and are of low pathogenicity. They are responsible for endocarditis. *Strep. milleri* may be classified

with this group but is now more often classified with pyogenic streptococci. It may cause liver, lung, or brain abscesses.

Streptococcus pneumoniae (Pneumococcus):   Strep. pneumoniae consists of diplococci capsulated with a carbohydrate antigenic capsule, which is correlated with its virulence. Virulence correlates with the presence of a capsule probably because this prevents or inhibits phagocytosis. Eighty-four capsular types are recognised. The organism is responsible for the following:

- lobar pneumonia
- chronic bronchitis
- meningitis
- sinusitis
- conjunctivitis
- septicaemia (especially in splenectomised patients).

Antibiotic sensitivity   All strains are sensitive to penicillin and erythromycin.

GRAM POSITIVE RODS

Anaerobic Gram positive rods are mainly soil saprophytes but a few are pathogens. The surgically important ones include species which produce powerful toxins, e.g. *Clostridium perfringens* (gas gangrene), *C. tetani* (tetanus), *C. botulinum* (botulism) and *C. difficile* (diarrhoea in association with antibiotic-induced colitis). Gas gangrene, tetanus and antibiotic-induced colitis will be dealt with later in the chapter.

GRAM NEGATIVE COCCI

They include *Neisseria gonorrhoea, Neisseria meningitidis* and *Moraxella catarrhalis, N. gonorrhoea* and *N. meningitidis* are intracellular Gram negative diplococci. *N. gonorrhoea* is especially important as it may cause fever and severe lower abdominal pain in females or be the cause of a urethral discharge in males. A Gram stain of a smear from a high vaginal swab in the female or from a urethral discharge in the male may confirm the diagnosis by demonstrating the presence of Gram negative intracellular diplococci.

GRAM NEGATIVE BACILLI

This is a large group of microorganisms of surgical importance. They may be divided into facultative anaerobes, e.g. *E. coli* and *Klebsiella*, and aerobes, of which *Pseudomonas* is the most commonly encountered in surgical practice.

Facultative anaerobes (Enterobacteria, Coliforms)

Escherichia coli

This is a normal inhabitant of the human intestine. Some strains produce powerful toxins. *E. coli* is an important cause of sepsis and diarrhoea. Examples of sepsis include:

- UTIs
- wound infection, especially after surgery on the lower gastrointestinal tract
- peritonitis
- biliary tract infection
- septicaemia.

Examples of diarrhoeal illnesses include:

- infantile gastroenteritis
- traveller's diarrhoea
- haemorrhagic diarrhoea, e.g. haemolytic uraemic syndrome.

Klebsiella

Klebsiella spp. inhabit the human intestine. Some strains are saprophytic in soil, water and vegetation. They are responsible for:

- UTIs
- septicaemia
- endocarditis
- pneumonia (rare).

Proteus

Proteus spp. are responsible for:

- UTIs
- wound infections, e.g. burns, pressure sores
- septicaemia.

Salmonella

They inhabit animal gastrointestinal tract. They are predominantly animal pathogens which can cause disease in humans. *Salmonella typhi* and *Salmonella paratyphi* differ from other species in that man is the only natural host. Foodstuffs from animal sources are the usual source of transmission of infection. They are responsible for:

- enteric fever, typhoid or paratyphoid; these are due to *S. typhi* and *S. paratyphi A, B, C*
- gastroenteritis (food poisoning), usually due to *S. enteritidis* or *S. typhimurium*
- osteomyelitis (rare)
- septic arthritis (rare).

S. typhi may survive in symptomless carriers and persist in the gall bladder. Faecal carriage may occur by contamination with bile, and epidemics may occur especially if the carrier is a food handler.

Shigella

They are intestinal parasites in man. They cause dysentery. *Sh. dysenteriae* which produces exotoxins causes the most severe illness. Other shigellae may cause a milder form of dysentery, *Sh. sonnei* being the most common cause in the UK.

Yersinia

These are animal parasites which occasionally cause disease in humans. *Yersinia pseudotuberculosis* and *Yersinia enterocolitica* are the most common, causing food poisoning and mesenteric adenitis.

Other enterobacteria

These include *Enterobacter*, *Citrobacter*, *Providencia*, *Morganella* and *serratia*. They are human and animal intestinal parasites but some strains are saprophytes. Moist hospital environments may act as reservoirs. They are often multiresistant to antibiotics. They may cause the following:

- UTIs
- wound infections after abdominal surgery
- respiratory infections in hospitalised patients
- septicaemia

Antibiotic sensitivity

Sensitivities should be determined, as some strains may be resistant to the more commonly used antibiotics. Antibiotics used against enterobacteria include ampicillin, amoxycillin, trimethoprim, aminoglycosides, ciprofloxacin, cephalosporins (second and third generations) and chloramphenicol. For UTIs the antimicrobial drugs nalidixic acid and nitrofurantoin may be appropriate.

Aerobic Gram negative bacilli

Pseudomonas aeruginosa

This inhabits human and animal gastrointestinal tracts, water and soil. The organism survives in moist environments in hospitals and may also survive in aqueous antiseptics and other fluids. It is an important cause of hospital-acquired infections. It particularly affects patients with serious underlying conditions, e.g. burns and malignancy, or as a result of therapeutic interventions, e.g. urinary catheters, endotracheal tubes. It is a frequent cause of infection in the immunocompromised patient. It is a pathogen in the following conditions:

- UTIs, especially within indwelling catheters
- burns
- wound infections
- septicaemia

- pressure sores
- venous stasis ulcers
- chest infections, especially patients on mechanical ventilation and those with cystic fibrosis
- eye infections (it may contaminate certain types of eye drops).

Antibiotic sensitivity

The presence of *Ps. aeruginosa* is not necessarily an indication for antibiotic therapy especially if it is isolated from a superficial site. Clinical and bacteriological assessment in the individual patient is appropriate before prescribing antibiotics. *Ps. aeruginosa* is resistant to most common antibiotics. The most suitable antibiotics are aminoglycosides, certain beta-lactams, e.g. penicillins (ticarcillin, piperacillin), ciprofloxacin and cephalosporins (ceftazidime).

Other Gram negative bacilli

Campylobacter

These are curved or spiral rods which are micro-aerophilic. They are found in various animal species, including chickens, domestic animals and seagulls. Campylobacter is the most common cause of bacterial food poisoning in the UK.

Haemophilus influenzae

This is mainly found in the respiratory tract, often as part of the normal flora but may also cause respiratory disease, especially community-acquired respiratory disease. It exists in non-capsulated and capsulated strains.

Non-capsulated strains are responsible for exacerbation of chronic bronchitis and bronchiectasis. Capsulated strains often cause severe infections in young children, e.g. meningitis, acute epiglottis, osteomyelitis, arthritis and orbital cellulitis. Septicaemia may occur especially as part of postsplenectomy sepsis. A vaccine is available against *H. influenzae* Type B (HiB).

Antibiotic sensitivity

These include ampicillin, tetracycline, erythromycin, ciprofloxacin, cephalosporins (second and third generations) and septrin. Chloramphenicol should be reserved for severe infections, e.g. meningitis and acute epiglottis.

Pasteurella multocida

This is a small ovoid gram negative bacillus. It inhabits the respiratory tract of many animals, notably dogs and cats. In man it may cause septic wounds after animal bites. It is sensitive to penicillin, tetracycline, erythromycin and aminoglycosides.

SPECIFIC ANTIBIOTICS AND ANTIMICROBIALS

This section deals with antibiotics particularly as they are used for the surgical patient. The list is not meant to be comprehensive.

PENICILLINS

Benzyl penicillin

This is active against streptococci, pneumococci, clostridia, *N. gonorrhoea* and *N. meningitidis*. Few staphylococci are now sensitive. The main surgical indications are for the prophylaxis of gas gangrene and tetanus and for streptococcal wound infections. It may be given parenterally either i.v. or i.m.

Phenoxymethyl penicillin (penicillin V)

This is administered orally. It may follow a course of intravenous benzyl penicillin to complete a course of treatment. It is used prophylactically following splenectomy to prevent pneumococcal septicaemia, especially in children where it is used long term. It may also be used for prophylaxis in patients with rheumatic heart disease.

Flucloxacillin

This is administered either orally, i.m, or i.v. for penicillinase-resistant *Staphylococcus aureus*. It is often used as an adjunct to drainage of abscesses, especially in diabetics or immunosuppressed patients.

Amoxycillin and ampicillin

These may be administered either orally, i.m. or i.v. Their use in the surgical context is largely for chest infections or urinary tract infections. Many staphylococci and coliforms produce β-lactamase and are therefore resistant. Amoxycillin and ampicillin are active against *Streptococcus faecalis* and *Haemophilus influenzae*.

Co-amoxyclav (augmentin)

This contains amoxycillin and potassium clavulanate. It may be administered either orally or i.v. The clavulanate is inhibitory to β-lactamase and extends the spectrum of amoxycillin. It is active against coliforms, staphylococci and bacteroides. It is also useful in surgery as prophylaxis in bowel, hepatobiliary and GU surgery.

Piperacillin

This may be administered i.m. or i.v. It is active against bacteroides, coliforms, *Klebsiella* and *Pseudomonas aeruginosa*. It is often used in combination with an aminoglycoside for life-threatening infections.

When administering penicillins, care should be taken to check for previous sensitivity. Caution should be particularly exercised in asthmatics and others with a history of allergic conditions. Hypersensitivity reactions are usually manifested by an urticarial rash, although anaphylaxis may occur. Cross-sensitivity occurs between different penicillins. Most penicillins are relatively nontoxic, and therefore large doses may be given. Caution must be exercised in patients with renal and/or cardiac failure, as injectable forms contain potassium and sodium salts. Rarely, convulsions may occur after giving high doses i.v. or following intrathecal injection.

CEPHALOSPORINS

These drugs are assigned to three generations. Specific examples of each generation in surgical usage is described below.

Cephradine

This is a first generation cephalosporin which may be given orally, i.m. or i.v. In practice it is most commonly used orally. Cephradine is active against a wide range of Gram positive and Gram negative organisms, including *E. coli*, *Klebsiella*, *Proteus*, and *Staph. aureus* (unless methicillin-resistant). It is not active against *Strep. faecalis*, *Ps. aeruginosa* or bacteroides. It is useful as a second line drug for the treatment of urinary tract infections, respiratory tract infections, skin and soft tissue infections.

Cefuroxime

This is a second generation cephalosporin which may be given orally, i.m. or i.v. In practice it is used most commonly i.v. It is a broad spectrum antibiotic against Gram positive and Gram negative organisms. It is only moderately active against bacteroides and not at all against *Pseudomonas*. It is widely used in prophylaxis, especially in combination with metronidazole in colorectal and biliary tract surgery.

Cefotaxime and ceftazidime

These are third generation cephalosporins which are administered i.m. or i.v. They have a broad spectrum similar to second generation drugs but are also active against *Pseudomonas*. They are normally reserved for use in serious sepsis due to susceptible aerobic Gram negative bacilli.

About 10% of patients who are sensitive to penicillin are also sensitive to cephalosporins. Rashes and fever may occur. In patients with renal failure, dose reduction is required. Mild transient rises in liver enzymes may occur.

SULPHONAMIDES AND TRIMETHOPRIM

Co-trimoxazole (sulphamethoxazole + trimethoprim)

This may be given either orally, i.m., or i.v. It is used for treatment of urinary tract infections and respiratory infections. It is active against Gram positive and Gram negative organisms. *Ps. aeruginosa* is resistant. It may be used for *Salmonella* septicaemia and *Pneumocystis* pneumonia. Nausea, vomiting, rashes and mouth ulcers may occur. Leucopenia and thrombocytopenia may also occur occasionally.

Trimethoprim

This may be administered orally or i.v. by slow infusion. It is used for urinary tract infections and respiratory infections. It should be avoided in pregnancy. Nausea, vomiting, rashes, stomatitis and marrow suppression may occur. It potentiates the action of warfarin and phenytoin.

MACROLIDES

Erythromycin

This is usually administered orally or i.v. by slow infusion. Its use in surgical patients is limited. It is usually used as a second-line drug in patients sensitive to penicillin. It is active against streptococci, staphylococci, clostridia and *Campylobacter*. It is used for skin and soft tissue infections and respiratory tract infections. It is valuable in atypical pneumonia, Legionnaire's disease and *Campylobacter* enteritis. The chief side effect when given orally is diarrhoea. When given i.v., phlebitis at the site of infusion is a common side effect. It may potentiate warfarin and cyclosporin.

AMINOGLYCOSIDES

These are the first choice drugs for severe Gram negative infections, usually given in combination with a β-lactamase antibiotic. The most commonly used are gentamicin and amikacin.

Gentamicin

This is usually given i.v. but can also be given i.m. It is active against coliforms, *Ps. aeruginosa* and staphylococci. Streptococci and anaerobes are resistant.

Amikacin

This is reserved for life-threatening infections with gentamicin-resistant organisms with proven amikacin sensitivity.

The major side effects of aminoglycosides are ototoxicity (vertigo or deafness) and nephrotoxicity. Therapeutic levels depend on renal function. Serum levels must be monitored. Accurate monitoring of levels is essential in patients with impaired renal function and patients on long term therapy.

QUINOLONES

Ciprofloxacin

This is usually given orally or i.v. It is a broad spectrum antibiotic against Gram negative bacteria, including *Ps. aeruginosa*, and staphylococci. Anaerobes are resistant. Its uses in surgery include urinary tract infections, especially those that are catheter related, prostatitis and skin and soft tissue infections with *Ps. aeruginosa*. It is also useful for chest infections, especially those due to Gram negative organisms. The side effects include nausea, diarrhoea and vomiting. CNS side effects include anxiety, nervousness, insomnia and rarely convulsions. Ciprofloxacin potentiates warfarin.

OTHER ANTIBIOTICS AND ANTIMICROBIALS

Metronidazole

This is widely used in surgery both prophylactically and therapeutically. It may be given orally, i.v. or rectally. It is active against anaerobic bacteria, e.g. bacteroides and clostridia. It is also active against the protozoal organisms *Entamoeba histolytica* and *Giardia lamblia*. It is used for intraperitoneal sepsis and gynaecological sepsis.

It is used prophylactically in appendicitis against wound infection (usually given rectally) and in colorectal surgery, where it is given i.v. with induction of anaesthesia. It is also administered for giardiasis, intestinal amoebiasis and amoebic liver abscess. The side effects include anorexia, a sore tongue and an unpleasant metallic taste. It potentiates warfarin.

Tetracycline

This is of limited use in surgery. It may be used in chronic bronchitis, non-specific urethritis and atypical pneumonia.

Fusidic acid

This is usually used for penicillin-resistant staphylococcal infections and staphylococcal osteomyelitis. Tissue concentrations are good. It may be administered orally or i.v.

Vancomycin

This may be given orally or i.v. It is active against staphylococci (including methicillin-resistant strains), streptococci and clostridia. Its chief use is for severe infections. Recently its use has increased due to intraperitoneal administration in CAPD peritonitis. Side effects include phlebitis when given i.v., ototoxicity and

nephrotoxicity. Serum levels must be monitored to control dosage.

Teicoplanin

Teicoplanin is a bacteriocidal glycopeptide active against both aerobic and anaerobic Gram positive bacteria. It is usually administered i.v. but may be given i.m. It is active against *Staph. aureus* and coagulase positive staphylococci (sensitive or resistant to methicillin), streptococci, enterococci, *Listeria monocytogenes*, micrococci and Gram positive anaerobes, including *Clostridium difficile*. Teicoplanin is chemically related to vancomycin, with similar activity and toxicity.

ANTIBIOTICS IN SURGERY

Antibiotics are never a substitute for sound surgical technique. Pus, dead tissue and slough need removing. Antibiotics should be used carefully and only with positive indications. Prolonged or inappropriate use of antibiotics may encourage resistant strains of organisms to emerge. Except in straightforward cases, advice should be sought from a microbiologist .

PRINCIPLES OF ANTIBIOTIC THERAPY

Selection of antibiotic

The decision to prescribe antibiotics is usually clinical and is based initially on a 'best guess' policy, i.e. based on experience of the particular condition, what the organism is likely to be, and to which antibiotic it is most likely to be sensitive.

The following sequence of events usually occurs in selection of an antibiotic:

1. A decision is made on clinical grounds that an infection exists.
2. Based on signs symptoms and clinical experience, a guess is made at the likely infecting organism.
3. The appropriate specimens are taken for microbiological examination, i.e. culture and sensitivity.
4. The cheapest and most effective drug or combination of drugs effective against the suspected organism is given.
5. The clinical response to treatment is monitored.
6. The antibiotic treatment is altered if necessary in response to laboratory reports of culture and sensitivity.

Occasionally the response of the infection to an apparently appropriate antibiotic is poor. Possible causes for this include:

- failure to drain pus, excise necrotic tissue, or remove foreign bodies
- failure of the drug to reach the tissues in therapeutic concentration, e.g. ischaemic limb
- the organism isolated is not the one responsible for the infection
- after prolonged antibiotic therapy, new organisms develop
- inadequate dosage
- inappropriate route of administration.

Treatment with a combination of antibiotics

There are several reasons why it may be appropriate to use two antibacterial drugs in combination. These include:

- as a temporary measure during the investigation of an undiagnosed illness
- to achieve a synergistic effect
- to prevent the development of bacterial resistance
- the treatment of mixed infections
- to allow reduction in the dosage of a potentially toxic drug.

Although not a hard and fast rule, it is generally accepted that to use a bacteriocidal and a bacteriostatic drug together may be antagonistic. Two bacteriostatic drugs used in combination may be simply additive, but the use of two bacteriocidal drugs may achieve a synergic effect.

Route of administration

Antibiotics should be given intravenously in severe infections in seriously ill patients. Some antibiotics, e.g. gentamicin, can only be given by the parenteral route. When the patient has had gastrointestinal surgery, antibiotics are best given parenterally until GI function is resumed, and then the drugs may be given orally. It is best to avoid the intramuscular route if possible, as it is uncomfortable for the patient and, in shocked patients, absorption would be inadequate.

Duration of therapy

This depends upon the individual's response and laboratory investigations. For most infections which show an appropriate response to treatment after 48 h, a suitable 'course' should be for 5–7 days. A clinical cure is the most appropriate response, and this should be taken in conjunction with microbiological data.

Dosage

The dosage of a drug may need to be modified in renal and liver disease. In renal failure the dosage of drugs eliminated by the kidney may require major adjustment, e.g. aminoglycosides or vancomycin, whereas those eliminated by the liver, e.g. erythromycin, can usually be given in normal dosage.

Penetration of tissue

The drug must penetrate to the site of the infection: e.g. in meningitis the antibiotic must pass into the CSF. Deep abscesses are a particular problem and an important cause of antibiotic failure. An antibiotic cannot penetrate through the wall of the abscess to a collection of pus but may allow healing around the pus and may create an antibioma. The importance of draining pus cannot be overemphasised.

Hypersensitivity

This is most often due to penicillin and may manifest itself merely in the development of a rash but may also manifest in the form of life-threatening anaphylaxis. A clear history of sensitivity to antibiotics must be sought.

Drug toxicity

Some antibiotics are toxic, e.g. ototoxicity and nephrotoxicity with aminoglycosides, bone marrow depression with chloramphenicol.

Super infection

Super infection may occur with antibiotic-resistant microorganisms, e.g. yeasts. This is probably most common in immunosuppressed patients. Antibiotic-associated pseudomembranous colitis may occur in any patient taking antibiotics. Initially this was thought to be due specifically to clindamycin, but it is now realised that broad spectrum β-lactam antibiotics are most often involved.

PROPHYLACTIC ANTIBIOTICS

Despite aseptic techniques, some operations carry a high risk of postoperative wound infection, bacteraemia, or septicaemia. Administration of antibiotics in the perioperative period will reduce the risks.

Indications for prophylactic antibiotics

- implantation of foreign bodies, e.g. cardiac prosthetic valves, artificial joints, prosthetic vascular grafts
- patients with pre-existing cardiac disease who are undergoing surgical procedures, including dental procedures, e.g. patients with mitral valve disease, as prophylaxis against subacute bacterial endocarditis
- amputation, especially for ischaemia or crush injuries where there is dead muscle. The risk of gas gangrene

is high, especially in contaminated wounds. Penicillin is the antibiotic of choice

- diabetics
- immunosuppressed patients
- organ transplantation
- compound fractures and penetrating wounds
- surgical incisions where there is a high risk of bacterial contamination, i.e. clean contaminated wounds or frankly contaminated wounds (e.g. bowel preparation for colonic surgery).

Most prophylactic antibiotics are given to prevent wound infection. In some cases they are given prior to instrumental procedures in potentially infected sites, e.g. when performing cystoscopy, when they are given to prevent bacteraemia. Any patients with congenital heart disease, rheumatic heart disease, or prosthetic valves should be given antibiotics before an elective procedure which may result in bacteraemia. Procedures include dental procedures (including scaling and polishing), GU instrumentation, GI endoscopy, respiratory tract instrumentation, and open surgery. In most cases one dose is given preoperatively, either orally if the procedure is under local anaes-

thetic (1 h preoperatively) or intravenously if the procedure is under general anaesthetic. There is variable practice, but it is usual for 1–4 doses to be given postoperatively. The aim is to achieve therapeutic levels at the time of surgery. Table 7.1 shows some indications for prophylactic antibiotics, the likely organism involved, and a recommended prophylactic regime.

SURGICAL SEPSIS

The term sepsis covers several purulent infections which the surgeon may encounter in surgical practice.

SKIN INFECTIONS

Boils, styes and carbuncles

A boil (furuncle) is an infection of a hair follicle. A stye (hordoleum) is an infection of a hair follicle on the eye lid. A carbuncle is a group of boils interconnecting in the subcutaneous tissue by tracts. These infections are painful but not serious. Antibiotics are rarely indicated

Table 7.1 Prophylactic antibiotics		
Clinical situation	Likely organism(s)	Prophylactic regime
Appendicectomy	Anaerobes	Metronidazole (single dose pr 1 h preop)
Biliary tract surgery	Coliforms	Cephalosporin (i.v. immediately preop and for 24 h postop)
Colorectal surgery	Coliforms Anaerobes	Metronidazole + cephalosporin or gentamicin (i.v. immediately preop and for up to 48 h postop)
GU surgery Open surgery	Coliforms	Gentamicin (single i.v. dose pre-procedure). Cephalosporin (i.v. immediately preop and for 24–48 h post-op) or gentamicin (single i.v. dose immediately preop)
Insertion of prosthetic joints	*Staph. aureus* *Staph. epidermidis*	Flucloxacillin (i.v. immediately preop and for 24–48 h postop)
Amputation of limb	*C. perfringens*	Penicillin (i.v. immediately preop and for 24 h postop)
Vascular surgery with prosthetic graft	*Staph. aureus* *Staph. epidermidis* Coliforms	Cephalosporin (i.v. immediately preop and for 24 h postop)
Prevention of tetanus in contaminated wound (+ immunoprophylaxis)	*C. tetanus*	Penicillin (i.v. or i.m. on presentation)
Prophylaxis of endocarditis		
Minor dental procedure under LA	Oral streptococci	Amoxycillin (single oral dose 1 h preop; clindamycin if allergic)
Major dental procedure under GA		Low risk: amoxycillin (oral dose 4 h preop and one dose postop) High risk: amoxycillin & gentamicin (i.m. or i.v. immediately preop; vancomycin if allergic)
GU instrumentation	Coliforms	Amoxycillin + gentamicin (i.v. immediately preop)

for boils and styes but may be appropriate for carbuncles. Infection is usually due to *Staph. aureus*, which is usually an endogenous strain carried in the nose or on the skin. Boils may be recurrent, appearing in crops over several weeks or several months. They may be a presenting sign of diabetes. Antibiotic therapy is indicated only in certain cases: e.g. boils on the 'dangerous area' of the face where venous drainage is to the cavernous sinus and where cavernous sinus thrombosis may result; and also in the immunocompromised patient.

Erysipelas

This is a spreading infection of the skin due to *Streptococcus pyogenes*. It presents as a raised, red, indurated area of the skin which is sharply demarcated. The patient may present with high fever and appear toxic. It is a rare condition at the present time but responds well to penicillin.

CELLULITIS

Cellulitis is a spreading infection of the subcutaneous tissues.

Acute pyogenic cellulitis

This is due to *Strep. pyogenes* and presents as a red, painful swelling, usually of a limb, being commonly associated with lymphangitis and lymphadenitis. It is particularly likely to occur in the lymphoedematous limb. Treatment is with penicillin.

Anaerobic cellulitis

This is rare and is usually due to anaerobes or clostridia but more often is due to synergistic infection with both aerobes and anaerobes. The causative organisms are usually a combination of anaerobes (bacteroides, anaerobic cocci) and aerobes (coliforms, *Pseudomonas aeruginosa* and *Strep. pyogenes*). Clinically, redness and oedema present around a wound (surgical or traumatic). This may progress in two ways, as follows.

Bacterial gangrene

The skin becomes purple and ischaemic and eventually undergoes necrosis. Fournier's gangrene of the scrotum is an example.

Necrotising fasciitis

In this condition the skin remains normal in the early stages whilst the infection spreads along fascial planes, causing extensive necrosis. Later the overlying skin becomes deprived of its blood supply, loses its sensation and eventually becomes purple, black and undergoes

necrosis. This is a life-threatening condition in which the patient is seriously ill with fever, toxaemia and, occasionally, septic shock. Wide excision of the area of necrosis and infection, together with treatment with appropriate antibiotics is indicated. The mortality rate is high.

LYMPHANGITIS AND LYMPHADENITIS

Lymphangitis is a non-suppurative infection of lymphatic vessels that drain an area of cellulitis. Lymphadenitis is infection of the regional lymph nodes as a result of infection in the areas which they drain. It usually, but not always, results from cellulitis and lymphangitis. Occasionally the nodes suppurate and form an abscess. Lymphangitis produces red tender streaks along the line of lymphatics extending from the area of cellulitis towards the regional lymph nodes. Lymphadenitis is represented by enlarged, tender, regional lymph nodes. Occasionally the overlying skin is red and the glands may be fluctuant. Treatment of both lymphangitis and lymphadenitis depends upon isolation of the appropriate infecting organism.

GAS GANGRENE

Gas gangrene is a rare disease in peace time but is closely associated with grossly contaminated wounds due to war injuries. However, there remains a problem in civilian surgical practice in that clostridial infection can occur after elective surgery especially on the gastrointestinal tract (*Clostridium perfringens* is a normal bowel inhabitant), lower limb amputation, or vascular surgery on the ischaemic limb. In the case of trauma it is due to contamination of wounds by dirt and soil which contain clostridia derived from animal faeces. Infection is favoured by extensive wounds with the presence of necrotic tissue which provides an anaerobic environment for clostridia to proliferate. An anaerobic environment initiates conversion of spores to vegetative, toxin-producing pathogens. Clostridia proliferate and produce toxins that diffuse into the surrounding tissue. The toxins destroy the local microcirculation. This allows further invasion which can advance extremely rapidly. The α toxin of *Clostridium perfringens* kills muscle cells and destroys fat. Gas formation occurs with local crepitus. As the disease advances, toxins are released into the systemic circulation, causing the clinical features of pallor, restlessness, delirium, tachycardia, jaundice and ultimately septic shock and death. With gas gangrene the surface oedema, necrosis, and discoloration of the skin are less extensive than the underlying myositis. Diagnosis is confirmed by examining a specimen of exudate or tissue after Gram staining, when the typical Gram positive bacilli are seen.

TETANUS

This is a rare condition in the UK, because of widespread immunisation. It is caused by *Clostridium tetani*, an anaerobic Gram positive bacillus which produces a neurotoxin. It is found in soil and faeces. The neurotoxin enters the peripheral nerves and travels to the spinal cord where it blocks inhibitory activity of spinal reflexes, resulting in the characteristic features of the disease. The disease follows the implantation of the spores into deep, devitalised tissues.

There is usually a history of a wound which may be as minor as the prick of a rose thorn. The incubation period is 1–30 days. Muscle spasm usually occurs first at the site of inoculation and is followed by trismus resulting in the typical risus sardonicus (lockjaw). Stiffness in the neck, back and abdomen follow, together with generalised spasms which may cause asphyxia. The muscles remain in spasm between convulsions. Opisthotonos (arching of the back and neck due to spasm) may occur. This stage is followed by convulsions which are extremely painful and during which the patient is conscious. Death may occur from asphyxia due to involvement of respiratory muscles or from inhalation of vomit with aspiration pneumonia. The diagnosis is usually clinical. Attempts at bacteriological confirmation often fail. Tetanus is rare in the UK because of an active immunisation programme in childhood with tetanus toxoid. All children should be immunised, and this repeated at 6 weeks and 6 months after the initial dose. Booster doses should be given at 5 yearly intervals. All patients attending an Accident and Emergency department with new trauma, however mild, should have booster unless one has been given within the previous year. Contaminated and penetrating wounds should be debrided and prophylactic penicillin administered. A tetanus toxoid booster should be given to the previously immunised patient. Those not previously immunised should be given human antitetanus immunoglobulin.

ABSCESSES

An abscess is a local collection of pus. Abscesses are walled off by a barrier of inflammatory reaction (pyogenic membrane), and fibrosis occurs, 'encapsulating' the abscess. It is therefore impossible to treat abscesses satisfactorily with antibiotics alone. Surgical drainage is also necessary.

Without treatment abscesses tend to 'point' spontaneously to the nearest epithelial surface: e.g. skin (boil), gut (pelvic abscess to rectum), and bronchus (lung abscess). Spontaneous drainage often leads to healing provided the initiating stimulus has been eliminated. If spontaneous drainage does not eliminate the initiating stimulus, a chronic abscess may form, resulting in a continuously discharging sinus or abscess which intermittently develops, discharges and heals. A good example of this is a stitch abscess or a stitch sinus which does not heal until the stitch is removed. Treatment of an abscess, inappropriately, with antibiotics alone, may actually halt the expansion of the abscess and sterilise the pus, giving rise to a sterile abscess or antibioma.

Pyogenic abscesses are caused by a wide variety of bacteria and occur at many different sites (Table 7.2). They may be clinically obvious such as in the breast, perianal region, or axilla, or they may be cryptic or hidden, e.g. subphrenic or pelvic abscesses. Abscesses do not necessarily form at the site of primary infection but may form at a more distant site, e.g. pelvic or subphrenic

Table 7.2 Common sites of abscesses

Site	Source of infection	Organism
Skin (boil)	Hair follicle	*Staph. aureus*
Breast	Breast feeding	*Staph. aureus*
Pelvic	Abdominal or pelvic sepsis, e.g. salpingitis appendicitis	Coliforms Bacteroides *Strep. faecalis*
Subphrenic	Abdominal or pelvic sepsis, e.g. peritonitis	Coliforms Bacteroides *Strep. faecalis*
Tubo-ovarian	Pelvic sepsis Gonorrhoea	Genital flora *N. gonorrhoeae*
Ischio-rectal	Spread from perianal glands	Coliforms
Perinephric	Acute pyelonephritis	Coliforms
Hepatic	Cholangitis Portal pyaemia	Coliforms
Lung	Aspiration pneumonia Bronchiectasis Bronchial obstruction *Staph. aureus* pneumonia	*Strep. pneumonia* Anaerobes *Staph. aureus*
Cerebral	Haematogenous, e.g. bronchiectasis, infective endocarditis Sinusitis Otitis media	Streptococci *Staph. aureus* Bacteroides

abscesses after perforated appendicitis, due to tracking of infected material.

'Metastatic' abscesses may form as a result of haematogenous spread or 'pyaemic' spread of infected thrombi. Portal pyaemia following appendicitis may result in liver abscesses, and infective endocarditis may result in cerebral abscesses.

ASEPSIS AND ANTISEPSIS

Asepsis is the exclusion of organisms from the tissues. Antisepsis is the attempt at the prevention of growth and multiplication of microorganisms that cause sepsis.

RISK FACTORS CONTRIBUTING TO SEPSIS

These may be related to problems in the patient, problems related to treatment, the injury or the disease process itself, and the environment. These causes are shown in Box 7.2.

WOUND INFECTION

Classification of wounds

Wounds may be classified by their potential for infection:

1. *clean*: an operation carried out through clean non-infected skin under sterile conditions where the GI tract GU tract, or respiratory tract are not breached, e.g. hernia repair, varicose vein surgery; the risk of wound infection should be less than 2%

2. *clean contaminated*: an operation carried out under sterile conditions with breaching of a hollow viscus other than the colon, where contamination is minimal, e.g. cholecystectomy; the risk of wound infection should be less than 8%

3. *contaminated*: an operation carried out where contamination has occurred, e.g. by opening the colon, an open fracture, or animal or human bites; the risk of wound infection is around 12%

4. *dirty*: an operation carried out in the presence of pus, or a perforated viscus, e.g. perforated appendicitis, faecal peritonitis; the risk of wound infection is 25%.

Factors influencing the development of wound sepsis

These are shown in the Box 7.3.

HOSPITAL-ACQUIRED INFECTION

Hospital-acquired infections, or nosocomial infections occur in about 10% of hospitalised patients. The commonest are UTIs, wound infections, lower respiratory tract infections, and skin and soft tissue infections. Present-day pathogens are often resistant to antibiotics, a major problem being methicillin-resistant *Staph. aureus*

Box 7.2   Risk factors contributing to sepsis

- Patient-related
  Age
  Diabetes
  Intercurrent illness, e.g. cardiac, respiratory, renal
  Immunosuppression
  Nutritional status
  Obesity

- Injury or disease-related
  Location
  Extent

- Treatment-related
  Length of preoperative stay
  Duration of surgery
  Emergency vs elective surgery
  Poor surgical technique

- Environment related
  Contamination
  Super infection
  Long term stay on ITU

Box 7.3   Factors influencing the development of wound sepsis

- Type of surgery
  Clean or contaminated
  Prosthesis or foreign body
  Drain
  Duration of surgery
  'Place' on list

- Surgical team
  Skill of surgeon
  Aseptic technique
  Carriage of *Staph. aureus*

- Age and general condition of patient

- Precautions taken against possibility of infection
  Preoperative duration of stay
  Adequate antisepsis of hands
  Adequate skin preparation
  Preparation of the bowel
  Antibiotic prophylaxis
  Adequate ventilation

- Ward factors postoperatively

(MRSA). Predisposition to hospital-acquired infection includes:

- age — the extremes of life
- susceptible patients, e.g. immunosuppressed, diabetic, those with prosthetic implants
- modes of treatment, e.g. intravenous lines, indwelling catheters, etc.

The origin of bacterial infection may be divided into two main sources:-

- endogenous — with patient's normal flora
- exogenous — from other people or objects in the environment.

ENDOGENOUS INFECTION

This occurs where the organism is carried by the patient either as part of the normal flora or 'replacement' flora, i.e. 'replacement' organisms which colonise various sites when the patient is treated with antimicrobials. A knowledge of the normal flora present at various sites is important such that distinction may be made from 'replacement' organisms which have resulted from antibiotic therapy. The following are examples of normal flora:

- skin — coagulase negative staphylococci and diphtheroids
- upper respiratory tract — *S. viridans*, diphtheroids, anaerobes, commensal neisseriae
- lower gastrointestinal tract — coliforms, faecal streptococci, pseudomonas, anaerobes (bacteroides, clostridia)
- anterior urethra — skin flora (as above) or faecal flora (as above).

Commensal bacteria are potential pathogens, and infection may result if the balance is disturbed by a breach of the body defences or if an organism normally a commensal at one site gains access to another site where it is not a commensal: e.g. *E. coli*, which is part of the normal flora of the colon, gaining access to the urinary tract and giving rise to a UTI. Broad spectrum antibiotics alter the normal flora, inhibiting sensitive organisms and allowing overgrowth of resistant bacteria which may result in serious infection. A detailed knowledge of the normal flora is required to distinguish normal flora in culture from pathogens responsible for infection. 'Replacement' organisms resulting from antibiotic therapy may cause infection. *Klebsiella* may colonise the upper respiratory tract after a course of antibiotics and give rise to chest infections, particularly in the ventilated intubated patient. Although *Klebsiella* is not part of the normal

flora of the upper respiratory tract, it is part of a 'replacement' flora, and the infection is therefore endogenous in origin.

EXOGENOUS INFECTION

Exogenous infection is derived either from other people or objects in the environment:

1. *people*: this may be from medical, nursing, or other patients either from infection, subclinical infection, or asymptomatic carriers
2. *inanimate objects (fomites):* these include surgical instruments, anaesthetic equipment, ventilators, humidifiers, and parenteral fluids, particularly if drugs are added under non-sterile conditions
3. *other sources*: these include floors, blankets, urinary bottles, toilets, dust, air and air conditioning systems.

METHOD OF SPREAD OF INFECTION

Infection may spread by the following methods:

- contact — hands, clothing, etc.
- airborne — droplets and respiratory infection, dust, scales shed from skin, aerosols, nebulisers, air conditioning
- ingestion — food poisoning, overcrowded wards, especially psychiatric and geriatric, faecal–oral spread, poor kitchen hygiene, and carriers.

PREVENTION AND CONTROL OF HOSPITAL-ACQUIRED INFECTION

The following are important factors in the prevention and control of hospital-acquired infection:

- education of staff: hand washing; correct disposal of waste, e.g. soiled dressings; good nursing care; safe environment, e.g. appropriate space between beds, clean toilets, etc.; good theatre technique; good aseptic surgical technique
- skin infection and antisepsis
- sterilisation and disinfection
- prophylactic antibiotics
- protective clothing
- isolation of patients with established infection
- appropriate design of hospital buildings
- staff health: exclude staff suffering from infection from contact with patients; protect staff, e.g. hepatitis B immunisation
- surveillance: e.g. infection control; monitoring of infection rates; careful tracking of potentially dangerous bacteria; appropriate policy making.

CONTROL OF STAPHYLOCOCCAL OUTBREAKS

Patients with obvious skin sepsis or skin lesions should be excluded from the surgical team. Carriers of *Staph. aureus* should be excluded and treated. Personnel should wear protective theatre clothing, caps to cover the hair, clean theatre underdress, gowns and masks. Following adequate washing with antiseptics, gloves should be worn. Chlorhexidine, povidone-iodine or alcoholic chlorhexidine are suitable for hand preparation. The number of personnel in theatre should be reduced to a minimum. Theatre environment is important. The air flow should be in the correct direction. Floors should be kept clean and horizontal surfaces, e.g. trolleys, reduced to a minimum as these are dust traps. The walls and ceilings should be cleaned with antiseptic on a regular basis. Lights above the operating table should be kept dust free to prevent potentially bacteria-laden particles landing in the wound.

As far as the patient is concerned, the bed linen and clothes must not be allowed in the theatre area. Any shaving that is carried out should be carried out immediately prior to surgery and not some time before which may allow staphylococci to colonise small lacerations in the skin. Disinfection of the skin at or near the operation site should be carried out and the skin at or near the site of the wound separated from the rest by drapes or occlusive drapes, e.g. Opsite. Figure 7.1 shows how staphylococcal infection may spread.

METHICILLIN-RESISTANT *STAPHYLOCOCCUS AUREUS* (MRSA)

Patients and staff in whom colonisation or carriage of MRSA is suspected should be screened by taking swabs from the hairline, nose, axillae, groin and perineum. Eradication of the carriage of MRSA in a carrier involves application of antiseptics, e.g. mupirocin or chlorhexidine, to the nose and skin and use of antiseptic soaps and shampoos. Treatment may be required for up to 3 weeks. Nasal swabs are checked at 3 days after the last application of cream and again at 3 weeks. Patients with MRSA should be nursed in isolation. Vancomycin or teicoplanin may be the only agents available for treatment for MRSA. Strains of *Staph. aureus* resistant to methicillin are also resistant to virtually all beta-lactam agents. Many epidemic strains are multiresistant, exhibiting resistance to aminoglycosides, macrolides and other antistaphylococcal agents which include the topical agent mupirocin, which has been used to eradicate the organism from carriers.

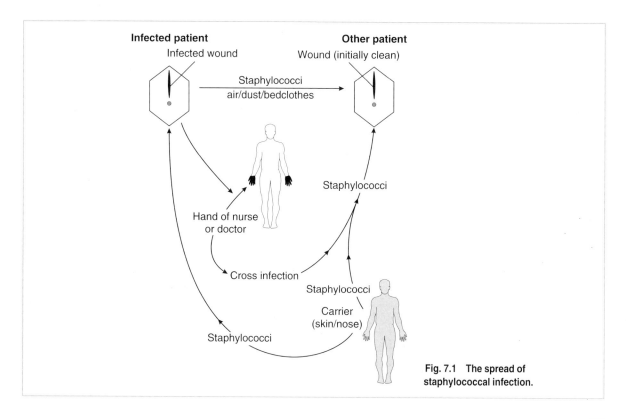

Fig. 7.1 The spread of staphylococcal infection.

TRANSMISSIBLE INFECTION AND THE SURGEON

The surgeon, as indeed any medical, nursing, or para-medical personnel, is at risk from three main viral infections: hepatitis B, hepatitis C and HIV.

HEPATITIS B

The hepatitis B virus (HBV) may be transmitted by:

- blood transfusion
- inoculation via sharps injuries from blood or blood products
- droplet transmission
- syringe and needle sharing in drug addicts
- sexual intercourse with an infected partner
- homosexual practices.

Antigen carriage is a risk for hospital staff, especially those in 'high risk' areas, e.g. theatre staff. Dialysis units are often quoted as being a 'high risk' area but, following outbreaks many years ago, all staff and patients are tested for HBsAg. Hepatitis vaccine is offered to all high risk health workers. These categories involve surgeons, theatre nurses, Pathology department staff, Accident and Emergency staff, staff in Liver Transplant units, workers in residential units for the mentally handicapped, staff of GI units, and staff of Infectious and Communicable Disease units.

The incubation period of HBV is between 6 weeks and 6 months. 5–10% of infected patients will develop a carrier state, and awareness of this is important for surgeons. A number of antigen–antibody systems occur relating to HBV. The three viral antigens are hepatitis B surface antigen (HBsAg), core antigen (HBcAg) and e-antigen (HBeAg).

Following infection, antibodies are formed against all three of the viral antigens, but there are important clinical consequences of their identification. Infected persons and carriers have HBsAg and anti-HBcAg but lack anti-HBsAg in their blood. On recovery from infection, HBsAg disappears from the blood and anti-HBsAg becomes demonstrable together with anti-HBcAg. The e-antigen is found only in HBsAg positive sera and appears during the incubation period. The presence of HBeAg (e-antigen) implies high infectivity. Carriers with a persistence of the e-antigen are much more likely to infect others. It has been shown that surgeons who possess the e-antigen may infect their patients during operative procedures.

HEPATITIS C

Hepatitis C virus (HCV) is present in blood and spreads in the same way as HBV by blood transfusion, intravenous drug abuse, and from mother to infant. Sexual transmission is uncommon. The incubation period is 2–4 months, at which stage a mild disease occurs in about one in ten individuals. Carriers are a source of infection. About 50% of infected patients develop chronic active hepatitis, and 20% progress to cirrhosis. Infection is also associated with liver cancer.

HIV

Infection with HIV is permanent, and it is likely that all carriers will eventually develop AIDS. Surgical personnel are a high risk. Infection from HIV results from the passage of infected body fluid (usually blood) from one person to another. Needle stick injuries and scalpel injuries are possible sources of infection. In the general population HIV may be transmitted by unprotected anal, vaginal and oral intercourse, by sharing needles in drug abuse, and by infected blood products: e.g. as has happened in the past with haemophiliacs. The following are at risk of becoming HIV positive:

- homosexual or bisexual males
- prostitutes (male and female)
- intravenous drug abusers
- haemophiliacs who were treated before routine testing became available, i.e. October 1995
- sexual partners of the above
- children of infected mothers.

HIV is a retrovirus which infects lymphocytes, macrophages and monocytes, i.e. cells that are found in all body fluids. HIV binds the CD4 receptors on T helper lymphocytes (CD4 cells). After a long latent period, up to 8–10 years, the CD4 cell counts begin to decline and the immunosuppression increases the risk of many opportunistic infections and also tumours. Diagnosis is based on the detection of anti-HIV antibodies in the serum. The majority of infected individuals develop antibodies within 3 months of exposure.

Care at surgery needs to be exercised with patients who are known to have AIDS or to be HIV positive. Patients with anorectal disease related to homosexuality, haemophiliacs, and sexual partners and children of the above should be treated with appropriate caution. Counselling is required and consent must be obtained for HIV testing. If a patient refuses and is suspected of being HIV positive then precautions must be taken with nursing care and any invasive procedures from simple venepuncture to major surgery.

PRECAUTIONS FOR THE CARE OF KNOWN AND SUSPECTED HBV, HBC AND HIV CARRIERS

- All personnel involved in patient care should be aware of the problem.
- Protection from contaminated body fluids should be arranged.
- Contaminated fluids, dressings, etc. should be disposed of correctly.
- Appropriate theatre technique should be adopted.
  1. Any patient considered as a risk should be indicated as belonging to a high risk category in the operating list. Under no circumstances should the actual disease causing the risk be placed upon the operating list.
  2. Only absolutely necessary personnel should be in theatre. There should be no spectators.
  3. Remove all but essential equipment.
  4. Use disposable scrub suits, footwear, gowns, and drapes.
  5. Use plastic aprons, two pairs of gloves, visors to prevent splashing in the eyes.
  6. The operation should be done with no-touch technique if possible, with meticulous attention to haemostasis. Stapling devices rather than needles should be used if possible.
  7. All disposable equipment should be removed in specifically marked containers.
  8. The theatre should be thoroughly cleansed with dilute bleach solution.
  9. Recovery staff must also be aware of the risk.

ACCIDENTAL INJURY TO STAFF

HBV positive patient   Let the stab site or laceration bleed. Wash the area well with soap and water. An accident form should be filled in and the incident reported to Occupational Health. If the recipient of the injury is not immunised, then a course of vaccine should be started immediately. Hepatitis B immune globulin should also be administered.

HIV positive patient   Let the injury bleed and wash it well. Report the incident to Occupational Health and fill in an accident form. Blood tests may be required in future to check for HIV following counselling of the recipient of the injury. These tests should be carried out at 3 months and 6 months. There is no gross evidence that chemoprophylaxis with zidovudine is effective. However, it

may be used, but the side effects are unpleasant. Nausea, malaise, fatigue, headache and vomiting have been reported, together with bone marrow suppression.

STERILISATION

Sterilisation is the complete destruction of all microorganisms including spores, cysts and viruses. Sterilisation may be achieved by physical and chemical methods.

PHYSICAL

Heat

Moist heat

Steam under pressure attains a higher temperature than boiling water, the final temperature being directly related to pressure. Sterilisation by steam under pressure is the most commonly used method in hospitals. This is carried out in autoclaves, where steam is heated to 121°C. Steam condenses on the surface of the instruments in the autoclave, giving up a large amount of latent heat of vaporisation required for its production. The sterilising cycle must be long enough to ensure adequate sterilisation. The 'hold time' at 121°C should be 15 min, but the entire cycle is longer, allowing for heating up and cooling down. A higher temperature of 134°C with a 'hold time' of 3 min may also be used. Continuous recordings should be made of the temperature in the autoclave, and all sterilisers should have a preset automatic cycle which cannot be interrupted until the cycle is completed. Monitoring of the efficacy of sterilisation is carried out by Browne's tubes placed among the instruments. These glass tubes contain fluid which changes from red to green after appropriate exposure. Sterile packs can be identified as appropriately sterilised by changing colour of heat sensitive inks on the pack (Bowie–Dick test). Bacteria, fungi, spores and viruses are destroyed in autoclaves at 134°C for a 'hold time' of 3 min or 121°C for a 'hold time' of 15 min. Slow viruses, e.g. Creutzfeld–Jakob's disease, are difficult to destroy and will need longer times. Moist heat is more effective than dry heat because it penetrates materials better and denatures proteins of the cell walls of microorganisms.

Dry heat

The efficacy of dry heat depends on the initial moisture of the microbial cells. Dry heat at 160°C with a 'hold time' of 2 h will kill all microorganisms. However, many articles will not withstand these high temperatures. The process is not suitable for materials that are denatured or damaged at the required temperature, e.g. plastics. It is not suitable for aqueous fluids, e.g. i.v. fluids. It may be used for solids, non-aqueous liquids, and to sterilise objects that will stand the heat in enclosed (airtight) containers. All items must be thoroughly cleaned and dried before they are placed in a hot air oven.

Irradiation

Sterilisation by ionising radiation is an industrial process and is used commercially for large batches of suitable objects. These are heat-labile articles and often single-use items, e.g. catheters, syringes and i.v. lines.

Filtration

Bacteria and spores may be removed from heat-labile solutions by filtration. Cellulose acetate (Millipore) filters with a small pore size can remove viruses. The efficiency of sterilisation is determined by pore size. This method is used by the pharmaceutical industry for sterilisation of drugs for injection.

Chemical

Ethylene oxide

This is a highly penetrative agent against vegetative bacteria, spores and viruses. It is a highly explosive gas and must be used under strictly controlled conditions. It is used to sterilise heat-labile articles. It is ideal for electrical equipment, fibre optic endoscopes, or for resterilisation of single-use items, e.g. dialysis lines. However, the resterilisation of dialysis lines is not to be condoned, but is necessitated by financial expediency in some countries. The gas penetrates well into rubber and plastics. It is toxic, irritant, mutagenic and may be carcinogenic.

Glutaraldehyde

Immersion in 2% glutaraldehyde can be used to sterilise endoscopes and other instruments containing plastic or rubber. Inactivation of microbes varies, and different times are required, TB organisms requiring at least 60 min. Glutaraldehyde may cause contact dermatitis in personnel involved in sterilising equipment, e.g. nurses preparing endoscopes.

Formaldehyde

Dry saturated steam in combination with formaldehyde kills vegetative bacteria, spores, and most viruses. It is suitable for many heat-labile instruments, e.g. cystoscopes, as sterilisation can be achieved at low temperature, i.e. 73°C for 2 h. Items contaminated with body fluids are excluded, as proteins will be fixed and deposited on the equipment.

DISINFECTION

Disinfection is a process used to reduce the number of viable microorganisms. It fails to inactivate some bacterial spores and some viruses. Disinfection has to be distinguished from cleaning, which is a process which physically removes contamination but does not necessarily inactivate microorganisms. The efficacy of disinfection depends on several factors: for example, the length of exposure, or the presence of blood, faeces, or other organic matter which may reduce the efficacy of the disinfection process. Some examples of disinfection are given below:

- *Hypochlorite* (Milton, Eusol). Hypochlorites have a wide antibacterial spectrum, including viruses. They are inactivated by organic matter.
- *Povidone-iodine* (Betadine). This has wide antibacterial spectrum. It is useful for preoperative skin preparation of the patient and as a surgical scrub solution.
- *Chlorhexidine* (Hibitane). This is active against Gram positive bacteria. It is usually used as a 0.5% solution in 70% ethanol or in water. Unlike iodine it is devoid of the risk of irritation of the skin and sensitisation.
- *Quaternary ammonium* salts (Cetrimide). Quaternary ammonium compounds are active against Gram positive bacteria. They have no action against *Pseudomonas*. They are weak disinfectants.
- *Formaldehyde*. Formaldehyde has a wide antibacterial spectrum, including viruses. Formaldehyde is a hazardous substance. It is irritant to the eyes, respiratory tract, and skin. Aqueous 10% formaldehyde can be used to disinfect contaminated surfaces. If used as a gas it needs to be used in an air-tight cabinet.
- *Glutaraldehyde* (Cidex). This has a wide antibacterial spectrum, including viruses. It kills spores slowly. Penetration is poor and it is irritant and may cause hypersensitivity.
- *Boiling water*. This is an efficient disinfection process which kills bacteria, including TB, some viruses, including HBV and HIV, and some spores. Items for disinfection must be thoroughly cleaned and totally immersed in the boiling water. It is suitable for proctoscopes and sigmoidoscopes.
- *Pasteurisation*. This can be used for foodstuffs such as milk which can be disinfected but not sterilised by moist heat. Milk is held at 63–66°C for 30 min. All non-spore-forming pathogenic bacteria, including *Mycobacterium tuberculosis*, brucellae, *Campylobacter* and salmonellae, are killed.

COMPLICATIONS OF INFECTION

PATHOPHYSIOLOGY OF THE BODY'S RESPONSE TO INFECTION

One of the most frequent and serious problems confronting the clinician is the management of the systemic response to infection. The incidence of sepsis has been increasing over the last 25 years and is the most common cause of death in ITUs. New terminology has arisen in an attempt to stratify the spectrum of sepsis and to introduce a universal definition of the various stages of sepsis. The Society of Critical Care Medicine and the American College of Chest Physicians, at a meeting held in 1991, produced a series of definitions for the systemic inflammatory response syndrome (SIRS), sepsis, and other clinical conditions related to sepsis. SIRS is defined as a characteristic clinical response manifested by two or more of the following criteria: (i) temperature above 38°C or below 36°C (rectal); (ii) heart rate above 90 bpm; (iii) respiratory rate above 20 breaths per minute or a $PaCO_2$ less than 4.3 kPa; (iv) WBC above 12 000 cells per mm^3, below 4 000 cells per mm^3 or 10% of immature forms. Sepsis is described as SIRS with a documented infection and severe sepsis as SIRS with documented infection and haemodynamic compromise. Multiple organ dysfunction syndrome (MODS) is a state of physiological derangement in which organ function is not capable of maintaining homeostasis.

There is a continuum from the development of SIRS to the onset of sepsis and progression to shock and multiple organ dysfunction. The identification of SIRS alone in a patient on ITU has a poor specificity for predicting the development of sepsis and septic shock. However, there is an increasing incidence of organ system failure as patients progress from SIRS to septic shock.

PATHOPHYSIOLOGY OF SYSTEMIC INFLAMMATORY RESPONSE SYNDROME

SIRS may be initiated by infection (bacterial, viral, fungal, protozoal) or non-infected causes, e.g. trauma, burns, cirrhosis and pancreatitis.

Three stages have been described in the development of SIRS

- *Stage I* — In response to a local insult, the local environment produces cytokines which provoke an inflammatory response, promote wound repair, and recruit cells of the reticulo-endothelial system.
- *Stage II* — Small quantities of cytokines are released into the circulation to enhance the local response. Macrophages and platelets are recruited, and growth factor production is stimulated. An acute phase response occurs which is controlled by a simultaneous decrease in pro-inflammatory mediators and release of endogenous antagonists. These mediators hold the initial inflammatory response in check. This continues until the wound is healed, the infection resolves and homeostasis is restored.
- *Stage III* — If homeostasis is not restored, stage III (SIRS) develops. A massive systemic reaction occurs, cytokines becoming destructive rather than protective. Inflammatory mediators trigger numerous humoral cascades, resulting in sustained activation of the reticulo-endothelial system with loss of integrity of the microcirculation and dysfunction of various distant end-organs.

The destructive systemic and regional responses to SIRS, i.e. increased peripheral dilatation, excessive microvascular permeability, accelerated microvascular clotting, and leucocytes/endothelial cell activation, contribute to pathological changes in various organs and are considered the major aetiological factors in the development of septic shock, ARDS and MODS. Changes associated with MODS include fever, hypermetabolism, anorexia, protein catabolism, cachexia, and altered fat, glucose and trace element mineral metabolism. These processes are accelerated in the presence of a second insult, e.g. shock, infection, ischaemia following the initial trauma. Mediators of SIRS include endotoxin, TNFα and interleukins, chiefly IL-1 and IL-6. Cells involved include endothelial cells and leucocytes, especially neutrophils. Secondary inflammatory mediators include arachidonic acid metabolites, nitric oxide, and platelet-activating factor (PAF).

Attempts to abrogate SIRS may be approached in three ways:

- eradication of the source of infection
- treatment of sepsis-associated cardiovascular, metabolic and multiorgan disturbances
- inhibitors of toxic mediators e.g. anti-TNFα, anti-interleukin 1.

It is now thought that SIRS, which is a pro-inflammatory response, is only one part of two-pronged response. The other part of the response is an anti-inflammatory response termed the compensatory anti-inflammatory response syndrome (CARS). Thus, at any one time there is a mixture of responses, each vying with the other, which may result in a predominance of SIRS or a predominance of CARS, or even an intermediate mixed inflammatory response syndrome (MARS). The result of these responses carries a variety of consequences known as CHAOS, i.e. *C*ardiovascular shock, *H*omeostasis, *A*poptosis, *O*rgan dysfunction and immune *S*uppression. However, as yet it has not been possible to diagnose the state of the systemic inflammatory response in a particular patient, i.e. whether at the time it is SIRS, CARS, or MARS. Until such time as this is achieved, it will not be possible to treat the systemic inflammatory response with any degree of certainty.

ADULT RESPIRATORY DISTRESS SYNDROME

The causes of ARDS are shown in Box 7.4. The condition is further discussed in Chapter 11.

SEPTICAEMIA

Bacteraemia is the presence of bacteria in the circulation, where they can be identified by blood culture. There is no sign of clinical infection. Septicaemia implies the presence of bacteria in the circulation, identified by blood culture, with clinical evidence of infection. In septicaemia there is multiplication of bacteria in the blood, with a failure of bacteriocidal mechanisms to stem the number of organisms released into the circulation.

Septicaemia is often a complication of a more localised infection, e.g. subphrenic abscess, peritonitis, or cholangitis. Clinical presentation is usually due to a worsening of the patient's condition with fever, confusion, agitation, rigors, tachypnoea, hypotension and organ failure. Consequences of septicaemia include SIRS and MODS and multiorgan failure. Some conditions predisposing to septicaemia and causative organisms are shown in Table 7.3.

Box 7.4   Causes of adult respiratory distress syndrome (ARDS)

- Shock
  Septic shock, especially Gram negative
  Haemorrhagic
  Cardiogenic
  Anaphylactic

- Trauma
  Major trauma
  Direct pulmonary trauma
    Lung contusion
    Near drowning
    Irradiation
    Smoke inhalation
    Aspiration of vomitus (gastric acid)
    Inhalation of chemicals, e.g. chlorine, ammonia

- Cerebral
  Head injury (neurogenic pulmonary oedema)
  Cerebral haemorrhage

- Embolism
  Fat
  Air
  Amniotic fluid

- Drugs
  Opiates
  Barbiturates

- Others
  Acute pancreatitis
  Disseminated intravascular coagulation
  Cardiopulmonary bypass
  Massive blood transfusions
  Eclampsia
  Oxygen toxicity

Table 7.3   Causes of septicaemia

Predisposing factor	Causative organism
Abdominal sepsis, e.g. peritonitis, abscess, cholangitis	Coliforms, bacteroides *Strep. faecalis*
Infected wounds Burns	*Staph. aureus* Coliforms, bacteroides *Strep. pyogenes*
Urinary tract infection	Coliforms
Chest infection	*Strep. pneumoniae*
Gynaecological infection, e.g. salpingitis	Coliforms, bacteroides *Strep. faecalis* *Staph. aureus* Toxic shock syndrome (tampons)
Indwelling vascular lines e.g. CVP lines, Hickman catheters	*Staph. epidermidis* *Staph. aureus* Coliforms
Postsplenectomy	*Strep. pneumoniae* *H. influenzae* *N. meningitidis*
Intravenous drug abuse	*Staph. aureus*
Immunocompromised, e.g. organ transplant recipients, AIDS	Coliforms *Pseudomonas* *Staph. aureus* *Strep. pneumoniae* Fungi

MULTIORGAN FAILURE

The pathophysiology of the response of the body to infection has been described above. Multiple organ failure is a final common pathway associated with the consequences of severe infection, severe tissue injury, or shock.

Infection and endotoxaemia are the most common causes of multiorgan failure, but hypovolaemic shock, if it lasts long enough and causes enough damage, may also cause multiorgan failure. Massive tissue injury, e.g. pancreatitis, burns, or crushing injury, may also result in multiorgan failure.

Factors leading to multi-organ failure include:

- excessive release of endogenous mediators, including TNFα, IL-1, IL-6
- impaired local microvascular perfusion interfering with delivery of oxygen to the tissues, with disruption of cellular metabolic functions
- impaired intestinal barrier function with bacterial translocation releasing endotoxins into the portal circulation and to the liver
- damage to reticulo-endothelial function
- immune depression with T and B cell depression, T suppressor cell stimulation, resulting in increased vulnerability to infection.

The target organs of cytokines include the lung, cardiovascular system, liver, kidney, brain, gastrointestinal tract, reticulo-endothelial system and immune system. Failure of individual organs in multiorgan failure often follows a predictable pattern with pulmonary failure occurring first, followed by hepatic, intestinal, renal and finally cardiac failure. The mortality of multiorgan failure is directly related to the number of organs that have failed. With one organ affected, the prognosis is fairly good, with about 70% of patients surviving. With two organs failing, it falls to 50%, and with four the mortality approaches 100%. The prognosis is also affected by the age of the patient and previous compromise of organ function.

Specific systems

Nervous system

Samuel Jacob, Andrew T Raftery

ANATOMY

CRANIAL CAVITY

The cranium, or the skull, consists of the cranial cavity and the facial skeleton. Most bones of the cranial cavity are flat bones having two plates of compact bone separated by a thin layer of trabecular bone, or the diploe. Both the inner and outer surfaces are lined by periosteum, the inner periosteum being the endosteal layer of dura mater. The bones of the cranial cavity are the frontal, occipital, sphenoid, ethmoid and the paired temporal and parietal bones.

The cranial cavity has a cranial vault and the base of the cranium with the three cranial fossae.

Cranial vault

The cranial vault, or the roof of the cranial cavity, is formed by the frontal bone anteriorly, the paired parietal bones laterally and the occipital bone posteriorly (Fig. 8.1). A midline sagittal groove marks the position of the superior sagittal sinus. The sinus and its groove widen as they pass posteriorly. The falx cerebri is attached to the lips of this groove. Irregular depressions along the groove lodge the arachnoid granulations.

The sagittal suture separates the two parietal bones in the midline. The coronal suture divides the frontal from the parietal bones, and the lambdoid suture divides the two parietal bones from the occipital and the temporal bones. Posterior to the coronal suture the middle meningeal vein and its tributaries, accompanied by the

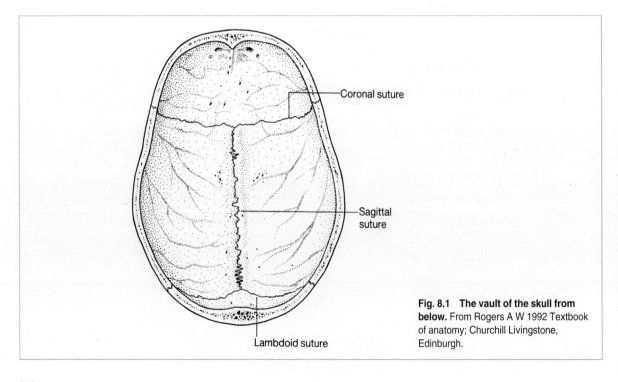

Coronal suture

Sagittal suture

Lambdoid suture

Fig. 8.1 The vault of the skull from below. From Rogers A W 1992 Textbook of anatomy; Churchill Livingstone, Edinburgh.

middle meningeal artery, groove the vault of the skull. The bony vault is thin in the temporal and the lower part of the occipital regions, where there are thick muscular attachments. A blow on the skull vault may cause internal injuries without fracture because of the plasticity of the skull bones.

The lambda is the junction between the lambdoid suture and the sagittal suture. It is the area of the posterior fontanelle in the infant. The bregma, where the anterior fontanelle was in the infant, is at the junction between the coronal and the sagittal sutures. The glabella is the prominence above the nasion which is the depression between the two supraorbital margins. The pterion is a thin part of the skull at the junction of the parietal, frontal and temporal bones and the greater wing of the sphenoid in the temporal region of the skull. The anterior branch of the middle meningeal artery and the accompanying vein traverse the pterion.

Three cranial fossae

The floor of the cranial cavity has three cranial fossae — the anterior, middle, and the posterior cranial fossae — each progressively lower than the one in front. The anterior cranial fossa overlies the orbit and the nasal cavities.

The frontal lobe of the brain lies in the anterior cranial fossa. The middle cranial fossa lies below and behind the anterior and contains the temporal lobes. Most posteriorly the posterior cranial fossa lies at the lowest level and contains the brainstem and the cerebellum.

Anterior cranial fossa

The anterior cranial fossa (Fig. 8.2) is largely formed by the orbital plate of the frontal bone supplemented posteriorly by the lesser wing of the sphenoid. The ethmoid bone with its cribriform plate and the crista galli occupies the gap between the two orbital plates. The orbital plate separates the anterior cranial fossa from the orbit. The cribiform plate roofs the nasal cavities.

The following structures pass between the anterior cranial fossa and the nasal cavities.

- The olfactory nerves — about 20–30 nerves arise from the olfactory mucosa of the nasal cavities, pass through the cribriform plate and enter the olfactory bulbs which lie on the cribriform plate.
- Emissary veins connecting the cerebral veins and veins in the nasal cavity also pass through the cribriform plate as well as the foramen caecum lying anterior to the crista galli.

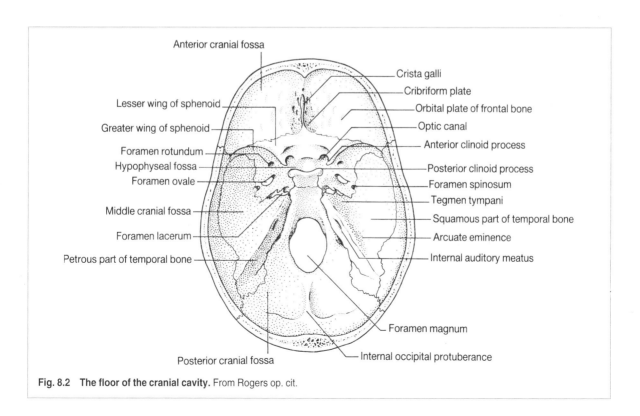

Fig. 8.2 The floor of the cranial cavity. From Rogers op. cit.

- The anterior ethmoidal nerves and arteries accompanied by veins pass through the anterior part of the cribriform plate into the nasal cavities.

A fracture of the anterior cranial fossa may cause bleeding into the nose and/or orbit and CSF rhinorrhea. Bleeding into the orbit may manifest as subconjunctival haemorrhage and/or proptosis.

Middle cranial fossa

The body of the sphenoid lies in the middle forming the floor of the pituitary (hypophyseal) fossa (Fig. 8.2). Laterally are the greater wings of the sphenoid and the squamous parts of the temporal bones. The petrous part of the temporal bone containing the middle and inner ear forms the posterior boundary of the fossa.

The pituitary fossa is bounded in front and behind by the anterior and posterior clinoid processes. It contains the pituitary gland and is roofed by the diaphragma sellae, a fold of dura mater.

Anteriorly the middle cranial fossa has the optic canal and the supraorbital fissure communicatiing with the orbit. The optic canal transmits the optic nerve and the ophthalmic artery. The supraorbital fissure transmits the:

- oculomotor nerve
- trochlear nerve
- abducens nerve
- ophthalmic division of the trigeminal nerve
- ophthalmic veins.

Lateral to the pituitary fossa the middle cranial fossa has a few important foramina:

- the foramen rotundum, transmitting the maxillary nerve
- the foramen ovale, posterolateral to the foramen rotundum, transmitting the mandibular nerve
- the foramen spinosum, posterolateral to the foramen ovale, for the middle meningeal artery
- the foramen lacerum — the upper opening of the carotid canal contains the internal carotid artery.

Fractures of the middle cranial fossa are common, as the bone is weakened by the foramina and canals. Fracture involving the tegmen tympani, the thin anterior surface of the petrous temporal bone, results in bleeding into the middle ear. Excessive bleeding ruptures the tympanic membrane, discharging blood from the ear. This can be associated with CSF otorrhoea. The seventh and eighth nerves also may be involved, as they run in the petrous temporal bone.

Posterior cranial fossa

The posterior cranial fossa has an anterior wall formed by the petrous temporal bone laterally and the body of the sphenoid and the basilar part of the occipital bone medially. The latter two form the clivus which extends from the foramen magnum to the dorsum sellae. The occipital bone mostly forms the floor and lateral walls of the fossa. The internal occipital protuberance is in the midline on the posterior wall. Above this the skull is grooved by the superior sagittal sinus. Running anterolaterally on either side from the internal occipital protuberance are the grooves for the transverse sinuses, which continue down beneath the petrous temporal bone as the sigmoid sinuses. The sigmoid sinus passes through the jugular foramen to become the internal jugular vein. The ninth, tenth and eleventh nerves as well as the inferior petrosal sinus pass through the jugular foramen anterior to the sigmoid sinus. The hypoglossal or anterior condylar canals transmitting the hypoglossal nerves lie on the anterior rim of the foramen magnum. Through the foramen magnum the medulla oblongata continues into the vertebral canal as the spinal cord. The vertebral arteries and the spinal accessory nerves enter the skull via the foramen magnum.

Anteriorly in the fossa on the medial aspect of each petrous temporal bone is the internal acoustic meatus conveying the seventh and eighth nerves and the labyrinthine arteries into the internal ear. Below the internal acoustic meatus in the anterior aspect of the jugular foramen is the cochlear canaliculus into which opens the aqueduct of the cochlea (perilymphatic duct) which brings the perilymph of the internal ear into communication with the CSF.

Fractures of the posterior cranial fossa may involve the basilar part of the occipital bone which separates the pharynx from the posterior cranial fossa. Bleeding may then occur into the pharynx. More lateral fractures can bleed into the back of the neck.

BRAIN AND MENINGES

Brain

The brain is subdivided into the forebrain, midbrain and hindbrain, comprising the major parts listed in Table 8.1.

Cerebral hemisphere

The cerebral hemisphere has a layer of grey matter on its external surface, the cerebral cortex, and white matter in the interior in which there are nuclei forming the basal ganglia. The cavity of the cerebral hemisphere is the lateral ventricle.

The cerebral hemisphere (Fig. 8.3) is divided into four lobes for descriptive purposes:

- The frontal lobe lies in the anterior cranial fossa, and its anterior end is the frontal pole.

Table 8.1	Major subdivisions and parts of the brain
Major subdivisions	**Parts**
Forebrain	Cerebral hemisphere, or telencephalon [lateral ventricle] Diencephalon containing thalamus and hypothalamus [third ventricle]
Midbrain	Mesencephalon [cerebral aqueduct] } Brainstem
Hindbrain	Pons, medulla and cerebellum [fourth ventricle]

The parts of the ventricular system are shown in brackets.

- The temporal lobe lies in the middle cranial fossa, with an anterior end the temporal pole and an upturned projection on its medial surface, the uncus.
- The parietal lobe lies above the temporal lobe between the frontal and the occipital lobes.
- The occipital lobe lies above the tentorium cerebelli, and its posterior end is the occipital pole.

The cerebral cortex has a large number of sulci (clefts) and gyri (folds). The lateral sulcus is the largest sulcus on the superolateral surface and separates the temporal lobe from the parietal and frontal lobes (Fig. 8.3).

The central sulcus separates the precentral and post-central gyri which contain the primary motor and sensory areas of the cortex. On the medial surface of the hemisphere the parieto-occipital sulcus separates the occipital lobe from the parietal lobe. The calcarine and post-calcarine sulci concerned with visual centres are also seen on the medial surface.

The corpus callosum which is seen between the two hemispheres carries commissural fibres linking one hemisphere to the other. Its anterior enlargement is the genu and the posterior end the splenium.

Major functional areas of the cortex

A number of major functional areas are located in the various lobes of the cerebral hemisphere (Fig. 8.4).

The olfactory impulses are linked with the temporal lobe in the region of the uncus. The auditory cortex lies on the superior temporal gyrus on the lateral surface of the hemisphere. The visual pathways reach the occipital cortex around the calcarine sulcus. The major motor area of the cortex is the precentral gyrus, from which fibres pass through the internal capsule to the motor nuclei of the cranial and spinal nerves. The somatic sensory cortex, which is mostly the postcentral gyrus, receives afferents from the thalamus carrying various sensory modalities. The motor elements of speech are centred on the Broca's area in the posterior part of the inferior frontal gyrus of the dominant hemisphere. Both pre- and postcentral gyri have somatotopic representation as shown in the homunculus in Figure 8.5.

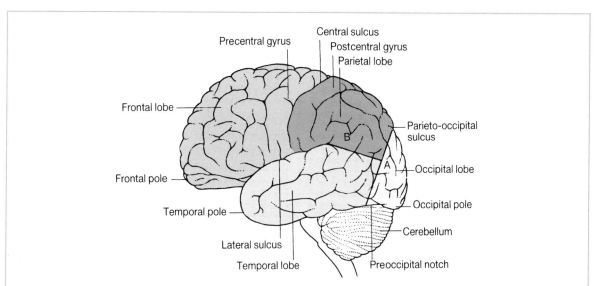

Fig. 8.3 The brain: lateral view. Line A indicates the posterior border of the temporal lobe; line B indicates the superior border of the temporal lobe (along with the lateral sulcus). From Rogers op. cit.

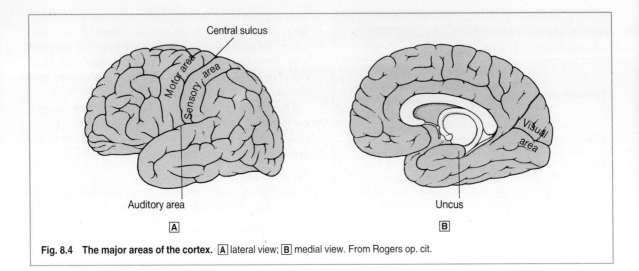

Fig. 8.4 The major areas of the cortex. [A] lateral view; [B] medial view. From Rogers op. cit.

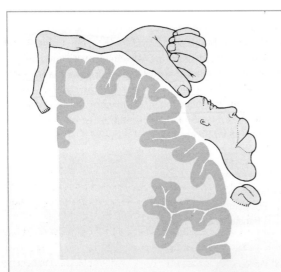

Fig. 8.5 The motor homunculus, showing proportional somatotopic representation in the precentral gyrus. From Rogers op. cit.

Basal ganglia

These nuclei are situated deep in the cerebral hemisphere and consist of the corpus striatum — containing the caudate nucleus, the putamen and the globus pallidus (Fig. 8.6) — and the claustrum and the amygdala. The putamen and the globus pallidus are together known as the lentiform nucleus. The lentiform nucleus is separated from the thalamus and the caudate nucleus by the internal capsule. The caudate nucleus and the putamen receive their afferent fibres mostly from the cerebral cortex and the thalamus and send their efferents to the globus pallidus. Efferents from the globus pallidus go to the thalamus, substantia nigra, red nucleus and the reticular formation in the brainstem. The basal ganglia and their connections form the major part of the extrapyramidal system.

The diencephalon is the middle portion of the forebrain. It consists of the thalamus, the hypothalamus and the third ventricle. A faint groove running from the interventricular foramen to the cerebral aqueduct separates the thalamus from the hypothalamus. The thalamus is the major relay centre in the sensory pathway. Most sensations are carried from lower levels through various sensory tracts to the thalamic nuclei, from where they are relayed to the sensory cortex. The hypothalamus, lying antero-inferior to the thalamus, is the coordinating area for visceral functions; it also contains centres for endocrine functions.

Midbrain

The midbrain connects the diencephalon to the pons of the hindbrain and contains a small canal, the cerebral aqueduct. The cerebral aqueduct extends from the third ventricle to the fourth ventricle. The part behind the aqueduct is the tectum containing the superior and inferior colliculi, which are respectively connected to the visual and auditory pathways. The two cerebral peduncles lying in front of the aqueduct are further divided into tegmentum and basis pedunculi by the substantia nigra. The basis pedunculi contain the descending fibre tracts which are continuations of the internal capsule. The tegmentum of the midbrain has the ascending tract as well

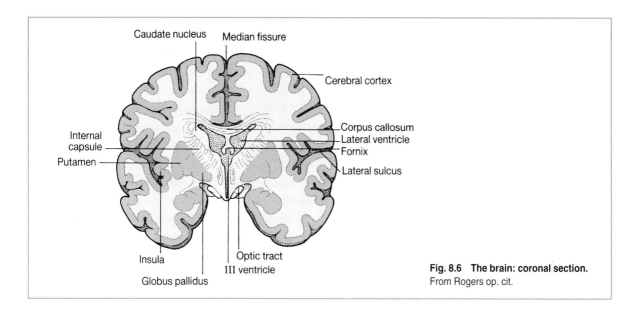

Caudate nucleus   Median fissure

Cerebral cortex

Corpus callosum
Lateral ventricle
Fornix

Lateral sulcus

Internal
capsule
Putamen

Insula

Optic tract
III ventricle

Globus pallidus

Fig. 8.6   The brain: coronal section.
From Rogers op. cit.

as nuclei for the oculomotor and the trochlear nerves. The oculomotor nerve nuclei are situated at the level of the superior colliculus and the trochlear nerve nucleus at the level of the inferior colliculcus. The substantia nigra is connected to the corpus striatum, providing the latter with its dopaminergic innervation.

The midbrain is contained in the gap between the free border and the tentorium cerebelli (the tentorial notch). An increase in cranial pressure above or below the tentorium can displace the midbrain and compress the structures surrounding it against the unyielding tentorium. The temporal lobe can be compressed and the uncus can herniate through the tentorial notch. Supratentorial lesions raising the intracranial pressure often compresses the oculomotor nerves at this level.

Hindbrain

The hindbrain (Fig. 8.7) lies below the tentorium cerebelli in the posterior cranial fossa. Its brainstem components, the pons and the medulla, lie on the clivus and extend from the midbrain downwards where it passes through the foramen magnum to become continuous with the spinal cord. The cerebellum projects posteriorly, occupying most of the posterior cranial fossa. The fourth ventricle, which is the cavity of the hindbrain, lies between the brainstem and the cerebellum.

The anterior part of the pons contains fibres largely composed of those descending from the higher centres to synapse in the pontine nuclei. These fibres are relayed to the cerebellum as the middle cerebellar peduncles. The

rest of the pons (the pontine tegmentum) contains a number of ascending and descending tracts as well as nuclei of the trigeminal nerve, abducens nerve, the facial nerve and the reticular formation. The facial colliculus is a bulge at the posterior aspect of the pons, where the facial nerve fibres wind round the abducens nerve nucleus. Most laterally in the pons is the nucleur complex associated with the vestibulocochlear nerve.

Medulla

The medulla extends from the pons downwards for about 2.5 cm, where it passes through the foramen magnum to become continuous with the spinal cord.

The anterior surface of the medulla is grooved by an anteromedial sulcus on either side of which are two elevations, the pyramids. The pyramid contains the corticospinal fibres a large proportion of which decussate at the lower part of the medulla in the pyramidal decussation. Lateral to the pyramid is another bulge, the olive, which contains the inferior olivary nucleus, which relays fibres to the cerebellum. The groove between the pyramid and the olive contains the rootlets of the hypoglossal nerve which originate from the hypoglossal nucleus in the substance of the medulla. Posterolaterally the medulla has the inferior cerebellar peduncle which connects the medulla to the cerebellum. The sulcus between the inferior cerebellar peduncle and the olive has the ninth (glossopharyngeal), tenth (vagus) and the eleventh (accessory) cranial nerves. The nuclei of these are also seen in the medulla.

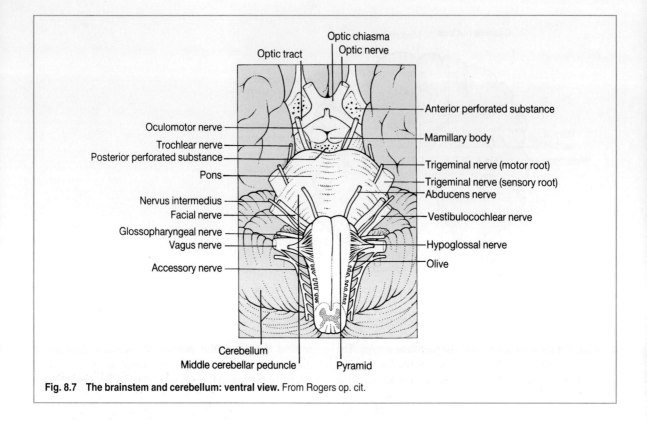

Optic chiasma
Optic nerve
Optic tract

Oculomotor nerve
Trochlear nerve
Posterior perforated substance
Pons
Nervus intermedius
Facial nerve
Glossopharyngeal nerve
Vagus nerve
Accessory nerve

Anterior perforated substance
Mamillary body
Trigeminal nerve (motor root)
Trigeminal nerve (sensory root)
Abducens nerve
Vestibulocochlear nerve
Hypoglossal nerve
Olive

Cerebellum
Middle cerebellar peduncle
Pyramid

Fig. 8.7   The brainstem and cerebellum: ventral view. From Rogers op. cit.

Cerebellum

The cerebellum (Fig. 8.8) is the largest part of the hind-brain. It is made up of two lateral cerebellar hemispheres separated by the vermis. The cerebellum is connected to the brainstem by the three pairs of cerebellar peduncles.

- The superior cerebellar peduncles connect the cerebellum to the midbrain and contain efferent fibres from the cerebellum to the midbrain and the thalamus.
- The middle cerebellar peduncles connect the pons and cerebellum and contain the axons of the pontine nuclei relaying impulses from the higher centres to the cerebellum.
- The inferior cerebellar peduncles form the connection between the medulla and the cerebellum and carry fibres connecting the vestibular nuclei, spinal cord and the inferior olivary nuclei to the cerebellum.

The most anterior and caudal part of the lateral lobe is the flocculus attached to the nodule in the midline. The flocculonodular lobe is an important part in the vestibular system, which maintains balance. The bulge of the lateral lobe that projects inferiorly posterolateral to the medulla is the tonsil. In cases where there is raised intracranial tension, the tonsils can herniate into the foramen magnum and compress the medulla oblongata following a lumbar puncture.

The structural organisation of the cerebellum is uniform and is similar to that of the cerebral hemisphere, i.e. a thin layer of cortex outside and the deeper white matter containing various cerebellar nuclei.

Meninges

The three layers of the meninges are:

- the dura mater
- the arachnoid mater
- the pia mater.

The three meningeal spaces are:

- the extradural (epidural) space between the cranial bones and the endosteal layer of dura; this is a potential space which becomes a real space when there is an extradural haemorrhage from a torn meningeal vessel
- the subdural space, a potential space that may enlarge after head injury
- the subarachnoid space between the arachnoid and pia, which contains CSF and the blood vessels of the brain.

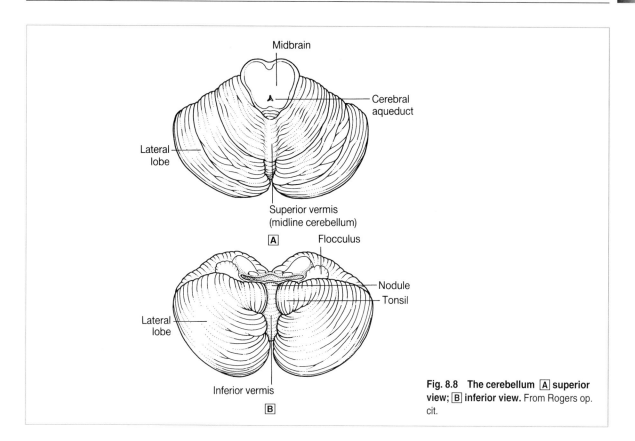

Fig. 8.8 The cerebellum $\boxed{A}$ **superior view;** $\boxed{B}$ **inferior view.** From Rogers op. cit.

Dura mater

The dura mater has an outer endosteal layer and an inner meningeal layer. The attachment of the endosteal layer to the floor of the cranial cavity is firmer than it is to its roof. A blow on the head can detach the endosteal layer from the skull cap without fracturing the bone. However, tearing of the meninges of the base of the skull is often associated with a fracture.

The meningeal layer of dura continues into the vertebral canal as the dura mater covering the spinal cord. The two layers of dura mater are fused together except in areas where they form walls of the dural venous sinuses.

The cranial cavity is divided into compartments by three folds of dura mater. These folds are (Fig. 8.9):

- falx cerebri
- tentorium cerebelli
- falx cerebelli.

Falx cerebri The falx cerebri lies between the two cerebral hemispheres, and is attached anteriorly to the crista galli and posteriorly to the tentorium cerebelli. The superior sagittal sinus lies along its superior border, and the inferior sagittal sinus lies along its inferior free margin. The straight sinus is seen where the falx cerebri meets the tentorium cerebelli.

Tentorium cerebelli The tentorium cerebelli is attached anteriorly to the posterior clinoid process of the sphenoid bone, and its attahcment runs posterolaterally along the superior border of the petrous temporal bone where the superior petrosal sinus is enclosed. Where the latter empties into the transverse sinus, the attached border turns posteromedially along the lips of the groove for the transverse sinus to reach the internal occipital protuberance and then continues on the opposite side of the skull to the other posterior clinoid process. The free border of the tentorium cerebelli is attached to the anterior clinoid process and, running posteriorly and then medially, it curves round the midbrain, forming the tentorial notch.

Just behind the apex of the petrous temporal bone the inferior layer of the tentorium prolongs into the middle cranial fossa as the trigeminal cave. This prolongation crosses inferior to the superior petrosal sinus to lie on the anterior surface of the petrous temporal bone in between the endosteal and the meningeal layers of the dura.

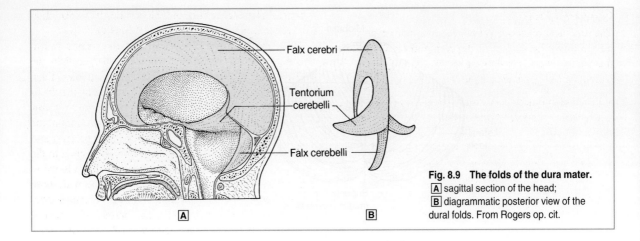

Fig. 8.9 **The folds of the dura mater.**
[A] sagittal section of the head;
[B] diagrammatic posterior view of the dural folds. From Rogers op. cit.

Falx cerebelli This is a small fold of dura below the tentorium in the posterior cranial fossa. It lies between the two lateral lobes of the cerebellum.

Diaphragma sellae This fold of dura mater forms the roof of the hypophyseal fossa. It covers the pituitary gland and has an aperture for the passage of infundibulum.

Meningeal arteries

There are several meningeal arteries which supply the meninges as well as the bones of the skull. The middle meningeal artery, a branch of the maxillary artery, enters the skull through the foramen spinosum and divides into an anterior and posterior branch. The anterior branch lies in the region of the pterion and is a usual source of extradural haemorrhage.

Surface anatomy: The middle meningeal artery enters the skull at a point level with the midpoint of the zygo-matic arch and divides 2 cm above it. The pterion, a point important for making a burr hole, is 4 cm above the zygo-matic arch and 3.5 cm behind the lateral angle of the eye.

Arachnoid mater

The smooth outer surface of the arachnoid mater is sepa-rated from the dura by the subdural space. The subarach-noid space between the arachnoid and the pia contains the cerebrospinal fluid and the major blood vessels. The arachnoid and the subarachnoid space extend into the vertebral canal and the sacral canal up to the level of the 2nd piece of sacrum. The deeper surface of the arachnoid gives delicate prolongations into the subarachnoid space. There are also prolongations, the arachnoid granulations which are the sites of reabsorption of CSF, into the superior sagittal sinus (Fig. 8.10) and probably into other venous sinuses.

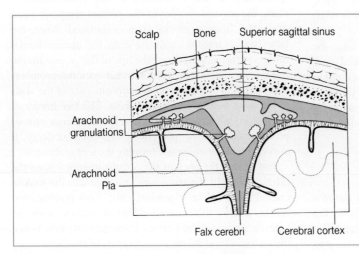

Fig. 8.10 **Cranial section through the skull.** From Rogers op. cit.

Subarachnoid cisterns

The subarachnoid space varies greatly in size as the arachnoid follows the surface of the dura and the pia follows that of the brain. The largest spaces are the cisterns, of which the following are important:

- the cerebellomedullary cistern (or cisterna magna), which lies posterior to the medulla below the cerebellum
- the pontine cistern, which lies anterior to the pons
- the interpeduncular cistern, which is in the space between the cerebral peduncles and the optic chiasma. It contains the circle of Willis and the oculomotor and the trochlear nerves.

Pia mater

The pia mater follows the surface of the brain closely, dipping down into all sulci except the finer ones of the cerebellum. Blood vessels entering the brain carry a sleeve of pia into the nervous tissue, which stops short at the capillary levels. At the choroid fissure of the lateral ventricle and at the roof of the third and fourth ventricles the pia mater is invaginated by blood vessels forming the telachoroidea and the choroid plexus.

Ventricular system and cerebrospinal fluid

Cerebrospinal fluid is produced in all four ventricles by the choroid plexus. It flows from the lateral ventricles into the third ventricle, from there through the cerebral aqueduct into the fourth ventricle and thence into the subarachnoid space. It is reabsorbed into the venous system through the arachnoid granulations along the dural venous sinuses. The total volume of CSF is about 100–150 mL in the adult; its pressure is about 8–10 cmH$_2$O.

The general shape of the ventricular system is shown in Figure 8.11. The lateral ventricles, larger than the others, are contained in the cerebral hemispheres. Each lateral ventricle has a body which is floored by the thalamus and the caudate nucleus. The corpus callosum forms its roof. The anterior horn projects forward in front of the interventricular foramen. The posterior horn projects into the occipital lobe, and the inferior horn projects into the temporal lobe. The choroid plexuses, which are found in the inferior horn and the body, are continuous with those on the roof of the third ventricle through the interventricular foramen. The interventricular foramen (foramen of Monro) is bounded by the anterior end of the thalamus and the fornix. It connects the lateral ventricle to the third ventricle.

The third ventricle is a narrow slit-like space between the two thalami and the hypothalami. It is roofed by the tela choroidea, a double layer of pia mater, containing choroid plexus. The third ventricle is connected to the fourth ventricle by the cerebral aqueduct.

The fourth ventricle is tent shaped with a diamond shaped floor or anterior wall formed by the pons and the medulla. It is roofed by the superior and inferior medullary vela connected to the superior and inferior cerebellar peduncles, respectively. The cerebellum lies posterior to the fourth ventricle. The fourth ventricle has three openings on its roof, which connect it to the subarachnoid space. The single foramen of Magendie is in the midline, and the paired foramen of Luschka more laterally.

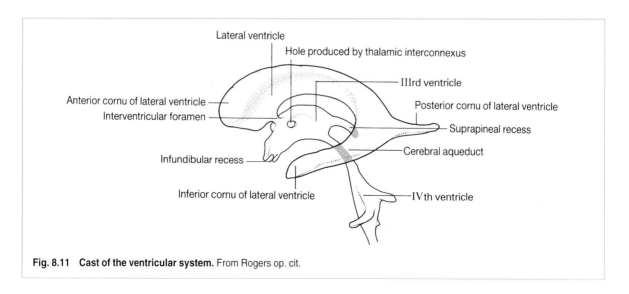

Fig. 8.11 Cast of the ventricular system. From Rogers op. cit.

Through these, CSF from the ventricular system enters the subarachnoid space.

BLOOD SUPPLY TO THE BRAIN

Arterial supply

The two vertebral arteries and the two internal carotid arteries supply the brain (Fig. 8.12).

Vertebral arteries

After entering the cranial cavity through the foramen magnum, the two vertebral arteries lie in the subarachnoid space and ascend on the surface of the medulla to the lower border of the pons where they unite to form the basilar artery. The basilar artery lies in the groove on the anterior surface of the pons and, at its upper border, divides into the two posterior cerebral arteries.

The following branches supplying the brain and spinal cord arise from the vertebral artery:

- the posterior spinal artery
- the anterior spinal artery
- the posterior inferior cerebellar artery.

The posterior spinal artery arises from the lower part of the vertebral artery, descends along the line of attachment of the dorsal roots of the spinal nerves and supplies the dorsal column of the white mater and the dorsal horn of the grey mater of the spinal cord. The artery often arises as a branch of the posterior inferior cerebellar artery.

The anterior spinal artery descends in front of the medulla and unites with the artery of the opposite side, forming a single artery lying in the anterior median fissure of the spinal cord. The anterior spinal artery supplies the anteromedial aspect of the medulla, including the pyramid and the medial lemniscus.

The posterior inferior cerebellar artery winds backward deep to the rootlets of the hypoglossal, vagus and the glossopharyngeal nerves to reach the cerebellum. The artery supplies the posterolateral aspect of the medulla, besides the cerebellum, and its blockage compromises the nucleus ambiguus and the nucleus of the spinal tract of the trigeminal, resulting in ipsilateral paralysis of the muscles of the palate and pharynx and anaesthesia for pain and temperature on the face.

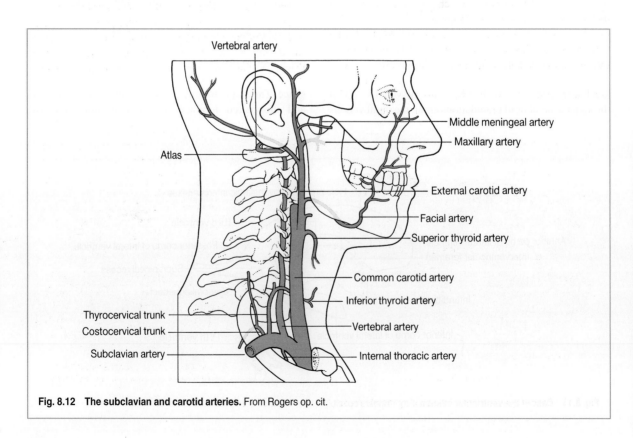

Fig. 8.12 The subclavian and carotid arteries. From Rogers op. cit.

Basilar artery

The following branches are given by the basilar artery:

- the anterior inferior cerebellar artery
- the labyrinthine artery
- the pontine arteries
- the superior cerebellar artery
- the posterior cerebral artery.

The anterior inferior cerebellar artery arises from the lower end of the basilar artery and supplies the cortex and white matter and the deeply lying nuclei of the cerebellum. It also supplies the upper part of the medulla and the lower end of the pons.

The labyrinthine artery accompanies the seventh and eighth cranial nerves and supplies the internal ear.

The pontine arteries supply the pons.

The superior cerebellar artery is given off very near the bifurcation of the basilar artery. It supplies the cerebellum and gives branches to the pons and midbrain. The oculomotor nerve lies between the superior cerebellar and posterior cerebral arteries.

The posterior cerebral arteries are the terminal branches of the basilar artery. Each posterior cerebral winds round the midbrain to reach the medial surface of the cerebral hemisphere and supplies the occipital lobe, including the visual area, as well as the temporal lobe (Fig. 8.13). Occlusion of the posterior cerebral artery causes blindness in the contralateral visual field.

Internal carotid arteries

The branches of the internal carotid artery supplying the brain are as follows:

- the posterior communicating artery
- the anterior cerebral artery
- the middle cerebral artery
- the anterior choroid artery.

The posterior communicating artery is a small artery running backwards from the internal carotid to join the posterior cerebral to form the circle of Willis.

The anterior cerebral artery is the smaller of the two terminal branches of the internal carotid artery. It crosses over the optic nerve and, near the midline, is connected to the opposite artery by the anterior communicating artery. The anterior cerebral artery supplies the medial part of the inferior surface of the frontal lobe, and courses along the upper surface of the corpus callosum, supplying the medial surface of the frontal and parietal lobes and the corpus callosum. It also supplies a narrow strip on the upper part of the lateral surface. The motor and sensory areas of the lower extremity, located in this area (Fig. 8.5), are supplied by the anterior cerebral artery, resulting in characteristic paralysis when the artery is occluded.

The middle cerebral artery is the larger of the terminal branches of the internal carotid artery. It lies in the lateral sulcus, and its branches supply the lateral surface of the frontal, parietal and temporal lobes, except the narrow

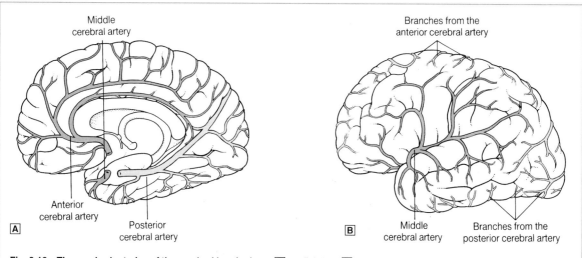

Fig. 8.13 **The cerebral arteries of the cerebral hemisphere.** [A] medial view; [B] lateral view. From Rogers op. cit.

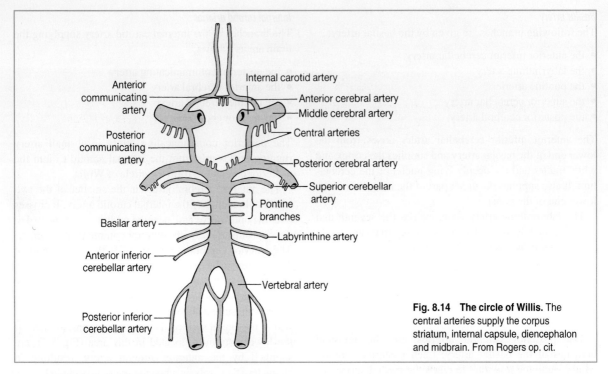

Anterior communicating artery

Internal carotid artery

Anterior cerebral artery

Middle cerebral artery

Posterior communicating artery

Central arteries

Posterior cerebral artery

Superior cerebellar artery

Pontine branches

Basilar artery

Labyrinthine artery

Anterior inferior cerebellar artery

Vertebral artery

Posterior inferior cerebellar artery

Fig. 8.14 The circle of Willis. The central arteries supply the corpus striatum, internal capsule, diencephalon and midbrain. From Rogers op. cit.

strip in the upper part supplied by the anterior cerebral. Occlusion of the artery results in contralateral motor and sensory paralysis of the face and arm.

The anterior choroid artery is given off from the internal carotid near its termination. It may also arise from the middle cerebral. It courses backward along the optic tract and supplies the interior of the brain, including the choroid plexus in the inferior cornu of the lateral ventricle.

Circle of Willis

The two internal carotids and the two vertebral arteries form an anastomosis known as the circle of Willis on the inferior surface of the brain (Fig. 8.14). Each half of the circle is formed by:

- the anterior communicating artery
- the anterior cerebral artery
- the internal carotid artery
- the posterior communicating artery
- the posterior cerebral artery.

Though the majority are thus interconnected, there is normally only minimal mixing of the blood passing through them. When one artery is blocked the arterial circle may provide collateral circulation.

Venous drainage of the brain

The veins of the brain, lying along with the arteries in the subarachnoid space, are thin-walled vessels without

valves. They pierce the arachnoid and drain into the dural venous sinuses. The major veins of the brain are as follows:

- the superior cerebral veins
- the superficial middle cerebral vein
- the basal vein
- the great cerebral vein.

The superior cerebral veins drain the lateral surface of the cerebral hemisphere. They open into the superior sagittal sinus. Veins lying posteriorly in this group are directed forward and join the sinus against the direction of the blood flow.

The superficial middle cerebral vein lies in the lateral sulcus. It runs downward and forward and drains into the cavernous sinus.

The basal vein is formed by the union of the deep middle cerebral vein, which lies in the depth of the lateral sulcus, and the anterior cerebral vein, which accompanies the anterior cerebral artery. The basal vein winds round the cerebral peduncle and ends in the great cerebral vein.

The great cerebral vein is formed by the union of the two internal cerebral veins which drain the interior of the cerebral hemisphere. It receives the basal veins and it drains into the straight sinus.

Cranial (dural) venous sinuses

The cranial venous sinuses (Fig. 8.15) are situated within

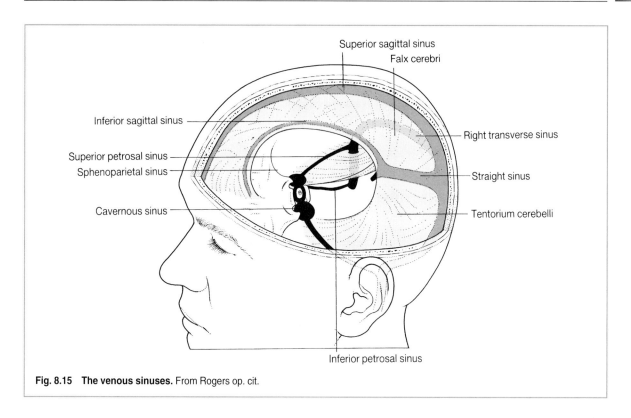

Fig. 8.15 The venous sinuses. From Rogers op. cit.

the dura mater. They are devoid of valves and drain eventually into the internal jugular vein.

The cranial venous sinuses are:

- the superior sagittal sinus
- the inferior sagittal sinus
- the straight sinus
- the transverse sinus
- the sigmoid sinus
- the confluence of sinuses
- the occipital sinus
- the cavernous sinus.

The superior sagittal sinus begins in front of the crista galli, courses backwards along the attached border of the falx cerebri, and usually becomes continuous with the right transverse sinus near the internal occipital protuberance. At its commencement it may communicate with the nasal veins. A number of venous lacunae lie along its course and open into the sinus. The sinus and the lacunae are invaginated by arachnoid granulations. The superior cerebral veins drain into the superior sagittal sinus (Fig. 8.16).

The inferior sagittal sinus lies along the inferior border of the falx cerebri and is much smaller than the superior sagittal sinus. It receives the cerebral veins from the medial surface of the hemisphere and joins the great cerebral vein to form the straight sinus.

The straight sinus, formed by the union of the inferior sagittal sinus and the great cerebral vein, lies in the attachment of the falx cerebri to the tentorium cerebelli. It usually becomes continuous with the left transverse sinus near the internal occipital protuberance.

The transverse sinus lies in the groove on the inner surface of the occipital bone along the posterior attachment of the tentorium cerebelli. On reaching the petrous temporal bone, it curves downwards into the posterior cranial fossa to follow a curved course as the sigmoid sinus.

The sigmoid sinus passes through the jugular foramen and becomes continuous with the internal jugular vein.

The confluence of sinuses is formed by two transverse sinuses connected by small venous channels near the internal occipital protuberance.

The occipital sinus, a small venous sinus extending from the foramen magnum, drains into the confluence of sinuses. It lies along the falx cerebelli and connects the vertebral venous plexuses to the transverse sinus.

Cavernous sinus

The cavernous sinus (Fig. 8.17), one on each side, situated

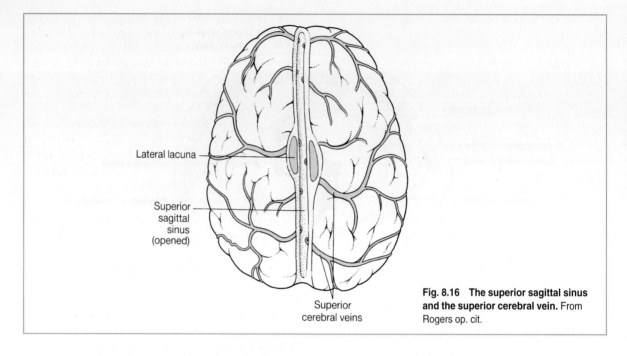

Lateral lacuna

Superior
sagittal
sinus
(opened)

Superior
cerebral veins

Fig. 8.16   The superior sagittal sinus and the superior cerebral vein. From Rogers op. cit.

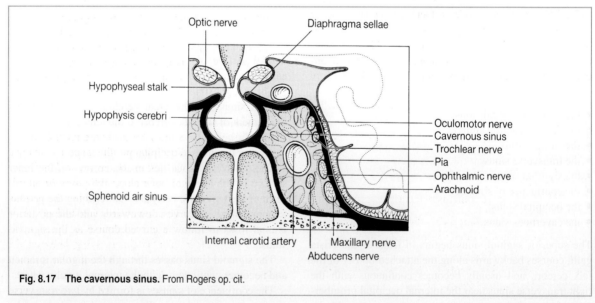

Optic nerve

Diaphragma sellae

Hypophyseal stalk

Hypophysis cerebri

Sphenoid air sinus

Internal carotid artery

Maxillary nerve
Abducens nerve

Oculomotor nerve
Cavernous sinus
Trochlear nerve
Pia
Ophthalmic nerve
Arachnoid

Fig. 8.17   The cavernous sinus. From Rogers op. cit.

on the body of the sphenoid bone, extends from the superior orbital fissure to the apex of the petrous temporal bone. Medially, the cavernous sinus is related to the pituitary gland and the sphenoid sinus. Laterally it is related to the temporal lobe of the brain. The internal carotid artery and the abducens nerve pass through the cavernous sinus. On its lateral wall from above downwards lie the oculomotor, trochlear and ophthalmic nerves. The maxil-

lary divisions of the trigeminal go through the lower part of the lateral wall or just outside the sinus. The endothelial lining separates these structures from the cavity of the sinus.

The connections of the sinus are illustrated in Figure 8.15. Posteriorly, the sinus drains into the transverse/sigmoid sinus through superior petrosal sinus and via the inferior petrosal sinus, passing through the jugular foramen, into the internal jugular vein. The ophthalmic veins drain into the anterior part of the sinus.

Emissary veins passing through the foramina in the middle cranial fossa connect the cavernous sinus to the pterygoid plexus of veins and to the facial veins. The superficial middle cerebral vein drains into the cavernous sinus from above. The two cavernous sinuses are connected to each other by anterior and posterior cavernous sinuses lying in front of and behind the pituitary.

CRANIAL NERVES

I: Olfactory nerve

See also Chapter 13. Axons from the olfactory mucosa in the nasal cavity pass through the cribriform plate of the ethmoid to end in the olfactory bulb. A cuff of dura, lined by arachnoid and pia, surrounds each bundle of nerves, establishing a potential communication and a route of infection between the subarachnoid space and the nasal cavity.

Bilateral anosmia due to severance of olfactory nerves may be produced in head injuries with a fracture of the anterior cranial fossa. Unilateral anosmia may be a sign of a frontal lobe tumour. The olfactory cortex consists of the uncus and the anterior perforated substance. An uncinate type of fit characterised by olfactory hallucinations and involuntary chewing movements associated with unconsciousness may be a sign of a tumour in the olfactory cortex.

II: Optic nerve

The optic nerve and the optic pathway are described in Chapter 13.

III: Oculomotor nerve

The oculomotor nerve contains two major components:

- somatic motor fibres supplying the superior, inferior and medial recti, the inferior oblique and the levator palpebrae superioris muscles
- parasympathetic fibres supplying the ciliary muscles and the constrictor pupillae (Ch. 13).

The somatic efferent nucleus (having five groups of cells, one for each muscle) and the Edinger–Westphal nucleus (parasympathetic) lie in the midbrain at the level of the superior colliculus. The oculomotor nerves emerge between two cerebral peduncles, pass between the posterior cerebral and superior cerebellar arteries and run forward in the interpeduncular cistern on the lateral side of the posterior communicating artery. Each nerve pierces the dura mater lateral to the posterior clinoid process to

lie on the lateral wall of the cavernous sinus. It then divides into a small superior and a large inferior division which enter the orbit through the superior orbital fissure. The superior division supplies the superior rectus and the levator palpebrae superioris, and the inferior division supplies the medial rectus, the inferior rectus, and the inferior oblique.

The parasympathetic fibres from the Edinger–Westphal nucleus leave the branch to the inferior oblique to synapse in the ciliary ganglion. Postganglionic fibres supply the ciliary muscles and sphincter (constrictor) pupillae via the short ciliary nerves.

Complete division of the third nerve results in:

- ptosis due to paralysis of levator palpebrae superioris
- divergent squint due to unopposed action of lateral rectus and superior oblique
- dilation of the pupil due to unopposed action of dilator pupillae which is supplied by the sympathetic fibres
- loss of accommodation and light reflexes due to paralysis of ciliary muscles and consrictor pupillae
- diplopia (double vision).

The oculomotor nerve can be paralysed by:

- aneurysms of the posterior cerebral, superior cerebellar or posterior communicating arteries
- raised intracranial pressure, especially associated with herniation of uncus into the tentorial notch
- tumours and inflammatory lesions in the region of the sella turcica.

IV: Trochlear nerve

The trochlear nerve is the smallest of the cranial nerves. Its somatic motor fibres supply the superior oblique muscle. The nucleus of the trochlear nerve lies in the midbrain at the level of the inferior colliculus. From this nucleus axons pass dorsally around the cerebral aqueduct to decussate in the superior medullary velum. Each nerve then winds round the cerebral peduncle and passes forward in the interpeduncular cistern lying between the superior cerebellar and posterior cerebral arteries lateral to the oculomotor nerve. The nerve pierces the dura posterolateral to the oculomotor nerve, near the point where the free margin of the tentorium crosses the attached margin, to enter the cavernous sinus. It then lies in the lateral wall of the cavernous sinus below the oculomotor nerve and above the ophthalmic division of the trigeminal nerve. The nerve enters the orbit through the superior orbital fissure lateral to the tendinous ring from which the four recti take origin. It then turns medially over the optic nerve and, passing over the levator palpebrae superioris, reaches the superior oblique muscle which it innervates.

When the trochlear nerve is injured, diplopia occurs on looking downwards. The patient complains of difficulty walking downstairs.

V: Trigeminal nerve

The trigeminal nerve (Fig. 8.18) is the principal sensory nerve of the head and it also innervates the muscles of mastication. Additionally, it is associated with four parasympathetic ganglia. Its distribution is as follows:

- sensory to — face, scalp, teeth, mouth, nasal cavity, paranasal sinuses and most of the dura mater
- motor to — muscles of mastication, mylohyoid, anterior belly of digastric, tensor tympani and tensor palati
- ganglionic connections to — the ciliary, sphenopalatine, otic and submandibular ganglia.

Nuclei of the trigeminal nerve

Motor nucleus   The motor nucleus of the trigeminal nerve, which gives rise to the branchial efferent fibres to the muscles of mastication and the other muscles listed above, is situated in the upper part of the pons near the floor of the fourth ventricle.

Sensory nuclei   There are three sensory nuclei in the brainstem which receive the general somatic afferent fibres of the trigeminal nerve.

- The mesencephalic nucleus, which is concerned with proprioception, is in the midbrain.
- The chief sensory nucleus, concerned with touch, tactile discrimination and position sense, is in the pons.
- The nucleus of the spinal tract, concerned with pain and temperature, is in the medulla and extends caudally into the upper segments of the spinal cord.

Within the nucleus of the spinal tract the fibres from the most anterior part of the face synapse in the caudal part of the nucleus, those from the posterior part most cranially, and the rest in the region of the nucleus in between. The central fibres from the nuclei decussate and ascend as the trigeminal lemniscus to the thalamus from where the impulses are relayed to the postcentral gyrus.

Sensory and motor roots of the trigeminal nerve

The two roots emerge from the pons, pass though the pontine cistern and enter the middle cranial fossa where the sensory root has the trigeminal ganglion.

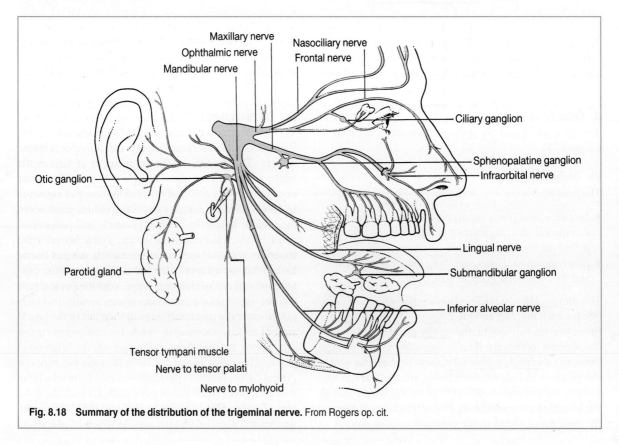

Fig. 8.18 Summary of the distribution of the trigeminal nerve. From Rogers op. cit.

Trigeminal ganglion

Most of the cell bodies of the sensory root are located in the trigeminal ganglion, which is also called the semilunar ganglion or the Gasserian ganglion. The ganglion lies near the apex of the petrous temporal bone inside the trigeminal cave, a pocket of dura invaginated from the posterior cranial fossa. Medially the ganglion is related to the internal carotid artery and the cavernous sinus. It can be blocked by introducing a needle through the foramen ovale, which is close to the ganglion. The motor root of the trigeminal nerve and the greater petrosal nerve lie deep to the ganglion. From the convex surface of the ganglion, which is pointing laterally, emerge the three peripheral divisions of the trigeminal nerve: the ophthalmic, the maxillary and the mandibular nerves.

Ophthalmic nerve

This nerve enters the cavernous sinus, lies on the lateral wall and passes to the orbit through the superior orbital fissure. Its branches supply the conjunctiva, cornea, the upper eyelid, the forehead, the nose and the scalp. The ciliary ganglion in the orbit is connected to the ophthalmic nerve

Maxillary nerve

From the middle cranial fossa, the maxillary nerve enters the pterygopalatine fossa through the foramen rotundum. It then passes through the inferior orbital fissure, lies on the floor of the orbit as the infraorbital nerve, and then passes through the maxillary sinus and emerges on the face through the infraorbital foramen. Its branches supply the cheek, the lateral aspect of the nose, the lower eyelid, the upper lip, the upper jaw and the teeth. The sphenopalatine ganglion is connected to the maxillary nerve in the pterygopalatine fossa.

Mandibular nerve

This nerve, which is both motor and sensory, leaves the skull through the foramen ovale. The sensory fibres innervate the auricle and the external acoustic meatus, the skin over the mandible, the cheek, the lower lip, the tongue and the floor of the mouth, the lower teeth and the gums. The motor fibres supply the muscles of mastication: the temporalis, masseter, medial pterygoid and the lateral pterygoid. Branches from the mandibular division also innervate the tensor tympani and tensor palati as well as the anterior belly of the digastric and the mylohyoid muscles. Proprioceptive fibres are also contained in the branches innervating the muscles.

The submandibular ganglion is connected to the lingual nerve (see Ch. 13, p. 385), which is a branch of the mandibular nerve.

VI: Abducent nerve

The abducent nerve has somatic motor fibres which supply the lateral rectus muscle. The nucleus of the abducent nerve lies in the floor of the fourth ventricle in the upper part of the pons. The fibres of the facial nerve wind round the nucleus to form the facial colliculus. The abducent nerve emerges on the brainstem at the junction between the medulla and pons. It then passes forward through the pontine cistern, pierces the dura mater to enter the cavernous sinus, where it lies on the lateral aspect of the internal carotid artery. The nerve enters the orbit through the tendinous ring at the superior orbital fissure and supplies the lateral rectus muscle.

VII: Facial nerve

The facial nerve (Fig. 8.19) supplies the muscles of the facial expression. It also conveys parasympathetic fibres to the lacrimal gland, glands in the nasal cavity, submandibular and sublingual glands, and transmits taste fibres from the anterior two thirds of the tongue.

The motor nucleus is situated in the lower part of the pons. From the nucleus, motor fibres loop around the abducent nerve nucleus (facial colliculus) and emerge at the cerebellopontine angle along with the nervus intermedius, which contains the sensory and parasympathetic fibres. The sensory fibres in the nervus intermedius are the central processes of the geniculate ganglion, and these fibres synapse in the nucleus of the tractus solitarius in the pons. The autonomic fibres originate from the superior salivatory nucleus in the pons. The nervus intermedius lies lateral to the motor fibres of the facial nerve, in between the latter and the vestibulocochlear nerve. The motor fibres of the facial nerve and the nervus intermedius pass through the pontine cistern and enter the internal acoustic meatus where the two join together to form the facial nerve. The nerve then passes through the facial canal in the petrous temporal bone. Here the nerve runs laterally over the vestibule to reach the medial wall of the middle ear, where it bends sharply backwards over the promontory. This bend, the genu, has the geniculate ganglion of the facial nerve. It passes downwards on the posterior wall of the middle ear to emerge though the stylomastoid foramen at the base of the skull.

In the petrous temporal bone, the facial nerve gives off three branches:

- the greater petrosal nerve
- the nerve to stapedius
- the chorda tympani nerve.

The greater petrosal nerve transmits preganglionic parasympathetic fibres to the sphenopalatine ganglion,

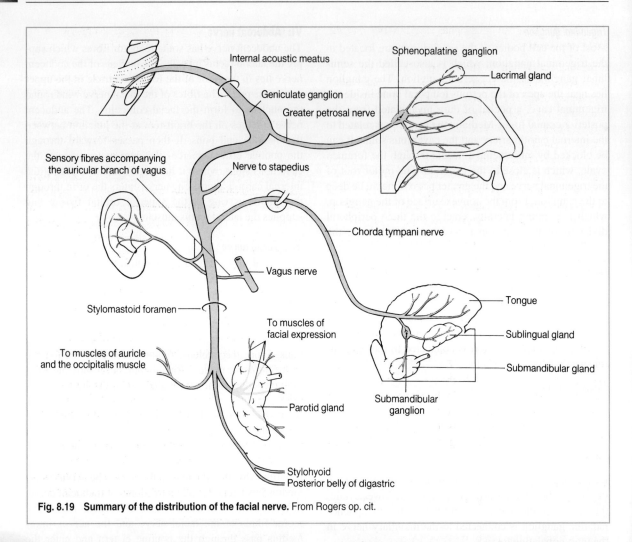

Fig. 8.19 Summary of the distribution of the facial nerve. From Rogers op. cit.

the postganglionic fibres from which supply the lacrimal gland and the glands in the nasal cavity. The chorda tympani nerve carries parasympathetic fibres to the submandibular and sublingual glands as well as taste fibres from the anterior two-thirds of the tongue.

After emerging from the stylomastoid foramen the nerve enters the parotid gland and divides into temporal, zygomatic, buccal, marginal mandibular and cervical branches. These supply the muscles of facial expression. Before entering the parotid gland the nerve supplies branches to the posterior belly of the digastric, stylohyoid and the muscles of the auricle.

Infranuclear paralysis of the facial nerve has a wide variety of causes such as acoustic neuroma and its surgery, viral infection producing inflammation and swelling of the nerve, fractures of the base of the skull, and tumours and surgery of the parotid gland. Bell's palsy is an infra-

nuclear paralysis of the facial nerve of unknown aetiology. The paralysis will affect all the muscles on the same side of the face. Supranuclear paralysis, which affects the contralateral facial muscles, spares the orbicularis oculi and the muscles of the scalp, since the part of the facial nerve nucleus supplying these has bilateral cortical connections.

VIII: Vestibulocochlear nerve
See Chapter 13.

IX: Glossopharyngeal nerve
The glossopharyngeal nerve contains sensory fibres (including taste) from the posterior third of the tongue and the oropharynx (tonsillar fossa). The nerve also supplies the stylopharyngeus muscle; its parasympathetic fibres innervate the parotid gland. It also innervates the carotid sinus and the carotid body.

In the medulla the glossopharyngeal nerve has the following nuclei:

- the nucleus ambiguus, which supplies nerve fibres to the stylopharyngeus muscle; this nucleus, through the branches of the vagus nerve, also innervates the muscles of the soft palate, pharynx and larynx
- the inferior salivatory nucleus, which innervates the parotid gland
- the nucleus of the tractus solitarius, which receives the taste fibres through the glossopharyngeal nerve
- the dorsal motor nucleus of the vagus, which the ninth nerve shares with the vagus for general sensation from the posterior third of the tongue and the oropharynx.

The glossopharyngeal nerve emerges on the brainstem in the groove between the olive and the inferior cerebellar peduncle. It goes forward and laterally and leaves the skull through the jugular foramen. In the jugular foramen the nerve has two ganglia which contain the cells of origin of its sensory fibres. On emerging from the foramen it gives off the tympanic branch which, after supplying the middle ear, continues as the lesser superficial petrosal nerve carrying parasympathetic fibres to the otic ganglion to supply the parotid gland. In the upper part of the neck the nerve accompanies the stylopharyngeus muscle and enters the pharynx by passing between the middle and superior constrictor muscles. Its terminal branches supply the posterior third of the tongue and the tonsillar fossa (oropharynx).

X: Vagus nerve

The vagus nerve (Fig. 8.20) contains the following sensory fibres:

- fibres from the mucosa of the pharynx and larynx and those transmitting visceral sensation of the organs in the thorax and abdomen
- fibres carrying general sensation from the dura, parts of the external auditory meatus, external surface of the tympanic membrane
- taste fibres from the epiglottis.

The vagus also contains preganglionic parasympathetic fibres to all the thoracic and abdominal viscera up to the splenic flexure. The cranial part of the accessory nerve which innervates the muscles of the soft palate, pharynx and larynx also is distributed via the vagus.

The following nuclei are associated with the vagus nerve in the brainstem:

- the dorsal nucleus of the vagus. This is situated in the floor of the fourth ventricle in the medulla and receives the general visceral sensation from the various organs supplied by the vagus. Its motor component gives rise to the preganglionic parasympathetic fibres in the vagus
- the nucleus of the tractus solitarius which the vagus shares with the facial nerve and the glossopharyngeal nerve for taste fibres
- the nucleus ambiguus from which originate the fibres of the cranial part of the accessory nerve, which is distributed along with the vagus nerve.

The vagus emerges on the brainstem in the groove between the olive and the inferior cerebellar peduncle, below the rootlets of the glossopharyngeal nerve, and passes through the jugular foramen. It bears two ganglia: the superior in the foramen and the inferior after emerging from it. Beyond the inferior ganglion the cranial part of the accessory nerve joins the vagus.

The branches and distribution of the vagus nerve

- meningeal branch — arises from the superior ganglion and supplies the dura of the posterior cranial fossa
- the auricular branch — also originates from the superior ganglion and supplies small areas on the medial aspect of the auricle, external auditory meatus and the outer surface of the tympanic membrane
- the pharyngeal branch — arises from the inferior ganglion and supplies muscles of the soft palate and pharynx
- the superior laryngeal nerve — this divides into external laryngeal nerve (supplies cricothyroid muscle) and internal laryngeal nerve (sensory nerve of the laryngeal part of the pharynx and the laryngeal mucosa above the level of the vocal cord)
- the recurrent laryngeal nerve
- the cardiac branches
- the pulmonary branches
- the branches to the abdominal viscera.

XI: Accessory nerve

The accessory nerve has a small cranial and a larger spinal root. The former arises from the nucleus ambiguus and emerges along with the fibres of the vagus from the brainstem. It then joins the spinal root for a short distance and branches off to rejoin the vagus to be distributed to the muscles of the soft palate, pharynx and larynx. The spinal root arises from the upper five segments of the cervical part of the spinal cord and enters the skull through the foramen magnum, where it joins the cranial root, and leaves the skull through the jugular foramen. Immediately below the jugular foramen the spinal root passes backwards to supply the sternocleidomastoid and trapezius.

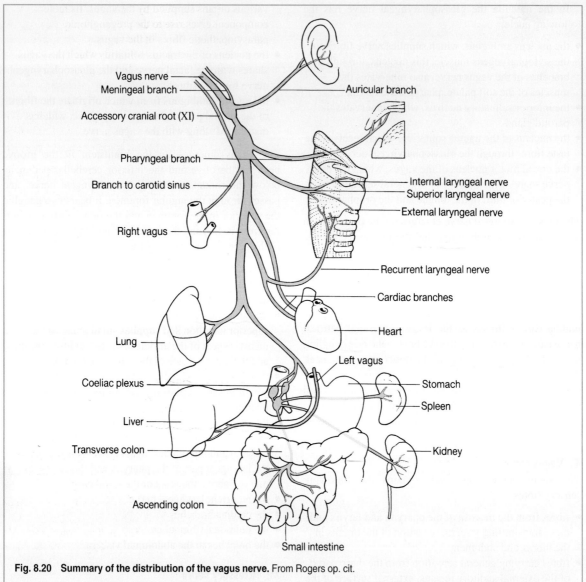

Fig. 8.20   Summary of the distribution of the vagus nerve. From Rogers op. cit.

Labels in figure: Vagus nerve; Meningeal branch; Accessory cranial root (XI); Pharyngeal branch; Branch to carotid sinus; Right vagus; Lung; Coeliac plexus; Liver; Transverse colon; Ascending colon; Small intestine; Auricular branch; Internal laryngeal nerve; Superior laryngeal nerve; External laryngeal nerve; Recurrent laryngeal nerve; Cardiac branches; Heart; Left vagus; Stomach; Spleen; Kidney

XII: Hypoglossal nerve

The hypoglossal nerve supplies all the extrinsic and intrinsic muscles of the tongue. Its nucleus, which gives rise to the somatic motor fibres, lies in the medulla in the floor of the fourth ventricle. The nerve emerges as rootlets in the groove between the pyramid and the olive; the rootlets unite to form the nerve, which leaves the skull through the hypoglossal canal. In the neck the nerve first lies between the internal jugular vein and the internal carotid artery, crosses superficial to the latter and the ex-

ternal carotid, and passes forward deep to the mylohyoid muscle to supply the muscles of the tongue.

SPINAL CORD

The spinal cord extends from the lower end of the medulla oblongata at the level of the foramen magnum to the lower border of the first or the upper border of the second lumbar vertebra. The lower part of the cord is tapered to form the conus medullaris from which a

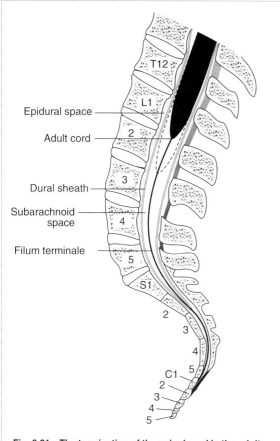

Epidural space

Adult cord

Dural sheath

Subarachnoid space

Filum terminale

T12
L1
2
3
4
5
S1
2
3
4
5
C1
2
3
4
5

Fig. 8.21 The termination of the spinal cord in the adult, showing its variation. The figure also shows the termination of the dural sheath.

prolongation of pia mater, the filum terminale, extends downwards to be attached to the coccyx. In the third month of intrauterine life the spinal cord fills the whole length of the vertebral canal, but from then on the vertebral column grows more rapidly than the cord. At birth the cord extends as far as the third lumbar vertebra and reaches its adult level gradually (Fig. 8.21).

The three layers of the meninges envelop the spinal cord. The dura mater, which is continuous with that of the brain, extends up to the second sacral vertebra. The arachnoid mater lines the inner surface of the dura, and the pia mater is adherent to the surface of the cord. The subarachnoid space with the CSF extends to the level of the second sacral vertebra. The epidural space outside the dura contains fat and the components of the vertebral venous plexus.

The spinal cord is suspended in the dural sheath by the denticulate ligaments (ligamentum denticulatum, Fig. 8.22).

These, having a serrated lateral edge, form a shelf between the dorsal and ventral roots of the spinal nerves.

The cord has on its surface a deep anterior median fissure and a shallower posterior median sulcus. It also has, on either side, a posterolateral sulcus along which the dorsal roots of the spinal nerves are attached.

The area of the spinal cord from which a pair of spinal nerves are given off is defined as a spinal cord segment. The cord has 31 pairs of spinal nerves and hence 31 segments: 8 cervical, 12 thoracic, 5 lumbar, 5 sacral and 1 coccygeal.

The dorsal (posterior) root of the spinal nerve which carries sensory fibres has a dorsal root ganglion which has the cells of origin of the dorsal root fibres. The ventral (anterior) root, which is motor, emerges on the antero-lateral aspect of the cord on either side. The anterior and posterior roots join together at the intervertebral foramen to form the spinal nerve which, on emerging from the foramen, divides immediately into the anterior and posterior rami, each containing both motor and sensory fibres. The length of the nerve roots increases progressively from above downwards. The lumbar and sacral nerve roots below the termination of the cord form the cauda equina.

Internal structure of the spinal cord

The grey matter containing the sensory and motor nerve cells is surrounded by the white matter with the ascending and descending tracts (Fig. 8.23).

In a transverse section the grey matter is seen as an H-shaped area containing in its middle the central canal. The central canal is continuous above with the fourth ventricle. The posterior (dorsal) horn of the grey matter has the termination of the sensory fibres of the dorsal root. The larger anterior (ventral) horn contains motor cells which give rise to fibres of the ventral roots. In the thoracic and upper lumbar regions there are lateral horns which have the cells of origin of the preganglionic sympathetic fibres.

(The grey matter is subdivided into a number of layers, the laminae of Rexed. Laminae I to VI are subdivisions of the dorsal horn, and laminae VII to IX are in the ventral horn. Lamina X is the central commissure connecting the two halves of the grey matter.)

The white matter is divided into the dorsal, lateral and ventral columns (funiculi), each containing a number of ascending and descending fibre tracts. A few of the major tracts are briefly described below:

Fasciculus gracilis (of Goll) and fasciculus cuneatus (of Burdach)

These two tracts form the major components of the dorsal column. The fasciculus gracilis lies medial to the fasci-

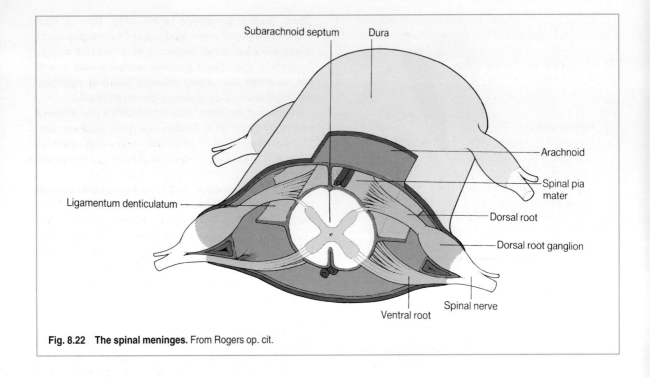

Fig. 8.22 **The spinal meninges.** From Rogers op. cit.

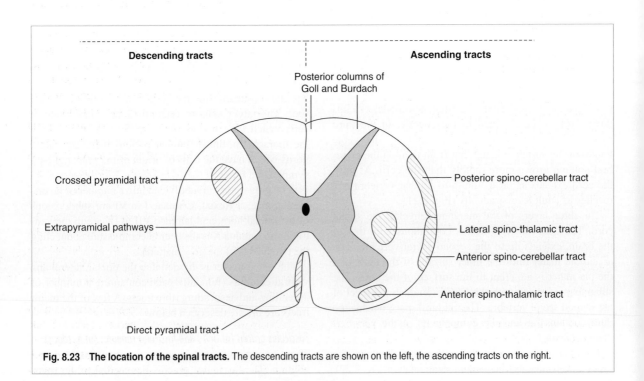

Fig. 8.23 **The location of the spinal tracts.** The descending tracts are shown on the left, the ascending tracts on the right.

culus cuneatus. They contain fibres subserving fine and discriminative tactile sensation as well as proprioception. As the spinal cord is ascended the fibres are added to the lateral part of the dorsal column. Hence the fasciculus gracilis deals mostly with sensation from the lower limb and the fasciculus cumeatus with the upper limb. Fibres in the dorsal columns are uncrossed, carrying sensation from the same side of the body. In the medulla the fasciculus gracilis synapses in the nucleus gracilis, and the cuneatus fasciculus synapses in the cuneate nucleus, from where second-order neurons proceed to the higher centres after crossing in the sensory decussation.

Lateral corticospinal tract (crossed pyramidal tract)

A major tract in the lateral funiculus is the lateral corticospinal tract. The corticospinal tracts control skilled voluntary movements and consist of axons of neurons in the frontal and parietal lobes. These descend through the internal capsule, the basis pedunculi of the midbrain, the pons, the pyramid of the medulla and then decussate in the motor decussation in the lower part of the medulla oblongata. The majority of fibres cross to the opposite side and descend as the lateral corticospinal tract. The lateral corticospinal tract thus contains axons of neurons of the controlateral cerebral hemisphere. These fibres terminate at different levels, forming synaptic connections with motor neurons. The fibres in the tract are somatotopically arranged, fibres for the lower part of the cord laterally and those for the upper levels medially.

Lateral spinothalamic tract

The lateral spinothalamic tract, conducting pain and temperature sensation as well as some tactile sensations, contains crossed ascending axons whose neurons lie in the grey matter of the opposite half of the spinal cord. Axons cross in the midline in the ventral grey commissure close to the central canal. Many of the fibres as they ascend give collaterals to the reticular nuclei in the brainstem and finally terminate in the thalamic nuclei. The fibres are somatotopically arranged, those for the lower limb superficial and those concerned with the upper limb deepest.

Fibres carrying pain and other sensations from the internal organs are carried in the spinoreticular tract, which terminates in the reticular formation in the medulla and pons.

Ventral corticospinal tract (direct pyramidal tract)

This tract, lying in the ventral part of the cord, has the corticospinal fibres which remain uncrossed in the motor decussation in the medulla. These fibres eventually cross the midline at segmental levels and terminate close to those in the lateral corticospinal tract.

Blood supply of the spinal cord

The blood supply of the spinal cord is derived from the anterior and posterior spinal arteries. The anterior spinal artery is a midline vessel lying in the anterior median fissure and is formed by the union of a branch from each vertebral artery. It supplies the whole of the cord in front of the posterior grey column. The posterior spinal arteries, usually one on either side posteriorly, are branches of the posterior inferior cerebellar arteries or directly from the vertebral arteries. They supply the posterior grey columns and the dorsal columns on either side.

The spinal arteries are reinforced at segmental levels by radicular arteries from the vertebral, ascending cervical, posterior intercostal, lumbar and sacral arteries. The radicular arteries enter the vertebral canal through the intervertebral foramina accompanying the spinal nerves and their ventral and dorsal roots. These arteries may be compromised in resection of segments of the aorta in surgery for aneurysms.

PERIPHERAL NERVOUS SYSTEM

The peripheral nervous system is formed by the cranial and spinal nerves carrying the somatic and autonomic nerve fibres. The cranial nerves have already been described (p. 175). The sympathetic nervous system is described on p. 184. This section describes the spinal nerves and their distribution.

Each spinal nerve is formed by the union of a dorsal and ventral root. The ventral root of the spinal nerve contains motor fibres whose cell bodies are in the ventral horn of the spinal cord. The sensory fibres in the dorsal root have their cells of origin in the dorsal root ganglion. The ventral and dorsal roots lie in the vertebral canal within the dural sac. They join together to form the spinal nerve in the intervertebral foramen, and immediately beyond the foramen the spinal nerve divides into the dorsal ramus and the ventral ramus. With the exception of the first two cervical spinal nerves the ventral rami are larger than the dorsal rami.

All dorsal rami pass backwards to innervate the muscles of the back, the ligaments and the joints of the vertebral column. They also supply cutaneous branches to the skin of the posterior aspect of the head, trunk and gluteal region. The dorsal rami of C1, L4 and L5 have no cutaneous branches.

The ventral rami in the thoracic region form the intercostal nerves. Each intercostal nerve innervates the muscles of its intercostal space and the overlying skin. The lower six intercostal nerves extend out to the anterior abdominal wall to innervate the muscles and the overlying skin in a segmental fashion. The ventral ramus of the first thoracic nerve gives off a small branch that constitutes the first intercostal nerve; it then crosses the first rib to join the C8 ventral ramus to form the lower trunk of the brachial plexus.

At cervical, lumbar and sacral levels the ventral rami form plexuses.

The cervical plexus is formed by the C1 to C4 ventral rami, and the nerves derived from it are distributed to the prevertebral muscles, levator scapulae, sternocleidomastoid, trapezius, the scalene muscles, the diaphragm as well as the skin of the anterior and lateral aspect of the neck, shoulder and the lower jaw and the external ear.

The brachial plexus is formed by C5 to C8 ventral rami along with the main branch of the T1 ventral ramus. The brachial plexus innervates the muscles and joints of the upper limb and shoulder girdle and the skin of the upper extremity.

The lumbar plexus is formed by L1 to L4 ventral rami with a contribution from the T12 ventral ramus. The femoral and obturator nerves formed from this plexus innervate the muscles and skin of the thigh (see below). Small nerves from the plexus innervate the muscles of the lower part of the anterior abdominal wall, skin of the foot, the lateral part of the hip and the external genitalia.

The sacral plexus is formed by S1 to S5 ventral rami with contribution from the ventral rami of L4 and L5. Branches of this plexus innervate the muscles and skin of the lower limb and the pelvic floor and the perineum.

The distribution of the major peripheral nerves is described in Chapter 12. The following is a summary of the innervation of the muscles to upper and lower extremities.

All muscles in the anterior compartment of the upper limb are innervated by the musculocutaneous nerve. All the muscles of the anterior compartment of the forearm are innervated by the median nerve except the flexor carpi ulnaris and the medial half of the flexor digitorum profundus; these are innervated by the ulnar nerve. Muscles in the posterior compartments to the arm and forearm are innervated by the radial nerve.

Of the intrinsic muscles of the hand, the median nerve supplies the abductor pollicis brevis, the flexor pollicis brevis, the opponens and the lateral two lumbricals. All the other intrinsic muscles of the hand are supplied by the ulnar nerve.

The obturator, femoral and sciatic nerves supply the three compartments of the thigh. The obturator nerve supplies the muscles in the medial compartment, the femoral supplies the anterior compartment, and the sciatic supplies the posterior compartment. Of the latter,

all the hamstrings originating from the ischial tuberosity are supplied by the tibial component of the sciatic nerve, and the short head of the biceps is supplied by the common peroneal component.

The deep peroneal nerve supplies all the muscles of the anterior compartment of the leg and the extensor digitorum brevis of the foot.

The superficial peroneal nerve supplies all the muscles in the lateral compartment of the leg, and the tibial nerve supplies the muscles in the posterior compartment.

Of the muscles of the foot, the medial plantar supplies flexor digitorum brevis, abductor hallucis, flexor hallucis brevis and the first lumbrical; all the rest of the muscles of the foot are supplied by the lateral plantar nerve.

SYMPATHETIC NERVOUS SYSTEM

The sympathetic nervous system plays a major rôle in regulating the internal environment of the body. When stimulated, it causes sweating, dilatation of the pupil, constriction of blood vessels, bronchial dilatation and diminished peristalsis. It is concerned with the stress reactions of the body. Stimulation of a part of the sympathetic nervous system produces a widespread response. Postganglionic sympathetic terminals release adrenaline and noradrenaline, except those of sweat glands, which are cholinergic in nature. Sympathetic efferents are accompanied by afferent fibres. These afferents conduct visceral pain impulses.

Sympathectomies are performed to increase circulation to the limbs, as in Raynaud's disease, acute embolisation and scleroderma; and also to relieve pain caused by phantom limb and causalgia; and to reduce excessive sweating (hyperhidrosis).

Spinal cord segments of origin of sympathetic fibres

The cell bodies of the preganglionic efferent fibres of the sympathetic nervous system lie in the lateral horns of grey matter of spinal cord segments T1–L2. The spinal cord segments involved in the innervation of the various regions of the body, and the detailed pattern of innervation, are shown in Figure 8.24. T1–T2 segments innervate the head and neck, T2–T7 the upper limb, T1–T4 the thoracic viscera, T4–L2 abdominal viscera, and T11–L2 the lower limb.

Sympathetic trunk (sympathetic chain)

The sympathetic trunk is a ganglionated chain extending from the base of the skull to the coccyx, lying on each side of the vertebral bodies approximately 2.5 cm lateral to the midline.

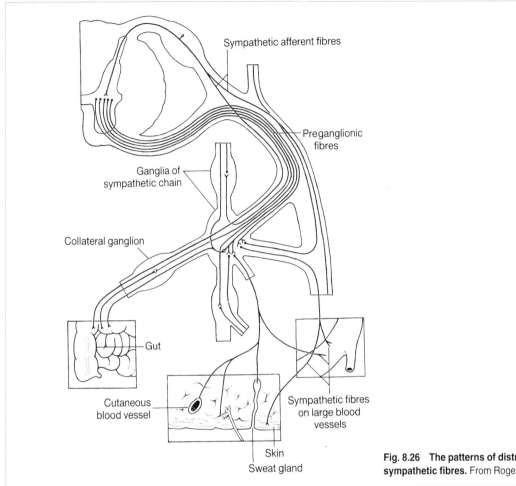

Sympathetic afferent fibres

Preganglionic
fibres

Ganglia of
sympathetic chain

Collateral ganglion

Gut

Cutaneous
blood vessel

Sympathetic fibres
on large blood
vessels

Skin

Sweat gland

**Fig. 8.26 The patterns of distribution of the
sympathetic fibres.** From Rogers op. cit.

first thoracic ganglion is not removed, as it would cause Horner's syndrome, and in any case preganglionic fibres to an upper limb usually do not arise above T2 level.

Lower limb

Preganglionic fibres from the T11–L2 spinal segments synapse in the lumbar and sacral ganglia, and the postganglionic fibres are distributed to the limb through the lumbosacral plexus.

For lumbar sympathectomy the third and fourth lumbar ganglia are removed. Preganglionic fibres do not arise below L2 level. The first lumbar ganglion is preserved to avoid compromising ejaculation.

Abdominal and pelvic viscera

The abdominal and pelvic viscera receive their sympathetic innervation through the following autonomic plexuses (Fig. 8.27):

- coeliac plexus
- aortic plexus
- hypogastric plexus.

The coeliac plexus is situated in front of the aorta in the region of the coeliac trunk. Its afferents come from the greater and lesser splanchnic nerves bilaterally. Branches of the vagus, especially the right vagus, also contribute to the coeliac plexus. The majority of preganglionic sympathetic fibres synapse in the two coeliac ganglia in the plexus, and postganglionic fibres accompany branches of the coeliac trunk and the superior mesenteric artery to supply the abdominal viscera.

The coeliac plexus continues downwards over the abdominal aorta as the aortic plexus, which in turn receives splanchnic nerves from lumbar sympathetic ganglia and distributes postganglionic fibres to viscera via plexuses accompanying branches of the abdominal

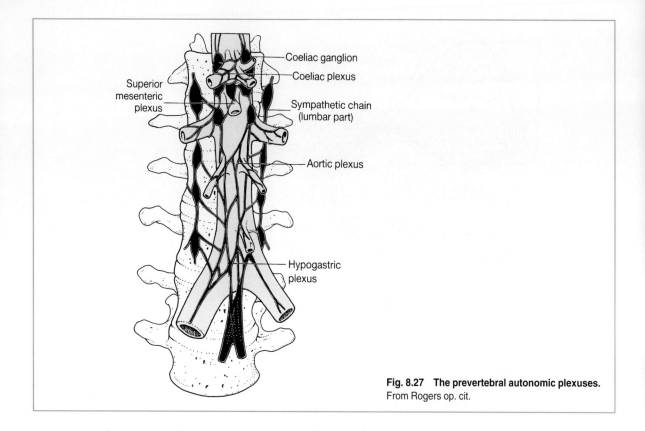

Fig. 8.27 The prevertebral autonomic plexuses.
From Rogers op. cit.

aorta. The hypogastric plexus, the continuation of the aortic plexus, lies in front of the fifth lumbar vertebra between the two common iliac arteries. It continues infero-laterally to both sides of the pelvis into the connective tissue medial to the internal iliac vessels. The plexus receives input from the splanchnic branches of the lumbar and sacral sympathetic ganglia. Resection of abdominal aneurysms and extensive dissection in the pelvis may remove aortic/hypogastric plexuses and hence may compromise ejaculation. The coeliac plexus can be blocked to relieve intractable pain in abdominal malignancies.

PARASYMPATHETIC NERVOUS SYSTEM

The parasympathetic nervous system functionally often antagonises the sympathetic system. Its stimulation constricts the pupils, reduces the heart rate, stimulates smooth muscle to contract (constricts bronchi, increases peristalsis) and stimulates a number of glands, including the salivary glands. It has a cranial and a sacral component. The cranial component accompanies the third, seventh, ninth and tenth cranial nerves, and the sacral component originates from the S2, S3, S4 segments of the spinal cord.

As with the sympathetic system, preganglionic parasympathetic fibres tend to be myelinated. The preganglionic fibres are long, and the associated ganglia are small and scattered near the viscera. Parasympathetic innervation is limited to the viscera and glands. There is no distribution to the skin and musculoskeletal tissues. Its distribution may be summarised as follows (Fig. 8.28):

- the oculomotor nerve supplying sphincter pupillae and ciliary muscles in the eye
- the facial nerve supplying the lacrimal, submandibular and sublingual glands, as well as glands in the nasal cavity and the mucosa of the palate
- the glossopharyngeal nerve supplying the parotid gland
- the vagus nerve supplying thoracic and abdominal viscera up to the left colic flexure
- S2–S4 sacral nerves supplying the pelvic viscera and the descending and sigmoid colon.

There are four ganglia associated with the parasympathetic nervous system in the head and neck. These are:

- the ciliary ganglion in the orbit, where preganglionic fibres accompanying the oculomotor nerve synapse.

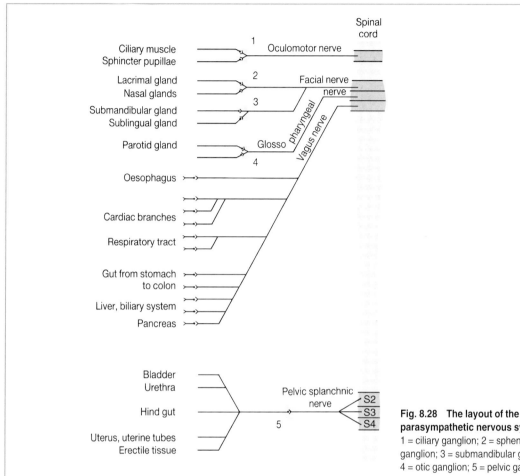

Fig. 8.28 The layout of the parasympathetic nervous system.
1 = ciliary ganglion; 2 = sphenopalatine ganglion; 3 = submandibular ganglion: 4 = otic ganglion; 5 = pelvic ganglion.

Postganglionic fibres, through the short ciliary nerves, supply the ciliary muscles and constrictor pupillae
- the sphenopalatine ganglion in the pterygopalatine fossa, where preganglionic fibres accompanying the facial nerve and then the greater petrosal nerve synapse. Postganglionic fibres accompany branches of the ganglion to supply the lacrimal glands in the nasal cavity and the palate
- the submandibular ganglion, attached to the lingual nerve in the submandibular region, where preganglionic fibres accompanying the facial nerve and then the chorda tympani nerve synapse. Postganglionic fibres supply the submandibular and sublingual glands and glands in the tongue and floor of the mouth
- the otic ganglion attached to the trunk of the mandibular nerve in the infratemporal fossa, where the preganglionic fibres accompanying the glossopharyngeal nerve and its branch, the lesser

petrosal nerve, synapse. Postganglionic fibres supply the parotid gland.

The ganglia of the vagus nerve and those of the sacral component of the parasympathetic system are very widely distributed and are in the wall of, or very near, the organs they supply.

PHYSIOLOGY

CEREBRAL BLOOD FLOW

Of the body tissues, brain is the least tolerant of ischaemia. Interruption of the cerebral blood flow for 5 s will cause loss of consciousness, and ischaemia of longer than 3 min results in irreversible brain damage.

The brain receives about 12% of the cardiac output. Cerebral blood flow remains remarkably constant, being held within a relatively narrow range, averaging 55 mL/min/100 g of brain tissue in humans. Regulation of the cerebral circulation is largely under the direction of the brain itself. Local mechanisms tend to maintain cerebral circulation relatively constant despite potential adverse extrinsic effects, e.g. sympathetic vasomotor activity, changes in mean arterial blood pressure, and circulating vasoactive substances.

Control of cerebral blood flow

Myogenic autoregulation

In the brain, arteriolar smooth muscle spontaneously contracts when the arteriolar wall tension is passively increased by an increase in arterial blood pressure. Conversely, the arterioles relax when the pressure decreases. The reduction in radius caused by contraction matches the increase in perfusion pressure such that there is no change in blood flow over a certain pressure range.

The term myogenic autoregulation is applied to this response, which is limited in extent. If mean arterial pressure falls below 50 mmHg, the vasodilatation is no longer sufficient to maintain flow. Conversely there is an upper limit to autoregulation above which the cerebral blood flow (CBF) rises sharply with arterial hypertension — the cerebral vessels becoming abnormally permeable, resulting in cerebral oedema. The normal upper limit of mean arterial blood pressure is around 150 mmHg. Thus, myogenic autoregulation maintains CBF remarkably constant in a range of mean arterial blood pressure of 50–150 mmHg.

Myogenic autoregulation may be impaired by a number of cerebral insults:

- hypoxia
- ischaemia
- trauma
- haemorrhage
- tumour
- infection.

CBF will then alter in a manner which is more passively related to changes in mean arterial blood pressure.

Under certain conditions, the brain may regulate its blood flow by initiating changes in systemic arterial blood pressure. This is caused by stimulation of the vasomotor centre in the medulla by ischaemia. This is known as Cushing's phenomenon and aids in maintaining CBF in certain cerebral conditions, e.g. expanding intracranial tumours.

Metabolic autoregulation

This leads to alteration of local blood flow to maintain a constant supply of oxygen to individual regions of the brain according to their level of activity. All organs receive a blood flow which can vary in proportion to metabolic requirements. During increased organ metabolism there is local decrease in PaO_2, an increase in $PaCO_2$, and increase in H^+ concentration. These changes result in arteriolar smooth muscle relaxation, ensuring an increase in flow with little or no change in perfusion pressure, to meet the needs of increased metabolism. Metabolic autoregulation is well developed in the brain.

Neural factors

The cerebral vessels are innervated by cervical sympathetic nerve fibres which accompany the internal carotid and vertebral arteries. However, it is thought that neural regulation of the cerebral circulation is weak and that the contractile state of the smooth muscle of cerebral vessels depends mainly on local metabolic factors, i.e. metabolic autoregulation, and cannot be overridden by nervous control of arterioles.

Local factors

CBF is altered when partial pressures of O_2 and CO_2 change throughout the body. CBF is extremely sensitive to changes in arteriolar partial pressure of CO_2. Increases in $PaCO_2$ cause marked cerebral vasodilatation. CBF doubles as $PaCO_2$ rises from 40 to 100 mmHg (hypercapnia) and halves as $PaCO_2$ falls to 20 mmHg (hypocapnia). The cerebral vasoconstriction caused by hypocapnia can cause mild cerebral ischaemia. Hyperventilation is used as a means of reducing raised intracranial pressure by inducing hypocapnic vasoconstriction with a reduction in CBF and cerebral blood volume. This type of therapy needs to be used with care to avoid ischaemic brain damage.

The relationship between CBF and PaO_2 is not as marked as in the case of $PaCO_2$. CBF remains constant over a wide range of PaO_2 values until PaO_2 falls below 60 mmHg. There is then a rise in CBF which is progressive and may be as high as three-fold at PaO_2 of 30 mmHg. Since a reduced O_2 supply is usually accompanied by an increase in $PaCO_2$, CBF is regulated by hypercapnia rather than hypoxia to maintain a constant O_2 supply.

Increased PaO_2 causes mild cerebral vasoconstriction only. Indeed, hyperbaric oxygen therapy reduces CBF by only 25%.

These vascular responses to change in arterial blood gas tensions may become impaired in the following states:

- head injury
- cerebral haemorrhage
- shock
- hypoxia.

Under such circumstances the protective autoregulatory mechanisms ensuring adequate CBF and oxygen delivery are lacking.

CEREBROSPINAL FLUID

CSF is produced by the choroid plexuses of the lateral, third and fourth ventricles. It flows from the lateral ventricles through the interventricular foramina into the third ventricle, where more CSF is produced. It then passes through the cerebral aqueduct into the fourth ventricle, where further CSF is formed. From the fourth ventricle CSF passes directly into the subarachnoid space, either via the lateral foramina (of Luschka) or the midline foramen (of Magendie). CSF then circulates through the subarachnoid space that surrounds the brain and spinal cord. In certain areas the subarachnoid spaces are dilated and are called cisterns. Two examples of cisterns are the following.

- The cisterna magna (cerebellomedullary cistern), which lies posterior to the medulla and below the cerebellum, is continuous inferiorly with the subarachnoid space around the spinal cord. It is possible to pass a needle through the foramen magnum into the cisterna magna to obtain a specimen of CSF.
- The lumbar cistern, which surrounds the lumbar and sacrospinal routes below the level of termination of the spinal cord, is the usual target for a lumbar puncture.

Finally, CSF is reabsorbed through the arachnoid villi into the sinuses of the venous system (Fig. 8.29). The arachnoid villi may become aggregated into arachnoid granulations. These may grow quite large in the adult,

producing hollows on the inner surface of the parietal bone in particular. Some CSF (approximately 15%) is absorbed in the lumbar area through spinal villi similar to arachnoid villi, or along nerve sheaths into the lymphatics. CSF absorption is passive, depending on its hydrostatic pressure being higher than that of venous blood.

The volume of CSF in the adult is about 140 mL, about 40 mL in the cerebral ventricles, and 100 mL in the subarachnoid spaces. CSF is produced at a constant rate of about 0.35 mL/min, i.e. 500 mL/day. This rate allows for the CSF to be turned over approximately four times daily.

The pressure in the CSF column measured with the patient recumbent in the lateral position is between 120 and 180 mmH$_2$O. The rate at which CSF is produced is relatively independent of the pressure in the ventricles and subarachnoid space and of the systemic blood pressure. However, absorption of CSF is a direct function of CSF pressure. CSF pressure transiently increases during coughing and straining as a result of increase in central venous pressure.

BLOOD–BRAIN BARRIER

In the cerebral microcirculation the junctions between endothelial cells are very tight. They do not permit the passage of substances which would normally pass between the endothelial cells of capillaries in other tissues. Also, the capillaries of the brain are surrounded by the end-feet of astrocytes which are closely applied to the basal membrane of the capillaries. The astrocyte end-feet and the tight junctions between the endothelial cells constitute a blood–brain barrier. This barrier is quite permeable at birth, demonstrated by the fact that bilirubin

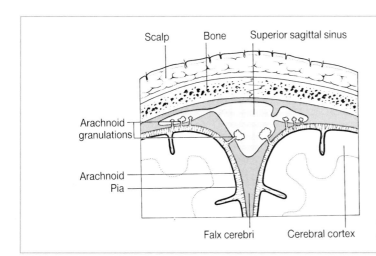

Fig. 8.29 Coronal section through the skull, showing the superior sagittal sinus and arachnoid granulations. From Rogers op. cit.

passes into the brain interstitial fluid if its concentration in plasma rises.

However, during infancy and childhood, permeability of the barrier decreases considerably. Certain substances are still able to cross the barrier, e.g. respiratory gases, glucose, and fat-soluble drugs like volatile anaesthetic agents. Hydrogen ions do not usually cross the barrier but can do so in chronic acidotic conditions. The existence of the barrier maintains a constancy of interstitial environment around the neurons, for these are sensitive to changes in K^+, Ca^{2+} and H^+ concentrations in the fluids surrounding them. Neurons are also protected from toxins which may be present in the systemic circulation. The barrier works in both directions, preventing the entry into the systemic circulation of large quantities of neurotransmitter substances released from the synapses of the CNS.

In some areas, the blood–brain barrier is absent. These include:

- circumventricular organs which abut on the third and fourth ventricles. At the area postrema, drugs such as morphine and digoxin, creatinine and ketones in diabetes mellitus pass through the capillaries to stimulate the chemoreceptor trigger area in the floor of the fourth ventricle, which is connected to the vomiting centre. Angiotensin II also passes through capillaries in this region to stimulate the vasomotor centre to increase sympathetic outflow, thus causing vasoconstriction and increasing peripheral resistance
- the posterior lobe of the pituitary gland. ADH and oxytocin are released from axon terminals in the posterior pituitary and pass into the circulation
- the median eminence of the hypothalamus. Here neurons within the hypothalamus pass releasing or inhibitory hormones into the capillaries of the hypothalamic–pituitary portal system. These control the secretion of hormones by the anterior pituitary.

NERVE CONDUCTION

Mixed peripheral nerves

A typical peripheral nerve consists of a number of fasciculi surrounded by the epineurium. Changes in electrical potential recorded from a peripheral nerve represent the sum of all potential changes in each individual axon. Stimulation thresholds and conduction velocities differ in different types of neuron.

No action potential is recorded if a subthreshold stimulus is applied to a nerve. As the intensity of the stimulus increases, nerve fibres are recruited and action potentials are recorded. The stimulus that recruits all nerve fibres

within an individual nerve is called the maximal stimulus. A supramaximal stimulus produces no increase in recorded potential changes, as all the nerve fibres have already been recruited and the action potential is an 'all or none' phenomenon.

Different nerve groups have different stimulation thresholds and different conduction velocities. The recorded action potential from a peripheral nerve therefore has a number of peaks, and this is termed the compound action potential. The compound action potential differs for different nerves and varies with stimulus strength until the maximal stimulus is applied and all nerve fibres are recruited.

Nerve fibres can be divided into different groups based on their morphology and function. Large myelinated fibres have faster conduction velocities than smaller non-myelinated fibres. A classification of nerve fibres is shown in Table 8.2.

Local anaesthesia

Local anaesthetics act on nerve fibres by altering the ionic permeability of the cell membrane. This is brought about by alterations in the membrane-binding of calcium, which prevent sodium influx which is necessary for production of an action potential. C-fibres, i.e. small unmyelinated patent fibres, are affected before A-fibres, i.e. large myelinated motor fibres.

PAIN

Pain is the sensation resulting from stimuli which are intensive enough to threaten or cause tissue injury. Painful stimuli may be:

- mechanical, e.g. pinprick
- chemical, e.g. acid, corrosive
- thermal, e.g. burn.

Pain may be considered to have two components: the sensation of pain itself and the emotional aspect of

Table 8.2	Types of nerve fibres	
Type	Function	Conduction velocity (mean m/s)
Aα	Motor proprioception	100
Aβ	Touch pressure	50
Aγ	Muscle spindles (motor)	30
Aδ	Pain, temperature, touch	20
B	Autonomic (preganglionic)	10
C	Pain	1

the suffering and distress associated with it. There are a number of different types of pain.

Somatic pain

The specific sense organs for pain, i.e. the peripheral pain detectors, are called nociceptors. In the skin they are probably free nerve endings. They are supplied by either small myelinated (Aδ) fibres or unmyelinated (C) fibres. The endings of Aδ fibres register high intensity mechanical stimuli (mechanical nociceptors), whilst the endings of C fibres register high intensity mechanical or heat stimuli (mechanothermal nociceptors). The latter are probably less selective in responding to mechanical, thermal, or noxious chemical stimuli. Nerves supplying mechanical nociceptors conduct at velocities as high as 30 m/s, while nerves supplying mechanothermal nociceptors conduct at velocities of less than 5 m/s. Stimulation of both types of fibres may give rise to a double sensation: an initial sharp pain caused by the fast-acting A fibres, followed by a longer lasting aching pain due to activity in C fibres.

Visceral pain

Visceral nociceptors are thought to be free nerve endings which occur in the walls of most hollow viscera and mesenteries. They are supplied by small myelinated and unmyelinated afferent fibres. Stimuli exciting a response in these nerves are usually stretching, distension, or ischaemia. Afferents have been identified in the ureter which respond specifically to overdistension, while afferents in the heart have been identified which respond to reduction in coronary blood flow. Excessive stretching or distension of many viscera give rise to colicky or intermittent pain, e.g. intestinal, biliary, or ureteric colic. Visceral pain can also occur with ischaemia, e.g. angina pectoris, or the colicky abdominal pain associated with mesenteric ischaemia. Visceral pains are commonly poorly localised and may be referred to other parts of the body. Most viscera are insensitive to stimuli which would cause intense pain if applied to the skin. Visceral peritoneum does not have pain receptors, whereas parietal peritoneum does. In the unanaesthetised patient, the viscera are:

- insensitive to the pain of cutting
- insensitive of the pain of burning
- sensitive to factors distending or stretching the wall
- sensitive to inflammation, probably due to spasm of the associated muscle.

Visceral pain is diffuse, poorly localised and may vary in intensity from a mild pain (the early stages of acute appendicitis where there is a mild central abdominal pain) to severe (biliary colic, ureteric colic).

The localisation of visceral pain in the abdomen depends upon the embryological derivation of the viscus involved:

- foregut-derived structures — poorly localised upper abdominal pain (e.g. biliary colic)
- midgut-derived structures — poorly localised across the central abdomen (e.g. early stages of acute appendicitis)
- hindgut-derived structures — poorly localised across the lower abdomen (e.g. left-sided obstructive colonic carcinoma).

Referred pain

Pain arising from a viscus is carried back to the CNS by visceral afferents of the autonomic nervous system. Visceral afferents enter the spinal cord at the dorsal root entry zone after entering the spinal canal in the white rami communicantes. Visceral afferents enter the dorsal root entry zone with other sensory fibres passing back from sensory areas, i.e. the dermatome supplied by a spinal nerve. The pain experienced by the individual is referred to the skin surface within the associated dermatome of the spinal nerve. A classical example of referred pain is that from the irritation of the undersurface of the diaphragm (nerve supply C4) referred to the cutaneous distribution of C4 (shoulder tip).

Pathophysiological basis of pain relief

There are two physiological mechanisms by which pain can be controlled:

- a peripheral afferent input system
- a central descending system.

Both of these systems act at a common site, i.e. the cells of the substantia gelatinosa in the grey matter of the dorsal horn.

A peripheral spinal gate control theory

The theory that antagonism exists between large cutaneous afferents and small pain fibres was based on the observation that counterirritation, e.g. heat or massage, will alleviate pain. Impulses in large fibres inhibit cells in the substantia gelatinosa of the dorsal grey matter, thus shutting the 'gate' to the ascent of impulses from the smaller pain fibres. Transcutaneous electrical nerve stimulation (TENS) is based on this theory. Skin electrodes activate the large fibres in peripheral nerves. This selective activation reduces the ability of nociceptive fibres (Aδ and C) to activate spinal neurons which transmit the pain signals to higher centres.

The central descending system

Analgesia can be produced by electrical stimulation of the periaqueductal grey matter in the midbrain or in the limbic system or thalamus. Descending fibres lie in the dorsolateral funiculus of the spinal cord, where control is exerted selectively on the pain input. Part of the descending control of pain may be due to release of endorphins or enkephalins. On the basis of these pathways a more invasive approach to neuromodulation of pain has been devised. Direct or percutaneous implantation of electrodes into the spinal canal to electrically stimulate the dorsal columns has been advocated. This is most effective for pain of the extremities, e.g. after nerve injuries or for peripheral neuropathies. In patients with ischaemic pain, spinal cord stimulation not only reduces pain but may also improve blood flow. Electrodes may also be placed stereotactically either into the periaqueductal grey matter or into the thalamus. Thalamic stimulation is useful for neuropathic pains, while periaqueductal grey matter stimulation is beneficial for nociceptive pain such as severe spinal pain.

Drug modulation of pain

Paracetamol

Paracetamol inhibits prostaglandin synthesis by a different action to that of NSAIDs (see below). Its action is related to local peroxide concentrations which act as a cofactor in prostaglandin synthesis. Paracetamol reduces peroxide levels. This effectively prevents prostaglandin biosynthesis where the peroxide concentration is low, e.g in brain, but not where it is high, e.g. in sites of inflammation or pus.

Non-steroidal anti-inflammatory drugs (NSAIDs)

Tissue injury results in the breakdown of cell wall lipid to arachidonic acid. Release of histamine and bradykinin initiates inflammation and stimulates nociceptors, a process sensitised by prostaglandins. NSAIDs limit the conversion of arachidonic acid to PGG_2, an intermediary in prostaglandin production, by inhibiting cyclo-oxygenase. This inhibition of production of prostaglandins by NSAIDs is responsible for their analgesic action.

Opioids

Opiates are drugs derived from the juice of the opium poppy. They exert their analgesic effects by binding to specific opiate receptors. This binding is stereospecifically inhibited by a morphine derivitive called naloxone. Compounds not derived from the opium poppy, but that exert direct effects by binding to opiate receptors, are called opioids. In practice, opioids are defined as directly acting compounds whose effects are stereospecifically antagonised by naloxone.

Opiates such as morphine, heroin and codeine are the most powerful analgesics known. They act by combining with the receptors in many areas of the CNS, including the periaqueductal grey matter, parts of the limbic system, and the substantia gelatinosa of the spinal cord. Certain endogenous analgesic peptides bind to these receptors. These may be divided into three groups:

- enkephalins
- dynorphins
- endorphins.

Opioid peptides are not effective when injected intravenously but are more potent than opiates when applied directly to certain areas of the brain and the spinal cord. Opioid peptides may play a role in the effects of acupuncture, as some of the effects of acupuncture can be blocked by the opiate analgesic naloxone. It has also been suggested that opioid peptides may be decreased in chronic pain states. As has been seen above, they can be increased by electrical stimulation of the periaqueductal grey matter.

Opioid peptides may act at the level of the spinal cord and in peripheral tissues. Substance P, a peptide present in the terminals of afferent fibres, has been suggested as the transmitter for nociceptive stimuli in the dorsal horn. Opioids may block the release of substance P presynaptically from these afferent fibres, thus reducing pain.

There are several types of opioid receptors: these are μ, κ, δ, σ.

Conventional opioids (e.g. morphine, pethidine) are agonists attaching to the μ receptors and produce:

- analgesia at a supraspinal level
- drug-induced euphoria
- respiratory depression
- drug dependency.

Opioid agonist-antagonists

The side effects of conventional opioids led to the development of antagonist analgesics. They are so named because they originated from the morphine antagonist nalorphine, which has analgesic properties of its own. These drugs antagonise opioid agonists (causing less respiratory depression and less addiction), but have analgesic properties. Pentazocine and nalbuphine are examples of opioid agonists–antagonists. The latter are antagonists at the μ receptors, but produce analgesia by attaching to the κ receptors. This would explain why nalorphine is unable to reverse (antagonise) the respiratory depression of pentazocine, but naloxone (a pure μ and κ antagonist) can.

BRAINSTEM DEATH

Many patients are maintained on artificial ventilation in Intensive Care Units. It is important to be able to decide between those who have the potential for survival and those who do not. It is therefore important to define the condition of brainstem death in which the heart and lungs function but there is no cerebral activity. Brainstem death is regarded as the legal equivalent of death as customarily defined by cessation of heart beat and spontaneous respiration. In order to make the diagnosis of brain death, certain preconditions must be satisfied:

- The patient's condition must be known to be due to irreversible brain damage of known aetiology.
- The patient must be in apnoeic coma, i.e. deeply unconscious and dependent on artificial ventilation.

There are certain exclusion criteria. There should be no doubt that other, potentially reversible, causes of the state of unconsciousness have been excluded, these include:

- residual drug effects — effects of narcotics, hypnotics, tranquillisers and muscle relaxants
- hypothermia — this must be excluded; the core temperature must be $> 35°C$
- circulatory, metabolic and endocrine disturbances, e.g. hypernatraemia, diabetic coma.

Once the preconditions and exclusions have been taken into account, there are certain clinical criteria which must be applied to confirm the absence of brainstem reflexes and the absence of spontaneous respiration. The following brainstem reflexes are tested for:

- Pupillary. There should be no pupillary response to light. The pupils do not respond either directly or consensually to sharp changes of the intensity of incident light. Cranial nerves involved in this reflex are II and III.
- Absent corneal reflexes. There should be no response to direct stimulation of the cornea. This would normally result in blinking of the eye. The cranial nerves tested are V and VII.
- No motor response to central stimulation. There should be no motor response within the cranial nerve distribution in response to adequate stimulation of any somatic area. The usual test is to apply supraorbital pressure.
- Absent gag reflex. The back of the throat is touched with a catheter. There should be no gagging. This tests cranial nerves IX and X.
- Absent cough reflex. There should be no response to bronchial stimulation by a catheter passed via the endotracheal tube. This tests cranial nerves IX and X.
- Absent vestibulo-ocular reflex. There should be clear access to the tympanic membrane which is confirmed by visual inspection with an auriscope. The head is flexed at 30°. There should be no eye movements following slow injection of 50 mL of ice cold water over 1 min into each external auditory meatus in turn. This tests cranial nerves VIII, III and VI.

Finally, spontaneous respiration must be demonstrated to be absent despite a stimulus that should provoke it. This is done by disconnecting the patient from the ventilator in the presence of a $PaCO_2$ above the threshold for respiratory stimulation. This is performed by preoxygenating the patient with 100% oxygen for at least 10 min. The $PaCO_2$ is allowed to rise to 5.0 kPa before testing. The patient is then disconnected from the ventilator. Oxygen is insufflated at 6 L/min via an endotracheal tube to maintain adequate oxygenation during the test, and the $PaCO_2$ is allowed to rise above 6.65 kPa. There should be no spontaneous respirations noted.

These tests should be carried out on two occasions, the time interval between the tests being a matter of clinical judgement. The tests should be carried out by two medical practitioners registered for more than 5 years, at least one of whom should be a consultant. They should be competent in the field and not members of the transplant team.

Death is pronounced and certified after completion of the second set of tests and not when ventilation is discontinued. The legal time of death is when the second set of tests indicate brainstem death.

PATHOLOGY
HEAD INJURY

In the United Kingdom approximately 250 per 100 000 population present to hospital each year with head injuries, most of which are due to road traffic accidents and falls. Head injury is one of the most frequent causes of disability and death, especially in young males. Head injuries may be classified according to their aetiology, i.e. missile or non-missile (blunt) injuries. Missile injuries have been referred to as penetrating injuries in the past, but in some cases the missile does not penetrate but causes a depressed fracture without penetrating brain substance.

Missile injury
These may be divided into three types:

- depressed injury, where the missile causes a depressed fracture but does not enter the brain

- penetrating injuries, where the missile enters the skull cavity but does not leave
- perforating injuries, where the missile enters and leaves the skull cavity. This type of injury is usually caused by high velocity bullet wounds, and the brain damage is extensive.

Non-missile injuries

These most commonly occur in road traffic accidents, falls and assaults. Damage may be minor or may result in severe injuries which are rapidly fatal. Brain damage occurs often as a result of acceleration/deceleration creating rotational and shearing forces which act on the mobile brain anchored within the rigid skull. Head injuries which may be fatal can occur without skull fractures.

Two main patterns of brain damage occur which are referred to as primary and secondary.

Primary brain damage

Contusions   These occur when the brain is crushed when coming into contact with the skull. They usually occur at the site of impact but may be severe on the side opposite the impact, i.e. *contre-coup* lesions. Large contusions may be associated with intracerebral haemorrhage.

Diffuse axonal injury   This occurs as a result of acceleration/deceleration and rotational movements. It may occur in the absence of a skull fracture. The majority of changes are usually only detectable on histology. Patients who have sustained diffuse axonal injury and survive are usually severely disabled.

Treatment cannot reverse primary brain injury. It is aimed at prevention, recognition and treatment of secondary brain damage.

Secondary brain damage

This occurs as a result of complications developing after the time of injury. Secondary brain damage may result from:

- intracranial haemorrhage
- cerebral hypoxia
- cerebral oedema
- intracranial herniation
- infection.

Sequelae of head injuries

Most patients make a satisfactory recovery unless the head injury is severe, when up to 10% may be severely disabled. Consequences of severe head injuries include:

- death (often diagnosed as brainstem death)
- persistent vegetative state

- post-traumatic epilepsy
- traumatic hemiplegia
- post-traumatic dementia
- cranial nerve palsies.

INTRACRANIAL HAEMORRHAGE

This may be extracerebral, which occurs in relation to coverings of the brain, or intracerebral, which occurs within the brain.

Intracerebral

This is usually an expansile haematoma within brain tissue. Most arise in hypertensive patients who have weak spots (microaneurysms) on their arteriosclerotic cerebral vessels. Other causes include bleeding into a tumour, vascular malformations, and bleeding associated with coagulopathies.

Extracerebral

These are divided into different types according to where they occur in relationship to the meninges. Extradural and subdural haemorrhages usually occur following trauma. Subarachnoid haemorrhage usually occurs following rupture of a 'berry' aneurysm and may also occur following trauma.

Extradural haemorrhage

This is bleeding into the extradural space between the skull and dura. It is caused by a head injury, usually with a skull fracture which causes tearing of an artery or a venous sinus. Classically the injury is to the middle meningeal artery following fracture of the temporal bone. The haematoma lies outside the dura and causes compression of the underlying brain as it expands. Clinically there is usually a lucid interval followed by a rapid increase in intracranial pressure. Transtentorial herniation may occur and manifest itself by reduction in conscious level and by brainstem compression. The condition is fatal unless diagnosed early and treated surgically by evacuation of the clot.

Subdural haemorrhage

This is bleeding into the subdural space between the dura and arachnoid mater. Bleeding is usually from small 'bridging' veins which cross the subdural space. Trauma is the usual cause. Two types are described as follows.

Acute subdural haematoma   This is commonly seen following head injury, often associated with a lacerated brain resulting from high speed injuries. The haematoma spreads over a large area. The patient usually has marked brain injury from the outset and is comatose, but the condition deteriorates further.

Chronic subdural haematoma This is usually seen in the elderly. Brain shrinkage makes the 'bridging' veins between cerebral cortex and venous sinuses more vulnerable. It may result from a trivial and forgotten head injury. It may occur weeks or months after the injury. Presentation is with personality change, memory loss, confusion, and fluctuating level of consciousness.

Subarachnoid haemorrhage

This is bleeding into the subarachnoid space between the arachnoid and pia mater. Causes include:

- trauma in association with head injury
- rupture of a 'berry' aneurysm
- rupture of a vascular malformation
- hypertensive haemorrhage
- coagulation disorders
- rupture of an intracerebral haematoma into the subarachnoid space
- tumours
- vasculitis.

Subarachnoid haemorrhage presents with sudden onset of severe headache. Blood spreads over the cerebral surface of the subarachnoid space. In approximately 15% of cases it is instantly fatal, a further 45% of cases dying later due to rebleeding. Blood accumulates in the basal cisterns and may block the egress of CSF, causing hydrocephalus. This can occur early or later in survivors where fibrous obliteration of the subarachnoid space occurs due to organisation of the clot.

SPACE-OCCUPYING LESIONS

These may result from a variety of causes. They cause an expansion in volume of the cranial contents and will eventually cause raised intracranial pressure. Intracranial space-occupying lesions may be either diffuse or focal. Diffuse brain swelling results from either vasodilatation or oedema. Focal brain swellings include tumours, abscess and haematomas. The consequences of intracranial space-occupying lesions include:

- raised intracranial pressure
- intracranial shift
- intracranial herniation
- hydrocephalus.

RAISED INTRACRANIAL PRESSURE

The skull contains brain, CSF and blood. At normal intracranial pressures (10–15 mmHg or 12–18 cmH$_2$O), these three components are in volumetric equilibrium. If one component is elevated, intracranial pressure will increase, unless the volume of the other two components decreases proportionately (Monro–Kellie doctrine). The compensatory properties among the intracranial contents follow a pressure/volume exponential curve. Increased volume of any of the three components can be balanced up to a certain level without any increase in the intracranial pressure. However, eventually a critical volume is reached when any further volume increase results in raised intracranial pressure. The effects of raised intracranial pressure are:

- hydrocephalus
- cerebral ischaemia
- brain shift and herniation
- systemic effects.

Hydrocephalus

This is common complication of space-occupying lesions of the posterior cranial fossa which compress the cerebral aqueduct and fourth ventricle.

Cerebral ischaemia

The effects of raised intracranial pressure are exerted on the vascular component and result in progressive reduction in cerebral perfusion pressure. (Cerebral perfusion pressure = blood pressure – intracranial pressure.)

Brain shift and herniation

These usually occur following a critical increase in intracranial pressure. Lumbar puncture is contraindicated in any patient with raised intracranial pressure, as there is a risk of precipitating a potentially fatal brainstem herniation. Herniations occur at some specific sites:

Transtentorial herniation A laterally placed supratentorial mass may push the uncus and hippocampus over the tentorium cerebelli. The oculomotor nerves, cerebral peduncles, cerebral aqueduct, posterior cerebral artery, and brainstem may be compressed by the displaced temporal lobe. Transtentorial herniation is frequently fatal because of the secondary haemorrhage into the brainstem. Clinical manifestations of transtentorial herniation are shown in Table 8.3.

Tonsillar herniation Herniation of the cerebellar tonsils into the foramen magnum causes compression of the medulla. Medullary compression results in decerebrate posture, respiratory failure, and subsequent death.

Systemic effects

Systemic effects of raised intracranial pressure are thought to result from autonomic imbalance and over-

Table 8.3 Clinical manifestations of tentorial herniation	
Affected (compressed) structure	Clinical manifestation
Oculomotor nerve (Cranial III)	Ipsilateral pupillary dilatation
Ipsilateral cerebral peduncle	Contralateral hemiparesis
Contralateral cerebral peduncle	Ipsilateral hemiparesis
Posterior cerebral artery	Cortical blindness
Cerebral aqueduct	Headache and vomiting from hydrocephalus
Reticular formation	Coma
Midbrain	Decerebrate rigidity, death

activity as a result of compression of the hypothalamus. They include:

- hypertension
- bradycardia
- respiratory slowing
- pulmonary oedema (often haemorrhagic)
- gastrointestinal ulceration (Cushing's ulcer).

Clinical manifestations of raised intracranial pressure

Once the phase of compensation between the three components, i.e. brain, CSF and blood, is passed, further increase in volume of intracranial contents will cause an increase in intracranial pressure. The clinical signs and symptoms are:

- headache — due to distortion and compression of pain receptors within the dura mater and around cerebral blood vessels
- nausea and vomiting — due to pressure on the vomiting centre in the pons and medulla
- papilloedema due to venous obstruction
- decrease in level of consciousness ranging from drowsiness to coma depending on the degree of raised intracranial pressure.

MENINGITIS

Bacterial meningitis is the only form of meningitis which the surgical trainee is likely to encounter. Bacteria gain access to the CNS by four main routes:

- direct spread from an adjacent focus of infection, e.g. middle ear, mastoid, paranasal sinuses, osteomyelitis of vertebrae or skull
- blood-borne as part of septicaemia or septic embolus from bacterial endocarditis or bronchiectasis
- penetrating wounds, including skull fractures
- iatrogenic, e.g. following lumbar puncture or spinal anaesthesia or following neurosurgical procedures.

Meningitis may affect predominantly the dura mater (pachymeningitis) or the arachnoid or pia mater (leptomeningitis). The latter is the more common.

Pachymeningitis

This is usually a consequence of direct spread of infection following otitis media or mastoiditis and is a complication of skull fractures. Common pathogens include haemolytic streptococci from the paranasal sinuses, or *Staph. aureus* from skull fractures. Epidural abscess (pus between skull and dura mater) or subdural abscesses (pus in the subdural space) may result.

Leptomeningitis

This is usually a result of blood-borne spread of infection or may arise from direct spread from the skull bones. Different organisms cause infection at different ages:

- neonates — *E. coli, Salmonella*
- children — *H. influenzae* type b, *Neisseria meningitidis, Streptococcus pneumoniae*
- adults — *Neisseria meningitidis, Streptococcus pneumoniae*
- elderly — *Listeria monocytogenes, Streptococcus pneumoniae.*

Meningococcal meningitis is the commonest variety. The organism is spread by droplets from asymptomatic nasal carriers. The organism reaches the CNS by haematogenous spread. Onset of the illness is rapid with a petechial rash related to disseminated intravascular coagulation, accompanied by adrenal haemorrhage (Waterhouse–Friderichsen syndrome) which is often fatal.

Complications

Complications of bacterial meningitis include:

- cerebral infarction
- cerebral abscess
- subdural abscess
- hydrocephalus
- epilepsy.

CEREBRAL ABSCESS

Cerebral abscesses usually develop following focal inflammation of the parenchyma of the brain. They usually occur as a result of:

- direct spread of infection from sepsis in the middle ear or paranasal sinuses

- septic cerebral sinus thrombosis due to spread of infection from the mastoid or middle ear via the sigmoid sinus
- blood-borne infection, e.g. from infective endocarditis or bronchiectasis. In immunocompromised patients, abscesses may be caused by fungal or protozoal organisms.
- trauma – following open skull fractures.

Abscesses may occur in preferential sites according to their aetiology:

- temporal lobe or cerebellum from otitis media
- frontal lobe from paranasal sinuses
- parietal lobe from haematogenous spread.

Complications
Complications of cerebral abscesses include:

- meningitis
- intracranial herniation
- focal neurological deficit
- epilepsy.

Cerebral abscesses often cause a dramatic increase in intracranial pressure because of massive surrounding oedema. Lumbar puncture should not be performed in the presence of cerebral abscess, as this may precipitate fatal intracranial herniation.

CEREBRAL TUMOURS

The constituent cells of the nervous system can be divided into five main groups:

- neurons
- glia
- microglial cells
- connective tissue
- blood vessels.

Glial cells are specialised supporting cells of the CNS and comprise four main cells: astrocytes, oligodendrocytes, ependymal cells and choroid plexus cells. Microglial cells belong to the macrophage/monocyte system of phagocytic cells. They are important in reactive states, for example in inflammation and demyelinating disorders. The connective tissue in the central nervous system is confined to two main types, i.e. the meninges and perivascular fibroblasts.

Cerebral tumours may be broadly classified into two types; glial and non-glial, depending on their cell of origin (Box 8.1).

Box 8.1   Classification of cerebral tumours

Primary
- Glial (gliomas)
  - Astrocytomas
  - Medullablastomas
  - Ependymomas
  - Oligodendrogliomas
- Non-glial
  - Meningiomas
  - Acoustic neuromas
  - Pituitary tumours

Secondary
  - Lung
  - Breast
  - Kidney
  - Melanoma

Types of cerebral tumour

Astrocytoma
The peak incidence of astrocytoma is in early middle age. They vary in malignancy and some are slow growing and infiltrative. Most malignant astrocytomas are radioresistant, and survival overall is usually less than 5 years. In children the tumour is often well differentiated and cystic and occurs in the cerebellum. This type is histological benign and may often be completely excised, with potential cure.

Glioblastoma multiforme
This is the most malignant brain tumour. It is rapid growing and occurs between 40 and 60 years. It is rarely removable surgically and is radioresistant. Most patients are dead within a year of diagnosis.

Medulloblastoma
This is the commonest glioma of childhood. It occurs in the first decade of life, arising in the roof of the fourth ventricle, and infiltrates into the cerebellum. It may cause obstructive hydrocephalus. Spread is by the CSF and it may seed on the spinal cord.

Ependymomas
Ependymomas arising from the choroid plexus of the ventricles may be totally removable. Those arising from the ventricular walls are difficult to remove. Most of them are well differentiated. The malignant forms, however, may seed via the subarachnoid space.

Oligodendrogliomas
These occur in the cerebral hemispheres and are slow growing. Treatment is by tumour debulking and radiotherapy. Most patients are dead within 5 years of diagnosis.

Meningiomas

Meningiomas arise from arachnoid cells. They usually occur in females in the 40–60 age group. They compress the cerebral cortex early in their growth, and therefore fits may be an early sign. They may rarely cause osteoblastic change in the overlying bone, giving rise to exostosis producing a palpable lump over the vault of the skull. The most frequent sites are the parasagittal region, sphenoidal wing, olfactory groove and foramen magnum. They are usually slow growing and do not invade brain tissue but compress it. Small tumours are usually curable by excision. Even with subtotal excision for large tumours the prognosis is good.

Acoustic neuroma

This arises from Schwann cells of the nerve sheath of the eighth cranial nerve at the internal auditory meatus. As the tumour grows, it expands the internal auditory canal, extends into the cerebellopontine angle, compressing the pons, the cerebellum and adjacent cranial nerves. It may be a feature of von Recklinghausen's disease. Acoustic neuroma should always be considered in a patient with unilateral sensorineural deafness with tinnitus. It usually occurs in the age range 30–60. Facial weakness with unilateral taste loss is a later manifestation. The corneal reflexes are lost relatively early when the trigeminal nerve is stretched by the tumour. Dysphagia, hoarseness and dysarthria may arise due to involvement of nerves IX, X and XI. Unilateral cerebellar signs and features of raised ICP may occur, but these are now a rare occurrence.

Secondary tumours

The CNS is a common site for metastases, which may occur by haematogenous or direct spread. The commonest neoplasms to metasasize to the CNS are carcinoma of the breast, bronchus, kidney, colon, and also malignant melanomas.

Clinical features of CNS tumours

CNS tumours may present clinically in two main ways:

- local effects — these may include cranial nerve palsies, epilepsy, or paraplegia with a spinal cord tumour
- mass effects — many tumours may present with non-specific signs of space-occupying lesions without any localising signs. These symptoms include confusion, drowsiness, headache and vomiting. Other features may relate to the development of hydrocephalus and intracranial herniation.

Pituitary tumours

These cause symptoms because of their endocrine capacity or their effects on the optic chiasma.

Secretory tumours (e.g. prolactinoma)   Many tumours contain a mixture of secretory cells. Presentation is influenced by the hormonal production and the size of the tumour. Secretory tumours are usually small.

Non-secretory tumours   These usually grow to a large size and present through local effects. The symptoms and signs depend upon whether they arise from the endocrine capacity or local pressure effects. Bitemporal hemianopia results from compression of the optic chiasma. Compression of secretory cells by non-secretory tumours may result in hypopituitarism. Symptoms include reduced libido, infertility, amenorrhoea, myxoedema, depression, loss of sex characteristics, and hypoadrenalism. In children, growth arrest may occur. Hormonally active tumours may result in the following:

- overproduction of growth hormone: before fusion of the epiphyses, this will cause gigantism; in adult life acromegaly results
- hyperprolactinaemia: this is characterised by amenorrhoea, infertility, galactorrhoea, and impotence
- Cushing's disease (see Ch. 14).

SPINAL CORD INJURIES AND COMPRESSION

Cord injuries

Over 80% of spinal injuries result from road traffic accidents, the remainder resulting from falls and other trauma, e.g. penetrating wounds. Penetrating trauma may result in incomplete cord transection which may manifest clinically as Brown–Séquard syndrome (see below). Closed injuries are responsible for most spinal cord trauma and are usually associated with fractures or fracture/dislocations of the vertebral column. As with brain injuries there is primary and secondary damage:

- primary damage — contusions, transections, haemorrhage, necrosis
- secondary damage — extradural haematoma, infarction, infection, oedema.

Contusion or laceration is the usual result of spinal cord injury. There is resulting oedema and increased tissue pressure, and this, together with cord haemorrhage, further limits the blood supply. The distribution of cord oedema, of haemorrhage and of infarction determines the neurological symptoms and the signs elicited at the time of evaluation. Spinal cord injuries may be complete or incomplete.

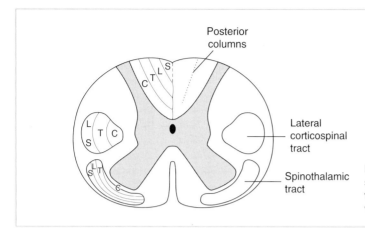

Posterior columns

Lateral corticospinal tract

Spinothalamic tract

Fig. 8.30 Cross-section of the spinal cord showing the representation of the cervical (C), thoracic (T), lumbar (L) and sacral (S) areas in the various spinal tracts.

Complete

When the spinal cord is transected there are three major and immediate effects:

- loss of voluntary movement in all parts innervated by the isolated spinal segment, i.e. distal to the level of transection; this loss is irreversible
- a loss of all sensation from those areas which depend on ascending spinal pathways crossing the site of injury
- spinal shock.

With complete cord transection there is no voluntary nervous function below the injury site. There is an initial phase of spinal shock with a loss of all reflexes below the injured cord. These include the bulbocavernosus and anal reflexes, and deep tendon reflexes. Spinal shock may last for a few hours to several weeks. The cessation of the spinal shock phase is marked by return of reflex activity in the spinal cord when the lesion is above the sacral segment, i.e. when there is an upper motor neuron lesion. The anal and bulbocavernosus reflexes are usually the first to return. The anal and bulbocavernosus reflexes both depend on intact sacral reflex arcs. The anal reflex is elicited by pricking the perianal skin with a pin when there is a visible contraction of the anal sphincter. The bulbocavernosus reflex is contraction of the anal sphincter in response to squeezing the glans penis.

Incomplete

In incomplete spinal cord injuries some function is present below the site of the injury. These injuries have a more favourable prognosis overall. There are recognised patterns of incomplete cord injury, although these are rarely 'pure' and variations may occur. The functional

anatomy of the tract of the spinal cord has already been described. The dorsal columns contain fibres serving fine and discriminative tactile sensation as well as proprioception. The lateral corticospinal tract (crossed pyramidal tract) controls skilled voluntary movement, and the fibres in these tracts are somatopically arranged, fibres for the lower part of the cord being lateral and those for the upper levels medial. The spinothalamic tracts conduct pain and temperature sensation. Pain and temperature fibres enter the posterior roots, ascend a few segments, relay in the substantia gelatinosa, then cross to the opposite site to ascend in these tracts to the thalamus, where they are then relayed to the sensory cortex. The fibres in these tracts are somatotopically arranged, those for the lower limb being superficial and those for the upper limb deepest in the cord. The arrangement of the fibres in the various tracts is shown in Fig. 8.30. The following are recognised patterns of incomplete cord injury (Fig. 8.31).

Anterior cord syndrome Damage to the anterior cord is particularly associated with flexion/rotation injuries to the spine, producing an anterior dislocation or by compression fracture of a vertebral body with bone encroaching on the vertebral canal. In addition to direct damage there is often compression of the anterior spinal artery so that the corticospinal and spinothalamic tracts are damaged by a combination of direct trauma and ischaemia. The result of this lesion is a loss of power as well as reduction of pain and temperature sensation below the lesion. Because the dorsal columns remain intact, touch and proprioception are unaffected.

Central cord syndrome This is typically seen in the older patient with cervical spondylosis who sustains a hyperextension injury. This may be from relatively minor trauma. The spinal cord is compressed between the osteo-

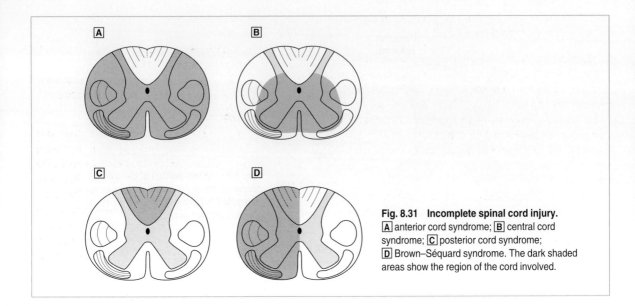

Fig. 8.31 Incomplete spinal cord injury.
A anterior cord syndrome; B central cord syndrome; C posterior cord syndrome; D Brown–Séquard syndrome. The dark shaded areas show the region of the cord involved.

phytes of the vertebrae and intravertebral disc in front and the thickened ligamentum flavum posteriorly. The more centrally situated cervical tracts supplying the arm tend to be more involved than the more peripherally placed tracts affecting the legs. Classically there is a flaccid (lower motor neuron) weakness of the arms but, because the distal leg and sacral motor and sensory fibres are located most peripherally in the cervical cord, peri-anal sensation and some lower extremity movement and sensation may be preserved.

Posterior cord syndrome This syndrome is most commonly seen in hyperextension injuries with fractures of the posterior elements of the vertebrae. The posterior columns are involved and therefore proprioception is affected. The patient usually has good power and sensation for pain and temperature below the lesion, but there may be profound ataxia due to the loss of proprioception which produces an unsteady and faltering gait.

Brown–Séquard syndrome This is hemisection of the cord. It may result from either stab injuries or fractures of the lateral mass of the vertebrae. The classical picture is paralysis on the affected side below the lesion (pyramidal tract), and also loss of proprioception and fine discrimi-nation (dorsal columns). Pain and temperature are normal on the side of the lesion but are lost on the opposite side below the lesion because the affected spinothalamic tract carries fibres which have decussated below the level of cord hemisection. The uninjured side therefore has good power but reduced or absent sensation to pin prick and temperature.

Cauda equina syndrome This syndrome may arise from bony compression or disc protrusions in the lumbar or sacral region, with compression of the lumbosacral nerve roots below the conus medullaris. This is a lower motor neuron lesion, and bowel and bladder dysfunction, as well as leg numbness and weakness, occur commonly with this syndrome.

Autonomic defects in spinal cord injuries

Vasomotor control Problems with hypotension arise in cervical or high thoracic lesions, i.e. those above the sympathetic outflow (T5). Because of interruption of sympathetic splanchnic control, the upright position results in hypotension secondary to impaired venous return, with consequent syncope. Adaptive mechanisms pos-sibly related to spinal reflexes occur with time. Control of the vasomotor system is labile during the first few days after a cervical spinal cord injury. There is a risk of sudden cardiac arrest following turning of the patient.

Temperature control The patient does not have the usual thermoregulatory mechanisms working below the level of the lesion. This is particularly so in quadriplegics. The mechanisms allowing for vasoconstriction to con-serve heat are lost. The patient is unable to shiver and consequently is unable to increase the body temperature. Also, the patient cannot sweat below the level of the lesion in response to hyperthermia. The quadriplegic patient therefore tends to assume the temperature of the environment.

Bladder control After a spinal injury the effect on the

bladder depends on the level of injury, degree of damage, and the time interval after the injury.

- Spinal shock. There is flaccid paralysis below the level of the lesion with absent reflexes. The patient develops acute retention of urine and requires catheterisation.
- Upper motor neuron lesion. If this is above the sacral segments, reflex activity returns after the phase of spinal shock passes and an automatic type of bladder results, i.e. the bladder empties involuntarily as it fills with urine. There is no sensation of bladder fullness.
- Lower motor neuron lesion. The reflex arc is interrupted and an autonomous bladder results. Bladder function is governed by a myogenic stretch reflex inherent in the detrusor muscle. There is a linear increase in intravesical pressure with filling until capacity is reached. Overflow incontinence then occurs.

Mixed types of lesions may occur with damage to the conus medullaris and cauda equina.

Bowel In a spinal cord lesion above the sacral segments the defaecation reflex is intact but automatic emptying of the lower bowel will occur because the normal control exercised by voluntary contraction of the external sphincter is lost and sensation is impaired. The external sphincter will be hypertonic in an upper motor neuron lesion. In a lower motor neuron lesion the reflex is interrupted but the autonomous bowel has intrinsic contractile mechanisms. The external anal sphincter is weak, and the anus is patulous with absent tone.

Autonomic dysreflexia This is seen in patients with cervical cord injuries above the sympathetic outflow but may also occur with high thoracic lesions above T5. It occurs after the period of spinal shock has worn off and results from distension of the bladder, which causes reflex sympathetic overactivity below the level of the spinal cord lesion, causing vasoconstriction and systemic hypertension. The carotid and aortic baroreceptors are stimulated and respond via the vasomotor centre with increased vagal tone, with resultant bradycardia. The peripheral vasodilatation which would have normally relieved the hypertension does not occur because the stimuli cannot pass distally through the severed cord. The patient develops a severe headache with profuse sweating and flushing of the skin above the level of the lesion. Intracranial haemorrhage may occur.

Spinal cord and nerve root compression

The following are the main causes of spinal cord and nerve root compression:

- prolapsed intravertebral disc
- trauma
- tumour, e.g. metastases, myeloma
- infection, e.g. tuberculosis, abscess
- skeletal disorders, e.g. osteoarthritis, Paget's disease
- vascular, e.g. haemorrhage, vascular malformation.

Prolapsed intravertebral disc

This usually occurs in the middle aged or elderly due to degenerative disc disease but may occur in young adults following strenuous exercise. A tear occurs in the annulus fibrosus, and the gelatinous nucleus pulposus herniates out both posteriorly and laterally. In the latter case it normally impinges on the nerve roots causing sciatica if it occurs in the lumbosacral region. Central herniation is less common but may cause direct cord damage and may occasionally compress the anterior spinal artery, leading to infarction. Disc prolapse occurs most commonly at C5/C6 and L5/S1 levels.

Osteoarthritis

Spondylosis occurs due to osteoarthritis. It becomes progressively more common over the age of 40 and is often accompanied by degenerative disc disease. Osteophytes occur at the upper and lower margins of the vertebral bodies, adjacent to the attachment of the annulus fibrosus. The osteophytes encroach on the spinal canal or intravertebral foramina and irritate the nerve roots.

PERIPHERAL NERVE LESIONS

Peripheral nerves contain sensory and motor axons (or both), most of which are myelinated. Each axon is surrounded by the endoneurium, a sheath of collagen fibres. Groups of axons, called fasciculi, are further surrounded by a connective tissue sheath called the perineurium. The fasciculi themselves are further surrounded by the epineurium, which is a thicker layer of connective tissue.

Nerve injury may be caused by one of the following:

- laceration
- contusion
- stretch
- compression.

Nerve injuries may be further classified according to the degree of damage:

- neuropraxia
- axonotmesis
- neurotmesis.

Neuropraxia

This results in temporary failure of conduction without

loss of axonal continuity. Recovery is rapid and complete and takes a few days to a few weeks.

Axonotmesis

This is complete division of an axon. If the axon is transected, that part of the axon no longer in continuity with the cell body dies (Wallerian degeneration). The axon distal to the site of injury degenerates. In myelinated fibres this is accompanied by breakdown of myelin around the degenerating axons. Degeneration commences at 3–4 days following injury. In axonotmesis the endoneurial tube remains intact and axonal regeneration can occur unless it is impeded by scar tissue at the site of injury (neuroma in continuity).

Neurotmesis

This would occur in a nerve laceration. There is complete break in the nerve fibres, i.e. axon, myelin sheath, and endoneurial tube. When a peripheral nerve is severed the distal nerve degenerates. The axon then regenerates from the nerve cell through the rejoined sheaths. The rate of the repair is approximately 1 mm/day. Unfortunately, individual nerves do not regenerate down their original nerve sheath, and motor axons may regenerate into a sensory distal sheath and vice versa. The functional results are therefore variable. The best results occur if the nerve is purely motor or purely sensory or in nerves rejoined by microscopical surgical techniques.

9

Cardiovascular system

Ken Callum, Andrew Dyson

ANATOMY

HEART

Development of the heart

The heart begins to develop towards the end of the third week of gestation as a pair of endothelial tubes which fuse to become the primitive heart tube. This develops within the pericardial cavity from which it is suspended from the dorsal wall by a dorsal mesocardium.

The primitive heart tube develops grooves which divide it into five regions: the sinus venosus, atrium, ventricle, bulbus cordis and truncus arteriosus (Fig. 9.1). The arterial and venous ends of the tube are surrounded by a layer of visceral pericardium. The primitive heart tube then elongates within the pericardial cavity, with the bulbus cordis and ventricle growing more rapidly than the attachments at either end, so that the heart first takes a U-shape and later an S-shape. At the same time it rotates

slightly anticlockwise and twists so that the right ventricle lies anteriorly and the left atrium and ventricle posteriorly (Fig. 9.1). Despite this, and an increase in the number of vessels entering and leaving, they still continue to be enclosed together in this single tube of pericardium.

As the tube develops, the sinus venosus becomes incorporated into the atrium and the bulbus cordis into the ventricle. Endocardial cushions develop between the primitive atrium and ventricle. An interventricular septum develops from the apex up towards the endocardial cushions.

The division of the atrium is slightly more complicated. A structure called the septum primum grows down to fuse with the endocardial cushions, but leaves a hole in the upper part which is termed the foramen ovale. A second incomplete membrane develops known as the septum secundum. This is just to the right of the septum primum and foramen ovale. Thus a valve-like structure

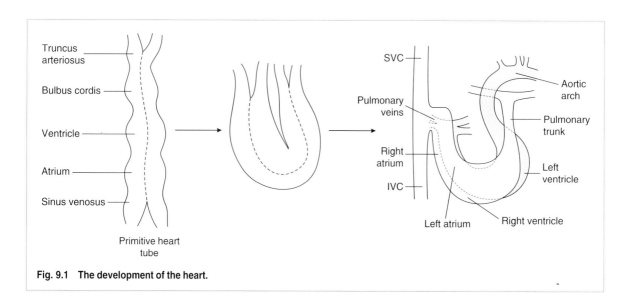

Fig. 9.1 The development of the heart.

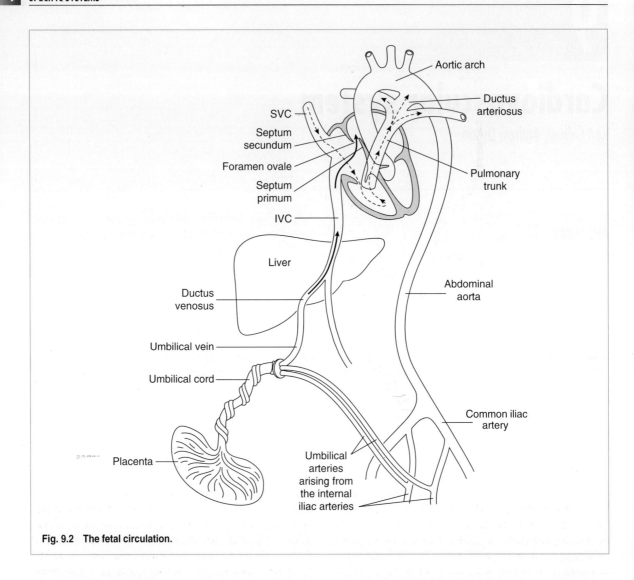

Fig. 9.2 The fetal circulation.

develops which allows blood to go from the right to the left side of the heart in the fetus (Fig. 9.2). At birth, when there is an increased blood flow through the lungs and a rise in the left atrial pressure, the septum primum is pushed across to close the foramen ovale. Usually the septa fuse, obliterating the foramen ovale and leaving a small residual dimple (the fossa ovalis). The sinus venosus joins the atria, becoming the two venae cavae on the right and the four pulmonary veins on the left (Fig. 9.1).

Development of the aortic arches

A common arterial trunk, the truncus arteriosus, continues from the bulbus cordis and gives off six pairs of aortic arches (Fig. 9.3). These curve around the pharynx to join to dorsal aortae which join together lower down as the descending aorta. These aortic arches are equivalent to those supplying the gill clefts of a fish. The first and second aortic arches disappear early, the third remains as the carotid artery, and the fourth becomes the subclavian on the right, and the arch of the aorta on the left, giving off the left subclavian. The fifth artery disappears early and the ventral part of the sixth becomes the right and left pulmonary artery, with the connection to the dorsal aortae disappearing on the right but continuing as the ductus arteriosus on the left connecting with the aortic arch.

In the early fetus the larynx is at the level of the sixth aortic arch, and when the vagus gives off its nerve to it

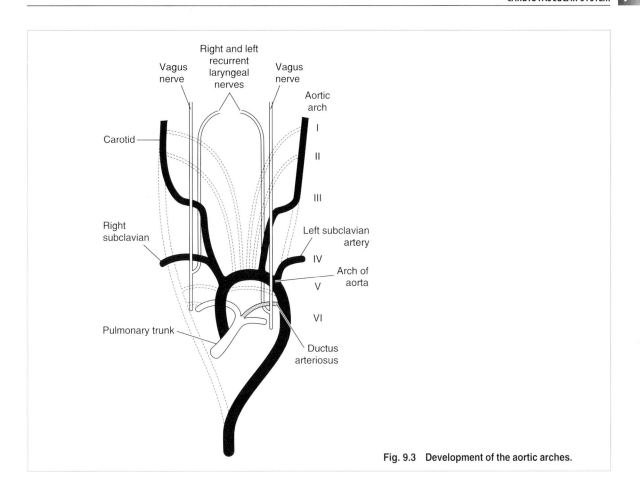

Fig. 9.3   Development of the aortic arches.

this is below the sixth arch. However, as the neck elongates and the heart migrates caudally, the recurrent nerves become dragged down by the aortic arches. On the right the fifth and sixth absorb leaving the nerve to hook round the fourth (subclavian) in the adult, while on the left it remains hooked around the sixth arch (the ligamentum arteriosum) of the adult.

Fetal circulation

Before birth the circulation (Fig. 9.2) obviously differs from that in the adult because oxygen and food must be obtained from maternal blood instead of from the lungs and the digestive organs. Oxygenated blood from the placenta travels along the umbilical vein, where virtually all of it bypasses the liver in the ductus venosus joining the inferior vena cava and then travelling on to the right atrium. Most of the blood then passes straight through the foramen ovale into the left atrium so that oxygenated blood can go into the aorta. The remainder goes through the right ventricle with the returning systemic venous blood

into the pulmonary trunk. In the fetus the unexpanded lungs present a high resistance to pulmonary flow, so that blood in the main pulmonary trunk would tend to pass down the low resistance ductus arteriosus into the aorta. Thus the best-oxygenated blood travels up to the brain, leaving the less well-oxygenated blood to supply the rest of the body. The blood is returned to the placenta via the umbilical arteries, which are branches of the internal iliac artery. At birth when the baby starts to breathe, there is a rise in the left atrial pressure, causing the septum primum to be pushed against the septum secundum and thus to close the foramen ovale. The blood flow through the pulmonary arteries increases and becomes poorly oxygenated, as it is now receiving the systemic venous blood.

The pulmonary vascular resistance is also abruptly lowered as the lungs inflate, and the ductus arteriosus becomes obliterated over the next few hours or days. This occurs by a prostaglandin-dependent mechanism which causes the muscular component of the ductal wall to contract when exposed to higher levels of oxygen at the time of birth. Closure of the ductus arteriosus is less likely to occur in very premature babies or those with perinatal asphyxia. Ligation of the umbilical cord causes thrombosis and obliteration of the umbilical arteries, vein and ductus venosus.

Congenital abnormalities of the heart and great vessels

Given the complex nature of the development of the heart, it is hardly surprising that there are a number of congenital abnormalities, which may be classified as follows.

Malposition

This includes dextrocardia, which is a mirror image of the normal anatomy, or situs inversus, where there is inversion of all the viscera. (Appendicitis may present as left iliac fossa pain in this condition.) These are very rare in normal life, but slightly more common in exams! In pure dextrocardia there is no intracardiac shunting and cardiac function is normal.

Left to right shunts (late cyanosis)

Atrial septal defect (ASD)   This may be from the ostium primum, secundum or sinus venosus and represents failure in the primary or secondary septa. Clinically important septal defects with intracardiac shunting should be differentiated from a persistent patent foramen ovale, where a probe may be passed obliquely through the septum, but flow of blood does not occur after birth, because of the higher pressure in the left atrium. This condition is said to occur in 10% of subjects, but it is not normally of any significance.

Ventricular septal defect (VSD)   This is the most common abnormality. Small defects in the muscular part of the septum may close. Larger ones in the membranous part just below the aortic valves do not close spontaneously and may require repair.

Patent ductus arteriosus (PDA)   Occasionally this normal channel in the fetus fails to close after birth and should be corrected surgically because it causes increased load to the left ventricle and pulmonary hypertension, and along with septal defects may later cause reverse flow and, therefore, late cyanosis.

Eisenmenger's syndrome   Pulmonary hypertension may cause reversed flow (right to left shunting). This is due to an increased pulmonary flow resulting from either an ASD, or VSD or PDA. When cyanosis occurs from this mechanism it is known as Eisenmenger's syndrome.

Right to left shunts (cyanotic)

Fallot's tetralogy   The four features of this abnormality are VSD, a stenosed pulmonary outflow tract, a wide aorta which overrides both the right and left ventricles, and right ventricular hypertrophy. Because there is a right to left shunt across the VSD there is usually cyanosis at an early stage, depending mainly on the severity of the pulmonary outflow obstruction.

Obstructive non-cyanotic abnormalities

Coarctation of the aorta   This is a narrowing of the aorta which is normally just distal to the ductus arteriosus and is thought to be an abnormality related to the obliterative process of the ductus. There is hypertension in the upper part of the body, with weak delayed femoral pulses. Extensive collaterals develop to try and bring the blood down to the lower part of the body, resulting in large vessels around the scapula, anastomosing with the intercostal arteries and the internal mammary and inferior epigastric arteries. These enlarged intercostals usually cause notching of the inferior border of the ribs, which is a diagnositic feature seen on chest x-ray.

Abnormalities of the valves   Any of these may be imperfectly formed and tend to cause either stenosis or complete occlusion (atresia). The pulmonary and the aortic valves are more frequently affected than the other two.

Anatomy of the heart

Surfaces and borders

The heart (Fig. 9.4) is a muscular organ which pumps the blood around the arterial system. It consists of four chambers: right and left atria and right and left ventricles. When viewed from the front it has three surfaces and three borders. The anterior surface consists almost entirely of the right atrium and right ventricle with a narrow strip of left ventricle on the left border and the auricle of the left atrium just appearing over the top of this. It lies just behind the sternum and costal cartilages. The posterior surface consists of the left ventricle and left atrium with the four pulmonary veins entering it, and the right edge is visible. The inferior or diaphragmatic surface consists of the right atrium with the inferior vena cava entering it and the lower part of the ventricles.

The three borders are the right, the inferior and the left. The right is made up entirely of the right atrium with the superior and inferior vena cava. This extends from the third to the sixth right costal cartilage approximately 3 cm from the midline. The inferior border consists of the right ventricle and the apex of the left ventricle. It extends from approximately 3 cm to the right of the midline at the level of the sixth costal cartilage to the apex which is in the fifth left interspace in the mid-clavicular line (approximately 6 cm from the midline). The left border extends from the apex up to the second left inter-

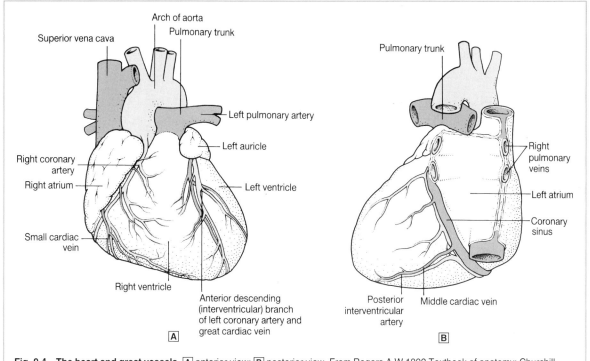

Fig. 9.4 The heart and great vessels. A anterior view; B posterior view. From Rogers A W 1992 Textbook of anatomy; Churchill Livingstone, Edinburgh.

space approximately 3 cm from the midline (Fig. 9.5). The outline of the heart can be seen clearly on a chest x-ray (Fig. 9.6). The apex of the heart is the lowest and most lateral point on the chest wall at which the cardiac impulse can be felt. As the heart is in contact with the diaphragm, it moves with each respiration. However, the anterior fibres of the diaphragm are short, so that the central tendon on which the heart rests moves relatively less.

Chambers of the heart

The heart (Fig. 9.7) consists of a right side which pumps blood through the lungs and the left side which pumps it through the systemic circulation. The atria collect blood from the veins and pump it into the ventricles during ventricular relaxation (diastole). When the ventricles are full they contract (systole), the valves between the atria and ventricles close, and the ventricles discharge their contained blood into the appropriate great vessel.

Right atrium This receives blood from the superior and inferior vena cava and from the coronary sinus. Running down between the venae cavae is a muscular

ridge, the crista terminalis, which separates the smooth walled posterior part of the atrium, which is derived from the sinus venosus, from the rougher area due to the pectinate muscles derived from the true atrium. The interatrial septum has an oval depression (the fossa ovalis) which marks the site of the fetal foramen ovale (Fig. 9.7).

Right ventricle The walls (Fig. 9.7) are much thicker than those of the atrium and there are a series of muscular thickenings, the trabeculae carnae. The tricuspid valve lies between the right atrium and right ventricle, and the three valve cusps are referred to as septal, anterior and posterior. The atrial surfaces are smooth, but the ventricular surfaces have a number of fibrous cords, the chordae tendineae, which attach them to the papillary muscles on the wall of the ventricle. These prevent the valve cusps from being everted into the atrium when the ventricle contracts.

The pulmonary valve lies just above the right ventricle at the beginning of the pulmonary trunk and consists of three semilunar cusps each with a thickening in the centre of its free edge. The pulmonary trunk has a dilatation or sinus alongside each of the cusps.

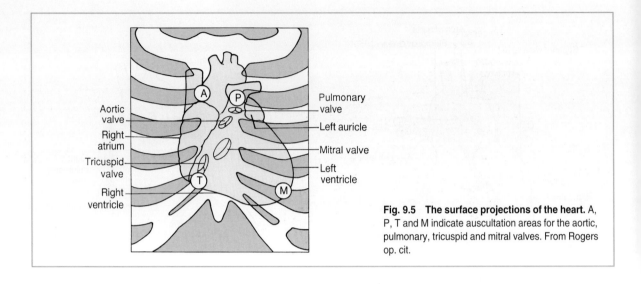

Fig. 9.5 The surface projections of the heart. A, P, T and M indicate auscultation areas for the aortic, pulmonary, tricuspid and mitral valves. From Rogers op. cit.

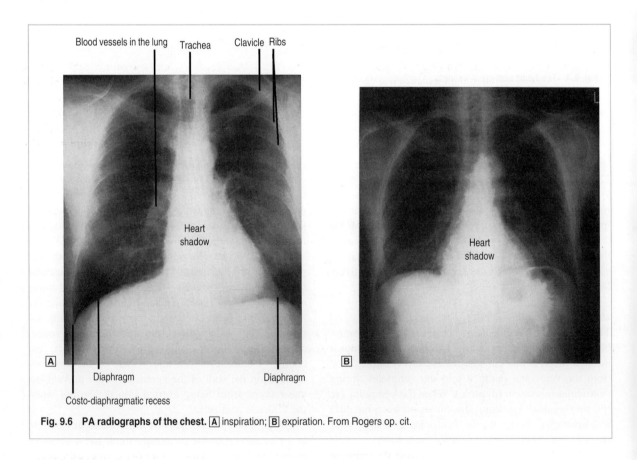

Fig. 9.6 PA radiographs of the chest. A inspiration; B expiration. From Rogers op. cit.

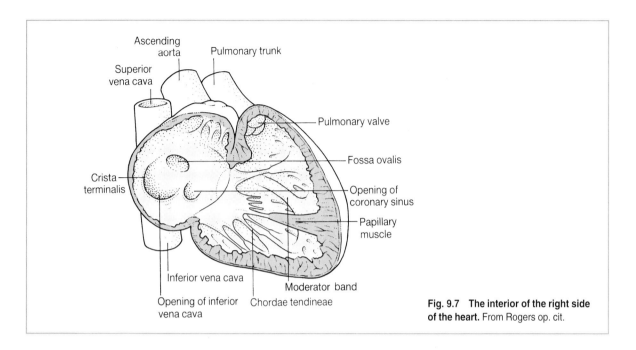

Fig. 9.7 The interior of the right side of the heart. From Rogers op. cit.

Left atrium The left atrium (Fig. 9.8) also develops both from a combination of the fetal atrium and the sinus venosus. There are four pulmonary veins, two from each side. On the interatrial surface there is again an impression representing the site of the fetal interatrial foramen.

Left ventricle The walls of the left ventricle (Fig. 9.8) are three times thicker than those of the right ventricle because the vascular resistance of the systemic circulation is so much greater than that of the pulmonary vasculature. The mitral valve lies between the atrium and ventricle and has two large cusps which were thought by early anatomists to look like a bishop's mitre. Chordae

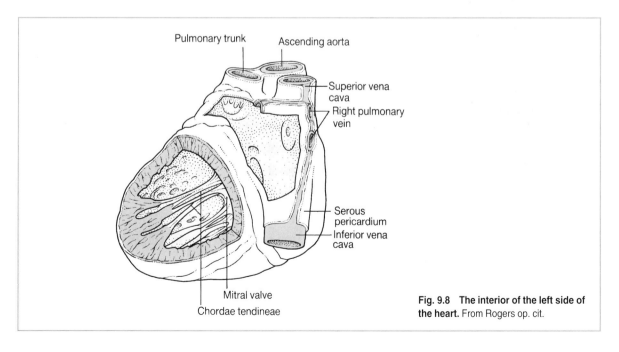

Fig. 9.8 The interior of the left side of the heart. From Rogers op. cit.

tendineae run from the ventricular surfaces and margins of these cusps to papillary muscles in the ventricular wall, as with the right ventricle.

The aortic valve is similar to the pulmonary valve but stronger to cope with the higher pressure. There are three cusps — right, left and posterior — and each also has a central nodule in the free edge and a sinus or dilatation in the aortic wall alongside each cusp. The left and right coronary arteries open from the left and right valves, respectively. In about 1% of the population the aortic valve is bicuspid, and these individuals are more likely to develop calcification and stenosis in later life.

Fibrous skeleton

The two atrioventricular orifices are bound together by a conjoined fibrous ring in the form of a figure of eight which acts as a fibrous skeleton to which the valves are attached and which also serves for attachment of the muscles of both the atria and the ventricles. This provides a tough yet flexible fibrous skeleton which helps to maintain the shape and position of the heart, but allows some change of shape during contraction.

Conducting system

Although cardiac muscle is similar to skeletal muscle in many ways, it does have certain differences. Cardiac muscle cells tend to be shorter and are frequently Y-shaped and are linked at each end to other muscle cells. At the sites of attachment there is an intercalated disc which, as well as anchoring the membranes of the cells, permits the spread of electrical activity. Cardiac muscle

cells are able to contract both spontaneously and rhythmically, and indeed isolated cells in culture contract regularly. As all the cells are in contact with each other and can all contract spontaneously, those with the fastest rate of contraction will drive the others. These are situated in the wall of the right atrium at the upper end of the crista terminalis (Fig. 9.9) and are termed the sinoatrial node (SA node or 'pacemaker of the heart'). From there the cardiac impulse spreads through the atrial muscles to reach the atrioventricular node, which lines the atrial septum close to the opening of the coronary sinus. From there the atrioventricular bundle (of His) passes through a channel in the fibrous skeleton of the heart to the membranous part of the interventricular septum, where it divides into a right and left bundle branch. The left bundle is larger than the right and divides into an anterior and posterior fascicle. These run underneath the endocardium to activate all parts of the ventricular musculature in such a way that the papillary muscles contract first and then the wall and septum in rapid sequence from the apex towards the outflow track, with both ventricles contracting together. The atrioventricular bundle is normally the only pathway through which impulses can reach the ventricles.

Blood supply to the heart

The arterial supply (Fig. 9.4) is of great clinical importance, as coronary occlusion is the chief cause of mortality in the western world. The right and left coronary arteries arise from the anterior and the left aortic sinuses, respec-

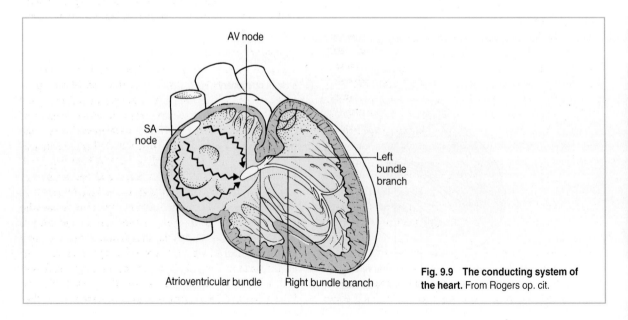

Fig. 9.9 **The conducting system of the heart.** From Rogers op. cit.

tively, just above the aortic valve, and the main branches lie in the interventricular and the atrioventricular grooves.

Right coronary artery   This passes between the pulmonary trunk and the right atrium and runs along the atrioventricular groove around the inferior border to the diaphragmatic surface. It ends by anastomosing with the terminal branch of the left coronary artery. The main branches are an artery to the SA node and adjacent atrium, the right marginal artery and the posterior interventricular which really runs inferiorly and is often called by clinicians the posterior descending artery. This branch also supplies the AV node and bundle, and parts of the right and left bundle branches.

Left coronary artery   Arising from the left aortic sinus the left coronary artery (the left main stem) varies from 4 to 10 mm in length and is the most important artery in the human body, in that occlusion will invariably lead to rapid demise! If stenosis of this artery is diagnosed, urgent operation is required to bypass it. It continues passing to the left behind the pulmonary trunk, reaching the atrioventricular groove. It is initially under cover of the left auricle, where it divides into two branches of equal size: the anterior interventricular (left anterior descending) and the circumflex artery. The circumflex artery continues around the left surface of the heart in the atrioventricular groove to anastomose with the terminal branches of the right coronary artery. The left anterior descending (also known as 'the widow maker'!) runs down to the apex of the heart in the anterior interventricular groove, supplying the walls of the ventricles down the interventricular septum. It gives off the diagonal branch and goes on to anastomose with the posterior interventricular artery.

There are some reasonably common variations. Firstly, the left coronary and circumflex artery may be larger and longer than usual and give off the posterior interventricular artery before anastomosing with the right coronary, which is smaller than usual. This occurs in approximately 10% of the population and is known as 'left dominance'. Another 10% have 'codominant' coronary circulation with equal contribution to the posterior interventricular branch. In approximately one third of individuals the left main stem may divide into three rather than two branches. The third branch, the intermediate, lies between the left anterior descending and the circumflex and may be of large calibre and supply the lateral wall of the left ventricle.

The blood supply to the conducting system is of clinical importance. In just under 60% of the population the SA node is supplied by the right coronary artery, while in just under 40% it is supplied by the circumflex (dual supply in 3%). The AV node is supplied by the right coronary artery in 90% and circumflex in 10%.

Venous drainage

There are three groups of veins of the heart (Fig. 9.4):

1. some tiny veins that drain directly into the chambers of the heart (venae cordis minimae)
2. the anterior cardiac veins, which are small and open directly into the right atrium
3. the coronary sinus, which is the main venous drainage; it lies in the posterior atrioventricular groove and opens into the right atrium just to the left of the mouth of the IVC. It has three main tributaries:
   - the great cardiac vein, which ascends in the anterior interventricular groove next to the left anterior descending artery
   - the middle cardiac vein, which drains the posterior and inferior surface and lies next to the posterior interventricular artery
   - the small cardiac vein, which accompanies the right marginal artery and drains into the termination of the coronary sinus.

Nerve supply to the heart

The sympathetic supply (cardio-accelerator) is from the upper thoracic segment of the spinal cord through the sympathetic trunk, and the parasympathetic supply is from the vagus (cardio-inhibitor), and the fibres of each go via the superficial and deep cardiac plexuses.

Pain fibres pass through sympathetic ganglia to spinal nerves via the white rami communicantes. The close proximity with the cervical and thoracic spinal nerves may explain the site of referred cardiac pain to the chest, neck and arm.

Pericardium

Fibrous pericardium   The heart and the roots of the great vessels are contained within the fibrous pericardium. It is fused with the adventitia of the great vessels. You will remember from the development of the heart that the pericardium surrounded the original primitive heart tube, which subsequently had two arteries and two veins at each end and then, as the heart enlarged, folded upon itself so that the arteries and the veins were close to each other. This still applies, and the two arteries become the aorta and the pulmonary trunk while the veins to the right atrium become the superior and inferior vena cava and to the left the four pulmonary veins, and these latter two structures become incorporated into their respective atria. Thus, the superior and inferior venae cavae and the four pulmonary veins are all invested with the same layer of fibrous pericardium, while there is another layer investing the aorta and the pulmonary trunk, and the gap between the two becomes the transverse sinus while the blind end coming up between the four pulmonary veins and the inferior vena cava becomes the oblique sinus.

The fibrous pericardium can stretch very gradually if there is a gradual enlargement of the heart, but if there was a sudden increase in the volume of its contents, such as from bleeding, then it cannot stretch and will embarrass the function of the heart (cardiac tamponade).

Serous pericardium This covers the heart and the origin of the great vessels and fuses with the fibrous pericardium at the sites around the great vessels just described. This is a very small space between the two layers, which normally has a small amount of fluid allowing lubrication for movement of the heart within the pericardium.

Clinical features

Cardiac arrest
Because the bulk of the heart and especially the ventricles is just behind the sternum, regular compression there can be used for external cardiac massage in cardiac arrest until more definitive treatment can be given.

Cardiac tamponade
A chronic pericardial effusion may be drained by inserting a needle just to the left of the xiphisternum, pointing upwards at an angle of about 45° and slightly laterally towards the tip of the left scapula. This is done under both ECG and image intensifier control. In an acute cardiac tamponade where there is not time to get imaging it is safer to make an incision just to the left of the xiphisternum and deepen the wound in the same direction as previously described, but using a combination of forcep and finger dissection. If the diagnosis is correct, a bulging pericardium will be felt; if it is not, no harm has been done.

Cardiac surgery
Thoracotomy The most common approach to the heart for cardiac surgery is the median sternotomy in which the sternum is split in the midline, the diaphragm detached and tissues behind dissected away carefully avoiding damaging the pleura, particularly on the right, as it may cross the midline a little. Other methods are lateral thoracotomy in which the approach is through the upper border of the chosen rib, trimming the periosteum off and thus avoiding damage to the intercostal nerve and vessels which run in a groove just below the rib.

Cardiopulmonary bypass The superior and inferior venae cavae are cannulated through the wall of the right atrium to take blood to the bypass machine which will oxygenate the blood, and this will then be brought back through a cannula in the aortic arch, usually proximal to the brachiocephalic trunk.

Coronary artery bypass grafts Traditionally the great saphenous vein has been used to anastomose from the ascending aorta to the relevant coronary vessel distal to the block. Alternatively the internal thoracic artery may be anastomosed directly to the relevant coronary artery.

Septal defects The atrium is approached through its right border, thus avoiding the SA node, whereas the right ventricle can be incised vertically or transversely, avoiding any obvious arteries or veins. The left atrium can be incised behind the interatrial groove and in front of the two pulmonary veins in order to approach the mitral valve.

Transplantation The patient's heart is removed, incising through the right atrium, leaving the two venae cavae, the posterior wall of the atrium and the region of the SA node intact. The posterior part of the left atrium with the four pulmonary veins is also left in situ. The incision continues through the aorta and pulmonary trunk, and the donor heart is trimmed in a similar way and anastomosed along this line described.

AORTA AND GREAT VESSELS

Introduction
The aorta can be divided into four parts:

- the ascending aorta
- the arch of the aorta
- the descending aorta
- the abdominal aorta.

Just above the aortic valve the diameter measures approximately 3 cm, but it gradually tapers as it gives off its branches, so that at the bifurcation of the aorta into common iliacs the diameter is less than 2 cm.

Ascending aorta
This measures approximately 5 cm, and the whole of it is within the fibrous pericardium along with the pulmonary trunk. It starts at the aortic valve and goes up and slightly to the right, ending to the right of the sternum at the level of the second right costal cartilage.

Branches
The left and right coronary arteries are the only branches; these have already been described on pages 212 and 213.

Relations
See Figure 9.4.

- Anteriorly lies the infundibulum of the right ventricle and the pulmonary trunk.
- Posteriorly lies the left atrium and the left main bronchus.
- To the right is the right atrium.
- To the left is the left atrium and pulmonary trunk.

The arch of the aorta

This is a continuation of the ascending aorta and travels first superiorly and to the left, and slightly posteriorly, crossing the anterior surface of the trachea and posteriorly over the root of the left lung, and finishing just to the left of the fourth thoracic vertebra where it becomes the descending aorta (Fig. 9.10). Its apex reaches the mid-point of the manubrium sterni.

Branches

There are three major branches:

- the brachiocephalic artery (which becomes the right common carotid and subclavian artery)
- the left common carotid artery
- the left subclavian artery.

Relations

On the left anterior surface the aortic arch is crossed by:

- the left phrenic nerve, which descends on the left surface of the pericardium just anterior to the root of the lung down to the diaphragm
- the left vagus nerve, which crosses the arch at the origin of the left subclavian, descending posteriorly to the root of the lung and giving off the left recurrent

laryngeal nerve just lateral to the ligamentum arteriosum.

Descending thoracic aorta

This is the continuation of the arch and starts opposite the lower border of the 4th thoracic vertebra and slightly to the left of it. It ends in the midline at the lower border of the 12th thoracic vertebra, where it passes behind the median arcuate ligament of the diaphragm.

Branches

These can be classified into three groups.

Lateral segmental branches   These are the posterior intercostal arteries that supply the lower nine of the eleven intercostal spaces. Each artery gives off a dorsal and a lateral cutaneous branch. The dorsal branch gives off a spinal branch to supply the spinal cord. The blood supply to the cord consists of the anterior and posterior spinal arteries, which descend in the pia from the intra-cranial part of the vertebral artery. They are reinforced by segmental arteries, and in the thoracic region these are the dorsal branches of the 2nd to 11th posterior inter-costal arteries. These supply the radicular arteries to the spine, which are a very important contribution to rein-force the longitudinal vessels. As a consequence they are known as 'booster' or 'feeder' vessels. These are very variable in size and position. The largest one is known as the arteria radicularis magna (or artery of Adamkiewicz), which most commonly arises at the 10th or 11th thoracic level but may arise anywhere upto the 4th thoracic level. Operations on the thoracic spine or thoracic aneurysms

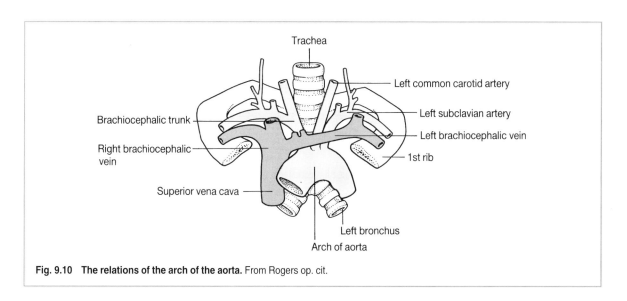

Fig. 9.10   The relations of the arch of the aorta. From Rogers op. cit.

may interfere with the parent stems of these radicular vessels, which may result in damage to the spinal cord, causing paraplegia.

Lateral visceral (bronchial)   These supply the bronchial walls and substance of the lung excluding the alveoli.

Midline branches   There are four or five oesophageal branches.

Relations

Anteriorly are the root of the lung, the pericardium of the left atrium, and below that the posterior fibres of the diaphragm. Anteriorly and to the right lie the oesophagus and trachea; lower down the oesophagus becomes anterior and then moves to its left as it descends. Posteriorly are the vertebral column and hemiazygos veins, to the right are the azygos veins and thoracic duct and pleura and lung, and on the left the pleura and lung.

Abdominal aorta

The abdominal aorta (Fig. 9.11) commences at the aortic opening of the diaphragm at the level of the 12th thoracic vertebra, descending to the 4th lumbar vertebra where it divides into the two common iliacs. It tapers as it gives off a number of large branches.

Branches

Posterior lateral branches to the body wall   There are five paired branches: the inferior phrenic artery and four lumbar arteries.

Paired to viscera   There are three paired visceral arteries: the suprarenal, the renal arteries and the testicular or ovarian arteries.

Midline unpaired branches to the viscera   There are three such branches, as follows.

- *The coeliac trunk* supplies the foregut and its derivatives which are the stomach, duodenum, liver, gallbladder and part of the pancreas. The coeliac trunk arises from the aorta, immediately below the aortic opening in the diaphragm.
- *Superior mesenteric artery* supplies the midgut, i.e. from the middle of the second part of the duodenum to the commencement of the left third of the transverse

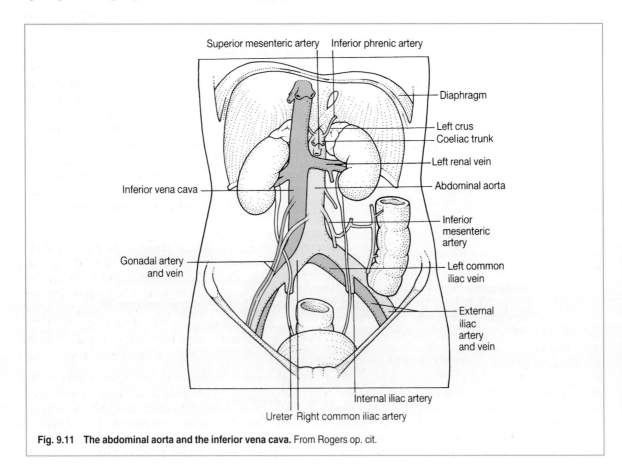

Fig. 9.11   The abdominal aorta and the inferior vena cava. From Rogers op. cit.

colon, and it arises a centimetre below the coeliac trunk.

- *Inferior mesenteric artery* supplies the hindgut from the left third of the transverse colon down to the rectum, where it terminates as the superior haemorrhoidal arteries. It arises from the lower third of the abdominal aorta, and is a much smaller artery than the coeliac and the superior mesenteric. It anastomoses with the superior mesenteric via the marginal artery (see Ch. 17).

Terminal branches   These are two common iliacs and the median sacral.

Relations

To the right from above downwards are the right crus of the diaphragm, the cisterna chyli and the commencement of the azygos vein. From the level of the superior mesenteric artery downwards, the inferior vena cava is closely applied to the right side of the aorta, although it gradually becomes more posterior at the lower end so that the iliac veins lie behind the iliac arteries.

To the left is the left crus of the diaphragm, the fourth part of the duodenum, the duodeno-jejunal flexure and the left sympathetic trunk.

Posteriorly are the upper four lumbar vertebrae.

Anteriorly at the level of the coeliac trunk, the lesser sac of peritoneum separates the aorta from the lesser omentum and liver. Below that, the left renal vein crosses the abdominal aorta immediately below the origin of the superior mesenteric artery. This is at the level of the neck of the vast majority of abdominal aortic aneurysms. It is usually possible to get a clamp on just below the renal vein, but occasionally the aneurysm extends high up, stretching the renal vein like a ribbon across it. Because the left renal vein has tributaries from the left adrenal and from the left ovarian or testicular, the left renal vein can be divided providing it is sufficiently far to the right not to impair the entrance of these vessels, which can then act as venous collaterals. The inferior mesenteric vein also runs quite close to the aorta at this level. In an elective aneurysm this is not a problem, but when there is a large haematoma following a leak, it is possible to damage it if one is not aware of its presence. Also the third part of the duodenum may be adherent to an aneurysm, which may be a particular problem if it is an inflammatory aneurysm. When the anastomosis between a graft and aorta has been done, it is important to have some tissue between it and the duodenum (usually the wall of the aneurysm sac is used). If this is not done there is a small risk of a fistula developing between the anastomosis and the duodenum (aortoduodenal fistula) which is an uncommon but serious cause of haematemesis and melaena. The pancreas lies anterior to the aorta with the third part of the duodenum below. Below this lie the parietal peritoneum and peritoneal cavity with the line of attachment of the mesentery to the small bowel.

It should be noted that in a slim person the aorta and inferior vena cava are remarkably close to the anterior abdominal wall. The lumbar vertebrae have a large body, spinal canal and spinous process. These vessels are thus at risk, for example, when inserting a needle to obtain a pneumoperitoneum. It is also worth noting that the bifurcation of the aorta is approximately at the level of the umbilicus, so that aneurysms of the abdominal aorta are normally above this level (although they may of course involve the common iliacs).

Other great vessels of the thorax

These are systemic arteries, namely the brachiocephalic, left common carotid and left subclavian artery, and veins: right and left brachiocephalic vein and the superior vena cava. In addition there are the pulmonary trunk, right and left pulmonary arteries and the four pulmonary veins which are the great vessels of the pulmonary circulation (see Ch. 11).

The brachiocephalic artery

This is the first and largest of the three great arteries arising from the aortic arch. It originates from the apex of the arch in the midline, travelling superiorly and posteriorly to the right, and it terminates behind the right sternoclavicular joint by dividing into the right subclavian and right common carotid artery.

There are normally no branches, though occasionally the thyroidea ima artery may arise from it, supplying the lower part of the thyroid. It lies behind the left brachiocephalic vein and in front of the trachea.

Right subclavian artery

This arises from the bifurcation of the brachiocephalic artery and courses to the outer border of the first rib where it becomes the axillary artery (Fig. 9.12). It arches laterally over the apex of the lung to reach the superior surface of the first rib, where it lies in a groove just behind the insertion of the scalenus anterior. It is divided into three parts by the scalenus anterior muscle. The first part is medial to it and gives off three branches.

- The vertebral artery is the most important branch of the subclavian. It crosses the dome of the cervical pleura and passes through the transverse foramina of the upper six cervical vertebrae. It then turns posteromedially over the posterior arch of the atlas through the foramen magnum, where it joins its fellow from the other side

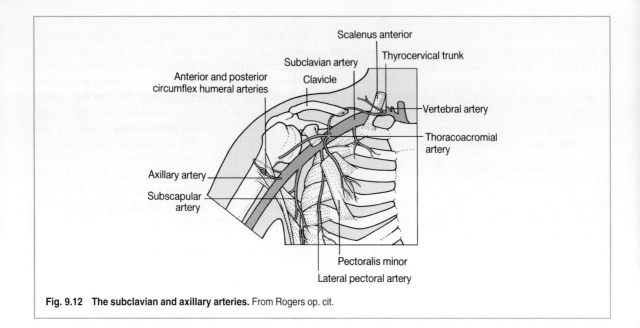

Fig. 9.12 The subclavian and axillary arteries. From Rogers op. cit.

in front of the pons to form the basilar artery. The vertebral artery gives off the anterior and posterior spinal arteries and the posterior inferior cerebellar arteries.

- The thyrocervical trunk gives off the inferior thyroid artery, the transverse cervical and suprascapular arteries.
- The internal thoracic artery (formerly known as internal mammary, Fig. 9.13) runs anteriorly and downwards over the pleura to reach the anterior ends of the intercostal spaces, giving off anterior intercostal branches, a musculophrenic artery, and finishing as the superior epigastric artery. Thus it supplies the whole of the anterior body wall down to the umbilicus. This artery is clinically important, because it can be used for coronary artery bypass grafts by mobilising it and anastomosing it directly to the coronary arteries beyond a stenosis or block. It may also be damaged in stab wounds of the chest.

The second part of the subclavian artery lies deep to the scalenus anterior muscle. This gives off the costocervical trunk which supplies the deep structures of the neck, and also the superior intercostal artery which gives off the first and second posterior intercostal arteries.

The third part is lateral to the scalenus anterior and normally has no branches.

Relations It is closely related to the pleura at the apex of the lung, being separated from the lung by the suprapleural membrane. The right vagus crosses the anterior surface of the artery at its medial end and gives off the recurrent laryngeal nerve which loops under the artery, travelling posteromedially, and then back up to the larynx between the oesophagus and trachea initially, and closely behind the thyroid higher up. The cervical sympathetic chain also divides into two branches which loop around the anterior and posterior surface of the artery, reuniting on the other side.

Behind the scalenus anterior muscle, the artery is closely related to the lower trunk of the brachial plexus posteriorly, and the upper and middle trunks are superior to it. The phrenic nerve runs down in front of the scalenus anterior, crossing it from lateral to medial. In surgical exploration of the subclavian artery, the scalenus anterior is divided to expose the artery, the phrenic nerve initially being retracted medially.

Cervical rib A cervical rib is a common abnormality occurring in approximately 1 in 200 of the population, and in half of these it is bilateral. However, they only rarely cause symptoms. These may be neurological, arising from pressure on the lowest trunk of the brachial plexus, resulting in paraesthesia along the ulnar border of the forearm and wasting of the small muscles of the hand (T1). This tends to occur with smaller cervical ribs and fibrous bands. When there is a large cervical rib with a bulbous end, this may cause pressure on the subclavian artery. This may result in poststenotic dilatation. The dilated part may develop thrombi in the wall and these may break off and occlude the distal vessels of the arm and hand, sometimes with very serious consequences.

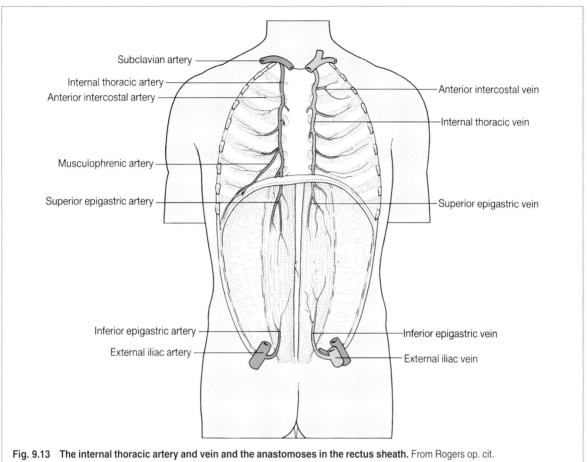

Fig. 9.13 **The internal thoracic artery and vein and the anastomoses in the rectus sheath.** From Rogers op. cit.

Left common carotid artery

The left common carotid artery is the second branch of the aortic arch arising slightly to the left of the midline. The trachea lies posteriorly, and the artery ascends to the thoracic inlet, passing behind and slightly to the left of the sternoclavicular joint, from where it continues up into the neck. There are no branches in its thoracic course.

Left subclavian artery

This is the third and most posterior branch of the arch of the aorta. It ascends posterior and to the left of the common carotid artery to the thoracic inlet, where it arches over with similar course and relations to those of the right subclavian artery, which have previously been described. There are no branches in the thoracic part of the left subclavian.

The great systemic veins of the thorax

The superior vena cava which carries blood into the right atrium is formed from the union of the right and left brachiocephalic veins (Fig. 9.10). These receive blood from the head and neck and upper limbs as well as from the upper half of the body wall of the trunk.

Right brachiocephalic vein

This is a short wide vein formed by the union of the right subclavian and the right internal jugular veins. This junction is just behind the medial end of the right clavicle. The vein runs down and joins the left brachiocephalic to become the superior vena cava behind the medial end of the right first costal cartilage.

Tributaries It receives three tributaries:

• the right vertebral vein
• the right internal thoracic vein
• the inferior thyroid veins.

Relations The vein lies anterior and to the right of the equivalent artery and to the right of the vagus nerve.

Left brachiocephalic vein

The vein starts behind the medial end of the left clavicle by the union of the left subclavian and internal jugular veins. It runs obliquely downwards and to the right to join the right brachiocephalic behind the first right costal cartilage. Thus the left brachiocephalic vein is considerably longer than the right.

Tributaries   These are the same as for those on the right but in addition the superior intercostal veins drain into it.

Relations   At its origin it lies anterior to the cervical pleura. As it passes to the right it lies anterior to the left internal thoracic artery, the left phrenic nerve, the left subclavian artery, the left vagus nerve and the left common carotid artery and then the trachea and the brachiocephalic artery. The manubrium sterni and the remnant of the thymus gland lie anteriorly, with the aortic arch inferiorly.

Superior vena cava (SVC)

This starts behind the first right costal cartilage by the union of the two brachiocephalic veins. It passes inferiorly to enter the right atrium behind the third right costal cartilage. It is important to be aware of these landmarks when inserting a central venous pressure line since the end should lie in the SVC, and this should be checked on x-ray. The lower part of the SVC is within the fibrous pericardium. It receives one other major tributary, which is the azygos vein, into which most of the venous drainage from the thoracic and abdominal walls drains (Fig. 9.14).

Relations   Anteriorly are the right lung and pleura, the right internal thoracic artery and the medial ends of the upper two intercostal spaces. Posteriorly are the trachea, the right vagus and lung and pleura lateral in the upper part. Laterally are the right phrenic nerve and right pleura and lung, and medially is the ascending aorta.

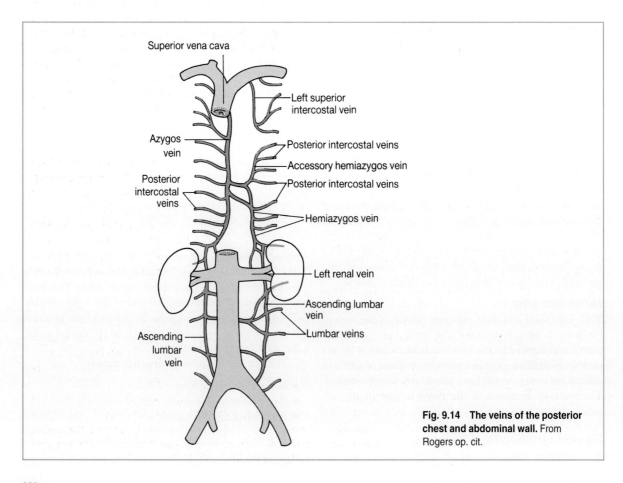

Fig. 9.14   The veins of the posterior chest and abdominal wall. From Rogers op. cit.

BLOOD SUPPLY TO THE TRUNK

Arterial supply to the body wall

This comes from three sources: firstly the intersegmental branches from the aorta, secondly the branches from the subclavian and axillary arteries, and thirdly the branches from the external iliac artery.

Segmental branches from the aorta

The segmental branches from the aorta which supply the body wall are:

- the posterior intercostal arteries, which have been described earlier
- the subcostal artery, the next vessel below the intercostal, and supplies the abdominal wall in the same manner
- lumbar arteries which continue in series with the posterior intercostal and subcostal arteries, and in the same way have a dorsal and ventral branch with the former giving a branch to the spinal cord
- the median sacral artery which is given off in the midline just above the bifurcation of the aorta and descends down in front of the sacrum.

Branches from the subclavian and axillary arteries

The internal thoracic artery has already been described and is shown in Figure 9.13.

Branches of the external iliac artery

These are:

- the inferior epigastric artery, which arises from the external iliac just above the inguinal ligament, and medial to the deep inguinal ring enters the rectus sheath to supply the rectus abdominis muscle and to anastomose with the superior epigastric artery.
- the deep circumflex iliac artery.

The superior and inferior epigastric vessels have a good anastomosis. They can each be used as the basis for plastic procedures. The so-called TRAM flap (Transverse Rectus Abdominus Myocutaneous flap) is sometimes used for breast reconstruction following mastectomy. A flap of upper rectus abdominis muscle and a transverse elliptical piece of skin attached to it are swung up to fill the defect in the breast region, being kept alive by blood from the internal thoracic artery and vein. Similarly the inferior epigastric artery and vein are such good vessels that a 'free flap' of the lower part of the rectus abdominus muscle and the overlying skin can be excised and moved to another part of the body, providing there is a suitable artery and vein to which they can be anastomosed using microvascular techniques.

Venous drainage of the body wall

This consists of the following.

Intersegmental veins

These are equivalent to the arteries described.

Azygos veins

These are three longitudinal veins lying on the bodies of the thoracic vertebrae (Fig. 9.14). There is a single azygos vein on the right, while on the left there are the hemiazygos and the accessory hemiazygos.

Vertebral venous plexus

This lies in the external surface of the vertebrae and is also known as Batson's plexus.

Veins in the anterior chest abdominal wall

These are equivalent to the arterial supply.

Iliac arteries

See Figure 9.11.

Common iliac artery

The aorta divides into the common iliac arteries to the left of the midline, at the level of the body of the 4th lumbar vertebra. They pass downwards and laterally to bifurcate into internal and external iliac in front of the sacroiliac joint at the level of the sacral promontory. The ureter passes just in front of the common iliac artery at its bifurcation. This is an easy site at which to identify the ureter at operation. There are normally no branches of the common iliac artery.

External iliac artery

This is a continuation of the common iliac artery which has travelled downward and laterally to reach the mid-inguinal point, where it passes deep to the inguinal ligament to enter the thigh as the femoral artery.

The branches are the inferior epigastric and the deep circumflex iliac artery. Remember it is the inferior epigastric which runs medial to the deep inguinal ring, so that a hernia lateral to it is an indirect hernia, whereas one medial to it is a direct hernia.

Internal iliac artery

This runs inferiorly to end opposite the upper margin of the greater sciatic notch by dividing into an anterior and posterior trunk. These supply the pelvic organs, perineum, buttock and anal canal. The internal iliac vein lies posteriorly and the ureter anteriorly.

In the fetus the internal iliac arteries are large, and each anterior trunk gives off an umbilical artery. These fibrose shortly after birth and subsequently become the medial umbilical ligaments, which are fibrous cords running up to the umbilicus.

Iliac veins

The external iliac veins (Fig. 9.11) run at first medially and, as they ascend and become common iliac veins, they run posterior to the iliac arteries. They join at the level of the fifth lumbar vertebra behind the right common iliac artery. Thus the left iliac vein is longer than the right. The tributaries of the internal and external iliac veins are equivalent to those of the arteries. The common iliac veins lie behind and slightly to the right of the common iliac arteries, to which they are very closely related. In aortoiliac operations, when the iliac arteries need to be clamped, great care is needed in dissecting to avoid damage to the iliac veins.

Inferior vena cava

From its origin at the level of the 5th lumbar vertebra to the right of the midline and behind the right common iliac artery, the IVC ascends vertically through the abdomen, piercing the central tendon of the diaphragm to the right of the midline to empty into the right atrium (Fig. 9.11). It is larger than the aorta, and as it ascends, is related anteriorly to the small intestine, the third part of the duodenum, the head of the pancreas with the common bile duct and then the first part of the duodenum. It lies in a deep groove in the liver before piercing the diaphragm. It receives the right and left hepatic veins from the liver. Sometimes these fuse to give one trunk going into the vena cava, but occasionally the central hepatic vein opens separately. In partial liver resections or in operations for transplantation, it is obviously important to know the precise anatomy prior to surgery. See Chapter 17.

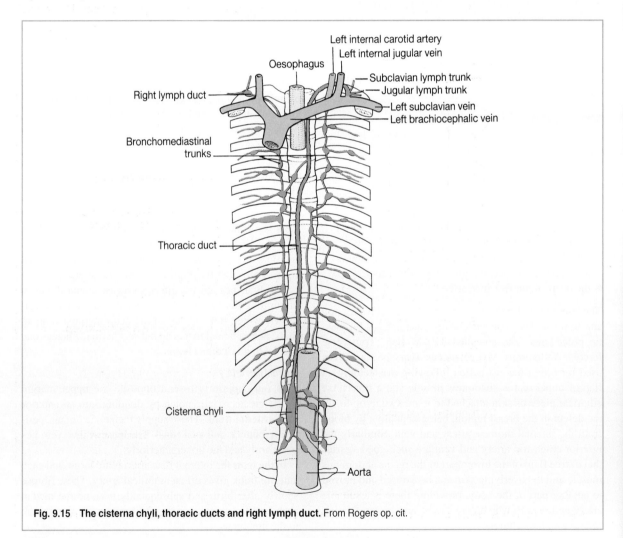

Fig. 9.15 **The cisterna chyli, thoracic ducts and right lymph duct.** From Rogers op. cit.

Lymphatics

The lymphatics (Fig. 9.15) from the abdomen and lower limbs drain into the cisterna chyli, which lies between the abdominal aorta and the right crus of the diaphragm. It passes through the aortic opening to become the thoracic duct, ascending behind the oesophagus. At the level of T5 it inclines to the left of the oesophagus and runs upwards behind the left carotid sheath. It then passes around and over the left subclavian artery and drains into the commencement of the brachiocephalic vein. The left jugular, subclavian and mediastinal lymph trunks, draining the head and neck, the left upper limb and the thorax, respectively, usually join the thoracic duct shortly before it enters the brachiocephalic vein, although they may open directly into it. The equivalent lymph vessels on the right join to become the right lymphatic duct which enters the origin of the right brachiocephalic vein.

It is important to be aware of the thoracic duct in operations on the neck in this area, particularly block dissection of the neck. If the thoracic duct is damaged and not ligated, then a troublesome chylous lymphatic leak will result. Damage to the thoracic duct in the thorax may occasionally occur from fractures of the thoracic spine, or at surgery, and may result in a chylothorax.

Blood supply of the head and neck

The brachiocephalic artery and the left common carotid artery in the chest have already been described (pp. 217–219). Each common carotid artery enters the neck (Fig. 9.16), from behind the sternoclavicular joint, and thereafter on both sides they have a similar course and relationships. They ascend in the carotid fascial sheath with the internal jugular vein lying laterally and the vagus nerve between and somewhat behind them. The cervical

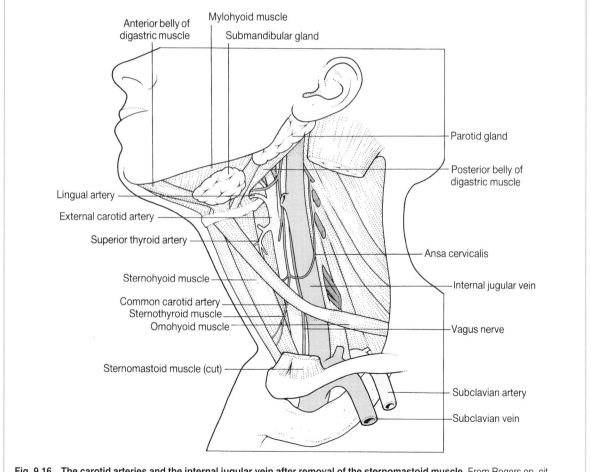

Fig. 9.16   The carotid arteries and the internal jugular vein after removal of the sternomastoid muscle. From Rogers op. cit.

sympathetic chain ascends immediately posterior to the carotid sheath, while the sternocleidomastoid muscle is superficial to it. The carotid sheath is crossed superficially by the omohyoid muscle. At the level of the upper border of the thyroid cartilage the common carotid artery bifurcates into the internal and external carotid artery. There are no other branches of the common carotid.

Internal carotid artery

This commences at the bifurcation of the common carotid artery, and at its origin is dilated into the carotid sinus which acts as a baroreceptor. In the bifurcation is the carotid body, a chemoreceptor. Both are supplied by the ninth cranial nerve. At first the internal carotid lies lateral and slightly more superficial to the external, but it rapidly passes medial and posterior to it, as it ascends to the base of the skull between the side wall of the pharynx and the internal jugular vein. The upper part of the internal carotid artery and the internal jugular vein are closely related to the last four cranial nerves (Fig. 9.17). The internal carotid is separated from the external in the upper part by the styloid process, the stylopharyngeus muscle, and the glossopharyngeal nerve and pharyngeal branch of the vagus.

At the base of the skull the internal carotid enters the petrous temporal bone in the carotid canal, and subsequently gives off the ophthalmic artery, the anterior and middle cerebral arteries and the posterior communicating artery. There are no branches of the internal carotid in the neck.

It should be noted that atheromatous emboli may arise from stenoses at the origin of the internal carotid. When they do so, they may cause transient attacks of blindness (amaurosis fugax) on the same side if emboli travel to the ophthalmic artery. However, if they go to the cerebral cortex, they will cause transient ischaemic attacks (sensory or motor) on the opposite side of the body due to the decussation of the nerve pathways.

External carotid artery

The external carotid (Fig. 9.18) extends from the upper border of the thyroid cartilage to a point midway between

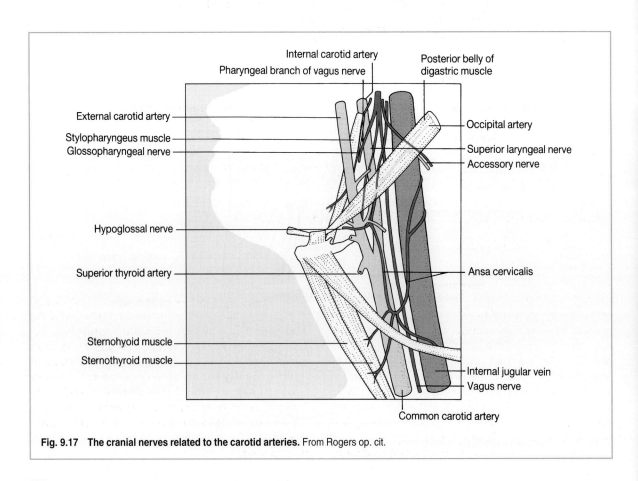

Fig. 9.17   The cranial nerves related to the carotid arteries. From Rogers op. cit.

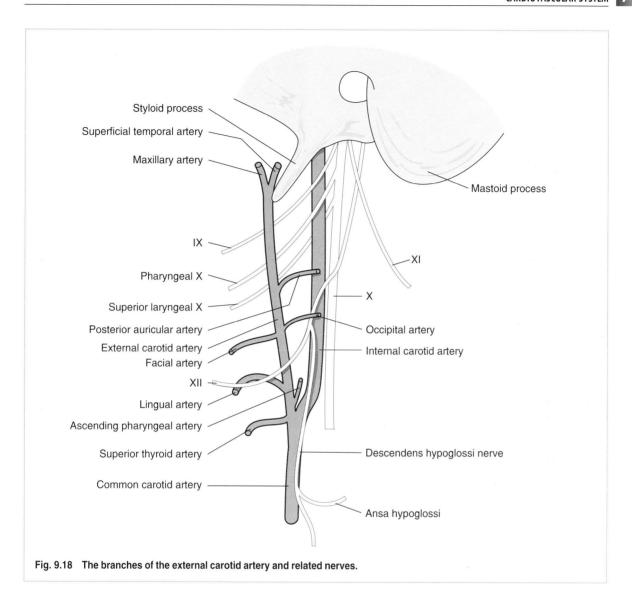

Fig. 9.18 The branches of the external carotid artery and related nerves.

Labels: Styloid process, Superficial temporal artery, Maxillary artery, Mastoid process, IX, XI, Pharyngeal X, X, Superior laryngeal X, Posterior auricular artery, Occipital artery, External carotid artery, Internal carotid artery, Facial artery, XII, Lingual artery, Ascending pharyngeal artery, Superior thyroid artery, Descendens hypoglossi nerve, Common carotid artery, Ansa hypoglossi

the angle of the mandible and the mastoid process. At its origin it is anteromedial to the internal carotid but, as it ascends, it becomes more superficial. Almost immediately it gives off two branches: the ascending pharyngeal and the superior thyroid. Shortly above, it gives off the lingual artery, and then the facial and occipital artery, with the hypoglossal nerve crossing the external carotid just beneath the occipital branch. It then gives off the posterior auricular artery and terminates by dividing into the maxillary and superficial temporal artery.

The common carotid artery is sometimes ligated for an intracranial aneurysm arising from the internal carotid. The external carotid artery is occasionally ligated for severe bleeding from the nose or the tonsillar bed. The level of the bifurcation of the carotid does vary, and at its lowest end the internal carotid is more accessible than the external, although within a centimetre or so the external becomes more superficial. The external carotid is the only one of the three that has any branches in the neck. To be sure of ligating the correct vessel the external carotid should be identified by finding the lowest one or two branches.

225

Venous drainage

External jugular vein

Superficial drainage of the head and neck is via the external jugular vein, which is formed from the junction of the superficial temporal and maxillary vein and posterior auricular vein. It runs obliquely downwards and backwards superficially over the sternomastoid muscle, piercing the deep cervical fascia 2.5 cm above the clavicle to enter the subclavian vein.

Internal jugular vein

This is formed at the jugular foramen and is a continuation of the sigmoid sinus. It lies behind the internal carotid artery but, as it descends, it become lateral to the lower part of the internal and to the common carotid artery, with the vagus nerve lying between the vein and the artery. It receives some pharyngeal veins, the common facial vein, the superior and middle thyroid veins, and the lingual vein. It then joins the subclavian vein to become the brachiocephalic vein; the left and right brachiocephalic veins then merge to form the superior vena cava. The deep cervical chain of lymph nodes is closely applied to the internal jugular vein.

In the operation of carotid endarterectomy, the sternomastoid muscle is dissected and retracted backwards, and the common facial vein is then doubly ligated and divided. When this has been done and the internal jugular is also dissected backwards, the common and internal carotid arteries are exposed.

The lymphatics of the head and neck are described in Chapter 13.

BLOOD SUPPLY OF THE UPPER LIMB (Fig. 9.19)

Axillary artery

The axillary artery is the continuation of the subclavian artery, extending from the outer border of the first rib to the lower border of teres major. It is divided into three parts by the pectoralis minor muscle. It is enclosed in the axillary sheath along with the axillary vein and the components of the brachial plexus. The vein lies medial to the artery, and the cords of the brachial plexus are arranged around the artery. The pectoralis major covers it apart from its distal end. It conveniently has one branch on the first part, two from the second and three from the third. These are:

- first part — superior thoracic artery
- second part — acromiothoracic and lateral thoracic artery
- third part — subscapular artery, anterior circumflex humeral and posterior circumflex humeral.

There is a rich arterial anastomosis around the scapula, which may be an important collateral channel in cases of obstruction of the distal subclavian artery.

Brachial artery

This is a continuation of the axillary artery commencing at the lower border of teres major and running along the medial borders of coracobrachialis and biceps accompanied by venae comitantes. At its lower end it runs under the bicipital aponeurosis dividing into the radial artery and ulnar artery at the level of the neck of the radius. It is crossed at the level of the middle of the humerus by the median nerve, which passes superficially from its lateral to medial side. Its branches are the profunda brachii, a nutrient artery to the humerus, and the superior and inferior ulnar collateral arteries.

The lower part of the brachial artery is susceptible to damage in supracondylar fractures of the humerus, particularly in children. Despite the anastomosis around the elbow, intense spasm of the arteries lower down may occur and if uncorrected may result in ischaemic damage of the forearm muscles (Volkmann's ischaemic contracture).

Radial artery

This commences at the level of the neck of the radius lying on the tendon of biceps. It travels down the forearm, and distally it may be found lying superficially between brachioradialis and flexor carpi radialis, and it is between these two tendons that it may be palpated at the wrist. It then passes distally, giving off a branch to assist in the formation of the superficial palmar arch before winding round the lateral border of the wrist to reach the 'anatomical snuffbox'. It then pierces the first dorsal interosseous muscle and enters the palm to form the deep palmar arch with a deep branch of the ulnar artery.

The ulnar artery

The ulnar artery extends from the bifurcation of the brachial artery to the superficial palmar arch in the hand. It accompanies the ulnar nerve, and together they descend along the lateral border of the flexor carpi ulnaris. It becomes palpable at the wrist and crosses superficial to the flexor retinaculum with the ulnar nerve on its medial side. It divides into a superficial and deep branch with the larger superficial branch forming the superficial palmar arch.

The radial artery is normally selected for insertion of a cannula for measuring intra-arterial pressure. There is a small risk of thrombosis of the artery, and it is therefore important to check for the integrity of the palmar arches, and in particular the ulnar inflow, before inserting the

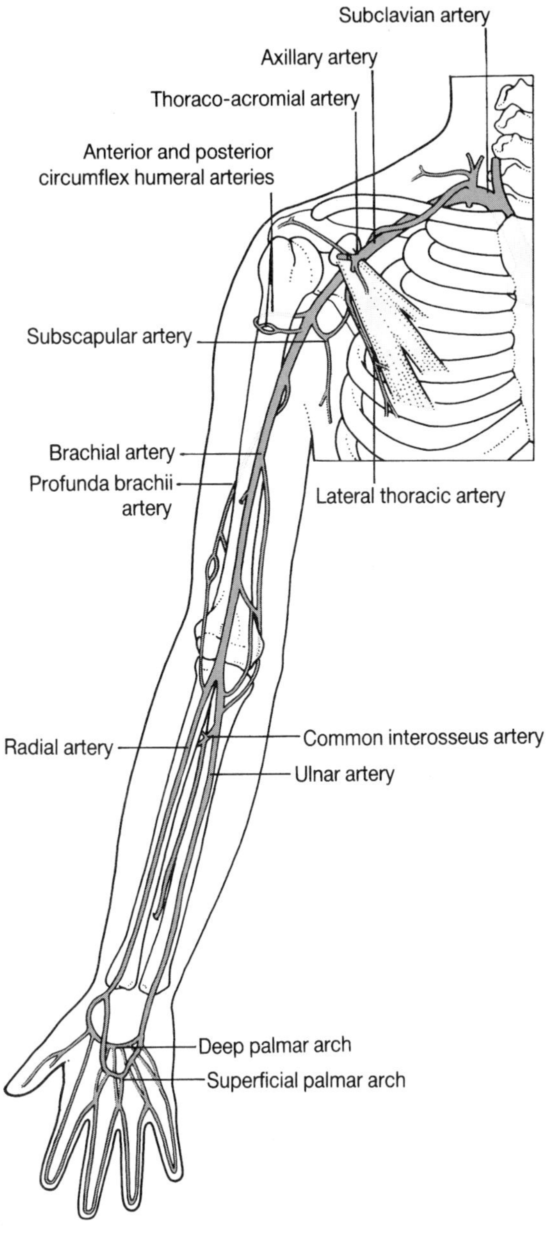
Subclavian artery
Axillary artery
Thoraco-acromial artery
Anterior and posterior circumflex humeral arteries
Subscapular artery
Brachial artery
Profunda brachii artery
Lateral thoracic artery
Radial artery
Common interosseus artery
Ulnar artery
Deep palmar arch
Superficial palmar arch

Fig. 9.19 The arteries of the upper limb. From Rogers op. cit.

arterial line. This is done by Allen's test in which both arteries are occluded by the examiner's firm finger pressure whilst the patient clenches their fist a few times to exsanguinate it. The pressure on the radial artery is maintained, while that on the ulnar is removed; if the palmar arch is satisfactory, it will rapidly flush again. Integrity of the radial artery input can be checked in the same way.

VENOUS DRAINAGE OF THE UPPER LIMBS (Fig. 9.20)

Superficial veins

The veins in the digit drain into a dorsal venous arch on the back of the hand. Two veins are formed from the dorsal and venous arch: the cephalic and the basilic.

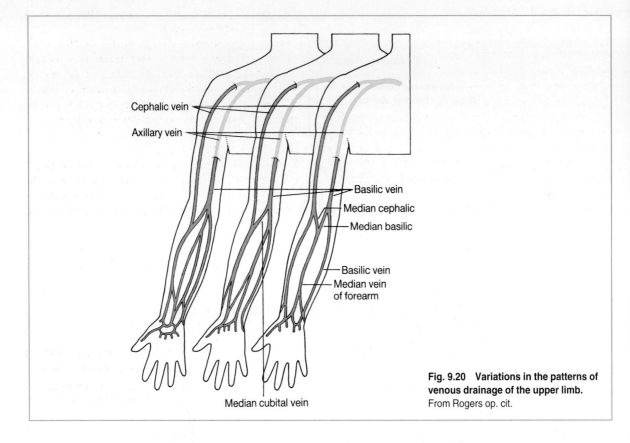

Cephalic vein

Axillary vein

Basilic vein

Median cephalic

Median basilic

Basilic vein
Median vein
of forearm

Median cubital vein

Fig. 9.20 Variations in the patterns of venous drainage of the upper limb.
From Rogers op. cit.

Cephalic vein

This starts in the anatomical snuffbox and courses upwards along the lateral aspect in front of the forearm. At the elbow it is lateral to the biceps tendon, and continues up the arm along the lateral border of the biceps and along the deltopectoral groove. It then pierces the clavipectoral fascia and drains into the axillary vein.

The cephalic vein at the wrist is the most popular site for intravenous cannulation. It should be noted, however, that it is also the most useful vein for creating an arteriovenous fistula for haemodialysis, because of its proximity to the radial artery. In patients with chronic renal failure who may require a fistula, it is appropriate to try to cannulate other veins to avoid thrombophlebitis occurring in the cephalic vein, which would make creation of a fistula difficult.

Basilic vein

This runs upwards on the posteromedial aspect of the forearm, passing to the anterior aspect of the arm just below the elbow. Above the elbow it continues along the medial border of the biceps. It pierces the deep fascia in the middle of the arm, ascending along the medial aspect of the brachial artery. At the lower border of teres major the basilic vein joins the venae comitantes of the brachial artery to form the axillary vein.

There are a number of veins in the cubital fossa, but it is best to avoid these for intravenous injection, as the brachial artery is close to them and separated only by the bicipital aponeurosis. An inadvertent injection of the artery can have disastrous consequences.

Deep veins

These run along the arteries as paired venae comitantes. At the lower border of teres major they are joined by the basilic vein to form the axillary vein, which continues up medial to the axillary artery.

The axillary lymphatics are described in Chapter 15. Suffice it to say that in block dissection of the axilla, one of the early steps is to divide the pectoralis minor muscle as high as possible. This exposes the axillary contents and in particular the axillary vein, which has to be dissected clean of lymph nodes.

BLOOD SUPPLY OF THE LOWER LIMBS

Femoral artery

This is a continuation of the external iliac artery after it has passed deep to the inguinal ligament at its midpoint (Fig. 9.21). The upper part lies in the femoral triangle and the lower part in the adductor canal. Anatomists talk about the whole artery from the inguinal ligament to the popliteal fossa as being 'the femoral artery'. However, vascular surgeons and radiologists describe the first inch or so as being 'the common femoral artery', which gives off two branches: the deep femoral or profunda femoris

artery, and the superficial femoral artery which is the main artery entering the adductor canal. The main branches are shown in Figure 9.21.

The common femoral artery is close to the skin and is normally an extremely easy pulse to feel. A Seldinger catheter can be passed either proximally or distally for selective radiology and angioplasty. It can also be used for inserting catheters for emergency renal dialysis and is a convenient site for arterial samples for blood gases.

The profunda femoris artery

This large branch supplies the muscles of the thigh, but also acts as an important anastomotic channel with the vessels around the knee joint. When the superficial femoral artery becomes blocked the branches of the

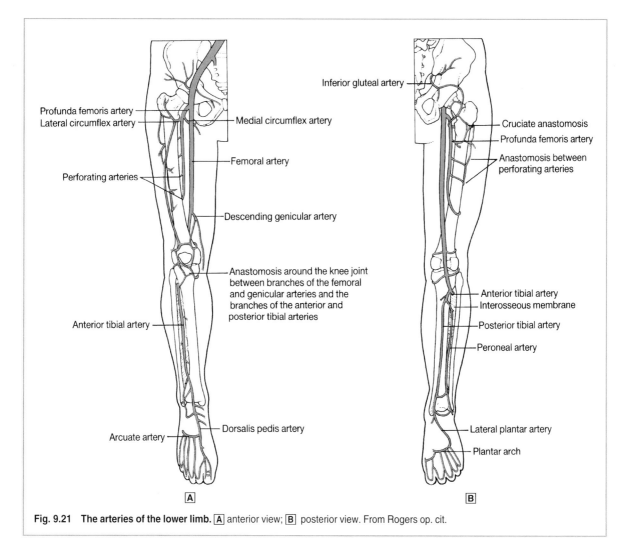

Fig. 9.21   The arteries of the lower limb. A anterior view; B posterior view. From Rogers op. cit.

profunda femoris can enlarge considerably, and with the passage of time many patients become symptom-free as this vessel can be such a good collateral. A branch of the profunda femoris vein crosses the profunda artery about a centimetre below its origin. Ligation and division of this vein exposes the profunda femoris artery.

Femoral triangle

This is bounded (Fig. 9.22):

- superiorly — by the inguinal ligament
- medially — by the medial border of the adductor longus
- laterally — by the medial border of the sartorius.

Its floor consists of the iliacus and psoas major, pectineus and adductor longus, and the roof is formed by the superficial fascia containing superficial inguinal lymph nodes and the great saphenous vein. The contents of the triangle are the femoral vein, artery and nerve together with deep inguinal lymph nodes. The femoral artery leaves at the apex of the triangle to enter the adductor canal.

The operation of block dissection of the groin is used to remove inguinal lymph nodes involved by malignant secondary deposits. The superficial and deep fascia at the roof of the femoral triangle are removed along with the saphenous vein and all its tributaries and the fatty and lymphatic contents of the triangle, leaving only the femoral artery, vein and nerve. The inguinal ligament is normally divided in its midpoint so that an extraperitoneal removal of external iliac nodes can be performed.

Adductor canal (subsartorial canal or Hunter's canal)

This passes from the apex of the femoral triangle to the hiatus in the adductor magnus muscle at the junction of lower and middle thirds of the thigh. The adductor magnus and adductor longus lie posteriorly, the vastus medialis anterolaterally, while the sartorius, which lies in a fascial sheath, forms the roof of the canal. The femoral artery runs through the canal with the femoral vein just behind it, and the saphenous nerve. It is known as Hunter's canal because John Hunter first described the exposure and ligation of the femoral artery for treatment of popliteal aneurysm.

Popliteal fossa

This is a rhomboid-shaped space (Fig. 9.23) whose boundaries are:

- superiorly and laterally — the biceps tendon
- superiorly and medially — the semimembranosus and semitendinosus
- inferiorly and both medially and laterally — the medial and lateral heads of the gastrocnemius.

The floor from above downwards is the popliteal surface of the femur, the posterior aspect of the knee joint, and the popliteus muscle covering the posterior surface of the tibia. The roof is formed by the deep fascia, which may be pierced by the small saphenous vein prior to its entry into the popliteal vein, although the level at which the small saphenous vein joins the popliteal vein is quite variable.

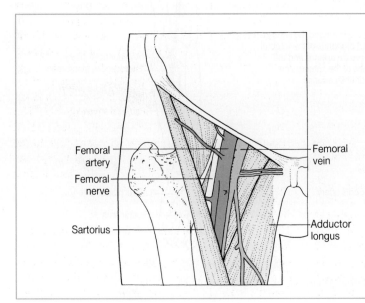

Femoral artery
Femoral nerve
Sartorius
Femoral vein
Adductor longus

Fig. 9.22 The femoral artery, the femoral vein and the femoral nerve in the femoral triangle.
From Rogers op. cit.

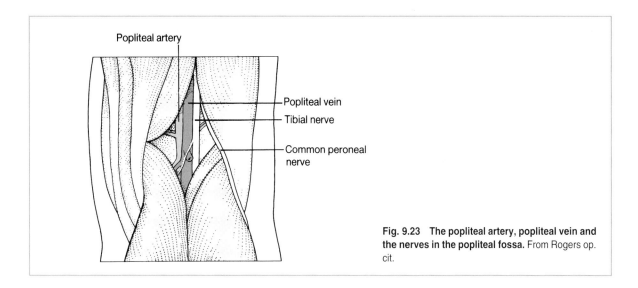

Popliteal artery

Popliteal vein

Tibial nerve

Common peroneal nerve

Fig. 9.23 The popliteal artery, popliteal vein and the nerves in the popliteal fossa. From Rogers op. cit.

The common peroneal nerve leaves the fossa at its lateral aspect, just medial to the biceps tendon. The popliteal artery lies deepest in the fossa with the popliteal vein immediately superficial to the artery. The tibial nerve lies at first lateral to the vessels and then passes superficial to them to lie on their medial side. The popliteal fossa also contains fat and lymph nodes.

Popliteal artery

This is a continuation of the femoral artery from the adductor hiatus to the lower border of the popliteus muscle, where the anterior tibial artery is given off. It may be exposed above the knee by a medial incision along the anterior border of the sartorius muscle. This is separated from the vastus medialis and retracted posteriorly, and after incising the fascial roof of Hunters' Canal, the popliteal artery is found emerging from the hiatus in the adductor magnus.

Below the knee, a medial incision is made along the course of the great saphenous vein which is preserved. The fascia over the medial head of the gastrocnemius is divided in the same line and deepened without difficulty, exposing the popliteal artery, vein and tibial nerve.

It may also be exposed by a posterior approach through the popliteal fossa by deep dissection in the midline, taking care not to damage the more superficial vein and nerve. The medial approach is better for bypass, whereas the direct posterior approach is better for procedures such as arterial cysts or popliteal entrapment. Anatomy books describe the popliteal artery as dividing into the anterior and posterior tibial artery. However, vascular surgeons

normally describe the upper part of the latter as the tibio-peroneal trunk. It is normally about 2 cm long and bifurcates into the posterior tibial and peroneal arteries. This part of the artery can be exposed by the same incision as for the popliteal below the knee and extending the exposure lower down by separating the medial head of the gastrocnemius from the tibia. At this level there is an extensive venous plexus around the artery which makes dissection considerably more difficult.

Anterior tibial artery

This arises at the bifurcation of the popliteal artery (Fig. 9.24). It passes forwards over the upper edge of the interosseus membrane between the tibia and fibula, descending on this membrane in the anterior compartment of the leg. It runs between the tibialis anterior and extensor hallucis longus muscles down to the front of the ankle. It can be exposed throughout its course by an incision between the tibia and fibula, separating these two muscles. It continues as the dorsalis pedis artery, which of course is normally easily palpable just lateral to the extensor hallucis longus tendon. It passes through the first interosseous space to the sole of the foot to join the plantar arch.

Posterior tibial artery

This descends deep to the soleus muscle, where it is surgically rather inaccessible (Fig. 9.24). However, in the lower third of the leg it becomes more superficial and can be dissected out by separating the flexor hallucis longus from the flexor digitorum longus muscles via a skin inci-

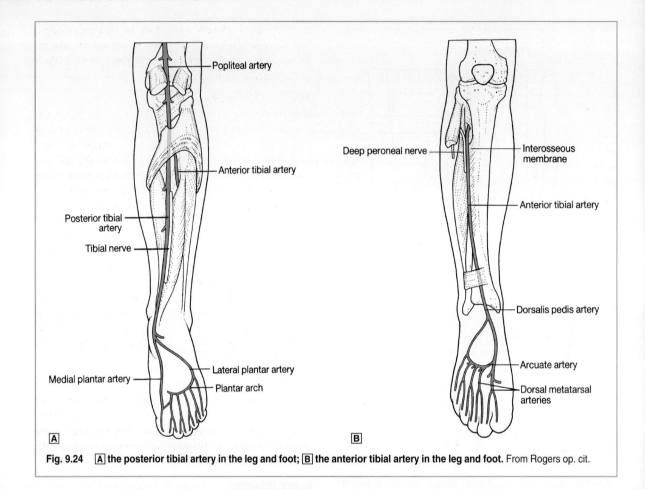

Fig. 9.24 [A] **the posterior tibial artery in the leg and foot;** [B] **the anterior tibial artery in the leg and foot.** From Rogers op. cit.

sion made along the course of the long saphenous vein. The posterior tibial artery is palpable behind the medial malleolus, midway between the latter and the tendo Achilles. The posterior tibial artery passes deep to the flexor retinaculum and ends by dividing into the medial and lateral plantar arteries, which provide the main blood supply to the foot.

Peroneal artery
This runs down the medial border of the fibula towards the lateral malleolus. It gives off a perforating artery which pierces the interosseous membrane to reach the anterior compartment, and ends by supplying the heel as the lateral calcaneal artery. It can be exposed by deepening the same incision used to expose the posterior tibial and feeling for the medial border of the fibula. The artery is found just medial to that. Alternatively, the peroneal artery can be exposed by removing a length of fibula. Rather surprisingly, it is most unusual to cause damage to

the peroneal artery using this approach. Although the peroneal artery is the smallest of the crural arteries, it assumes importance in vascular surgery because, of the three distal vessels, it is the one most frequently spared in atherosclerosis, particularly in diabetics.

The arterial supply to the sole of the foot is mainly by the medial and lateral plantar arteries reinforced by branches of the anterior tibial. An intact plantar arch is looked on as a good prognostic sign in assessing whether a distal bypass will be successful.

VENOUS DRAINAGE OF THE LOWER LIMB
Superficial veins

Great (long) saphenous vein
This arises from the dorsal venous arch of the foot and ascends immediately anterior to the medial malleolus (Fig. 9.25). The relation of the great saphenous vein to

the medial malleolus is a constant finding that proves useful in an emergency for performing a cut-down for venous access.

The vein then ascends on the medial side of the leg, passing a hands breadth behind the medial border of the patella to reach the saphenous opening, where it pierces the cribriform fascia to enter the femoral vein. The branches at the saphenofemoral junction are shown in Figure 9.25. The anatomy of this area is important because of the high incidence of varicose veins affecting the great saphenous vein which is treated by ligation and stripping of this vein. It should be noted that in the lower

calf the vein is closely applied to the saphenous nerve, and nowadays it is normally recommended to strip the vein to just below the knee, as going lower down is likely to damage the saphenous nerve.

Small (short) saphenous vein

This commences at the lateral aspect of the dorsal venous arch and ascends behind the lateral malleolus accompanied by the sural nerve. The small saphenous vein perforates the deep fascia about half way up the calf, and ascends lying deep to the deep fascia between the bellies of the gastrocnemius, to join the popliteal vein in the popliteal fossa. This feature of the small saphenous vein is described incorrectly in most anatomical textbooks, and failure to appreciate this point may result in an inadequate operation. The level at which the small saphenous joins the popliteal is quite variable. A duplex scan should be performed to show the level prior to operation, so that an incision can be made at an appropriate level for the operation of a short saphenous ligation. Stripping of this vein is also likely to cause nerve damage, this time to the sural nerve, giving numbness or paraesthesia in the outer side of the foot.

Deep veins

They are named after the arteries they accompany, and are present in the lower part as venae comitantes. However, as popliteal and femoral veins, they accompany the relevant arteries. The femoral vein continues in the pelvis as the external iliac vein.

Perforating veins

There are a number of perforating veins which pierce the deep fascia at different levels. There is usually a valve close to where these veins perforate the deep fascia. These valves only allow blood to pass deeply. Common sites are in the lower thigh as the perforating vein between the great saphenous and the femoral. There is similarly one in the upper calf. There is also a posterior arch vein which usually has three perforating veins in the medial part of the lower half of the calf. Venous ulcers are particularly likely to occur when these perforating veins become incompetent.

PHYSIOLOGY

The centre of the cardiovascular system is the heart. The function of this organ is to supply the body and its organs with sufficient oxygenated blood to meet everyday needs. In order to do this the heart pumps blood around the pulmonary and systemic circulations at a flow rate

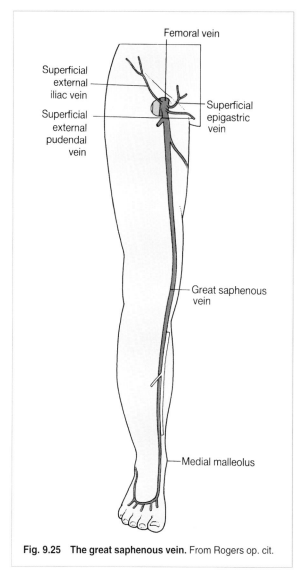

Fig. 9.25 The great saphenous vein. From Rogers op. cit.

that varies in adults from about 5 to 35 L/min and a frequency that varies in the range 50 to 200 beats/min. The generation of cardiac output and its control is a complex mixture of intrinsic (Starling's Law) and extrinsic factors (neurohumeral).

GENERATION OF CARDIAC OUTPUT

The key to the generation of cardiac output is the unique rhythmic muscular contraction of the heart. The word rhythmic is important. All cardiac muscle has the intrinsic capacity for rhythmic excitation: that is, independent of other influences, cardiac tissue will spontaneously depolarise until an action potential occurs and contraction is initiated. The fibres have differing rates of depolarisation, but since they form a functional syncytium with specialised conducting tissue, depolarisation spreads from cell to cell, and leads to coordinated contraction.

This rhythmic activity produces alternate contraction/relaxation (systole/diastole). Since atrial systole occurs fractionally before ventricular contraction, a final boost (15%) is given to ventricular volume before contraction of the ventricles.

Phases of the cardiac cycle

At a rate of 70 beats/min, the heart completes each cycle in less than 1 s (Fig. 9.26). Each cycle can be broken down into two phases each for diastole and systole:

- systole:
  — contraction (I) — mitral and tricuspid valve closure
  — ejection (IIa & b) — aortic and pulmonary valve opening
- diastole:
  — relaxation (III) — aortic and pulmonary valve closed
  — filling (IVa, b & c) — mitral and tricuspid valve open.

The phases and timing of events in the cardiac cycle are shown in Table 9.1. It is convenient to start when the ventricles are still in diastole at the beginning of atrial systole.

Phase IVc, atrial systole

The SA node depolarises and atrial musculature contracts (P wave on ECG). Atrial pressure rises and blood flows down the pressure gradient through the AV valves to the ventricles, completing the last 15% of ventricular filling. This is the end of diastole.

Phases I & II, ventricular systole

The electrical impulse from the atria now reaches the ventricles, which contract (QRS on ECG) — phase I. The

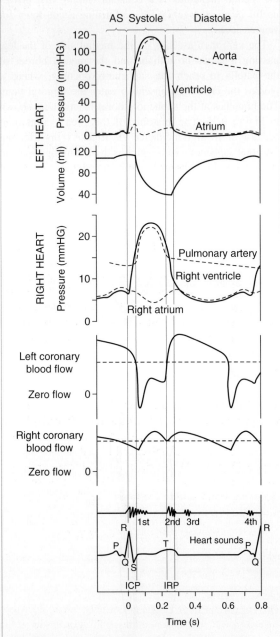

Fig. 9.26 The cardiac cycle. ICP = isometric contraction period; IRP = isometric relaxation period; AS = atrial systole.

pressure in the ventricles rises, closing the AV valves but not yet opening the semilunar (aortic and pulmonary valves). Thus all four valves are closed and the volume of blood in the heart remains constant as the pressure rapidly increases (isovolumetric contraction).

Phase	Name	Description	Timing (ms)
		Table 9.1 Phases and timing of events in the cardiac cycle (see diagram of pressures in the heart, Fig. 9.26)	
IVc	Atrial systole	Atria contract to fill last 15% of ventricles	60
I	Isovolumetric contraction	Ventricles contract with aortic and pulmonary valve closed	50
IIa	Ejection	Blood ejected into pulmonary artery and aorta	90
IIb	Ejection	Aortic/pulmonary pressures equalise with ventricles	130
III	Isovolumetric relaxation	Ventricular pressure falls Aortic/pulmonary valves close	120
IVa	Passive ventricular filling	Ventricles fill rapidly largely due to 'suction effect'	110
IVb	Passive ventricular filling	Rate of ventricular filling now declines	190

When the pressure in the ventricle exceeds that in the aortic (or pulmonary) artery the semilunar valves open. The pressure in the aorta and ventricle (and pulmonary artery and ventricle) is now the same, and both continue to rise rapidly. The opening of the valves marks the start of the ejection phase or phase II. A maximum pressure of 120 mmHg is reached on the systemic side and 18 mmHg on the pulmonary.

Phase III, diastolic relaxation

Having reached maximum pressure the ventricles now relax but maintain their volume for a short while (isovolumetric relaxation). The pressure inside drops below that of the aorta (and pulmonary artery) so the semilunar valves close. All four valves are closed again. The end of phase III is marked by the start of a fall in ventricular volume as the ventricles relax further. The ventricle ejects about 60% of its volume, the ejection fraction, which is defined as follows:

$$\text{ejection fraction} = \text{SV/LVEDV}$$

where SV = stroke volume; LVEDV = left ventricular end diastolic volume.

Phase IV, diastolic filling

The filling phase of diastole can now occur. It is important to realise that the downward displacement of the valves during ejection ensures a low atrial pressure (suction effect) and hence rapid initial filling (phase IVa). This rapid rate of filling declines as atrial volume increases (IVb). Finally active atrial contraction begins again (phase IVc). The ventricles are 'topped up' by about 15% at rest but much more at higher heart rates. Hence a failure of atrial contraction, especially at higher heart rates (e.g. fast atrial fibrillation, exercise) becomes more important and possibly life threatening.

Heart sounds

The first heart sound is caused by closure of the mitral (and much quieter tricuspid) valve. It is best heard at the apex. The second heart sound is produced when the aortic and pulmonary valves close and is best heard at the base of the heart.

A third heart sound may occur in early diastole if there is an abrupt end to ventricular filling. This occurs in an hyperdynamic circulation, such as pregnancy or anaemia.

A fourth heart sound may occur in late diastole and indicates a stiff (diseased) ventricle. It is only heard if the atria contract to augment filling and generally indicates heart failure or ventricular failure (Fig. 9.27).

Venous pulse

There are five waveforms that make up the jugular venous pulse. These can be clearly identified by physicians on inspection of the internal jugular vein in the semirecumbent position. Ordinary mortals are advised to inspect the central venous catheter trace as seen after modulation through a pressure transducer, where it looks as shown in Figure 9.28: a = active contraction and is positive; c = transmission of the carotid pulse; x = depression of the level of the valves during systole and is negative (suction effect); v = venous filling during ventricular systole; y = fall in atrial pressure as the tricuspid valve opens.

It is important to note that when quoting the jugular venous pressure, measurement should be taken from the same point, usually from the manubriosternal angle to the top of the venous wave (normally 3–4 cm at 45°). The pressure will be low in hypovolaemia and elevated in any form of right heart failure, cardiac tamponade, or obstruction of the superior vena cava.

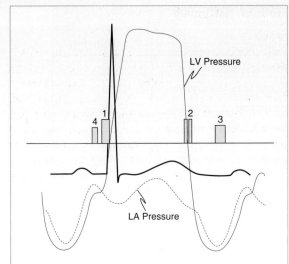

Fig. 9.27 Heart sounds. The diagram shows the heart sounds and left atrial / left ventricular pressure waveforms. (Note the splitting of the second sound.)

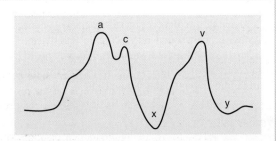

Fig. 9.28 Venous pulses. 'a' wave: atrial systole; not seen in atrial fibrillation; increased in tricuspid or pulmonary stenosis; heart block causes variable 'a' waves: and even 'cannon' waves. 'c' wave: leaflets of the tricuspid valve bulge into the right atrium during isovolumetric contraction. 'v' wave: right atrium is rapidly filled while tricupsid valve is closed. 'x' descent: atrium relaxes and tricuspid valve moves down. 'y' descent: tricuspid valve opens, and blood flows from right atrium to right ventricle.

Generation and conduction of cardiac impulse

Cardiac tissue has two types of cell:

1. cells that initiate and conduct impulses
2. cells that conduct and contract.

The latter form the muscles of the heart, which in turn form a functional syncytium.

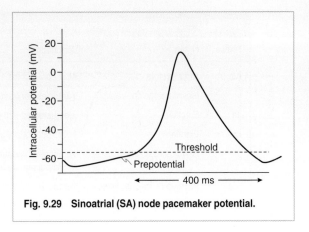

Fig. 9.29 Sinoatrial (SA) node pacemaker potential.

Generation of the cardiac impulse

The SA node and conducting system do not have a resting membrane potential. The cells are constantly depolarising at a slow rate after each repolarisation. This slow depolarisation continues until the threshold potential is reached and an action potential is triggered (Fig. 9.29).

The maximum transmembrane potential of the SA node is about –50 mV. The cell membrane is relatively permeable to sodium, so this ion gradually 'leaks in', lowering the transmembrane potential. When –50 mV is reached a sudden depolarisation occurs, and this is conducted to other cells, initiating a cardiac cycle. This is caused by a sudden dramatic and short-lived increase in permeability to sodium. The SA node has the fastest rate of depolarisation (i.e. the greatest permeability to sodium). This is increased by sympathetic activity and decreased by vagal (parasympathetic) activity. If the rate of spontaneous depolarisation of the SA node is slowed sufficiently, then the cardiac impulse will be generated from elsewhere in the conduction system (the second fastest pacemaker is the AV node).

The cardiac action potential, which is triggered by the pacemaker cells, has a unique shape that is vital to cardiac function. Once triggered, there is also a sudden short-lived increase in the permeability of the cell membrane to sodium. The ion diffuses into the cell and the transmembrane potential rapidly declines and overshoots to +50 mV. Potassium now diffuses out of the cell down the electronic gradient, rapidly reversing the situation and tending to restore the resting membrane potential (–80 mV). Before this can occur, however, the inward movement of calcium ions slows this process down and produces a plateau phase of about 200 ms (Fig. 9.30). During this period cardiac muscle cannot be stimulated further (it is inexcitable) and thus tetanic contraction

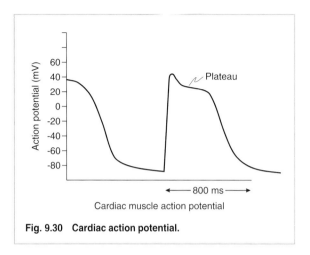

Fig. 9.30 **Cardiac action potential.**

is impossible. This plateau phase is unique to cardiac muscle; without it, rhythmic contraction would be impossible.

Excitation/contraction coupling

The force of myocardial contraction is proportional to the concentration of available calcium. The arrival of the action potential causes the release of calcium ions from the sarcoplasmic reticulum. These ions bind to troponin C and this in turn activates the actin–myosin interaction that results in contraction. The plateau phase of the action potential causes further calcium influx and prolongs and enhances contraction.

With so much ionic influx and outflux it is not surprising that acute changes in the ionic milieu have a profound effect upon the myocardium (Table 9.2).

CORONARY CIRCULATION

Arteries

Two arteries supply the myocardium: the right and left coronary arteries. The right provides one seventh of the circulation, the rest is provided by the left coronary artery. Each feeds the right and left ventricle, respectively, with a small degree of overlap. The arteries do not run within the muscle, rather over its surface. However, branches of the arteries do penetrate into the muscle to form a rich capillary network. This is of great importance since the wall tension of the myocardium can have a great bearing on coronary blood flow, especially in hypertension.

Veins

The venous drainage of the left ventricle is via the coronary sinus into the right atrium. Veins of the right ventricle also drain into the right atrium. 5% of total ventricular blood flow is into the Thebesian veins, which drain directly into the ventricles.

Blood flow

At rest the adult heart requires about 80 mL/min/100 g tissue — about 250 mL/min. (This will rise to about 1 L/min during exercise). From this blood flow the heart must extract the required amount of oxygen, which at rest is about 11 mL/min/100 g tissue (about 30% more than skeletal muscle).

Samples of venous blood from the coronary sinus show that extraction of oxygen is near maximal even at rest: in order to get more oxygen from the coronary circulation, the only option is increased flow.

One other feature of great importance distinguishes the coronary circulation: the cyclical nature of coronary blood flow. During systole the intramyocardial vessels

Table 9.2 The effects of various changes in the environment of the heart.		
Environment	Effect	Mechanism
Hypocalcaemia	Decreased contractility	Decreased calcium available from the sarcoplasmic reticulum
Hypercalcaemia	Initially increased contractility	Increased calcium available from the sarcoplasmic reticulum
Hypokalaemia	Initially positive chronotropic and inotropic effects	Decreased repolarisation of the myocardium, so more calcium may enter the cells
Hyperkalaemia	Decreased rate of conduction and slowing of the heart, dysrhythmias, reduced force of contraction (tall peaked T waves on ECG). Eventual cardiac arrest	Inactivation of the sodium channels. Accelerated repolarisation of the myocardium, so that less calcium can enter the cells
Low pH	Decreased contractility	Multiple factors

are compressed and so blood flow is curtailed, especially in the subendocardial region where wall tension is highest. This effect is exacerbated by hypertension (Fig. 9.31). Most coronary blood flow occurs in diastole. Unfortunately, during the high heart rates associated with exercise, diastole is shortened in comparison to systole, and the time for perfusion of the ventricles is shortened.

What then determines the coronary blood flow? The answer is the blood pressure (in this case diastolic) and the diameter of the coronary vessels. The latter is determined by tone of the vessels and the wall pressure exerted by the myocardial muscle. The tone of the vessels is determined by the presence of local metabolites, ade-

nosine, K^+ and oxygen lack (probably mediated by nitric oxide). Sympathetic innervation is certainly demonstrable but probably of little importance.

What does the heart use as an energy source? Less than 1% of energy can be derived anaerobically — less than required for contractions, but possibly enough to avoid immediate cell death, for example in ventricular fibrillation. Usually the heart uses the following substrates:

- 35% carbohydrates
- 5% ketones
- 60% fats.

These proportions change according to the nutritional state of the individual.

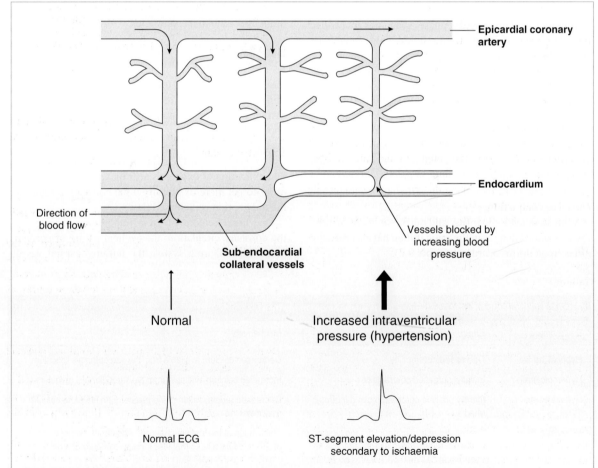

Fig. 9.31 Coronary circulation and wall tension. The diagram shows the effect of increasing ventricular wall tension on myocardial circulation. The effects are exacerbated by atheroma.

CARDIAC OUTPUT

Cardiac output is the volume of blood pumped out of the heart over a given time period and is usually expressed as follows:

$$Q = SV \times HR$$

where Q = cardiac output (L/min), SV = stroke volume (L), HR = heart rate (beats/min). For the average 70 kg example the figures would be:

- Q = 5 L/min
- SV = 70 mL
- HR = 70 beats/min.

Regulation of cardiac output

The regulation of the vascular system ensures that each organ receives its required minimum blood flow, that redistribution of blood occurs where appropriate, and that the heart is not overtaxed by providing maximal blood flow to organs which do not need it. Each organ has its own mechanisms for achieving these ends, and the heart has the capacity to increase or decrease its output according to demand. There are a number of mechanisms by which the heart achieves increases in output.

Starling's law of the heart

Loosely stated this states that the force of contraction is a function of the initial length of the muscle fibre (Fig. 9.32). If the initial fibre length is increased by greater venous return, then the heart can increase its output by as much as three fold compared with resting levels. It is also this mechanism which ensures that outputs of the left and right hearts are exactly matched. However, if the heart is overdistended, the force and rate of contraction quickly decline, leading to cardiac failure.

Increasing rate and force of contraction

Besides the Starling law, there are other mechanisms by which the heart can be made to work harder (Table 9.3). Sympathetic stimulation increases myocardial contractility and heart rate both by direct neuronal stimulation and by circulating catecholamines. As work is increased, so is oxygen consumption.

Heart rate is increased not only by increasing sympathetic stimulation but also by decreased vagal stimulation. Indeed the vagus nerve has an important role to play in controlling heart rate. This can be shown by denervation of the heart, where the resting rate increases to about 110 beats/min in the absence of both vagus and sympathetic nerves.

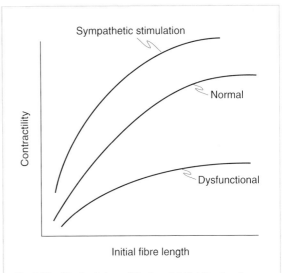

Fig. 9.32 Starling's law of the heart. Initial fibre length cannot be measured in humans, and so ventricular filling pressure is often used instead. The use of inotropic or vasodilator drugs moves the dysfunctional line towards the normal.

As the heart increases or decreases its output, simultaneously it must increase or decrease blood pressure, all things being equal.

CONTROL OF BLOOD PRESSURE

Pressure can be defined as the force per unit area, usually measured in newtons per square metre (N/m^2). The pressure exerted by a liquid is more simply defined as the height of a column of liquid that this pressure will support. By convention this is usually a column of mercury or water. The latter is more useful for lower pressures, as it is less dense.

$$P = h\,\delta\,g$$

where P = pressure, δ = density, g = gravitational constant of acceleration, h = height of liquid.

Blood pressure is somewhat more difficult to define since it is a dynamic variable and, in humans at least, not readily measurable by a column of fluid (which in the case of blood would be several metres high).

Blood pressure varies according to the phase of the cardiac cycle and the site at which it is measured (pulmonary, systemic, arterial, venous, etc.). It is also higher in the legs of a standing person than in the arms.

In common parlance the term 'blood pressure' refers to

Table 9.3   The effects of various agents on the rate and force of contraction of the heart

Stimulus	Effect	Mechanism
Catecholamines and sympathetic nerves	Increased contractility and rate	Stimulation and increased splitting of ATP
Calcium ions	Increased contractility	Increased actin–myosin interaction
Digoxin	Increased contractility and decreased rate	Shortens initial fibre length
Sympathomimetic drugs	Increased contractility and rate	Stimulation and increased splitting of ATP
Insulin	Increased contractility	Increased K^+ and glucose flux
Atropine	Increased rate	Blocks vagus (anticholinergic)
Parasympathetic (vagus nerve)	Decreased rate	Slows the SA node by increasing K^+ conductance
Beta-blockers	Decreased contractility and rate	Block receptors
Antiarrhythmic drugs	Decreased contractility	Various
Potassium ions	Decreased contractility	Accelerated repolarisation of the sodium channels, so that less calcium can enter the cells
General anaesthetic agents	Decreased contractility	Depression of actin–myosin interaction?

the systemic arterial pressure (other pressures dealt with elsewhere) and there are several terms, as follows.

- *Systolic blood pressure* is the maximum value during cardiac systole.
- *Diastolic blood pressure* is the minimum value during diastole.
- *Pulse pressure* is the difference between systolic and diastolic pressures.
- *Mean pressure* is the geometric mean, which can be calculated by adding one-third pulse pressure to diastolic pressure.

Measurement of blood pressure

This is best achieved with an arterial line when accuracy and continuous measurement are required, but for convenience an occlusion method using a Riva-Rocci cuff is used. The Korotkoff sounds are the noises heard over the brachial artery during deflation of the occluding, proximal cuff. There are five phases:

- Phase 1: Appearance of a tapping sound heard at systolic pressure.
- Phase 2: Sounds become muffled or disappear.
- Phase 3: Sounds reappear.
- Phase 4: Sounds become muffled again. In the UK this is taken as diastolic pressure.
- Phase 5: Sounds disappear. In the USA (and in most automated blood pressure monitors) this is taken as the diastolic pressure.

The sounds are thought to be caused by turbulent flow causing vibration of the arterial wall. A stethoscope amplifies the sound. How does this method compare with an arterial line? It should be noted that this is an occlusion technique and as such is fundamentally different from direct measurement with an arterial lines, which rarely reveals exactly the same pressures. Both phase 4 and 5 slightly over-read when compared with the direct method. In addition, phase 5 is a gradual process and hence can be more subjective. In high output states such as pregnancy or sepsis, these sounds may not disappear until the cuff is fully deflated. There are several potential errors.

1. A narrow cuff will give too high a reading. The cuff width should be two-thirds of the length of the forearm.
2. The inflating part of the cuff must lie over the artery so that the pressure within the cuff is the same as that transmitted to the vessel wall.
3. Mercury gauges are generally much more reliable than aneroid gauges, which need regular zeroing and calibration.
4. Atherosclerosis and calcification of the vessel wall will reduce vibration, sometimes below the audible range.
5. Hypotension will cause the sounds to be much quieter and more difficult to hear.

As a general rule, patients whose blood pressure is expected to change rapidly over many hours and/or who may need multiple arterial blood gas analysis are best provided with an arterial line which provides a constant indication of pressure.

How is blood pressure generated?

The circulatory system is best thought of as a long tube through which blood flows. In order for this to occur, pressure must be higher at one end than the other. In any flow system this pressure difference must be a function of resistance and flow:

$$\text{flow} = P \pi r^4 / 8 \eta l$$

where P = pressure, r = radius, η = viscosity, l = length. This is the Hagen–Poiseuille law.

However, this model is simplistic in that it applies only in systems where flow is laminar. If the flow becomes turbulent then the following equation applies:

$$P = kv*$$

where $v*$ = average velocity (not flow rate!) and k is a constant for turbulent flow. In this model, small increases in cardiac output cause great increases in pressure.

In summary, blood pressure increases as flow increases and, if flow is turbulent, this increase is marked. Vessel calibre has the most marked effect on pressure, with very small calibre change reflected in a large change in pressure. The system described above is an oversimplification inasmuch as there is no allowance for the pulsatile nature of blood flow nor the fact that fluids which obey these rules must be *Newtonian* (i.e. those whose viscosity is independent of flow rate).

Where does resistance occur in the circulation?

The arterioles and capillaries each account for about 25% of total peripheral resistance (TPR). Consequently these are often referred to as resistance vessels. Beyond this point in the circulation it follows that blood pressure must fall steeply.

Small radius capillaries are large in number (5×10^9). Their huge number, great length and enormous surface area, coupled with the low velocity of flow and high pressure drop, are vital factors in the capillary exchange mechanism.

The arterioles are endowed with much smooth muscle and hence can exert considerable control over resistance and flow through the capillaries. Furthermore they control the number of capillaries which are open to flow at any one time.

HOW IS BLOOD FLOW CONTROLLED?

The function of the circulatory system is to ensure that the entire body is provided with enough blood in all situations. This involves control at a *local* (organ) level and a general *systemic* level. The overall determinant of flow is cardiac output, but each organ in the body has regulatory mechanisms superimposed.

Local (organ) control

Regulation of blood flow in various organs is mainly achieved by alterations to the diameter of the vessels. This in turn is influenced by the smooth muscles of the vessel walls. The tone of these muscles is influenced by:

- neural activity
- hormones
- local control (autoregulation).

Neural activity

Most vessels have a resting muscle tone: when denervated some relaxation occurs. In general those vessels with least sympathetic innervation have greatest inherent tone (myocardium, skeletal muscle). The vessels of the skin have lowest tone and high innervation. The adrenergic fibres of the sympathetic nervous system are the predominant pathways whereby the systemic circulation is controlled. Vasomotor areas in the medulla have descending pathways to the thoracolumbar areas of the spinal cord. From here postganglionic fibres go from ganglia of the sympathetic chain to vascular smooth muscle. The major transmitter which acts on receptors to cause vasoconstriction is noradrenaline. The vasomotor centre discharges in response to afferent stimuli from baroreceptors, chemoreceptors and from the cortex itself, for example in anticipation of exercise. Because some tissues are not well innervated by this system, the effect of discharge from the vasomotor centre and increased adrenergic activity is a redistribution of blood from skin, muscle and gut to heart, brain and kidney areas, where there are fewer adrenergic receptors or thinner smooth musculature.

By contrast the cholinergic fibres of the sympathetic nervous system cause vasodilatation in skeletal muscle. Stimulation of these fibres results in a redistribution of blood from skin and viscera to skeletal muscle.

It follows that transection of the spinal cord above the thoracolumbar region will result in a loss of not only sensory and motor functions but also in loss of sympathetic vasomotor tone, contributing to the condition known as spinal shock. Very high transections of the cord not only allow profound falls in blood pressure but also result in the absence of sympathetic innervation of the myocardium, which can result in unopposed vagal stimulation and profound bradycardia (especially during endotracheal intubation, or the passage of a nasogastric tube to control an associated ileus).

Hormones

Adrenaline and noradrenaline from sympathetic nerve endings and the adrenal medulla pour into the circulation during stress (e.g. surgery). This appears to be their prime function: to give a boost during stress. They do not regulate day to day blood pressure and flow.

Angiotensin II is a powerful vasopressor produced by the action of renin on angiotensinogen. Renin is released when there is a decrease in the perfusion of the kidney. Whilst the vasoconstriction produced is great, it is more likely that this hormone acts mainly by increasing aldosterone concentrations, which in turn promote salt and water retention.

Local control

Many metabolites influence the calibre of blood vessels (but only in the presence of an intact endothelium). Amongst these are CO_2, K^+, H^+, bradykinins, prostaglandin and adenosine. Some tissues are more sensitive than others to various chemical changes: e.g. intense vasoconstriction occurs in the brain in response to hypocapnia. Hypoxia causes vasodilatation in almost all tissues (though not pulmonary).

The term *autoregulation* is used to refer to the mechanism by which blood flow is maintained at a constant rate over a wide range of perfusion pressures. This is most pronounced in the renal and cerebral circulation. There are two basic mechanisms:

1. A fall in blood pressure results in a reduction in blood flow. Local metabolites accumulate and these cause local vasodilatation, ultimately mediated by nitric oxide.
2. Myogenic response — this involves local neural reflex in response to stretch. It occurs at the level of the first-order arteriole.

The final common pathway for the relaxation of smooth muscle is via nitric oxide.

General systemic control of flow (and pressure)

Since a flow of blood is required for the circulation, a pressure must be maintained.

$$\text{mean arterial pressure} = CO \times TPR$$

where CO = cardiac output (L/min) and TPR = total peripheral resistance (usually expressed as N s/m^5). This is analogous to Ohm's law. Thus we see that the determinants of blood pressure are cardiac output and resistance. If we fill in typical values for an adult we find that:

$$TPR = \frac{80 \text{ mmHg}}{5 \text{ L/min}}$$
$$= 160\,000 \text{ N s/m}^5$$

TPR units are also expressed as dyne s/cm^5 (100 N s/m^5 = 1 dyne s/cm^5).

Baroreceptors

We have seen how cardiac output can vary. Regulation of cardiac output and vascular resistance in various vascular beds controls blood pressure. Superimposed on this is the baroreceptor system.

Baroreceptors are found in the wall of the aorta and carotid sinus. They are stretch receptors which, when stimulated (by increased blood pressure), lead to a reflex reduction in vasoconstriction, venoconstrictor tone, and to a lower heart rate. All of which, mediated by the autonomic nervous system and higher centres of midbrain, lead to a fall in TPR, cardiac output and blood pressure.

As blood pressure falls the baroreceptors become less stretched: vasoconstriction, venoconstriction and heart rate increase, and the fall in blood pressure is reversed.

The site of the baroreceptors, at the point of circulatory input to the brain, has obvious importance.

From a clinical point of view, it is possible that an autonomic neuropathy may render these reflexes ineffective for day to day regulation of, say, maintaining blood pressure in response to changes in posture. This can be investigated by use of the Valsalva manoeuvre, i.e. forced expiration against a closed glottis, causing a rise in intrathoracic pressure and a decreased venous return. The normal response is an initial reflex tachycardia and vasoconstriction in order to maintain blood pressure. On release of the elevated intrathoracic pressure, there is a transient increase in blood pressure and a fall in heart rate. This can all be measured at the bedside, but an accurate recording system should be used, e.g. an ECG.

In addition to the baroreceptors, there are other receptors to be found in the carotid and aortic bodies. These are chemoreceptors that respond to hypoxaemia and also to hypoperfusion. Stimulation results in an increase in sympathetic discharge and an increase in blood pressure.

Veins

The small veins have a large cross-sectional area, and they hold the bulk of the circulatory volume — much more blood than the great arteries and veins. In a resting, supine subject, return of blood to the heart is an entirely passive process, depending on the pressure in the capillaries (about 15 mmHg) being greater than that of the right atrium (near to zero).

When a subject stands up, return of blood to the heart must be augmented because the driving pressure in the capillaries is insufficient. Return of blood is helped by three mechanisms:

1. the pumping action of skeletal muscle on veins which contain valves
2. a reflex sympathetic constriction of the splanchnic arterioles and venous reservoirs
3. intrinsic and reflexive shutting down of arteriolar sphincters in the dependent limbs which greatly reduces the flow through those limbs.

The blood pressure within the veins when standing will normally be that which is required to return it to the heart, i.e. equivalent to a column of blood whose height is the same as the heart.

HAEMORRHAGE AND SHOCK

Shock is a general term that describes an inability of the circulation to meet the metabolic needs of the body. It is better to use the more accurate term 'acute circulatory failure'. This can occur, either because the body's metabolic needs have increased (septic shock), or because the heart is failing (cardiogenic shock), or because of a lack of circulatory fluid (hypovolaemic shock). Massive vasodilatation occurs as a component of septic shock or in high transection of the spinal cord, causing a relative lack of circulatory fluid. Oxygen is not stored in any significant quantity outside of the lungs, hence any decline in the circulation will manifest itself eventually as hypoxia.

The delivery of oxygen to the tissues, DO_2, is dependent upon the oxygen content of the blood multiplied by the cardiac output:

$$DO_2 = CaO_2 \times CO$$

where DO_2 = delivery of oxygen (mL/min), CaO_2 = oxygen content of arterial blood (mL/L arterial blood), CO = cardiac output (L/min).

The content of oxygen in the blood depends on the haemoglobin content, the saturation of the haemoglobin, and the small amount of oxygen dissolved in the plasma:

$$CaO_2 = (Hb \times 1.34 \times SaO_2) + (PaO_2 \times 0.0031)$$

where Hb = haemoglobin content (g/dL), SaO_2 = percentage saturation of haemoglobin with oxygen, PaO_2 = partial pressure of oxygen in the arterial blood (mmHg), 1.34 is the number of millilitres of oxygen which combine with each g/dL of haemoglobin for each percent saturation.

If we supply figures to this equation:

$$CaO_2 = (15 \times 1.34 \times 100) + (95 \times 0.0031)$$
$$= 20.4 \text{ mL } O_2/\text{dL blood}$$

If cardiac output is about 5 L/min then

$$DO_2 = 20.4 \times 5000/100$$
$$= 1020 \text{ mL/min}$$

At rest the body only requires about 200 mL/min but much more in times of stress. If a fall in cardiac output results in a decline in oxygen delivery then the tissues will switch to anaerobic metabolism. Whilst aerobic metabolism provides 36 moles of ATP for each mole of glucose, anaerobic metabolism produces just 2 moles, along with 2 moles of pyruvic acid which rapidly becomes lactic acid. Although vasoconstriction follows typical hypovolaemic shock, local acidosis will produce vasodilatation in affected tissues.

Experimental evidence suggests that oxygen transport must be increased above preshock values for survival.

Hypovolaemic shock occurs commonly and must be rapidly diagnosed and treated. As the circulatory fluid volume falls, tissue perfusion becomes increasingly impaired, leading to a loss of capillary integrity. Venous return declines, cardiac output falls, and the baroreceptors are stimulated to produce an increase in heart rate and arterial and venous constriction. At the same time, cardiac output is redistributed away from the less vital areas (skin, muscle and gut) to the brain and heart. The human body is able to maintain blood pressure until about 20% of the circulation is lost (and cardiac output has declined by a third), but beyond this any further fall in circulatory volume is matched by falls in cardiac output and blood pressure. The appearance of such a patient is pale and cold (less blood flow to the skin), but sweaty with a marked tachycardia (sympathetic discharge).

In addition to the baroreceptor reflexes, other mechanisms come into play. Increased aldosterone and ADH secretion result in salt and water retention. Capillary pressure falls, resulting in interstitial fluid exuding into the capillaries. The fall in tissue perfusion leads to a switch over to anaerobic metabolism and lactic acidosis. This adverse environment can cause depression of the myocardium, worsening the situation. The delivery of oxygen from the blood to the lung declines as a result of increased dead space and increased ventilation/perfusion mismatch. Hyperventilation occurs as a response to acidosis and hypoxaemia. Gasping, deep (Kussmaul) respiration may be seen, because of the chemoreceptor response.

If the situation continues, or is exacerbated, organ failure may develop. If, for example, the heart is faced with a sudden 50% reduction in circulating haemoglobin it must double its output to maintain the status quo, and in doing twice as much work will require twice as much oxygen. Since the blood now carries only half the oxygen it did, the coronary blood flow must increase four-fold. An atheromatous heart may quickly become ischaemic and fail. In becoming ischaemic, the bowel wall may become permeable to endotoxin, resulting in a superimposed septic shock. Generalised cell death may result in the release of toxic metabolites, interleukins and tumour necrosis factor (TNF). The respiratory rate increases in the face of hypoxia and acidosis. The lungs may develop a state of increased capillary permeability with the development of oedema (adult respiratory distress syndrome, ARDS). Without a rapid reversal of fortune, the kidneys may fail. Poor cerebral perfusion results in confusion followed by unconsciousness. The coagulation system of the blood may become activated, with micro-clots forming in the capillaries and generalised bleeding as coagulation factors become consumed (disseminated intravascular coagulation, DIC).

The treatment of hypovolaemia is by early infusion of intravenous fluid of the sort that stays in the circulatory space. Of these, colloids such as blood and plasma protein fraction will produce rapid results and will stay in the circulatory space for many hours. Crystalloid solutions such as Hartmann's solution and normal saline can be used but will expand both the circulatory and interstitial spaces, so that larger volumes must be used. Five percent dextrose and dextrose/saline are not suitable, since these fluids freely cross into all body compartments with little being retained in the intravascular space. Severe fluid loss requires close monitoring of the circulation to ensure speed and adequacy of diagnosis and treatment.

Features of acute circulatory failure

Features of acute circulatory failure ('shock') are:

- heart rate > 100 beats/min
- blood pressure < 100 mmHg
- elevated or reduced central venous pressure (see text)
- skin cold and clammy (sweaty)
- respiration rapid (often shallow)
- conscious level decreased (often drowsy and confused)
- urine output < ½ mL/kg/h.

MONITORING THE CIRCULATION

It is important to clarify that there is no easily performed single measure which defines a problem with the cir-

culation, be it hypovolaemia, hypervolaemia or a failing ventricle. Rather a series of measurements of more than one parameter over a period of time is required. Each measurement forms a part of the assessment of the circulation. Where hypovolaemia is suspected, although it is possible to measure the blood volume with great accuracy in the laboratory using radioisotope indicator dilution techniques (e.g. chromium-labelled red blood cells), in the hospital setting this is impractical. In general the amount of monitoring required increases with the infirmity and the complexity of the clinical problem. From simple non-invasive measurements of pulse and blood pressure we progress to more invasive measurements such as the central venous pressure and pulmonary artery pressure. It should be remembered that much information can be derived from simply taking the pulse and blood pressure and observing the patient's skin for temperature, colour and sweat. However, intermittent measurements may not always suffice, and continuous monitoring may be necessary.

ECG

The electrocardiogram can provide information on the following:

- the site of the pacemaker and the nature of cardiac rhythm
- disorders of conduction or excitation
- the size and muscle mass of the heart
- the viability and state of metabolism of the heart.

Crucially the ECG does not provide evidence of adequate (or inadequate) filling of the circulation: for example, a tachycardia sometimes combined with ST segment changes can imply hypovolaemia, but both these changes may occur in left ventricular failure.

For continuous monitoring purposes, an ECG is generally configured in the CM_5 configuration (leads are placed on the manubrium, left shoulder and 5th space midclavicular line), roughly equivalent to V_5 where 90% of ischaemic episodes can be detected by the observation of ST segment depression. (See Figures 9.33, 9.34 and 9.35.) A fuller account of the ECG follows on page 248.

Blood pressure

This should be measured at regular intervals. Where rapid changes in blood pressure are expected, or regular monitoring of blood gases is required, it is sensible to use an arterial line. Further information can be deduced from continuous observation of the pressure trace:

- The rate of pressure increase (up-slope) is proportional to myocardial contractility.

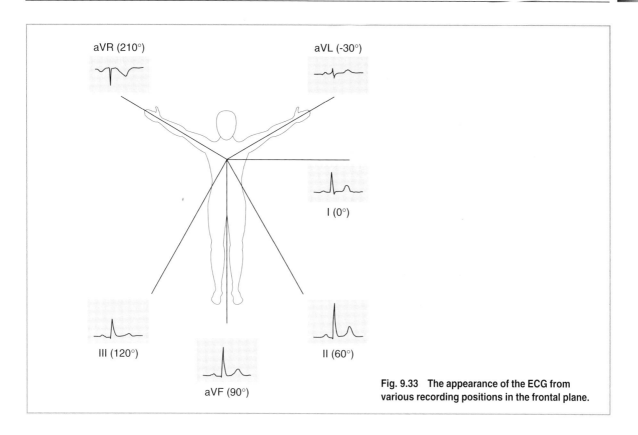

aVR (210°)

aVL (-30°)

I (0°)

III (120°)

aVF (90°)

II (60°)

Fig. 9.33 The appearance of the ECG from various recording positions in the frontal plane.

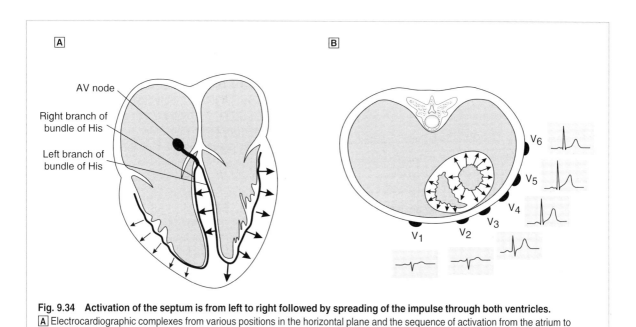

A

B

AV node

Right branch of bundle of His

Left branch of bundle of His

V6
V5
V4
V3
V2
V1

Fig. 9.34 Activation of the septum is from left to right followed by spreading of the impulse through both ventricles.
A Electrocardiographic complexes from various positions in the horizontal plane and the sequence of activation from the atrium to ventricles B.

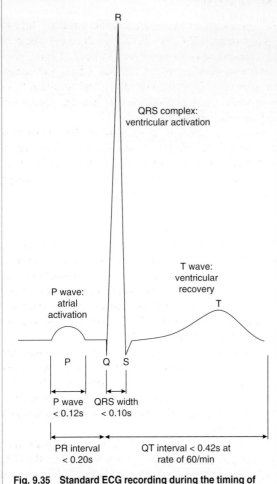

QRS complex:
ventricular activation

T wave:
ventricular
recovery

P wave:
atrial
activation

R

P

Q   S

T

P wave
< 0.12s

QRS width
< 0.10s

PR interval
< 0.20s

QT interval < 0.42s at
rate of 60/min

Fig. 9.35 Standard ECG recording during the timing of the various events.

• The area under the waveform is proportional to stroke volume.

The pulse oximeter

This measures saturation of haemoglobin with oxygen. It has rapidly established itself as an invaluable aid to managing seriously ill patients. It relies on measurement of the different absorption of oxyhaemoglobin and deoxy-haemoglobin at different wavelengths. The device emits pulses of infrared light at 940 nm, and 660 nm, every 10 μs. It then finds the points of maximum absorption (systole) and minimum absorption (diastole). The pulsatile component of absorption is measured, and from this is subtracted the constant component which is not due to arterial blood. The ratio of absorption at the two wavelengths is then compared with values obtained from an algorithm derived from experimental findings. The principle depends on oxygenated haemoglobin absorbing more infrared light at 940 nm than at 660 nm. The accuracy of these devices drifts down rapidly below 90% saturation since accurate calibration in healthy volunteers is not acceptable below this level. Low pressure, vaso-constriction, hypotension and venous pulsation can all interfere. Abnormal haemoglobins such as carboxy- and methaemoglobin and dyes such as methylene blue will all affect the pulsatile component and hence the accuracy of the algorithm used by the machine. Bilirubin gives falsely low readings, while carboxyhaemoglobin gives falsely high readings. Methaemoglobin has similar absorption at the two wavelengths and tends to show a consistent saturation of about 85%. Irregular pulse rhythms make prediction of maximum and minimum absorption difficult. Other factors that detrimentally affect performance are nail varnish, flickering lights, electrical interference (e.g. diathermy) and patient movement.

Urinary output

This is directly related to renal perfusion and should be monitored in all critically ill patients. A minimum flow of 0.5 mL/kg/h is essential.

Central venous pressure

It has already been mentioned that the monitoring of the CVP simply by inspection of the neck can give information regarding the state of the circulation and more specifically the right ventricular end diastolic pressure. Where continuous monitoring is required, there is no substitute for a transduced catheter with an oscilloscopic display.

For such a system to be of any use, then, two factors must be borne in mind. Firstly, the absolute value of the CVP is not useful in isolation; rather more important is the response to a fluid challenge. Secondly, the value of the CVP will depend on the patient's posture, and must be standardised for the readings to have any meaning: i.e. it should always be measured with the patient in the same posture — at, say, 45° or supine.

Why are isolated values of the CVP of little use? Firstly, because there is a degree of individual variation in the condition of the heart. Secondly, because even in the presence of severe hypovolaemia, some patients can compensate to a remarkable degree with vasoconstriction — so much so that the CVP can actually become transiently elevated. This is especially true in the young, fit subject. In such patients, continuous readings of the CVP during small and rapid infusions of fluid, will often reveal a decreasing CVP as vasoconstriction declines.

In patients with a failing heart, rapid boluses of fluid further elevate the CVP and may worsen cardiac failure.

There is another reason why isolated CVP readings may be unhelpful. There can be a marked disparity between the function of the left and right ventricles; indeed, one can fail independently of the other. Pulmonary vascular disease may render the CVP a very poor guide to filling pressures of the left heart. In such cases it may be useful to measure the left ventricular end diastolic pressure (LVEDP) or more accurately the pulmonary capillary wedge pressure (PCWP) from which the left atrial pressure can be inferred.

Pulmonary capillary wedge pressure

This measurement is essentially the 'CVP of the left heart'. Information obtained from its value needs to be interpreted in the same way, i.e. by continuous measurement in the light of fluid challenges and other measurable parameters. The principle is to pass a flotation balloon-tipped catheter (PA catheter) through the right heart into a pulmonary artery. Once inserted, inflation of the balloon occludes the flow from the right, allowing a fluid bridge to complete the connection to the left atrium. The pressure at the tip of the catheter at this stage will be the same as in the left atrium and thus will be closely related to left ventricular filling pressure. The normal PCWP is 6–12 mmHg and should usually be kept below 15 mmHg to minimise the risk of pulmonary oedema.

The major advantage of the catheter is that the measurement of cardiac output becomes possible.

Cardiac output

Again this can be useful as *part* of an overall assessment of the circulation. By injecting dye down a proximal orifice in the PA catheter and measuring its concentration against time at the distal end of the catheter, the cardiac output can be derived. In practice a temperature dilution technique is used today, with cold glucose solution injected proximally. The temperature change is measured distally by a thermistor. Computerised integration of the temperature curve can provide an instantaneous derivation of the cardiac output.

Once the cardiac output is known, then it is possible to derive values for the resistance of the circulation, the amount of work that the heart is performing, and oxygen delivery and oxygen consumption. Specific pharmacological therapy can then be given to optimise the circulation.

In the future it is increasingly likely that non-invasive measurements using ultrasound will provide for a detailed assessment of the circulation without the need for PA catheters.

CARDIAC ARREST

The term cardiac arrest refers to the complete loss of cardiac output. This may be due to abnormal electrical conduction within the heart (ventricular fibrillation, asystole) or to sudden loss of venous return (pulmonary embolus or shock). The loss of cerebral perfusion leads to immediate loss of consciousness and the cessation of respiration. There is no pulse.

Without a supply of oxygen the tissues switch over to anaerobic respiration. There is a rapid build up of acid metabolites that further depress myocardial contractility. At normal temperatures the brain cells undergo irreversible damage within 3 min.

Causes of cardiac arrest

The commonest cause of cardiac arrest in adults is ischaemic heart disease. A much smaller subgroup develops cardiac arrest as a result of special circumstances such as drug overdose, trauma, or hypothermia. Cardiac arrest can be subdivided into three common distinct scenarios: ventricular fibrillation (VF), asystole, and electromechanical dissociation (EMD).

Ventricular fibrillation This is the commonest and most easily treatable form of arrest. It is usually caused by myocardial infarction, but can also be caused by hyperkalaemia and electric shock. The rapid uncoordinated contractions of the ventricle produce no output but fortunately consume little oxygen.

Asystole This is fortunately less common. It carries a much graver prognosis and is characterised by a flat ECG indicative of absent electrical activity. A disconnected monitor may also cause this.

Electromechanical dissociation This also carries a poor prognosis but may occasionally indicate a remedial cause that must be excluded (e.g. severe hypovolaemia). The heart continues to produce electrical activity, indicative of contractions, but there is no discernible output.

Treatment of cardiac arrest

The treatment of cardiac arrest involves two distinct principles: restoration of the flow of oxygenated blood to the brain as soon as possible, and treatment of the underlying cause.

Restoration of oxygenated blood flow requires cardiac compression and decompression, while oxygenation of the blood requires inflation and deflation of the lungs.

External cardiac compression

This has been shown to be reasonably effective in producing a cardiac output but, even in expert hands, will not produce a cerebral perfusion greater than 30% of normal. A suitably hard mattress (or the floor) will be required. Effective compressions of the lower sternum will prolong survival time provided that blood is oxygenated. The rate depends on the size of the patient and varies from 60 to 100 compressions/min. The term cardiac compression is a simplification. Echocardiography studies have shown that all the heart valves are incompetent during resuscitation. It is thoracic compression that propels blood out of the thorax. Forward blood flow occurs because the veins at the thoracic inlet collapse during compression, while arteries remain patent. It has also been shown that the simple act of coughing can produce a life-sustaining circulation.

Inflation of the lungs

This can be achieved with expired air (mouth to mouth) but this contains only about 18% oxygen. The lungs are much better inflated with 100% oxygen from a suitable device (e.g. an Ambu bag). It has been shown that cardiac outputs are potentially higher in the intubated subject, because the increased airway pressure results in more blood being forced into the left heart from the pulmonary circulation.

Defibrillation

This is the depolarisation of the myocardium by the passage of direct electric current and is required when the ventricles are fibrillating. This is the single most treatable cause of cardiac arrest, and so delay must not be allowed (for every 1 min delay, survival rates decrease by 2–7%). If a sufficient mass of myocardium is depolarised, then defibrillation will be successful. This depends on the current passed through the muscle (amperes) not the total energy of the shock (joules). This will depend on transthoracic impedance, skin resistance, body size, electrode position and the energy of the shock. Excessive shocks may damage the myocardium, while too small a shock will not depolarise sufficient myocardium. 200 joules is the usual starting point for an adult.

Electrode position is only important inasmuch as it reflects the current passed through the heart. The best position is right of the upper sternum and 5th left intercostal space in the midclavicular line. An alternative is to place one electrode in front of the heart and one behind. This is ideal for defibrillation but interrupts cardiac massage.

Electric shock will not only treat VF but will also convert atrial or ventricular dysrhythmias when applied to coincide with the R wave of the ECG. This is called synchronised defibrillation. This can be achieved automatically with some machines. It is essential that the shock does not fall on the T-wave (part of the relative refractory period), which will result in VF.

Other forms of cardiac arrest carry a grave prognosis and depend upon the diagnosis of a treatable cause. The UK Resuscitation Council now publishes a single algorithm for the treatment of cardiac arrest, and this is reproduced in Figure 9.36.

CARDIAC FUNCTION TESTS

There are times when it is necessary to derive specific diagnostic information about the heart: for example, to estimate the degree of failure of a ventricle, or of stenosis of a valve. These tests can be divided into invasive and non-invasive.

Electrocardiography

The ECG is used to elucidate problems with the conduction system, such as arrhythmias, and to diagnose myocardial hypertrophy, ischaemia and infarction. The principle on which the ECG is based is that the depolarisation of the myocardium can be measured from the surface, and when amplified can be displayed on an oscilloscope or a printed trace (see Figs 9.33, 9.34, 9.35). Twelve leads are commonly used so that the heart can be 'looked at' from every angle. The six standard or limb leads (aVR, aVL, I, II, aVF and III) look at the heart from the sides or the feet. The chest leads (V1–6) look at the heart from the front (horizontal) plane. Thus V1–2 view the right ventricle, V3–4 the septum and V5–6 the left ventricle.

As the myocardium depolarises, beginning at the SA node, through the atria to the AV node and then down the bundle of His, it does so along a coronal axis which runs from 11 o'clock to 5 o'clock. Those leads which look at the heart from the patient's right will see an overall negative deflection (e.g. aVR), whilst those looking from the left will see an overall positive deflection (e.g. lead II). This axis may change if, for example, the left ventricle becomes hypertrophied and the greater bulk of the electrical depolarisation moves away from lead II towards lead I.

Although an ECG may suggest the presence of ischaemia, there may be no evidence of this at rest. Exercising the heart may provoke ECG changes that reflect ischaemia. The ST segment becomes depressed as workload increases and it is said to be significant if > 1 mm.

Some patients require continuous ambulatory monitoring in order to detect episodic ischaemia, and this is usually referred to as Holter monitoring.

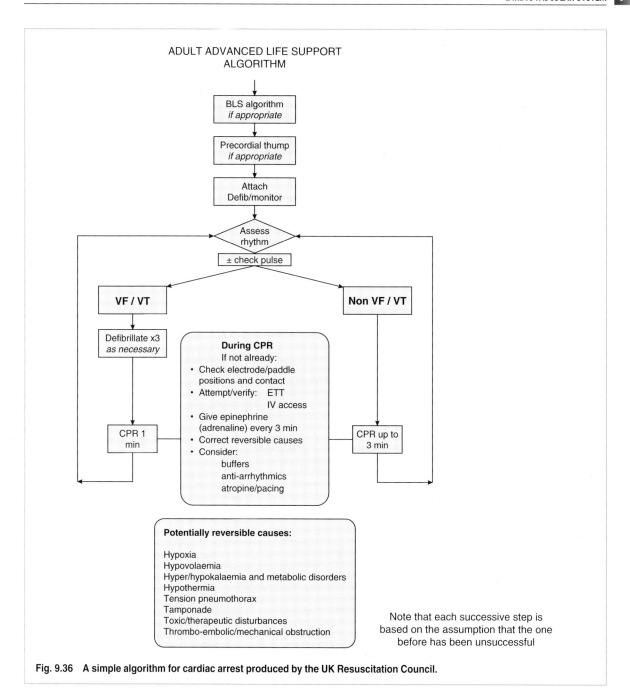

ADULT ADVANCED LIFE SUPPORT
ALGORITHM

BLS algorithm
if appropriate

Precordial thump
if appropriate

Attach
Defib/monitor

Assess
rhythm

± check pulse

VF / VT

Non VF / VT

Defibrillate x3
as necessary

During CPR
If not already:
• Check electrode/paddle
  positions and contact
• Attempt/verify: ETT
                     IV access
• Give epinephrine
  (adrenaline) every 3 min
• Correct reversible causes
• Consider:
      buffers
      anti-arrhythmics
      atropine/pacing

CPR 1
min

CPR up to
3 min

Potentially reversible causes:

Hypoxia
Hypovolaemia
Hyper/hypokalaemia and metabolic disorders
Hypothermia
Tension pneumothorax
Tamponade
Toxic/therapeutic disturbances
Thrombo-embolic/mechanical obstruction

Note that each successive step is
based on the assumption that the one
before has been unsuccessful

Fig. 9.36   A simple algorithm for cardiac arrest produced by the UK Resuscitation Council.

Echocardiography

Information about the structure of the heart, integrity of the valves, blood flow and movement of the myocardium can be detected by use of reflected sound.

There are several types of analysis, and it is possible to visualise heart movement in real time. Using Doppler techniques it is possible to estimate the ejection fraction of the left ventricle and pressure gradients across the valves.

Cardiac catheterisation

The insertion of a catheter from a peripheral vein or artery into the heart under radiographic control permits very accurate measurement of pressures within the heart. It also permits the analysis of blood samples for oxygen saturation in left-to-right or right-to-left shunts. The injection of radio-opaque dye can reveal information about the state of the coronary arteries.

Radio-isotopic scanning

This method relies on the detection of gamma radiation as it is emitted from radionuclides as they pass through the heart. The advantage of this technique is that it is non-invasive and therefore safe. There are two methods used. One relies on the circulating blood containing the isotope being repeatedly imaged as it passes through the heart (blood pool scanning). The other technique uses the different rates of absorption of thallium by ischaemic and non-ischaemic myocardium to demonstrate inadequately-perfused areas of the heart.

CARDIAC SUPPORT

It may be necessary to support the heart and circulation for a variety of reasons. These can be classified into situations where the heart itself is failing (e.g. cardiogenic shock) and situations in which the heart is unable to meet the extra demands made upon it by changes in the requirements of the peripheral circulation (e.g. septic shock).

The goal of support is to enable the heart to meet the needs of the circulation, without increasing workload to the point at which the oxygen demand of the myocardium exceeds its supply. In order to achieve this it may be necessary to use invasive monitoring techniques described above in addition to intensive pharmacological manipulation. As a final resort, the use of a mechanical support device may be required.

Pharmacological support

In general there are three types of agent used: inotropes, vasoconstrictors and vasodilators. Many of the drugs used have more than one of these properties (Table 9.4). Most have very short half-lives and so must be given by a reliable infusion method.

Dopamine

This is a stimulant of dopaminergic receptors at low doses (< 4 μg/kg/min). Stimulation of these receptors results in an increase in renal blood flow, glomerular filtration rate (GFR) and sodium excretion. As the dose increases, β_1 receptors are also stimulated, resulting in an increased heart rate and contractility. Even higher doses (> 10 μg/kg/min) stimulate α_1 receptors, which may result in decreased tissue perfusion (and GFR) despite a higher blood pressure. About 50% of the action of dopamine is mediated by the release of noradrenaline from nerve terminals.

Dobutamine

This is a β_1 (and to a lesser extent β_2) agonist and a synthetic derivative of isoprenaline. Doses of 2.5 μg/kg/min and above result in an increased heart rate, contractility, cardiac output and coronary blood flow combined with afterload reduction. At higher doses the tachycardia may well result in a disadvantageous effect on the myocardial oxygen supply/demand ratio and limit therapy. Its main advantage over isoprenaline is that it causes less tachycardia and it does not cause the release of noradrenaline.

Adrenaline

This has both α and β effects. It is used mainly as a bronchodilator and in the treatment of acute anaphylactic reactions. It has a great potential for causing arrhythmias and so must be infused with caution. This propensity to cause arrhythmias is put to use in cardiac arrest situations where it can be used to provoke ventricular fibrillation, which may then respond to DC shock.

The effect of an infusion of adrenaline depends on the dose. Adrenaline is most effective on α_1 receptors, which are vasodilatory and found mainly in skeletal muscle.

Table 9.4	The effects of various inotropes on cardiovascular receptors					
Receptor	Dopamine	Dobutamine	Adrenaline	Noradrenaline	Isoprenaline	Effect
α_1	++	−	++	+++	−	Vasoconstriction
α_2	+	−	++	+++	−	Vasoconstriction
β_1	+	+++	+++	++	+++	Increased cardiac rate and force
β_2	−	+	+++	+	+++	Vasodilatation
D_1	+++	−	−	−	−	Renal and splanchnic vasodilatation
D_2	++	−	−	−	−	Suppression of release of noradrenaline

However, as the dose increases, effects become more pronounced, increasing cardiac output and TPR. Unfortunately vasoconstriction is most pronounced in the skin and kidneys and can lead to acute renal failure. The combination of vasodilatation in the muscle beds and vasoconstriction elsewhere leads to a characteristic widening of the pulse pressure (systolic blood pressure increased more than diastolic). Because of its effect on renal blood flow the role of adrenaline in circulatory support is reserved for refractory hypotension with a low peripheral vascular resistance.

Noradrenaline

This is a powerful α_1 stimulant (although it does increase myocardial contractility). Infusions result in vasoconstriction and an increase in TPR with increased systolic and diastolic blood pressure. Renal blood flow declines with increasing infusion rates. Cardiac output is unchanged or decreased, but an increased workload results in a higher oxygen demand. Its use is largely restricted to the treatment of shock where there is a very low peripheral vascular resistance (e.g. sepsis).

Isoprenaline

This is exclusively a β stimulant affecting receptors of the heart, bronchi, skeletal muscle and gut vasculature. Infusion of isoprenaline reduces TPR by vasodilatation in skeletal muscle, kidney and mesentery. It has positive inotropic and chronotropic actions and produces an increased cardiac output. Tachycardia limits the clinical use of isoprenaline.

Nitrates

These can be used where vasodilatation may be required: e.g. pulmonary oedema or left heart failure. The principle is to reduce TPR and to venodilate, reducing afterload and preload respectively. Nitrates are predominantly venodilators. Where arterial vasodilatation is required (reduced afterload) hydralazine may be used. Close supervision and monitoring of the circulation, e.g. with arterial lines, CVP, PCWP and cardiac output measurement, are often required.

Phosphodiesterase inhibitors

These work by decreasing the rate of breakdown of cAMP by phosphodiesterase III (conversely β stimulation increases production of cAMP). The effect is to increase myocardial contractility. Amrinone is a potent inotrope with marked vasodilator effects that reduce SVR and PVR with reductions in afterload to the left and right heart. It has little chronotropic effect, but may cause significant hypotension.

The choice of inotrope or vasodilator depends on the nature and severity of the problem, and any underlying complication such as ischaemic heart disease. It may become necessary to perform repeated assessments of the circulation using pressure and cardiac output measurements to calculate TPR and myocardial workload (see above). The practitioner must not lose sight of more basic clinical observations such as urine output and skin temperature in all of this.

Circulatory assist devices

At the present time the role of mechanical devices in augmenting (or completely generating) cardiac output is restricted to temporary support preceding or following cardiac surgery. This will change in the near future as technology advances.

Ventricular assist devices can be used to increase the output and decrease the workload of the heart. The most commonly used device today, however, is the intra-aortic balloon counter-pulsation device. This is inserted into the femoral artery until it resides in the descending aorta. The balloon is rapidly inflated during diastole to increase coronary and cerebral blood flow. It is deflated during systole, decreasing afterload and increasing the ejection fraction of the left ventricle.

Cardiopulmonary bypass

Cardiopulmonary bypass (CPB) is a complex subject, which could easily occupy an entire chapter on its own. There are several systems in use today, most commonly for cardiac surgery, but also as a last resort in respiratory failure, where it has enjoyed good success in neonates.

Two basic types of oxygenators are used: *bubble oxygenators* and *membrane oxygenators*. The former work by bubbling gas into blood directly, whilst the latter, as their name suggests, use a membrane to separate oxygen from blood. Bubble oxygenators are cheaper but cause a greater degree of turbulence and foaming which disrupts blood cells. With prolonged CPB this could be disadvantageous.

The damage to blood cells during CPB is an inherent part of the technique, necessitating the use of filters on both the venous and arterial sides of the loop. These filters cause depletion of circulating platelets. In addition the risk of large and small air emboli is ever present.

Blood must be pumped around the system, and in most cases a non-occlusive roller pump is used to reduce trauma to the cells and to provide a pulsatile flow.

Technique

This consists of taking blood from a major vein, usually the vena cava, and pumping the arterialised blood back into the ascending aorta. In dire emergencies it is possible to institute CPB via the femoral artery and vein.

CPB can be total — that is, all blood is excluded from the cardiac chambers (e.g. for cardiac surgery) — or partial. In this case some venous blood is allowed to flow past the cannula to the right atrium. This can be useful in distending the heart to its normal size for estimating the length of a graft and to provide a degree of pulsatile flow. It also facilitates the washout of cardioplegic components from the coronary circulation. The existence of incompetent valves may require venting of the left ventricle (for example) to prevent undue distension. Indeed it is usual to monitor pulmonary artery pressures during bypass.

The extracorporeal circulation must be primed with a suitable solution prior to bypass, and it is vital that air is excluded at all times from the patient's circulation. A solution of heparinised balanced salts to which a colloid is added to make it of normal colloid osmotic pressure is the norm. Mannitol is sometimes added to produce a diuretic effect and act as a free radical scavenger. A low Hb or electrolyte deficit can be corrected by altering the final solution appropriately. Of all the additives the most critical by far is heparin, absence of which is invariably fatal. Its presence and correct level of activity must be checked throughout.

It is usual to institute hypothermia by means of a heat exchanger during CPB. This will increase the viscosity of blood but will allow a lower flow rate. There is no absolute agreement about the maintenance of blood pressure during CPD but, as a guide, a mean range of 50 to 100 mmHg is acceptable. Judicious use of vasopressors or dilators may be necessary. Too high a blood pressure may cause cerebral haemorrhage, too low will result in progressive metabolic acidosis and oliguria. The preservation of the myocardium is achieved with hypothermic CPB, and surface cooling with iced saline. The coronaries are perfused with cold cardioplegia solution (or by direct hypothermic perfusion from the CPB). The heart can be arrested for the duration of surgery by use of a hyperkalaemic cardioplegic solution to which mannitol is usually added. At the end of surgery this solution is washed out with oxygenated blood and the heart restarted with direct application of DC shock.

PATHOLOGY

ATHEROSCLEROSIS

Introduction

Atherosclerosis is by far the most common disorder leading to death and serious morbidity throughout the developed world and is responsible for more deaths than all forms of cancer. Although any artery in the body may be affected, the most frequently involved arteries are those to the heart and brain, leading to myocardial infarction and stroke. The aorta and the lower limb vessels are also commonly diseased, which may cause a variety of problems, including gangrene of the legs.

Definition

Because our understanding of its aetiology and pathogenesis is incomplete, it is difficult to define. The basic lesion is the fibro-fatty plaque in the intima of medium sized and large arteries. This consists of a core of tissue debris rich in lipids with a covering fibrous cap of connective tissue with varying degrees of cellular proliferation.

The word comes from the Greek word 'athere', meaning gruel or porridge, and 'sclerosis', meaning hardness! The atheromatous fatty core is 'porridge-like', but, with the passage of time, increasing fibrosis and calcification surrounding sclerosis results to a variable degree.

Lesions of atherosclerosis

Fatty streaks

These are common in the young, even infants, and consist of intracellular lipid deposits, mainly in smooth muscle and macrophages. They are seen initially in the aorta and subsequently in smaller arteries. At necropsy they appear to be slightly raised, subendothelial yellow streaks, but when the artery is distended, as in life, they do not cause any narrowing. They are thought to be precursors of atherosclerotic plaques, and yet there is indirect evidence that the fatty streak can resolve.

Gelatinous plaques

These are small, soft, blister-like elevations which are mainly translucent, but the central areas may be pale pink or grey. They occur commonly in the aorta and larger vessels. They have a high fluid content and twice as much albumin and four times the fibrinogen and lipoprotein content as the normal intima. As with the fatty streak, their relationship to subsequent atherosclerotic plaques remains unproven.

Fibro-lipid plaques

These are the characteristic lesions of atherosclerosis (Fig. 9.37). Most commonly they have a lipid rich core with overlying fibrous cap on the luminal surface. However, there is great variation: from the basal accumulation of lipid being very large with only a thin overlying layer, to the opposite extreme where the cellular and con-

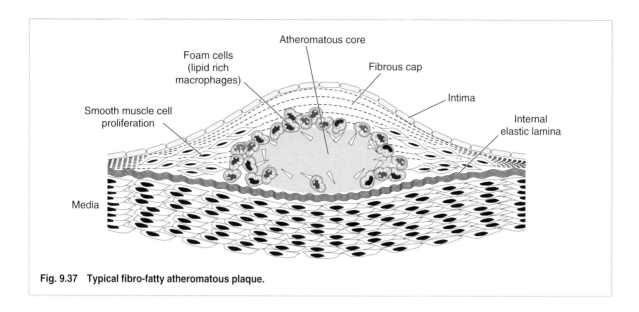

Fig. 9.37 Typical fibro-fatty atheromatous plaque.

nective tissue elements predominate. This gives a pearly white lesion which, if cut into, may have little or no lipid (fibrous plaque). The fibro-fatty plaque may cause the intima to be thicker than the media, which is frequently abnormally thin. This medial thinning may subsequently lead to aneurysm formation.

Plaques tend to be found at certain sites, but especially the lower abdominal aorta, coronary arteries, renal arteries, distal superficial femoral and popliteal, descending thoracic aorta, internal carotid and circle of Willis and internal iliac arteries. Other arteries tend to be spared, especially those to the upper limbs.

Microscopically, plaques have three components:

1. cells, mainly vascular smooth muscle cells (SMCs), macrophages and lymphocytes
2. connective tissue fibres of collagen, elastin and proteoglycans
3. lipids, mainly cholesterol and oxidised cholesterol in the form of low density lipoproteins. These are quite irritant and have been shown to cause severe inflammatory reactions in connective tissue and probably involve a similar response in the arterial wall, resulting in periarterial inflammation, fibrosis and lymphocyte infiltration.

It is interesting to note that fibrous plaques do not cause narrowing of the lumen until they are quite thick; it has been shown in vivo that coronary plaques must occupy 40% of the arterial wall before they can be detected radiologically.

Complicated plaques

The typical fibro-lipid plaque may undergo several complications, mainly as late developments, as follows.

1. Rupturing or ulceration of the luminal surface may occur. This may result in the fatty part discharging into the blood stream as so called 'cholesterol emboli'.
2. Thrombosis may occur over ulcerated or fissured plaques, which may extend, leading to arterial occlusion, particularly in the coronary circulation.
3. Haemorrhage may occur into a plaque because of breakdown of the overlying fibrous cap. This may balloon the plaque, narrowing the lumen or leading to its rupture.
4. Calcification frequently occurs, which may be patchy or extensive.
5. Extensive necrosis of the plaque may occur, which may also cause embolism of plaque material and may leave large areas of ulceration.
6. There may be thinning and weakening of the media, with associated loss of elastic tissue, which may result in aneurysmal dilatation.

Risk factors

Constitutional factors

There are four constitutional factors which play a part: age, sex, familial tendency and race.

Age This is the strongest and most constant factor associated with atherosclerosis. The risk of myocardial infarction, and especially stroke, increases with each decade right up to advanced age.

Sex Males are more prone to atherosclerosis, while females appear to be protected by their hormones until after the menopause, except in diabetics. With advancing age the difference gradually diminishes until the incidence becomes the same in both sexes by the seventh to eighth decades.

Familial tendency The definition of a positive family history is when a first degree relative develops vascular symptoms before the age of 50 in the absence of major risk factors such as smoking and hypertension. Thus it implies a true genetic predisposition.

Race Although there is wide geographical racial variation in the incidence of atherosclerosis, this seems to lose its effect in immigrant populations. They seem to acquire a risk for atherosclerosis more similar to that of the host population than that of the country from whence they came.

Acquired (correctable) risk factors

There are at least a hundred different clinical or biochemical 'risk factors' that have been associated with atherosclerotic vascular disease. These range from major risk factors such as smoking, hypertension, diabetes and raised cholesterol to minor risk factors such as type A personality, waist–hip ratio, plasma fibrinogen, plasma insulin levels and various lipoprotein subfractions. A risk factor is identified when population studies show a relationship between a marker, such as plasma cholesterol, and the incidence of coronary heart disease (CHD) or stroke. The largest study to identify a clear relationship between plasma cholesterol and coronary heart disease was the American Multiple Risk Factor Intervention Trial (MRFIT). Similar epidemiological data from the Framingham study showed a linear relationship between blood pressure and CHD.

Such epidemiological studies identify 'risk factors', but these data alone do not provide evidence that intervention to lower the risk factor will necessarily reduce CHD. For example, lowering cholesterol in isolation may be ineffective if numerous other risk factors are not addressed simultaneously. Observational studies provide hypotheses upon which intervention trials are based. Large intervention trials were undertaken in the 1970s and 1980s which demonstrated that a small sustained reduction in diastolic blood pressure of only 6 mmHg produces a 40% reduction in the incidence of stroke and a 10–15% reduction in CHD mortality. Effective drug therapy of hyperlipidaemia with statins (e.g. simvastatin and pravastatin) have only been available for the last 10

years. Recent trials have shown considerable benefits, especially in the form of secondary prevention for patients who already have vascular symptoms.

Thus a working clinical definition of a correctable risk factor is 'that level of blood pressure or cholesterol above which treatment has been shown to do more good than harm'. For continuous variables, such as blood pressure and cholesterol, intervention trials have set the cut-off point for routine intervention. The level of cholesterol above which treatment is indicated depends upon the clinical context of the individual patient. In premenopausal women, with no previous vascular disease or associated risk factor, cholesterol levels of 8 mmol/L would not require drug treatment, based on present evidence. In contrast, a male with a previous myocardial infarction and other risk factors of atherosclerosis would merit intervention at cholesterol levels greater than 5.5 mmol/L.

In the case of cholesterol-lowering trials, the cost–benefit ratio is strongly in favour of secondary prevention rather than primary. Secondary prevention is treatment of patients with existing symptomatic vascular disease, whereas primary prevention involves treatment of asymptomatic (albeit high risk) individuals.

These risk factors are described in more detail below.

Smoking There is a strong correlation between cigarette smoking and occlusive arterial disease of both the coronary arteries and those to the lower limbs. British data show that middle aged men who smoke have three times the risk of dying from coronary artery disease, and that the risk increases with the number smoked and is reduced in those who give up.

The precise way in which smoking causes damage is still not known for sure, but smoking causes endothelial changes, can reduce the production of prostaglandins, impair vasodilatation, increase the level of low density lipoproteins (LDL), and increase platelet aggregation. The problem of finding the mechanism of damage of cigarette smoking is complicated by the fact that approximately four thousand chemical compounds can be found in cigarette smoke!

Hypertension High blood pressure is a major risk factor for atherosclerosis at all ages and is associated with an increased risk of death from coronary and cerebrovascular disease. It would appear to be the actual level of blood pressure that causes the damage rather than any other factor: in coaractation of the aorta, atherosclerosis develops in the high pressure vessels proximal to the stenosis, but not distally; and, in the rare congenital anomaly in which the left coronary artery arises from the pulmonary artery, atherosclerosis, develops in the right coronary artery but not the left.

Diabetes This is a powerful risk factor which increases the risk of myocardial infarction five times, the risk of amputation of the lower limb 25 times and of blindness 40 times. The pattern of arterial disease is different in diabetes, tending to involve the infrageniculate arteries (although the foot vessels are often spared, which may have implications for limb salvage procedures). Diabetics tend to have higher levels of low density lipoproteins (LDL) and triglycerides (TGs) and lower levels of high density lipoproteins (HDL). Diabetics have also been shown to have endothelial dysfunction. These factors together are the major cause of premature vascular disease in diabetic patients.

Diminished sensation with impaired autonomic function and vasomotor control and loss of pain reflex along with blunted inflammatory response and altered capillary dynamics may mean that relatively moderate ischaemia is poorly tolerated.

Hyperlipidaemia There are essentially five important lipoproteins in the body, as follows.

1. Chylomicrons are only found in plasma after a fatty meal and are composed mainly of triglycerides.
2. Very low density lipoproteins (VLDL) mainly transport triglycerides and some cholesterol from the liver.
3. Intermediate density lipoproteins (IDL) are transient and derived from VLDL after it has been acted on by lipase.
4. Low density lipoproteins are derived from VLDL via the intermediate IDL. The level of LDL in the plasma is most strongly correlated with the development of atherosclerosis. LDL plays an important part in the transport of endogenous cholesterol *into* body cells. In the presence of activated monocytes and endothelial cells, free radicals oxidise LDL. Oxidised LDL is itself toxic to endothelial cells, which compounds the endothelial injury; it is also chemotactic to monocytes and immobilises macrophages, which, along with smooth muscle cells, take it up preferentially. Thus oxidised LDL makes up the greater part of the lipid content of atheroma. There is both theoretical and some experimental evidence to suggest that anti-oxidants may inhibit the formation of atherosclerosis and cause some reduction of lesions already present.
5. High density lipoproteins. There is an inverse relationship between the level of HDL and symptomatic atherosclerosis. This is because HDL is involved in a 'reverse transport' of cholesterol *from* cells and tissues to the blood stream, and then to the liver, where it is converted to free cholesterol. This is excreted in the bile, converted to bile acids or re-incorporated into plasma lipoproteins. Thus the higher the level of HDL the better ('high helps!').

It should be noted that these 'risk factors' simply increase the likelihood of atherosclerosis, but a small proportion of individuals develop ischaemic heart disease or strokes in the absence of any of these risk factors. However, the Framingham study shows that the possession of:

- one of the four major risk factors doubles your chance of a heart attack
- two major risk factors quadruples the likelihood
- three risk factors increases the risk seven-fold.

Pathogenesis

With atherosclerosis being such a common and lethal disease an enormous amount of research has been done, which has resulted in numerous claims as to the cause. Theories of the pathogenesis need to account for:

- the focal nature of the lesions
- the place of risk factors in causation, especially hyperlipidaemia
- the presence of lipids in most lesions
- smooth muscle proliferation which is both an early and characteristic feature of atherosclerosis (AS).

The various theories of pathogenesis are as follows.

1. *Response to injury.* This may occur from chronic or repeated endothelial injury such as endotoxins, carbon monoxide or other chemicals from cigarette smoke, viruses and other substances such as homocysteine (which causes premature AS in homocysteineurics). However, the shear stress and turbulence resulting from haemodynamic disturbances in the complex branching arterial system is a more likely cause, probably in combination with other factors. These mechanical effects are likely to be exaggerated by hypertension.
2. *Increased permeability to lipids.* The endothelial damage results in increased permeability, so that there is an increase in lipid absorption into the intima.
3. *Raised lipids.* This increased lipid absorption is more likely in hyperlipidaemia, and the LDL is likely to be oxidised by free radicals at the site of injury where they are absorbed into the intima. Oxidised LDL is itself toxic to endothelial cells and attracts monocytes and macrophages.
4. *Smooth muscle proliferation.* Monocytes migrate subendothelially, where they become macrophages, absorb oxidised LDL and become foam cells. Smooth muscle cells, mainly from the media, migrate to these areas and thereafter take up lipids. These smooth

muscle cells tend to proliferate under the influence of growth factors, in particular platelet-derived growth factor (PGDF) which may come from platelets themselves, but also from macrophages. This then is the beginning of the fibrous plaque, which may grow and undergo the complications previously described on page 253.

5. *Thrombogenic theory*. This is that plaques arise from mural thrombi formed at sites of endothelial injury, with subsequent organisation and re-endothelialisation. While it is unlikely that this is how atheromatous plaques first develop, it does almost certainly play a part in the growth and development of plaques which are already present, particularly when they are ulcerated.

Platelets in health and disease

So far, platelets have barely been mentioned, and yet they play a very important role in the progression of atherosclerosis. They are formed from megakaryocytes (*mega*, large; *karyo,* nucleus) in the bone marrow. Each megakaryocyte can produce about three thousand platelets, which are actually released from circulating megakaryocytes in the lung. Platelets are discoid, measuring 2–4 μm (i.e. a quarter to a half the size of red cells), and when quiescent they have a lifespan of 7–10 days. They have numerous surface pores which connect with a canalicular system and serve to increase the surface area. The platelet membrane has glycoproteins which act as receptors that assist in adhesion, and phospholipids which interact with coagulation factors.

Platelets have a key role in haemostasis and interact with the blood vessel wall, other platelets and the coagulation proteins. They can change shape and put out pseudopodia, which is part of the process of platelet activation and helps with adhesion. They have no nucleus but they do have granules and lysosomes and can produce enzymes, adhesive proteins, growth factor and coagulation factors.

Adhesion

Adhesion is the platelets' first response to vessel injury. When the subendothelial surface is exposed, platelets adhere, especially to the collagen, but not, at this stage, to each other.

Change of shape

With a strong stimulus (agonist) such as thrombin, collagen, trypsin or the slightly weaker stimuli such as thromboxane A, adrenaline or platelet-activating factor, platelets can change shape to an irregular surface and put out pseudopodia. If the stimulus is strong enough, aggregation and secretion will ensue; if not, the platelets can revert back to the normal discoid shape.

Aggregation

In the normal resting phase, platelets do not interact with each other. Stimulation by the agonists already mentioned causes platelets to stick together. This aggregation uses energy and fibrinogen and calcium. There are two phases of aggregation:

- primary aggregation — the platelet aggregates are small and, if the agonist is weak or dilute, they can break up again.
- secondary aggregation — the aggregates are larger and are associated with secretion from the platelets.

Secretion (release action)

This marks the final phase of platelet activation and accompanies secondary aggregation; it consists of the extrusion of the contents of the storage organelles. It usually starts because of the presence of thromboxane, although thrombin can also initiate the process. Secretion includes four platelet specific proteins, including platelet-derived growth factor (PDGF). This is chemotactic for connective tissue cells such as fibroblasts and smooth muscle cells, and its mitogenic influence causes cell doubling in 36 h. The concentrations of PDGF required for chemotaxis vary between neutrophils, monocytes and fibroblasts, resulting in an orderly sequence of cellular infiltration into a wound, according to the concentration gradients.

Inhibition of platelet activation

There are a number of substances that inhibit platelet activation by raising intracellular cyclic AMP; these include papaverine, dipyridamole and several prostaglandins. Aspirin and to a lesser extent NSAIDs prevent platelet aggregation (but not adhesion) by inhibiting platelet cyclo-oxygenase which prevents the conversion of arachidonic acid to thromboxane. These effects are irreversible for the life of each platelet (7–10 days).

In summary, platelets, by adhering to the site of vascular injury, focus and localise the coagulation mechanism where it is needed. However, where they adhere and aggregate at atherosclerotic plaques, they may exacerbate the process by stimulating the proliferation of smooth muscle cells.

Alcohol

In moderation (1–2 units per day) alcohol has been shown to reduce the incidence of CHD. This is thought to be predominantly by inhibiting platelet aggregation in a similar way to aspirin. There is some evidence that it may also be associated with higher levels of HDL, though this is controversial. There is some evidence that it may also inhibit the oxidation of LDL. Red wine is thought to be more effective in these two aspects than other forms of alcohol, though this too is controversial and may be associated with other aspects of the lifestyle of wine drinkers, especially those in Mediterranean countries. However, consumption of larger doses of alcohol increases the risk of coronary artery disease, probably because the increased calorie intake causes a rise in lipids, in addition to all the other harmful effects that it may have on the liver and pancreas!

ISCHAEMIC HEART DISEASE

Introduction
Ischaemic heart disease (IHD) is the term used for several closely related conditions where the supply of oxygenated blood to the heart is inadequate. In the vast majority, atherosclerotic narrowing of the coronary arteries is the main cause, although it may be aggravated by increased demand due to ventricular hypertrophy or impaired oxygen transport, as in severe anaemia, advanced lung disease and carbon monoxide poisoning.

Four ischaemic syndromes may result, depending on the severity and speed of onset:

1. stable angina
2. acute coronary syndromes (unstable angina and acute myocardial infarction)
3. sudden cardiac death
4. ischaemic cardiomyopathy.

Incidence
Ischaemic heart disease remains the principal cause of death in the developed world and accounts for the consumption of vast economic health care resources. Coronary atherosclerosis accounts for 1.5 million heart attacks per year in the United States of America and approximately half a million of these will result in death. Mortality from coronary heart disease is high in the United Kingdom when compared with other European countries. The highest rates are in Scotland where, for men aged between 35 and 65, the mortality is 30–40% higher than in England. In 1997 nearly four thousand men and women in Scotland died from coronary heart disease before reaching the age of 65.

Pathogenesis
This is the same as that for atherosclerosis and its complications (p. 252). The vast majority of patients with stable angina have stenoses of 70% or more of one, two or three of their major coronary vessels. However, most patients who develop an acute myocardial infarction have plaques which are causing 40–50% narrowing of the lumen,

which develop plaque fissuring or rupture with secondary thrombosis leading to coronary occlusion. Bleeding may occur into the soft lipid centre with rapid platelet aggregation and the formation of a 'dumb-bell' shaped thrombus. This may be non-occlusive, causing crescendo angina, or occlusive, resulting in myocardial infarction. The fragmented plaque may heal with no increase in the stenosis, or it may leave a residual tight stenosis, or recanalisation of a complete occlusion may subsequently occur.

It would be very useful to know what causes the fissuring of the fibrous cap of the plaque which allows the process to start. At present this is not known, though matrix metalloproteases have been suggested.

Haemodynamic factors such as hypotension following haemorrhage, spinal anaesthesia, or operation may result in reduced coronary blood flow, especially where there is pre-existing atheroma.

Clinical varieties of ischaemic heart disease

Angina of effort
This is characterised by central chest pain, which may radiate, most commonly down the left arm. It is caused by a shortage of oxygenated blood supplying the heart muscle, due to increased demand during exercise, in the presence of narrowed coronary arteries, perhaps accompanied by spasm of these vessels at times of stress.

Acute coronary syndromes (unstable angina and acute myocardial infarction)
Acute myocardial infarction is the leading cause of death in the developed world. 60% of all deaths in males over the age of 50 are due to this cause. It is the most important clinical challenge in affluent societies.

Myocardial infarction may be subendocardial or transmural.

- *Subendocardial (partial thickness or non-Q-wave infarct).* The inner third of the heart muscle is the least well perfused and therefore more vulnerable to reduced coronary flow. In subendocardial infarct, although there is usually diffuse coronary atherosclerosis, there is less commonly superimposed thrombosis. Frequently there are S-T/T wave changes but no Q wave.
- *Transmural infarction (full thickness or Q-wave infarct).* This is more common and more serious and usually involves the left ventricle. This is the variety of infarction that may follow disruption of a plaque with superimposed thrombosis. The platelet activation and aggregation responsible for this may be reduced if the patient is on antiplatelet drugs such as aspirin. There are normally Q waves on ECG.

The arteries involved tend to be the left circumflex coronary in just under 20%, the right coronary in approximately 30%, and the left anterior descending in approximately 50%. About a third of patients have disease in one vessel, a third have two vessels involved, while a further third have disease in all three vessels. Coronary angiograms after MI have occasionally shown evidence of spontaneous clearing of vessels between 4 h after the infarct and 12–24 h. This is presumably due to natural thrombolysis. In many patients there is a 'window of opportunity' between the onset of ischaemia and the development of irreversible changes, when fibrinolysis and/or balloon angioplasty may be able to restore the blood supply. The time interval is probably 6–12 h. After 12 h myocardial necrosis has begun and thrombolysis is unlikely to help.

In the evolving myocardial infarction, reduced myocardial perfusion leads to an accumulation of metabolites, hypoxia and the formation of oxygen free radicals. This may cause damage which is either reversible or irreversible depending on the extent, duration and severity of the ischaemia, and also on the collateral circulation and the metabolic demand of the myocardium. After successful thrombolysis, reperfusion occurs, but myocardial function is initially impaired due to 'stunned' myofibres which may not function well for a while but subsequently recover. Where there is an area of irreversible damage which is reperfused, there may be haemorrhage into the necrosed myocardium (myomalacia cordis or 'raspberry ripple heart') causing worsening cardiac function.

There are a number of pathological complications of an acute transmural infarct which may develop:

1. arrhythmia – both superventricular and ventricular arrhythmias occur, the most serious being ventricular tachycardia and fibrillation
2. acute heart failure due to myocardial dysfunction, which may take the form of cardiogenic shock or of pulmonary oedema due to left ventricular failure
3. papillary muscle infarct causing stretching or rupture with acute mitral regurgitation; when papillary muscle rupture has occurred the regurgitation is usually very severe with cardiac failure
4. pericarditis, which may be fibrinous or fibrinohaemorrhagic
5. mural thrombus which may result in subsequent peripheral arterial embolism causing stroke, acutely ischaemic limbs or mesenteric ischaemia
6. scarring of the heart muscle, which subsequently stretches, resulting in ventricular dilatation with dysfunction and occasionally formation of a discrete ventricular aneurysm
7. rupture of the myocardium, causing interventricular septal defect or bleeding into the pericardium with cardiac tamponade, depending on the site of the rupture.

All these complications are much less common since the advent of fibrinolytic therapy.

Sudden cardiac death

This is defined as an unexpected death from cardiac cause within an hour of the onset of acute symptoms. Although other types of heart disease such as aortic stenosis, hypertrophic cardiomyopathy or primary ventricular fibrillation may cause it, the overwhelming majority are due to ischaemic heart disease. In a small percentage no definite cause is found. The final cause of death is almost always a lethal arrhythmia.

Of all the clinical manifestations of coronary heart disease sudden death is most strongly related to cigarette smoking. Smoking causes an increase in catecholamines, increases heart rate, blood pressure and cardiac output, and at the same time may cause generalised vasoconstriction which may include the coronary arteries. It also increases platelet aggregation. Carbon monoxide levels rise in heavy smokers because of the greater affinity for haemoglobin of carbon monoxide compared with oxygen. Thus smoking could trigger cardiac arrest in a patient with pre-existing coronary artery disease by increasing the demand of the myocardium for oxygen at the same time as reducing the delivery.

Ischaemic cardiomyopathy

This tends to occur in the elderly, with insidious and gradually deteriorating congestive cardiac failure and ECG changes. There is often a history of angina or myocardial infarction. It may be due to multiple small infarcts or chronic myocardial ischaemia or a combination of both. Histologically the main finding is diffuse myocardial atrophy and interstitial fibrosis. The clinical course is one of gradually deteriorating heart failure, and although they may die of an acute cardiac event, more commonly it is merely a contributory factor to some other unrelated cause of death.

It is important to differentiate ischaemic cardiomyopathy from 'hibernating myocardium'. In this condition the myocardial cells are viable, but are chronically hypoxic. They have reduced function which causes heart failure, but they are potentially reversible with successful revascularisation. Differentiation between the two is by stress echocardiography and myocardial perfusion scintigraphy. This will show whether or not there are multiple areas of myocardial scarring due to previous small infarctions, which is an irreversible change.

VALVULAR HEART DISEASE

Introduction

This may be congenital or acquired. Congenital aortic stenosis is uncommon, while congenital disease of the other valves is very rare. Acquired valvular disease may be stenosis, where the valve fails to open enough, or regurgitation, where it fails to close. The functional effect is very variable: from trivial to devastating. The degree of stenosis or regurgitation is obviously important, but in addition the rate of development affects the amount of compensation which may occur. Thus patients with gradual development of mitral stenosis may be symptom free with quite marked stenosis, until eventually a state of decompensation is reached.

Disease of the tricuspid and pulmonary valves is rare in each case. Of surgical interest is that carcinoid syndrome can occasionally cause stenosis of either of these. In practice the mitral and aortic valves are more commonly affected by disease.

Mitral valve disease

Stenosis

This may be caused by rheumatic endocarditis secondary to an immune response to β-haemolytic streptococci. It is much less common than many years ago but does still occur occasionally. It gradually causes left atrial hypertrophy, and then chronic passive congestion of the lungs (brown induration), with pulmonary oedema. Treatment is now usually by balloon valvuloplasty; otherwise, surgical valvotomy or valve replacement may be required.

Regurgitation

This may also be caused by rheumatic heart disease or endocarditis, but is more commonly due to mitral valve prolapse. This is also known as 'floppy valve'. It is due to a myxomatous degeneration of the mitral valve, and the enlarged mitral valve leaflets prolapse back into the atrium during systole. This is a common condition which gradually deteriorates with age. The cause of the myxoid degeneration is not known but seems to be a connective tissue disorder which occasionally is one feature of Marfan's syndrome. In the majority it is a chance finding on auscultation or echocardiogram and is of no clinical significance. However, as it gets more severe, mitral regurgitation can develop with resultant congestive cardiac failure, arrhythmias, thrombosis behind the valve cusps and subsequent embolism. Arrhythmias can occasionally cause sudden death.

Mitral valve repair or replacement may be required. It is the operation done for mitral prolapse if technically feasible.

Aortic valve disease

Stenosis

This too may be caused by rheumatic heart disease, when it is almost always accompanied by rheumatic mitral valve disease. The vast majority of cases are due to age-related calcification with stenosis. This tends to come on in the 70s or 80s but may develop at a younger age in individuals with congenital bicuspid valve. Nodules of calcium develop on the valve cusps and within the sinuses of Valsalva. Initially the left ventricle compensates by hypertrophy but, as the stenosis becomes more marked, patients may develop angina or syncopal attacks. The reasons for the latter are poorly understood but when they occur there is an increased risk of sudden death; thus when these symptoms develop, treatment is required urgently, with valve replacement.

Regurgitation

This may be caused by the same factors as aortic stenosis but in addition may be due to dissecting aortic aneurysm, Marfan's syndrome, endocarditis, ankylosing spondylitis, Still's disease, and also rarely to tertiary syphilis.

Artificial heart valves

These are used sufficiently commonly that most general or orthopaedic surgeons will have patients, referred with other conditions, who have artificial heart valves. There are two types: bioprostheses (usually made from porcine aortic valves) or mechanical valves constructed from metal and plastics. There are a number of complications such as thromboembolism or infective endocarditis. Thromboembolism is more likely with mechanical valves, and these patients require long term warfarin anticoagulation. When warfarin is stopped prior to surgery these patients should have intravenous heparin until shortly before surgery, which should be restarted as soon after as is considered safe. In addition there may be haemorrhagic complications from the anticoagulation!

Infective endocarditis may be a particular worry when treating patients with a variety of septic conditions such as abscesses, peritonitis, etc., and prophylactic antibiotics may be needed.

REPERFUSION SYNDROME

Introduction

The re-introduction of oxygenated blood after a period of ischaemia causes more damage than the ischaemia alone.

The vascular endothelium is the site of damage, and neutrophils have been shown to be the prime mediator. It may occur after embolectomy, thrombolysis, repair of abdominal aortic aneurysm, or any vascular reconstruction.

How and why does this occur?

Pathophysiology

Under normal circumstances, 98% of oxygen is broken down by the mitochondria, undergoing tetravalent reduction and producing high energy phosphate groups. Approximately 2% of oxygen metabolism takes place by univalent reduction, and as a result a series of highly reactive, toxic, oxygen free radicals are formed. A free radical is an atom or molecule with an unpaired outer electron which is very unstable and tends to react with the first atom or molecule with which it comes into contact, to achieve stability. The free radical super oxide (O_2^-), the hydroxide radical (OH^-) and hydrogen peroxide (H_2O_2) are the free radicals which occur commonly in the body. Neutrophils in the act of phagocytosis produce large amounts of free radicals which facilitate the 'killing process'. If this process were unregulated an overwhelming amount of tissue damage would occur. An enzyme, superoxide dismutase (SOD), catalyses the reduction of superoxide radicals to hydrogen peroxide, and this too is removed by a series of enzymes. Cell cytoplasm also has a number of antioxidants such as ascorbic acid and cystine which further limit free radical activity. Under normal aerobic conditions very few oxygen free radicals will be available to cause tissue damage.

During ischaemia there is an increased generation of highly reactive metabolites. These may initiate a cascade of reactions which release other oxygen free radicals within the endothelial cells and may overcome the cells' protective mechanisms. The main pathological effect of oxygen free radicals is the generation of chemotactic agents resulting in direct migration of activated neutrophils into the reperfused tissue, with consequent injury. The damaged endothelial cells become more permeable.

The role of the neutrophil

When neutrophils enter reperfused tissue they become activated and increase their synthesis of oxygen free radicals and proteolytic enzymes. They induce injury by adhering to the endothelium at two sites: firstly, the precapillary sphincter, which may result in the capillaries becoming blocked by white cells, and secondly, post-capillary venules, where they induce injury by secretion of proteolytic enzymes such as elastase. For vascular injury to occur, neutrophils must be present and must adhere to the endothelium.

Local effects of reperfusion syndrome

The local effects are:

- limb swelling due to increased capillary permeability
- compartment syndrome as a result of the swelling
- impaired muscle function due to ischaemia
- muscle contracture — may develop later if the muscle infarcts.

Effects of reperfusion syndrome

Immediate   Immediate effects are:

- hyperkalaemia due to leakage of potassium from the damaged cells; this may result in cardiac arrhythmias
- acidosis due to the buildup of acidic metabolites
- myoglobinaemia due to breakdown of muscle cells, which can result in acute tubular necrosis.

Within 48 hours   When the area of ischaemic tissue is large there may be serious widespread consequences:

- lung neutrophil sequestration, which may lead to pulmonary oedema and subsequently to ARDS
- renal neutrophil sequestration, which may lead to increased vascular permeability and to acute renal failure
- gastrointestinal endothelial oedema, which may lead to increased gastrointestinal vascular permeability and endotoxic shock.

Management

Experimental evidence has shown that oxygen free radical scavengers such as mannitol and allopurinol can limit the reperfusion injury. Unfortunately, they need to be administered well before reperfusion for maximum benefit. In practice at the present time the important thing is to identify patients at risk. Lower limb fasciotomy at the time of revascularisation may help. In patients with more extensive and prolonged ischaemia it may be safer to perform primary amputation.

ANEURYSMS

Types of aneurysms are shown in Figure 9.38.

Definition

An aneurysm is an abnormal localised dilatation of an artery or chamber of a heart due to weakening of the wall. They can be classified as:

1. true — where the wall is formed by one or more of the layers of the affected vessel
2. false — where the wall is formed by connective tissue which is not part of the vessel wall.

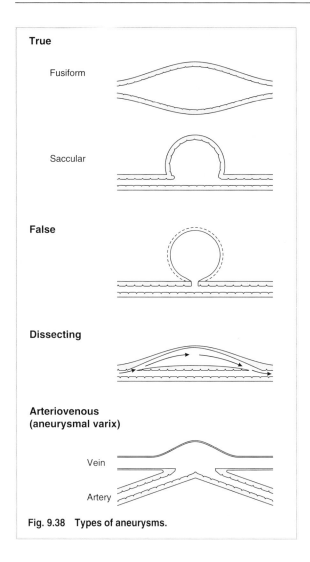

Fig. 9.38 Types of aneurysms.

Under the figure, labels within:
True
Fusiform
Saccular
False
Dissecting
Arteriovenous
(aneurysmal varix)
Vein
Artery

True aneurysms

True aneurysms may be:

1. fusiform — which is a dilatation due to a segment of the vessel wall affected around the whole circumference
2. saccular — where only part of the circumference is involved. It is thought these may be slightly more likely to rupture.

Congenital aneurysms

'Berry' aneurysms These are due to a congenital defect in the media at the junctions of vessels around the circle of Willis. They are the most common cause of subarachnoid haemorrhage, and although they can occur in young people the commonest age of presentation is about 50 years. There is an increased incidence in patients with hypertension.

Acquired aneurysms

Atheromatous aneurysms The most common site is the abdominal aorta, and the next most common sites are popliteal and femoral arteries.

Abdominal aortic aneurysm (AAA) There was a sevenfold increase in the incidence of this condition between the years 1950 and 1980, and the incidence is still rising. This is more than can be accounted for simply by increased lifespan. Risk factors are smoking and hypertension, but although these commonly occur in association with aortic aneurysms, there are some patients who have neither. The main complication is rupture, which may be intraperitoneal and accompanied by rapid death or retroperitoneal. Here they may leak, the blood pressure falls and a haematoma forms, holding the situation for anything from a few hours to a few days or even weeks. This situation is frequently described as a leaking abdominal aortic aneurysm. There is a familial tendency in some patients but by no means all. Histologically the main findings are atrophy of the medial smooth muscle cells and destruction of the elastic fibres and replacement with collagen. Much research has gone into trying to find the basic cause of this destruction of elastic tissue. Although this is not yet known for certain, the matrix metalloproteases have been implicated.

Although the destruction of elastin is the cause of the initial development of aneurysms, it is thought that damage to collagen may be the reason why they finally rupture. Some patients whose aneurysms have ruptured have been found to have increased levels of collagenases. Patients having any form of major surgery tend to have a rise in collagenases, and there is known to be an increased risk of rupture of abdominal aortic aneurysms in the few weeks following major surgery for some other reason.

About 25% of patients with AAA also have aneurysmal common iliac arteries. There is also an increased incidence of femoral and popliteal aneurysms.

While popliteal aneurysms may rupture, they far more commonly develop thrombus on the walls of the aneurysm, and repeated small emboli may break off. This tends to destroy the runoff vessels gradually, so that, when the aneurysm finally thromboses, there is quite frequently no suitable runoff to which to perform a bypass. Femoral aneurysms cause fewer problems.

Mycotic aneurysms These are most commonly associated with subacute infective endocarditis, although they may be due to any bacteraemia. *Salmonella* is one of

261

the more common organisms responsible. In the major vessels, they are more likely to occur at sites where the vessel is already diseased with atheroma. They tend to be saccular, with weakness of the wall at the site of infection. They may thrombose or rupture and should therefore be treated if the patient is fit enough.

Syphilitic aneurysms Although these were common many years ago, they are very rare now. They tend to involve the thoracic aorta. Microscopically, there is endarteritis of the vasa vasorum, with the inflammatory process extending into the media and causing ischaemia which damages the vessel wall.

Dissecting aneurysms (acute aortic dissection) The thoracic aorta is the most common artery affected. Blood enters the diseased media which splits into two layers. Blood may then enter this false lumen, which tends to cut off the blood supply to branches along its route. The condition is caused by medionecrosis — which may be associated with Marfan's syndrome, but by no means all the patients have this. There is a strong association with hypertension.

Once the dissection has occurred, it tends to rupture — either back into the main lumen of the artery, in which case the patient may survive for some time, or externally with rapid demise of the patient. When this condition involves the ascending aorta, it may dissect across a coronary ostium, leading to myocardial infarction, or across the aortic valve, causing aortic regurgitation.

False aneurysm (pulsating haematoma) This results from a small tear in the artery which is followed by haematoma the wall of which becomes organised and will hold the aneurysm for some time before it ruptures. These are due to injury with a small defect and usually they can be repaired simply by controlling the artery, closing the defect and evacuating the haematoma.

Arteriovenous aneurysms These are sometimes known as aneurysmal varices. These may be traumatic, or more commonly may follow formation of an AV fistula for renal dialysis. Here an artery is anastomosed to a vein in order to get a fast flow of blood in a superficial vessel suitable for needling to put blood through the kidney machine. Occasionally the flow is so good that aneurysmal dilatation gradually develops. They are associated with a raised venous pressure distally and may also result in a degree of distal ischaemia due to 'steal' of the blood back up the veins.

VARICOSE VEINS

A varicose vein is one which is tortuous and dilated and associated with local valvular incompetence. Varicose veins of the legs are extremely common, occurring in 10–20% of the population, with an increased incidence over the age of 50. They are said to be commoner in women, although a recent survey for the Vascular Surgical Society showed they were more common in men but that women consulted their doctors about them more often!

Varicose veins may be associated with:

1. poor support of the venous wall, which may be due to a familial tendency (approximately 40% of patients have a family history); in addition obesity and advancing age tend to result in loss of support of the vein; also prolonged dependent position as in patients with jobs that involve sitting or standing still for long periods
2. increased pressure within the lumen, which may be caused by a venous thrombosis, pregnancy, or tumour masses pressing on the veins.

Clinical features

By far and away the most common vein affected is the great saphenous, with incompetence, initially at the saphenofemoral junction, which gradually works its way down as the vein stretches and affects the next valve down. The next most common site is the short saphenous followed by incompetent valves in the veins which perforate the deep fascia connecting the superficial with the deep venous system (see anatomy section, p. 233).

Complications

These include:

- superficial thrombophlebitis
- venous eczema (mild irritation and rash)
- lipodermatosclerosis
- venous pigmentation due to haemosiderin deposition
- haemorrhage, which will be made worse by a proximal tourniquet and should be treated by local pressure and elevation
- venous stasis ulcer (longstanding venous stasis ulcers may become malignant – Marjolin's ulcer).

Venous lipodermatosclerosis

The skin in the gaiter area around the ankle becomes pigmented, indurated, tender and inflamed, most commonly on the medial side. The condition is produced by persistently high venous pressure in the surface veins, which distends the capillary bed and results in fibrin and other large molecules being deposited around the capillaries. These prevent diffusion of oxygen and other nutrients into the tissue. This results in necrosis of the subcutaneous fat, which subsequently turns to fibrous tissue (sclerosis). Thereafter, the skin and subcutaneous tissues break down very easily and form ulcers and are slow to heal.

LYMPHOEDEMA

Lymphoedema can be defined as an accumulation of tissue fluid due to defective lymphatic drainage. In the majority of cases, lymphoedema principally affects the lower limbs, although the arms, face and genitalia can all be involved.

Lymphoedema must be differentiated from other causes of oedema:

- cardiac failure
- renal failure
- hypoproteinaemia
- venous, such as post-thrombotic syndrome
- arteriovenous fistula.

Lymphoedema is described further in Chapter 10.

10

Haemopoietic and lymphoreticular system

Andrew T Raftery

HAEMOPOIESIS

Haemopoiesis is the production of blood cells. In the fetus, blood is formed in the bone marrow, spleen and liver. At birth the marrow is the main site of haemopoiesis, but eventually the red marrow of the long bones is replaced by fat such that, in the adult, red marrow remains only in the axial skeleton, ribs and skull, and in the proximal ends of the humerus and femur.

RED BLOOD CELL (ERYTHROCYTE)

Erythrocytes are non-nucleated blood cells which are biconcave and deformable. They are the most abundant blood cell and form 45% of the total blood volume, i.e. the haematocrit or packed-cell volume (PCV). Their function is to carry oxygen. About 1% of red cells stain purplish because of residual RNA. They are called reticulocytes. The proportion of these cells in the blood stream increases when bone marrow production of erythrocytes increases, e.g. after haemorrhage. Production of red cells in the bone marrow requires mitosis and maturation, the cells being derived from a pluripotent stem cell. The earliest red cell precursor is the proerythroblast, a large nucleated cell. By a series of divisions, the proerythroblast develops into a non-nucleated cell containing haemoglobin, i.e. an erythrocyte. At the stage of extrusion of the nucleus a reticulocyte is formed which contains remnants of RNA and ribosomes and continues to make haemoglobin. Reticulocytes mature for 1 or 2 days in the marrow before being released into the blood where, after a further 1 or 2 days, they lose their remaining ribosomes and become mature erythrocytes. Mature erythrocytes survive for 18–120 days in the circulation before being removed by macrophages in the spleen, and to a lesser extent in the bone marrow and liver. Within the macrophage the erythrocyte is broken down into haem and globin. The amino acids of the latter enter the general

amino acid pool of the body, while the haem group is broken down with the release of iron which attaches to transferrin. Transferrin is an iron-binding beta-globulin responsible for iron transport and delivery to receptors on erythroblasts, or to iron stores. The remainder of the haem group is converted to bilirubin. Renal secretion of erythropoietin stimulates red cell production to keep pace with the rate of destruction. Erythropoietin is secreted by the kidneys in response to local hypoxia and acts on red marrow, causing an increased output of erythrocytes until the rise in haemoglobin concentration in the blood restores normal delivery of oxygen to the tissues. Erythropoiesis requires an adequate dietary intake of iron, vitamin B_{12} and folate. Depletion of stores of these will reduce erythropoiesis.

ANAEMIA

Anaemia is the reduction of the concentration of haemoglobin in the circulation below the normal range. There are three main causes of anaemia: blood loss, haemolysis, and impairment of red cell formation/function.

Blood loss

Immediately after acute haemorrhage the haemoglobin level is normal. In the absence of intravenous fluid replacement, there is a slow expansion in plasma volume over the next 2–3 days. The result is a normochromic, normocytic anaemia. There is also a reticulocytosis, which is maximal at 1 week, together with a mild neutrophil leucocytosis. Occasionally metamyeloyctes are present in the blood film. Chronic blood loss leads to hypochromic, microcytic, iron deficiency anaemia.

Haemolysis

Haemolytic anaemias are a group of diseases in which red cell life span is reduced. Haemolysis is usually associated with increased erythropoiesis. Laboratory evidence of increased red cell destruction is demonstrated by:

(i) increased serum unconjugated bilirubin; (ii) reduced serum haptoglobin; (iii) morphological evidence of red cell damage, e.g. spherocytes, red cell fragments, or sickled cells; (iv) reduced lifespan of red cells, e.g. demonstrated by tagging with radioactive chromium. Laboratory evidence of increased erythropoiesis depends on demonstrating a reticulocytosis in the peripheral blood and erythroid hyperplasia in the bone marrow.

Clinical features of haemolytic states

These result from red cell destruction and compensatory erythropoiesis. Pallor and mild jaundice occur. Pigment stones may form in the gall bladder and bile ducts as a result of increased haemolysis, and splenomegaly may occur. In congenital forms, erythroid hyperplasia causing expansion of marrow cavities with thinning of cortical bone may also occur. Frontal bossing of the skull may occur due to widening of the marrow space between inner and outer tables of the skull.

There are a number of haemolytic conditions described, but only two, which are surgically relevant, will be discussed here: sickle cell anaemia and hereditary spherocytosis.

Sickle cell anaemia

This is due to the presence of a haemoglobin variant, HbS, in the red cells. Recurrent painful crises and chronic haemolytic anaemia occur relating to sickling of red cells on deoxygenation. Deoxygenated HbS is 50 times less soluble than deoxygenated HbA and polymerises on deoxygenation into long fibres which deform the red cell into the typical sickle shape. The presence of HbS is the result of a defect in the gene coding for glutamic acid, the latter being replaced by valine. When an individual is heterozygous for this defect, both HbA and HbS are formed, and they are individually said to have sickle cell trait. These individuals are usually haematologically normal and are usually asymptomatic. When only the trait is present the red cells do not usually sickle until the oxygen saturation falls below 40%, which is rarely reached in venous blood. In surgical practice the anaesthetist needs to be aware of the trait so that hypoxia is avoided intraoperatively. When the individual is homozygous, HbA is not formed. The red cells readily deform and sickle cell anaemia develops. Cells sickle at the oxygen tension normally found in venous blood. The increased rigidity of the cells causes them to plug small blood vessels, with resulting infarction and painful crises. Patients may develop acute abdominal and chest pain that mimics other intra-abdominal and thoracic catastrophes. Bone pain may occur and also the patient may develop priapism. The anaemic patient responds poorly to infection,

and septicaemia and osteomyelitis may develop, the latter being attributable on occasions to *Salmonella*. The spleen may calcify and atrophy due to repeated infarction. Pigment gall stones may occur.

Hereditary spherocytosis (congenital acholuric jaundice)

This is due to a defect in the red cell membrane. Clinical features include a family history, pallor, mild jaundice, and splenomegaly. Spherocytes are identified in the blood film. There is a raised serum bilirubin and an increased reticulocyte count. Cholecystitis may occur as a result of pigment stones. Splenectomy is the treatment of choice, being delayed until after the age of 10 years as postsplenectomy sepsis is less after this age. Splenectomy does not cure the spherocytosis but prevents the abnormally shaped cells being destroyed in the spleen. Following splenectomy the haemoglobin level rises, the jaundice disappears, and the lifespan of the red cells increases to near normal levels.

Impairment of red cell formation/function

This may arise as a result of: (i) deficiency of essential haematinics, e.g. iron, folate, vitamin B_{12}; (ii) chronic disorders, infections (TB), renal disease, liver disease, neoplasia, collagen disease; (iii) marrow infiltration, e.g. carcinoma, myeloma, lymphoma, myelofibrosis; (iv) endocrine disease, e.g. hypothyroidism; (v) cytotoxic and immunosuppressive agents.

Classification of anaemia

Anaemias may be classified by the morphological appearance of erythrocytes in a stained blood smear. Normocytes are red cells with a normal diameter, microcytes are those with a reduced diameter, and macrocytes are those with an increased diameter. Normochromic is a term applied to normal staining of the red cell with a central area of pallor, while hypochromic indicates reduced staining with a larger central area of pallor. Classification also depends on other criteria. The haematocrit or PCV is expressed as the percentage of packed red cells in relation to the total volume of blood and is normally approximately 45%. Other important parameters in assessing anaemia are:

- mean corpuscular volume (MCV), measured in femtolitres (FL)

$$\frac{\text{haematocrit (L/L)}}{\text{red cell concentration (L}^{-1})} = 78\text{–}98 \text{ FL}$$

- mean corpuscular haemoglobin (MCH), in picograms (pg)

Table 10.1   Morphological classifications of anaemia

Morphology	Values	Causes
Microcytic } Hypochromic }	MCV < 78 MCH < 26	Iron deficiency Thalassaemia
Macrocytic	MCV > 98	Folate deficiency, B$_{12}$ deficiency, alcoholism
Normocytic } Normochromic }	MCV normal MCH normal	Acute blood loss Haemolytic anaemia Chronic disorders Leucoerythroblastic anaemias

$$\frac{\text{haemoglobin concentration (g/dL)}}{\text{red cell concentration (L}^{-1})} = 26\text{--}33 \text{ pg}$$

- mean corpuscular haemoglobin concentration (MCHC), in grams per decilitre (g/dL)

$$\frac{\text{haemoglobin concentration (g/dL)}}{\text{haematocrit (L/L)}} = 30\text{--}35 \text{ g/dL}$$

A morphological classification of anaemia is shown in Table 10.1.

POLYCYTHAEMIA

Polycythaemia is an increase in the concentration of red cells above the normal level. There is a rise in both total blood volume and PCV; the latter may be as high as 60%. The Hb concentration rises to about 18 g/dL and, because of the increased proportion of erythrocytes, blood viscosity is high. Polycythaemia may be a primary condition, i.e. polycythaemia rubra vera, or may be secondary or relative, or due to inappropriate secretion of erythropoietin (Box 10.1). Polycythaemia, especially the true and secondary forms, increases whole blood viscosity. This leads to sluggish blood flow through the heart, brain and limbs, leading to myocardial infarction, stroke and ischaemic limbs. The spleen is enlarged in about 75% of cases. Haemorrhagic lesions may be a feature especially in the gastrointestinal tract. Peptic ulceration is common in polycythaemia rubra vera, but the reason is unknown.

WHITE BLOOD CELL (LEUCOCYTE)

White blood cells form part of the body's defence mechanism. They are divided into two main groups: phagocytes, which engulf and destroy bacteria and foreign matter, and lymphocytes, which are responsible for the

Box 10.1   Causes of polycythaemia

- true
  — polycythaemia rubra vera

- secondary — chronic hypoxia stimulates erythropoietin
  — high altitude
  — respiratory disease
  — cyanotic heart disease
  — smoking
  — haemoglobinopathy

- relative — reduced plasma volume, normal red cell mass
  — vomiting
  — diarrhoea
  — burns
  — inadequate fluid intake

- inappropriate — increase of erythropoietin
  — kidney disease, e.g. cystitis, carcinoma
  — renal transplantation
  — hepatocellular carcinoma
  — giant uterine fibroids
  — cerebellar haemangioblastoma

immune response. Granulocytes and monocytes develop in red bone marrow from a common stem cell. The granulocyte precursor is a myeloblast which subsequently differentiates and matures, acquiring characteristic granules, to become either a neutrophil, basophil, or eosinophil granulocyte. Precursors do not normally circulate but may do so in case of bone marrow disease or severe infections.

Neutrophils   Neutrophils have a scavenging function and are most important in defence against bacterial infection. They possess a segmented nucleus and abundant cytoplasmic granules containing enzymes e.g. alkaline phosphatase and lysosyme. They spend 14 days in the bone marrow, whereas their half-life in the blood is only 6–12 h. They enter tissues by penetrating the endothelium.

Lymphocytes   The role of lymphocytes is described in Chapter 6.

Monocytes   These are the largest blood cells. Their function is similar to that of the neutrophils. They enter the tissues and phagocytose and digest foreign and dying material.

Eosinophils   The eosinophil is important in the mediation of the allergic response and the defence against parasitic infections.

Basophils   They are the least frequent leucocytes in blood. They have a similar function to tissue mast cells. They are thought to be important in immediate hypersensitivity reactions, when they release histamine.

Changes in white cells in disease

Leucocytosis

Leucocytosis is an increase in the number of circulating white cells. The normal reference range is shown in Table 10.2. It may involve any of the white cells, but a polymorphonuclear leucocytosis is the most common, i.e. neutrophilia (see Table 10.3).

Leucopaenia

Leucopaenia is a reduction in circulating leucocytes. In practice the most common form is neutropaenia — a deficiency of neutrophil granulocytes. Neutropaenia may be selective or part of a pancytopaenia (Table 10.4).

Neutropaenia with counts of less than 0.5×10^9/L may result in severe sepsis, e.g. oral and oesophageal candida, septicaemia, opportunistic infection. This type of disease is seen in patients receiving chemotherapy for malignant disease or immunosuppressive therapy for organ transplantation.

Table 10.2   Reference range for white cell concentrations

Cell	Count (10^9/L)
Total white cell count	4–11
Neutrophils	2.0–7.5
Lymphocytes	1.0–3.0
Monocytes	0.15–0.6
Eosinophils	0.05–0.35
Basophils	0.01–0.10

Table 10.3   Causes of leucocytosis

Cell	Cause
Neutrophils	Sepsis, e.g. acute appendicitis Trauma, e.g. major surgery Infarction, e.g. myocardial infarction, mesenteric infarction Malignant disease Acute haemorrhage Steroid therapy
Monocytes	Sepsis Chronic infection, e.g. TB Malignant disease
Eosinophils	Allergy, e.g. asthma Parasitic infection Malignant disease, e.g. Hodgkin's

Table 10.4   Causes of neutropaenia

Type	Cause
Pancytopaenia	Bone marrow depression, e.g. cytotoxic drugs, malignant infiltration Severe vitamin B_{12} or folate deficiency Hypersplenism
Selective	Overwhelming sepsis, e.g. septicaemia Autoimmune Drug-induced, e.g. indomethacin, chloramphenicol, co-trimoxazole

PLATELETS

Platelets are discoid non-nucleated granule-containing cells that are formed in the bone marrow by fragmentation of the cytoplasm of megakaryocytes. Their concentration in normal blood is $160–450 \times 10^9$/L. They survive in the circulation for 8–10 days. Platelets are contractile and adhesive cells which are important in haemostasis. They adhere to exposed subendothelial tissues, aggregate, and form a haemostatic plug. Platelets may also take part in the repair process after vascular injury. Platelet-derived growth factor is mitogenic for smooth muscle and fibroblasts; it may also be involved in the development of atherosclerosis. The function of platelets is discussed further in the section on haemostasis. A reduction in the number of platelets is called thrombocytopaenia (Table 10.5).

HAEMOSTASIS

Haemostasis is the physiological process by which bleeding is controlled. It consists of four components: vasoconstriction, platelet activation, the coagulation mechanism and the fibrinolytic system.

Vasoconstriction

This is due to smooth muscle contraction mediated by local reflexes, thromboxane A2 and serotonin released by activated platelets.

Platelet activation

Vascular damage promotes haemostasis if the endothelial lining of blood vessels is disrupted. Platelets adhere to, and aggregate at, the sites of disruption, ultimately forming a platelet plug.

Adherence   Following injury to the vessel wall, loss of endothelium exposes subendothelial collagen, allowing adhesion of platelets to the damaged area and activation

Table 10.5	Causes of thrombocytopaenia
Type	**Cause**
Reduced production	Aplastic anaemia
	Drugs, e.g. tolbutamide, alcohol, cytotoxic agents
	Viral infections, e.g. EBV, CMV
	Myelodysplasia
	Bone marrow infiltration, e.g. carcinoma, leukaemia, myeloma, myelofibrosis
	Megaloblastic anaemia
	Hereditary thrombocytopaenia
Decreased platelet survival	
Immune	Idiopathic thrombocytopaenic purpura
	Drugs, e.g. heparin, quinine, sulphonamides, penicillins, gold
	Infections
	Post-transfusion
Non-immune	Disseminated intravascular coagulation
	Thrombotic thrombocytopaenic purpura
Hypersplenism	Sequestration of platelets

of the intrinsic pathway of coagulation. Damaged endothelial cells release von Willebrand factor, which is necessary for platelet adhesion, and also release tissue thromboplastin which activates the intrinsic pathway of coagulation. Simultaneously platelet granules release ADP, which initiates platelet aggregation.

Aggregation Thromboxane A2 is produced from arachidonic acid released from platelet phospholipids. Thromboxane A2 induces further ADP release, causing further platelet aggregation.

Platelet plug The aggregated platelets act as catalysts of coagulation with local generation of thrombin and conversion of fibrinogen to fibrin. The aggregated platelets, thrombin, and fibrin fuse to form the platelet plug.

Coagulation mechanism

The end-stage of blood coagulation is the conversion of soluble fibrinogen to insoluble fibrin by the protease thrombin. The coagulation mechanism is complex and involves two interacting systems: the intrinsic and extrinsic pathways. Activation of factor X is the result of preceding enzyme reactions in the two pathways. The intrinsic pathway involves normal blood components; the extrinsic pathway requires tissue thromboplastin released by damaged cells. The pathways are shown in Figure 10.1. All the soluble coagulation factors are manufactured in the liver with the exception of Factor VIII (endothelium), calcium, platelet factors and thromboplastin.

Fibrinolytic system

During the repair process in blood vessels and healing wounds, fibrin is removed by the fibrinolytic system (Fig. 10.2). Fibrin is broken down to soluble fibrin degradation products by plasmin. Plasmin is derived from the inactive precursor plasminogen by the action of plasminogen activators. Tissue plasminogen activator is released from endothelial cells. Control of the activation of plasminogen is provided by plasminogen-activator inhibitor I, which is released by endothelial cells and rapidly inactivates tissue plasminogen activator.

ASSESSMENT OF COAGULATION SYSTEM

Platelet count The normal range is $160–450 \times 10^9$/L. Thrombocytopaenia exists with counts of less than 100×10^9/L. Counts of 70×10^9/L are usually adequate for surgical haemostasis. Spontaneous bleeding usually occurs with counts of less than 20×10^9/L.

Bleeding time This is tested by measuring the time for a small puncture wound in the skin, made by a standard technique, to stop bleeding. The time varies from 1 to 8 min. A time within this normal range implies an adequate platelet count, normal platelet function, and a normal vascular response to injury. A prolonged bleeding time implies thrombocytopaenia, a platelet defect, or failure of vascular contraction.

Whole blood clotting time Blood clots in a glass tube in 5–15 min. A clotting time within this range requires integrity of the intrinsic system, an adequate final common pathway, and normal platelet function.

Prothrombin time (PT) This tests the integrity of the extrinsic pathway and final common pathway. Deficiencies of factor I, II, V, VII, X will be detected.

Activated partial thromboplastin time (APTT) This reflects the intrinsic mechanism, i.e. all factors except factor VII.

Kaolin–cephalin clotting time (KCCT) This test is independent of the platelet count. It tests the intrinsic pathway and common pathway.

Thrombin time (TT) This is increased if there is an inadequate concentration of fibrinogen. It is prolonged by heparin and by the presence of fibrin split products.

Fibrin degradation products (FDPs) These are products released from fibrinogen and fibrin by plasmin. They are increased in disseminated intravascular coagulation.

Assessment of the different pathways involved in coagulation may be made with two simple tests: the APTT for the intrinsic system and the PT for the extrinsic system.

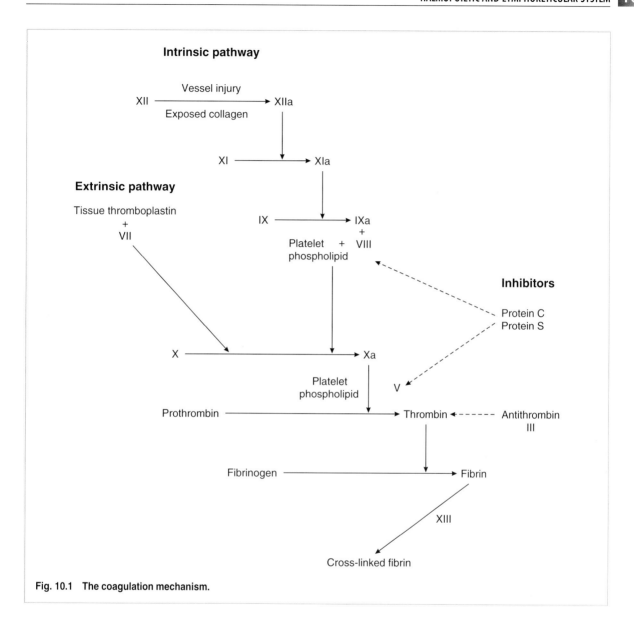

Fig. 10.1 The coagulation mechanism.

The test results and the conclusions that may be drawn from them are shown in Table 10.6.

DISORDERS OF HAEMOSTASIS

Platelet disorders

Thrombocytopaenia

This may be due to a failure of platelet production or increased destruction or sequestration of platelets, and

Table 10.6 Assessment of bleeding states (APTT tests the intrinsic system; PT tests the extrinsic system)	
Test result	Conclusion
APTT and PT normal	Platelet or vessel defect
APTT and PT abnormal	Deficit in common pathway
APTT normal and PT abnormal	Factor VII deficiency
APTT abnormal and PT normal	Deficit in intrinsic system

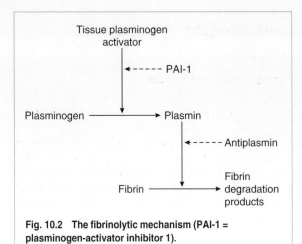

Fig. 10.2 The fibrinolytic mechanism (PAI-1 = plasminogen-activator inhibitor 1).

abnormal platelet function. The causes of thrombocytopaenia are shown in Table 10.5.

Abnormal platelet function may cause bleeding despite a normal platelet count. Abnormal platelet function may occur with: drugs, e.g. aspirin, non-steroidal anti-inflammatory drugs, carbenicillin, and ticarcillin; uraemia; septicaemia; and von Willebrand's disease.

Blood vessel wall abnormalities

These are rare and may be due to scurvy, steroids, Cushing's syndrome, or Henoch–Schonlein purpura.

Disorders of coagulation

Congenital coagulation disorders

These are uncommon, the commonest being haemophilia A and von Willebrand's disease.

Haemophilia A This is due to an inherited deficiency of Factor VIII. It is an X-linked recessive disorder affecting males and carried by females. Severity of the disease depends on the degree of factor VIII deficiency. The PT is normal but the APTT is prolonged.

von Willebrand's disease This is due to deficiency of von Willebrand's factor. It is transmitted as an autosomal dominant condition. Vascular endothelium releases decreased amounts of factor VIII. Although the platelet count is usually normal, platelet interaction with the endothelium is defective because of deficiency of von Willebrand's factor.

Acquired disorders of coagulation

Vitamin K deficiency Vitamin K is present in green vegetables and is synthesised by intestinal bacteria. It is fat soluble and requires bile for its absorption. It is required for the formation of factors II, VII, IX, X. Vitamin K deficiency may occur in the surgical patient as the result of obstructive jaundice, antibiotic therapy which alters the normal intestinal flora, or prolonged parenteral nutrition without vitamin K supplements.

Liver disease This is commonly associated with coagulation defects due to failure of clotting factor synthesis and the production of abnormal fibrinogen. Vitamin K will not help if there is hepatocellular failure. In addition, there may be thrombocytopaenia due to hypersplenism.

Disseminated intravascular coagulation (DIC) This results from simultaneous activation of coagulation and fibrinolytic systems. Activation of the coagulation system leads to the formation of microthrombi in many organs, with the consumption of clotting factors and platelets, in turn leading to haemorrhage. DIC may arise as a result of the following disorders: septicaemia, malignancy, trauma, shock, liver disease, acute pancreatitis, obstetric problems, e.g. toxaemia, amniotic fluid embolism. Clinically there is widespread haemorrhage. The presence of thrombocytopaenia, decreased fibrinogen, and elevated fibrinogen degradation products confirms the diagnosis.

NATURAL ANTICOAGULANTS

Antithrombin III

This is an inhibitor of thrombin, its action being potentiated by heparin. Congenital antithrombin III deficiency is inherited as an autosomal dominant. Heterozygotes may suffer from recurrent deep vein thrombosis, pulmonary embolism, and mesenteric thrombosis. Homozygotes present in childhood with severe arterial and venous thrombosis.

Protein C and protein S

These are synthesised in the liver and are dependant on vitamin K. Protein C degrades factors Va and VIIIa and promotes fibrinolysis by inactivating plasminogen-activator inhibitor I. Protein S is a cofactor for protein C and enhances its activity. Hereditary protein C deficiency may occur, patients being more susceptible to DVT, PE, superficial thrombophlebitis, and cerebral venous thrombosis.

ANTICOAGULANT DRUGS

The two used most commonly in surgical practice are heparin and warfarin.

Heparin

Heparin potentiates the action of antithrombin III. Standard unfractionated heparin is administered i.v. or s.c. and has a half life of about 1 h. Low molecular weight heparin is used subcutaneously and has a longer biological half life. Intravenous heparin is used in patients with DVT or PE, and the dosage is monitored by performing the KCCT, which should be maintained at 2–2.5 times the normal value. Subcutaneous heparin is given to reduce the risk of DVT or PE in patients undergoing major surgery or patients who are on prolonged bed rest, e.g. post-myocardial infarction or orthopaedic patients. Heparin does not cross the placenta and is therefore the drug of choice when anticoagulation is required during pregnancy. Bleeding due to overdose is managed by stopping the heparin and administering protamine sulphate intravenously. Side effects of heparin include thrombocytopaenia, hypersensitivity reactions, alopecia, and osteoporosis when used long term.

Warfarin

Warfarin is a coumarin derivative which is administered orally. It is a vitamin K antagonist and in effect induces a state analogous to vitamin K deficiency. It interferes with the activity of factors II, VII, IX and X. It delays thrombin generation, thus preventing the formation of thrombi. It is usual to give a loading dose (10 mg) and to determine the INR (the prothrombin ratio standardised by correcting for the sensitivity of the thromboplastin used) about 15–18 h later. Subsequent doses are based on the INR. Warfarin is usually administered for 3–6 months following DVT or PE. Lifelong warfarin is required for recurrent venous thromboembolic disease, some prosthetic heart valves, congenital deficiency of antithrombin III, deficiency of protein C or protein S, patients with lupus anticoagulant, and valvular heart disease complicated by embolism or atrial fibrillation. Bleeding is controlled by stopping warfarin and administering either fresh frozen plasma or vitamin K, depending upon the degree of urgency. If vitamin K is used there is a period of resistance to warfarin, and control may be difficult initially when the patient is restarted on warfarin. A number of drugs may interfere with the control of warfarin. These include antibiotics, laxatives (interfere with vitamin K absorption), phenylbutazone (interferes with binding of warfarin to albumin) and cimetidine (inhibits hepatic microsomal degradation). Warfarin crosses the placenta and is teratogenic. It should be avoided particularly in the first trimester of pregnancy.

LYMPHOID SYSTEM

LYMPH NODES

Normal structure and functions

Lymph nodes are discrete encapsulated structures, usually kidney-shaped, and range in diameter from a few millimetres to several centimetres. They are situated along the course of lymphatic vessels and are numerous where these vessels converge, e.g. the root of the limbs, the neck, the pelvis and the mediastinum. A lymph node has an outer capsule of connective tissue from which trabeculae pass into the deeper tissue (Fig. 10.3). Beneath the capsule is a space, the subcapsular sinus into which the afferent lymphatics drain after penetrating the capsule. Lymph from the subcapsular sinus passes via the medullary cords to the hilum of the lymph node from which the efferent lymphatics drain. Both afferent and efferent vessels have valves which allow only forward flow. The node itself consists of an outer cortex and an inner medulla and contains lymphatic sinuses. There are three distinct microanatomical regions within a lymph node. These are:

1. the cortex, which contains either primary or secondary lymphoid follicles
2. the paracortex, which is the T-cell-dependent region of the lymph node
3. the medulla, which contains the medullary cords and sinuses and also contains lymphocytes which are much less densely packed than in the cortex, together with macrophages, plasma cells and a small number of granulocytes.

Cortex

The cortex consists of primary lymphoid follicles which are unstimulated follicles, spherical in shape, containing densely packed lymphocytes. Secondary follicles are present after lymphocytes have been stimulated antigenically. These follicles have an outer ring of small B lymphocytes surrounding the germinal centre, which contains largely dividing lymphoblasts, macrophages and dendritic cells. Antigen is trapped upon the surface of the dendritic cells and presented to 'virgin' B lymphocytes in the presence of T helper cells, and these B cells subsequently undergo a series of morphological and functional changes. The function of germinal centres is to generate immunoglobulin-secreting plasma cells in response to antigenic challenge.

Paracortex

The paracortex is the T-cell-dependent region of the lymph

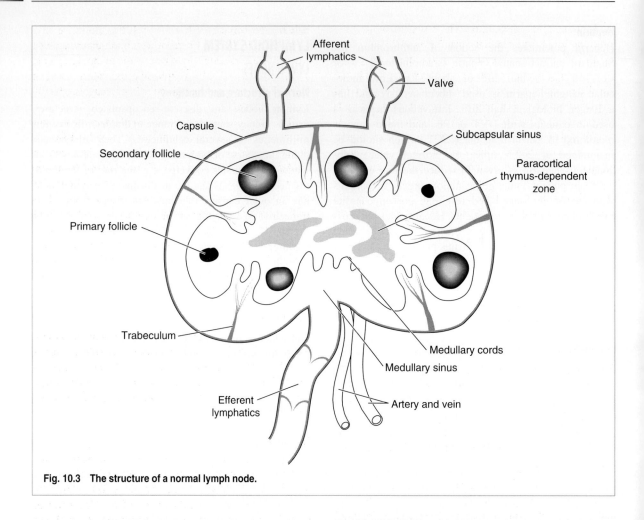

Fig. 10.3 The structure of a normal lymph node.

node. When a T cell response occurs there is marked proliferation of cells in this area. The paracortex contains large number of T lymphocytes with a predominance of helper/inducer cells. The cluster of differentiation (CD4) is expressed by helper/inducer T cells.

Medulla

Lymph enters the marginal sinus of the node and drains to the hilum through the sinuses which converge into the medullary region. The sinuses are lined by macrophages which phagocytose foreign or abnormal particles from the lymph passing through the node, i.e. the filtering function. Between the sinuses in the medulla lie the medullary cords which contain numerous plasma cells and are one of the main sites of antibody secretion within the lymph node. The immunological function of lymph nodes is discussed in greater detail in Chapter 6.

LYMPHATIC SYSTEM

The lymphatic system consists of a network of blind-ending lymphatic capillaries lining the interstitial space near the blood capillaries. Compared with blood capillaries, the spaces between the endothelial cells in lymphatic capillaries are larger, making them readily permeable to protein and fluid. Lymph collects in the thin-walled lymph vessels which eventually drain on the right side into the lymphatic duct and on the left side via the thoracic duct into the subclavian veins. Lymph is composed of fluid (plasma) and lymphocytes, many of which are stored in lymph nodes which are found along the course of the larger lymph vessels. Plasma proteins that leak out of the capillaries and fluid that is not reabsorbed into the capillaries are returned to the circulatory system via the lymphatics. The lymphatic system also acts as a pathway of absorption of fat from the gut and also is involved in the immune response (Ch. 6). The efflux of fluid at the arteriolar end of the capillary usually exceeds the influx of fluid at the venous end. This extra lymphatic fluid enters the lymphatic vessels and is returned to the blood via these vessels. Lymph flow is aided by rhythmical contractions of smooth muscle in the wall of the lymphatic vessels, retrograde flow being prevented by valves similar to those found in veins. During exercise, lymph flow can increase 5–15 times, firstly because of increased capillary pressure causing increased interstitial fluid formation and secondly because striated muscle contracts and helps to move the lymph onwards in the lymphatic vessels and to prevent stagnation in the tissues.

Obstruction to lymphatics (lymphoedema)

Lymphoedema is the accumulation of tissue fluid due to lymphatic obstruction or defective lymphatic drainage. If the lymphatics are obstructed the protein and excess fluid in the interstitial fluid cannot return to the vascular system and accumulate behind the obstruction, producing local oedema.

Lymphoedema may be primary or secondary.

Primary lymphoedema

This is a condition due to aplasia or hypoplasia of lymphatics. There are three types: congenital lymphoedema or Milroy's disease, which presents shortly after birth; lymphoedema praecox, which presents at puberty; and lymphoedema tarda, which presents around the age of 30.

Secondary lymphoedema

Lymphoedema may be secondary to result of damage to lymphatic channels by infection, surgery, radiotherapy, malignant infiltration, or trauma. Blockage of inguinal lymphatics by filarial parasites frequently causes gross oedema of the legs and, in the male, the scrotum. The resulting deformity is called elephantiasis.

Blockage of the lymphatic drainage from the small intestine usually occurs because of tumour involvement causing malabsorption of fats and fat-soluble substances. Blockage of lymphatic drainage at the level of the thoracic duct causes chylous effusions in the pleural and peritoneal cavities. At paracentesis or thoracocentesis, the fluid is opalescent because of the presence of numerous tiny fat globules (chyle).

SPLEEN

NORMAL STRUCTURE AND FUNCTION

The spleen is an encapsulated, purplish, friable organ situated in the left hypochondrium. It forms the left lateral extremity of the lesser sac. It lies along the long axis of ribs 9, 10 and 11, from which the diaphragmatic surface of the spleen is separated by the diaphragm, lung, and pleura. It normally weighs approximately 150 g in the adult but atrophies in old age, when it may weigh only approximately 50 g.

The visceral surface of the spleen is related to the stomach anteriorly, left kidney posteriorly, and the splenic flexure of the colon near its inferior pole. The anterior border of the spleen is notched. The hilum of the spleen lies between the gastric and renal surfaces and contains the vessels and nerves entering or leaving the spleen, as well as the splenic group of lymph nodes and the tail of the pancreas. Passing to the spleen are the gastrosplenic ligament to the greater curvature of the stomach which carries the short gastric and left gastroepiploic vessels, and the lienorenal ligament which carries the splenic vessels and the tail of the pancreas.

Blood supply

The arterial blood supply is via the splenic artery, which is a branch of the coeliac axis. The splenic vein is joined by the superior mesenteric vein to form the portal vein. The splenic artery and vein, the lymph nodes, and the tail of the pancreas are enclosed in the lienorenal ligament.

Embryology

The spleen develops from several masses of mesenchyme in the dorsal mesogastrium. These masses coalesce and develop into lymphoid tissue and move to the left with the dorsal mesogastrium. By the end of the third month of gestation the spleen is formed. The point at which the spleen remains attached to the dorsal mesogastrium becomes the gastrosplenic ligament. Congenital abnormalities in the form of accessory spleens or splenunculi are relatively common and occur in about 10% of the population. They are usually rounded encapsulated structures up to several centimetres in size and are usually located in the region of the spleen. They are clinically important in that, if they are left behind following splenectomy for such conditions as congenital acholuric jaundice (hereditary spherocytosis) or idiopathic thrombocytopaenic purpura, they may result in persistent symptoms.

MICROSCOPICAL STRUCTURE AND FUNCTION

The structure of the spleen (Fig. 10.4) is related to its two major functions, i.e. (i) production of antibodies and (ii) filtration of the blood and disposal of the defective blood cells.

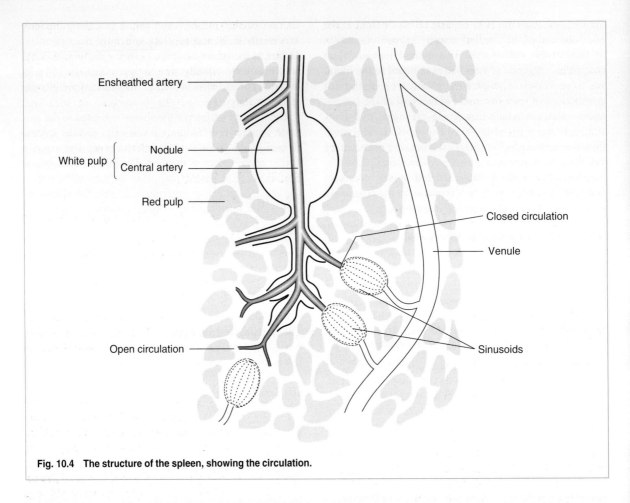

Fig. 10.4 The structure of the spleen, showing the circulation.

Structure

Deep to its peritoneal covering the spleen is enclosed in a thin connective tissue capsule. The connective tissue extends into the splenic pulp as trabeculae. These serve to support the pulp of the spleen and also transmit blood vessels into it. When a fresh spleen is cut across, two areas can be identified on the cut surface: firstly, islands of pale areas 1–2 mm in diameter which are white and are known as the white pulp, and secondly a deep red background which is known as the red pulp. The white pulp is composed of lymphatic nodules, mostly B lympho-cytes. The red pulp acts as a filter, removing effete red cells and particulate matter, and thus contains a large amount of red blood cells.

The splenic artery enters the spleen at the hilum, branches and follows the trabeculae of the fibrous cap-sule into the spleen. The branches leave the trabeculae as central arteries and arterioles and become ensheathed in lymphoid cells. Localised extensions of the lymphatic sheath form lymphatic nodules, each having an eccentri-cally placed arteriole which is a branch of the ensheathed artery.

White pulp

The white pulp consists of ensheathed arteries and lym-phoid nodules. The lymphocytes within the white pulp show distinct microarchitectural segregation of different functional subsets.

T lymphocytes are located in the immediate vicinity of the central artery, while the nodules contain mostly B lymphocytes. Activated lymphocytes migrate to the periphery of the nodule, to the marginal zone between red and white pulp, and differentiate into plasma cells capable of producing antibodies. The plasma cells circu-late in the red pulp and enter the sinusoids.

Red pulp

Most of the spleen is occupied by the red pulp, which

consists of cords of cells separated by sinusoids. The red pulp has a dual circulation with a closed circulation via sinusoidal pathways and an open circulation through the splenic pulp cords. These cords contain a large number of red cells which give the spleen its characteristic appearance. They also contain lymphocytes, granulocytes, platelets and macrophages. In the red pulp, macrophages phagocytose senescent red cells and particulate matter. The red pulp is drained by sinusoids, i.e. narrow channels with a discontinuous endothelial cell lining, cells being able to pass between the space between endothelial cells. The spaces between the endothelial cells allow normal pliable and deformable cells to pass. Red cells, plasma cells, granulocytes and platelets leave the spleen by passing through the spaces into the sinusoids.

Defective or effete cells are trapped as they attempt to enter the sinusoids through the spaces and are destroyed by adjacent macrophages. The open circulation, where the cells percolate slowly through the cords, leaves cells in prolonged contact with rows of macrophages before they enter the splenic sinusoids. Any abnormal cells are rapidly phagocytosed. The sinusoids join together as venules which leave the spleen as the trabecular veins eventually forming the splenic vein.

FUNCTION

The spleen has several functions, the two main ones being the production of antibodies and the filtration of blood and the disposal of defective blood cells. These two functions of the spleen are architecturally distinct. The lymphoid function occurs in the white pulp and the phagocytic activity in the red pulp.

Filtering function

1. Removal of old or abnormal red cells
2. Removal of abnormal white cells, normal and abnormal platelets and cellular debris. In splenectomised individuals, cells with inclusion bodies, e.g. Howell–Jolly bodies, are seen. Normally any intracytoplasmic inclusions, such as Howell–Jolly bodies, are removed by macrophages in the pulp cords (a process known as 'pitting'). In the absence of a functioning spleen there are characteristic changes in red cell morphology. Howell–Jolly bodies, which are remnants of nuclear material from developing erythrocytes, occur.

Immunological function

1. Opsonisation. While opsonised bacteria can be removed from the circulation by the entire reticulo-endothelial system, the spleen is well suited to removing poorly opsonised or encapsulated pathogens.
2. Antibody synthesis. This occurs chiefly within the white pulp. Blood-borne antigens stimulate B cells which proliferate and differentiate to form plasma cells which produce large amounts of antibodies (immunoglobulins).
3. Protection from infection. Splenectomy leaves some patients more prone to infection (see below).

DISORDERS OF THE SPLEEN

Hypersplenism

This is a term applied to splenomegaly associated with the following:

1. any combination of anaemia, leucopaenia, or thrombocytopaenia
2. compensatory bone marrow hyperplasia
3. improvement after splenectomy.

There is an exaggerated destruction or sequestration of circulating blood elements, which can affect red cells, white cells and platelets. The condition may be either primary or secondary.

Primary hypersplenism

This is essentially a diagnosis of exclusion where all causes of secondary hypersplenism have been excluded. It is a rare condition of unknown aetiology, mainly affecting women. There may be massive splenomegaly and an accompanying pancytopaenia, especially leucopaenia. There may be recurring fevers and infection. Splenectomy results in a good haematological response, although some patients may remain leucopaenic. Secondary splenomegaly may also be associated with hypersplenism.

Splenomegaly

The causes of splenomegaly are numerous but may be grouped together under the following headings:

1. congestion
2. infection
3. haematological disorders
4. immune disorders
5. storage disorders
6. amyloid

Congestion

Conditions leading to elevation of splenic venous pressure are capable of causing splenomegaly. Causes may be prehepatic, hepatic, or posthepatic. Prehepatic causes include thrombosis of the extra hepatic portion of the portal vein or splenic vein thrombosis. Hepatic causes include longstanding portal hypertension associated with cirrhosis. Posthepatic causes are usually associated with a raised pressure in the inferior vena cava, which is transmitted to the spleen via the portal system. There is usually coexisting ascites and hepatomegaly. Decompensated right-sided heart failure and pulmonary or tricuspid valve disease are the usual causes.

Infection

The spleen may enlarge in several infectious diseases but particularly in chronic malaria, typhoid and some viral diseases, particularly infectious mononucleosis.

Haematological disorders

Splenomegaly may occur in haemolytic anaemias, hereditary spherocytosis, idiopathic thrombocytopaenic purpura, and polycythaemia rubra vera. Splenic infiltration is a common feature of a variety of haematological neoplasms, including leukaemias, myeloproliferative disorders, Hodgkin's disease and non-Hodgkin's lymphoma. In chronic myeloid leukaemia and myeloproliferative syndromes, splenomegaly may be massive and the spleen may be palpable in the right iliac fossa.

Immunological disorders

A variety of immunological disorders may lead to splenomegaly, chiefly rheumatoid arthritis and systemic lupus erythematosus.

Storage disorders

Several storage disorders may cause splenomegaly. These include Niemann–Pick disease, Gaucher's disease and the mucopolysaccharidoses.

Amyloidosis

In systemic amyloidosis, amyloid is deposited in a wide variety of organs and virtually no organ is exempt. Clinical features suggesting amyloidosis include generalised diffuse organ enlargement, e.g. hepatomegaly or splenomegaly, and evidence of organ dysfunction, e.g. cardiac failure or renal failure.

EFFECTS OF SPLENECTOMY

Haematological effects

Loss of splenic tissue reduces the capacity of the spleen to remove immature or abnormal red cells from the circulation. The red cell count does not change, but red cells with cytoplasmic inclusions, e.g. Howell–Jolly bodies, may appear. Target cells, reticulocytes and siderocytes appear within a few days of operation. Granulocytosis occurs immediately after splenectomy but is replaced in a few weeks by lymphocytosis and monocytosis. The platelet count is usually increased and may stay at levels of $400\,000-500\,000 \times 10^9/L$ for over a year. Occasionally there may be a thrombocytosis in excess of $1000 \times 10^9/L$. This is not an indication for anticoagulation, but antiplatelet agents such as aspirin may help prevent thrombosis.

Postsplenectomy sepsis

Individuals are susceptible to fulminant bacteraemia after splenectomy. The risk is greatest in young children, especially in the first 2 years after surgery, accounting for 80% of all cases. The risk is also greater when splenectomy is undertaken for disorders of the reticulo-endothelial system rather than for trauma. In general, the younger the patient undergoing splenectomy and the more severe the underlying condition, the greater is the risk of developing overwhelming postsplenectomy sepsis. There is a small but significant risk of infection even in otherwise healthy adults following splenectomy. The risk is much higher in the first 2 years than in subsequent years. Lethal sepsis is more common in children and indeed is very rare in adults.

Streptococcus pneumoniae, Haemophilus influenzae and meningococci are the most common pathogens. There is a distinct clinical syndrome starting with mild non-specific symptoms followed by a high pyrexia and septicaemic shock which may ultimately be fatal. The risk of fatal sepsis is less after splenectomy for trauma. This may be due to splenosis, i.e. multiple small implants of splenic tissue which result from dissemination and autotransplantation of splenic fragments following splenic rupture. Presumably this results in areas of splenic tissue which function well enough to protect against septicaemia.

Prophylactic vaccinations should be given against pneumococcal septicaemia. For planned procedures a polyvalent pneumococcal vaccine should be given prior to splenectomy. Evidence exists that splenic function may be important in the immune response to the vaccine. Antipneumococcal IgM titres are lower when patients are vaccinated after splenectomy. The vaccine is only effective against 80% of pneumococcal organisms; therefore it is recommended that prophylactic penicillin be given for 2 years after splenectomy, when the risk of sepsis is at its greatest. Antibiotic prophylaxis is essential in children under 2 years of age. Some authorities believe that antibiotic prophylaxis should be continued for life. Vaccination against *H. influenzae* type b (HiB) and meningococci A and C should also be given.

THYMUS

STRUCTURE AND FUNCTION

The thymus develops from the third and fourth pharyngeal pouches and descends into the anterior superior mediastinum. It is an encaspulated structure, the capsule extending into the thymus as trabeculae dividing into a number of lobules. Each lobule has a cortex and medulla. The cortex contains densely packed lymphocytes which stain darkly. The medulla contains a few lymphocytes, macrophages but chiefly epithelial cells. The medulla also contains thymic (Hassall's) corpuscles, which are epithelial cells arranged concentrically, the centre of which may be keratinised. Their function is unknown. It is relatively largest at birth in comparison to body weight. It is absolutely at its largest at puberty but thereafter declines in size such that in the elderly it is atrophied and composed largely of fat. It lies behind the manubrium sterni, anterior to the large veins draining its venous blood into the left brachiocephalic vein. It extends slightly into the neck and also along the surface of the pericardium and may abut on the pleura. Its arterial blood supply is derived from the internal mammary artery or the peri-cardiophrenic arteries. Occasionally the lower para-thyroids may be related to the thymus, both structures developing from the third pharyngeal pouch.

The thymus is responsible for the induction of cell-mediated immune function in developing lymphoid cells (see Ch. 6).

DISORDERS OF THE THYMUS

Agenesis may occur, resulting in immunodeficiency syndromes. Histological abnormalities of the thymus such as lymphoid hyperplasia or tumours may be seen in association with certain autoimmune diseases such as myasthenia gravis, systemic lupus erythematosus, dermatomyositis, and aplastic anaemia.

Thymic tumours

Thymoma is a rare tumour of the epithelial elements of the thymus. Many are asymptomatic and are detected on chest x-ray performed for other reasons. Some are detected when myasthenia gravis develops. Others may present with signs of local disease such as cough, dyspnoea, stridor, or superior vena caval obstruction. The majority of thymomas are benign and well encapsulated. Malignant tumours are locally invasive, spreading by direct invasion of adjacent structures. Distant spread is exceedingly rare.

Other tumours of the thymus include Hodgkin's disease, non-Hodgkin's lymphoma, teratoma, thymolipoma and, rarely, thymic carcinoid.

Respiratory system

Andrew Dyson, Andrew T Raftery

ANATOMY

TRACHEA

The trachea is about 11 cm long, commencing at the lower border of the cricoid cartilage at the level of the 6th cervical vertebra, and terminating by dividing into the right and left main bronchi at the level of the 5th thoracic vertebra. The trachea is composed of fibroelastic tissue and is prevented from collapsing by a series of cartilaginous rings numbering 15–20. The rings are U-shaped, open posteriorly, where they are flattened, the posterior free end of the cartilaginous rings being covered by smooth muscle (trachealis). The trachea is lined by columnar ciliated epithelium containing numerous goblet cells.

Relations

Neck
- anteriorly — the isthmus of the thyroid gland, the inferior thyroid veins, sternohyoid, sternothyroid
- laterally — lobes of the thyroid gland, the carotid sheath
- posteriorly — oesophagus and recurrent laryngeal nerves running in the groove between the trachea and the oesophagus.

Thorax
- anteriorly — the brachiocephalic and left common carotid artery; the left brachiocephalic vein; thymus
- posteriorly — oesophagus and recurrent laryngeal nerves
- on the right — vagus nerve; azygos vein; pleura
- on the left — aortic arch, left common carotid artery, left subclavian artery, left recurrent laryngeal nerve, and pleura.

BRONCHI

The trachea terminates at the level of the sternal angle by dividing into the right and left main bronchi (Fig. 11.1).

The right main bronchus is wider, shorter and more vertical than the left. It is approximately 2.5 cm long and passes downwards and laterally behind the ascending aorta and superior vena cava to enter the hilum of the lung. The azygos vein arches over it from behind to enter the superior vena cava, while the pulmonary artery lies first below it and then anterior to it. The right main bronchus gives off an upper lobe bronchus just before it enters the lung. It then proceeds into the lung where it divides into the bronchi to the middle and inferior lobes.

The left main bronchus is approximately 5 cm long and passes downwards and laterally below the arch of the aorta, in front of the oesophagus and descending aorta. The pulmonary artery lies at first anteriorly and then above the bronchus. On the left side the main bronchus terminates by dividing into the bronchi to the upper and lower lobes of the left lung shortly after entering the lung.

LUNGS

The lungs (Fig. 11.2) are conical in shape. They conform to the shape of the pleural cavities. Each lung has a blunt apex which reaches above the sternal end of the first rib, a base related to the diaphragm, a convex parietal surface related to the ribs, and a mediastinal surface which is concave and related to the pericardium.

Each lung is subdivided by an oblique fissure into upper and lower lobes, the right lung being further divided by the horizontal fissure to produce a middle lobe. The surface marking of the oblique fissures is best represented by the line of the vertebral border of the scapula with the arm fully elevated. The horizontal fissure of the right lung passes horizontally and medially from the oblique fissure at the level of the fourth costal cartilage. The equivalent of the middle lobe in the left lung is the lingula which lies between the cardiac notch and the oblique fissure.

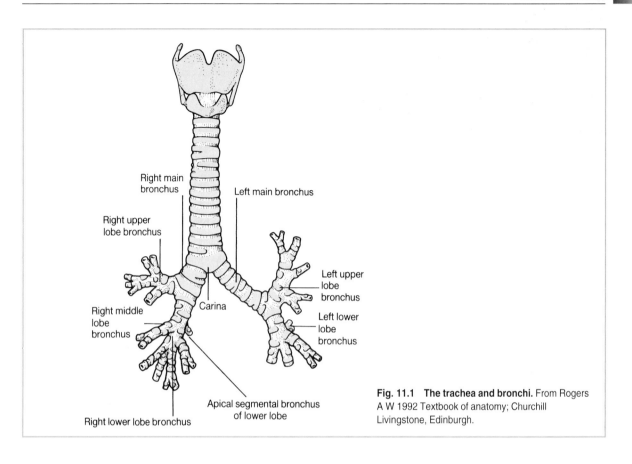

Fig. 11.1   The trachea and bronchi. From Rogers A W 1992 Textbook of anatomy; Churchill Livingstone, Edinburgh.

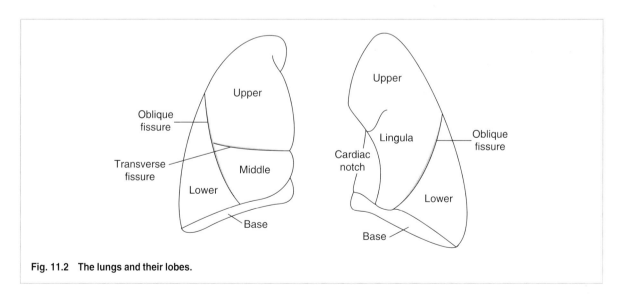

Fig. 11.2   The lungs and their lobes.

Bronchopulmonary segments

Each lobar bronchus divides to supply the broncho-pulmonary segments of the lung. Each lung has 10 segments. These are shown in Figure 11.3. Each of the bronchopulmonary segments is supplied by a segmental bronchus, artery and vein. There is no communication with adjacent segments. It is thus possible to remove an individual segment without interfering with a function of adjacent segments. Each segment takes its name from that of the supplying segmental bronchus.

Blood supply

The pulmonary trunk arises from the right ventricle of the heart behind the third left costal cartilage. It is directed upwards in front of the ascending aorta. It then passes backwards on the left of the ascending aorta and, beneath the aortic arch, it divides into the right and left pulmonary arteries.

Right pulmonary artery

This passes in front of the oesophagus to the root of the right lung, behind the ascending aorta and superior vena cava. Here it lies in front of and between the right main bronchus and its upper lobe branch.

Left pulmonary artery

This is connected at its origin with the arch of the aorta by the ligamentum arteriosum. It runs in front of the left main bronchus and descending aorta. The left recurrent

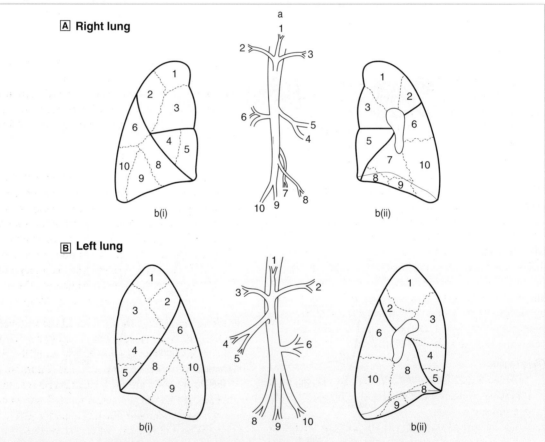

Fig. 11.3 **Bronchi and bronchopulmonary segments.** [A] Right lung: (a) the divisions of the right main bronchus; (b) bronchopulmonary segments: (i) lateral surface, (ii) medial surface. Upper lobe: 1, apical bronchus; 2, posterior bronchus; 3, anterior bronchus. Middle lobe: 4, lateral bronchus; 5, medial bronchus. Lower lobe: 6, apical bronchus; 7, medial basal (cardiac) bronchus; 8, anterior basal bronchus; 9, lateral basal bronchus; 10, posterior basal bronchus. [B] Left lung: (a) the divisions of the left main bronchus; (b) bronchopulmonary segments: (i) lateral surface; (ii) medial surface. Upper lobe: 1, 2, apicoposterior bronchus; 3, anterior bronchus. Lingula: 4, superior bronchus; 5, inferior bronchus. Lower lobe: 6, apical bronchus; 8, anterior basal bronchus; 9, lateral basal bronchus; 10, posterior basal bronchus.

laryngeal nerve loops below the aortic arch in contact with the ligamentum arteriosum.

PLEURA

Each pleural cavity is composed of a thin serous membrane invaginated by the lung. The visceral layer of pleura is intimately related to the surface of the lung and is continuous over the root of the lung with a parietal layer which is applied to the inner aspect of the chest wall, the diaphragm and the mediastinum. The two pleural cavities are totally separate from each other. Below the root of the lung the pleura forms a loose fold known as the pulmonary ligament which allows for distension of the pulmonary veins. The lungs conform to the shape of the pleural cavities but do not occupy the full cavity, as they would not be able to expand as in full inspiration.

Surface anatomy

The cervical pleura extends above the sternal end of the first rib. It follows a curved line drawn from the sterno-clavicular joint to the junction of the inner third and outer two thirds of the clavicle, the apex of the pleura arising about 2.5 cm above the clavicle. The line of the pleura on each side passes from behind the sternoclavicular joint to meet in the midline at the level of the second costal carti-lage. The right pleura then passes vertically down to the 6th costal cartilage before crossing the 8th rib in the mid-clavicular line, the 10th rib in the midaxillary line, and 12th rib at the lateral border of the erector spinae. On the left side the pleural edge reaches the 4th costal cartilage, where it arches out lateral to the border of the sternum, the pleura being separated from the chest wall by the protrusion of the pericardium. The medial ends of the 4th and 5th intercostal spaces are therefore not covered by pleura. Apart from this, its relationships are the same as those on the right side. The pleura actually descends below the 12th rib at its medial extremity.

Clinical points

1. The pleura rises above the clavicle and into the neck. It may be injured by a stab wound, a surgeon's knife, or a subclavian line.
2. A needle passed through the 4th and 5th intercostal spaces immediately lateral to the sternum will enter the pericardium without traversing the pleura.
3. The pleura descends below the medial extremity of the 12th rib. It may be inadvertently opened in the loin approach to the kidney or adrenal gland.

Nerve supply

The pleura receives its nerve supply from the nerves that supply the structures to which it is attached. The visceral pleura receives an autonomic supply from branches of the vagus nerve that supply the lung. It is sensitive only to stretching. The parietal pleura receives a somatic inner-vation from the adjacent intercostal nerves as they run round the chest wall. The diaphragmatic pleura is sup-plied by the phrenic nerve. The parietal pleura is there-fore sensitive to pain, and this may be referred via the intercostal nerves to the abdomen: i.e. diseases of the chest wall and pleura may present as abdominal pain.

THORACIC CAGE

The thoracic cage is formed by the vertebral column behind, the ribs and intercostal spaces on either side, and the sternum and costal cartilages in front.

Ribs

There are 12 pairs of ribs (Fig. 11.4). The first seven pairs are connected anteriorly via their costal cartilages to the sternum. The 8th, 9th and 10th ribs articulate with their costal cartilages, each with the rib above. The 11th and 12th ribs remain free anteriorly and are known as 'floating ribs'.

A typical rib comprises:

1. a head with two articular facets for articulation with the corresponding vertebra and the vertebra above
2. a neck giving rise to the costotransverse ligaments
3. a tubercle with a smooth facet for articulation with the transverse process of the corresponding vertebra
4. a shaft which is flattened from side to side and possesses an angle. The shaft possesses a groove on its lower surface, the subcostal groove. The intercostal vessels and nerves lie in this groove.

The first, 2nd, 10th, 11th and 12th ribs are atypical. Only the first and 12th are clinically important. The first rib is the shortest, flattest and most curved of the ribs. It is flattened from above downwards. The features of the first rib are shown in Figure 11. 4. The 12th rib is short, has no tubercle, and has only a single facet. There is no angle and no subcostal groove. Its only importance is in the loin approach to the kidney, where its relationship to the pleura is important. The pleura descends below the 12th rib at its medial extremity.

Clinical points

Rib fractures These may damage underlying or related structures. Fracture of any rib may lead to trauma to the lung and the development of a pneumothorax. Fracture of the left lower ribs may traumatise the spleen.

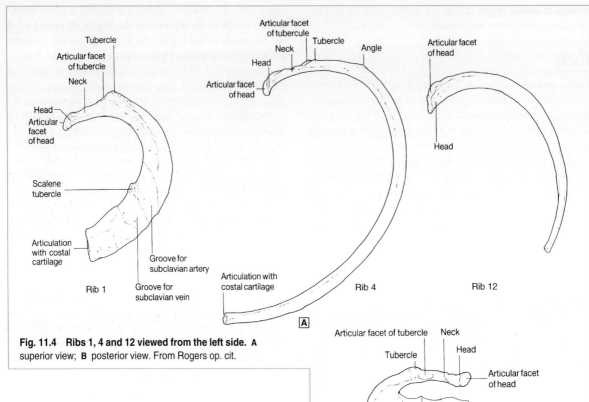

Fig. 11.4 Ribs 1, 4 and 12 viewed from the left side. A superior view; **B** posterior view. From Rogers op. cit.

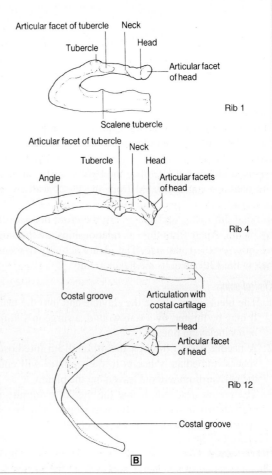

Fractures of the ribs may also traumatise the related intercostal vessels, leading to bleeding into the chest, i.e. haemothorax.

Coarctation of the aorta In this condition collateral vessels develop between the vessels above and below the block. The superior intercostal artery, derived from the costocervical trunk of the subclavian artery, supplies blood to the intercostal arteries of the aorta, thus bypassing the narrowing in the aorta. As a consequence, the intercostal vessels dilate and become tortuous because of the increased flow and erode the lower border of the ribs, giving rise to notching which may be seen on a chest x-ray.

Cervical ribs These occur with an incidence of 1:200 and may be bilateral in 1:500 cases. The rib may be complete, articulating with the transverse process of the 7th cervical vertebra behind and with the first rib in front. Occasionally, a cervical rib may have a free distal extremity and, in some cases, is merely represented by a fibrous band. A cervical rib may cause vascular or neurological symptoms. Vascular consequences include post-stenotic dilatation of the subclavian artery, caused by local turbulence, and therefore the risk of distal emboli. A subclavian aneurysm may also result. It is also associated with Raynaud's phenomenon. Pressure on the vein may result in subclavian vein thrombosis. A cervical rib may also cause pressure on the lower trunk of the brachial plexus which arches over it. This results in paraesthesia in the dermatomal distribution of C8/T1 together with wasting of the small muscles of the hand (myotome T1).

Sternum

This consists of three parts: the manubrium, the body and the xiphoid process.

Manubrium This is approximately triangular in shape. The medial end of the clavicle articulates with it, as do the first costal cartilage and the upper part of the second costal cartilage on each side. It articulates with the body of the sternum at the angle of Louis (manubriosternal joint).

Body The body of the sternum is composed of four pieces often known as sternebrae. The lateral margins of the body are notched to receive most of the second and the third to the seventh costal cartilages.

Xiphoid This is usually small and remains cartilaginous well into adult life. It may become more prominent when the patient loses weight (either naturally or due to disease). The patient may present to the clinic because he/she has noticed a lump which was previously covered with fat.

Relations

The manubrium forms the anterior boundary of the superior mediastinum. Its lowest part is related to the arch of the aorta and its upper part to the left brachiocephalic vein and the brachiocephalic, left common carotid, and left subclavian arteries. Its lateral portions are related to the lungs and pleura.

The body of the sternum is related on the right side of the median plain to the right pleura and the thin anterior border of the right lung which intervenes between it and the pericardium. To the left of the median plane, the upper two pieces are related to the left pleura and lung but the lower two are directly related to the pericardium. Clinically, sternal puncture is used to obtain bone marrow. A needle is passed through the cortical bone into the marrow. One should be aware of the posterior relations! The sternum is split for access for open heart surgery, and occasionally a split of the manubrium is required for access to the thymus, retrosternal goitre, or ectopic parathyroid tissue.

Costal cartilages

These connect the upper seven ribs to the sternum and the 8th, 9th and 10th ribs to the cartilage immediately above.

They are composed of hyaline cartilage and add resilience to the thoracic cage, protecting it from more frequent fractures. With increasing age they ossify and may be seen as irregular areas of calcification on a chest x-ray.

Intercostal spaces

Typically each intercostal space contains three muscles, comparable to those of the abdominal wall, and an associated neurovascular bundle which runs between the middle and the innermost layers of muscle. The three layers of muscle are: (i) the external intercostal, whose fibres pass downwards and forwards from the rib above to the rib below; the muscle is deficient in front where it is replaced by the anterior intercostal membrane; (ii) the internal intercostal, which runs downwards and backwards and is deficient behind where it is replaced by the posterior intercostal membrane; and (iii) the innermost intercostal, which may cover more than one intercostal space.

The neurovascular bundle runs between the internal intercostal and the innermost intercostal. It consists, from above downwards, of vein, artery and nerve, the vein lying directly in the groove on the undersurface of the corresponding rib. The arrangement of muscles, vessels and nerve is shown in Figure 11.5.

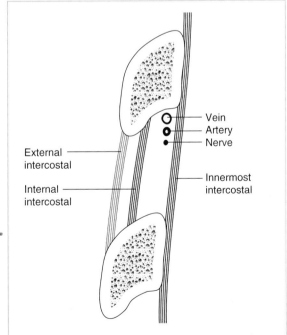

Vein
Artery
Nerve

External intercostal

Innermost intercostal

Internal intercostal

Fig. 11.5 An intercostal space. A needle passed into the chest immediately above a rib will avoid the neurovascular bundle.

DIAPHRAGM

The diaphragm (Fig. 11.6) is a dome-shaped septum separating the thorax from the abdomen. It is composed of a peripheral muscular part and a central tendon.

The muscular fibres arise from several sources: the crura, the arcuate ligaments, the ribs and the sternum. The right crus of the diaphragm arises from the front of the bodies of the first three lumbar vertebrae and the intervening intervertebral discs. The left crus arises from the first and second lumbar vertebrae and the intervening disc. The arcuate ligaments are a series of arches, the lateral being a condensation of the fascia overlying quadratus lumborum and the medial of the fascia overlying psoas major. The medial borders of the medial arcuate ligaments join anteriorly over the aorta as the median arcuate ligaments. The costal part of the diaphragm arises from the inner aspect of the lower six ribs and the sternal portion as two small slips from the posterior surface of the xiphisternum.

The central tendon is trefoil in shape and receives the insertion of the muscular fibres. Above, it fuses with the lower part of the pericardium.

There are three main openings in the diaphragm, although strictly speaking the aortic 'opening' is not in the diaphragm but lies behind it. The aortic 'opening' transmits the abdominal aorta, the thoracic duct, and often the azygos vein. The oesophageal opening lies in the right crus of the diaphragm and transmits the oesophagus, the vagus nerves, and branches of the left gastric artery and vein. The opening for the inferior vena cava lies in the central tendon of the diaphragm and transmits, in addition to the IVC, the right phrenic nerve.

The greater and lesser splanchnic nerves pierce the crura, and the sympathetic chain passes behind the medial arcuate ligament lying on psoas major.

Nerve supply

The diaphragm is supplied by the phrenic nerves (C3, 4, 5) which have long course in the neck and the thorax. Damage to the nerve leads to paralysis of the diaphragm, which results in elevation of the diaphragm seen on x-ray and paradoxical movement on respiration. The phrenic nerve also gives a sensory supply to the central part of the diaphragm. Irritation of the diaphragm, e.g. in peritonitis or pleurisy, results in referred pain to the cutaneous

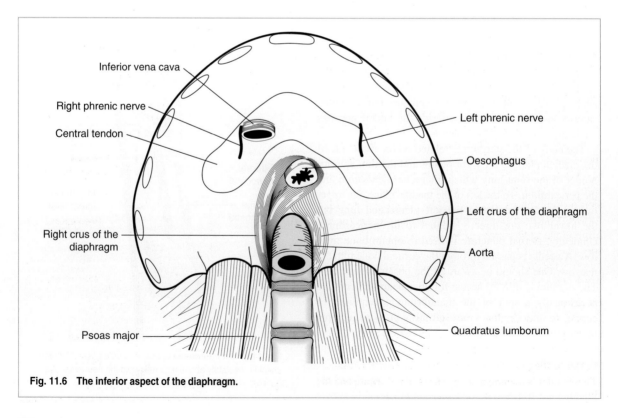

Fig. 11.6 The inferior aspect of the diaphragm.

- Inferior vena cava
- Right phrenic nerve
- Central tendon
- Left phrenic nerve
- Oesophagus
- Left crus of the diaphragm
- Right crus of the diaphragm
- Aorta
- Psoas major
- Quadratus lumborum

area of supply, i.e. the shoulder tip via dermatome C4. The peripheral part of the diaphragm receives sensory innervation from the lower six intercostal nerves.

ANATOMY OF RESPIRATION

There are two main mechanisms for increasing the volume of the thorax:

- movements of the rib cage, thoracic breathing
- contraction of the diaphragm, abdominal breathing.

Thoracic breathing

During inspiration, the ribs are elevated, and this occurs in two ways, as follows.

1. The anterior ends of the ribs are raised in the so-called pump handle action. Since the anterior ends are normally below the posterior ends, this increases the anteroposterior diameter of the thorax.
2. The most lateral and lowest parts of ribs 4–7 are raised in the so-called bucket handle action. Since the centre of these ribs is normally below the anterior and posterior ends, the transverse diameter of the chest is increased when they move upwards.

Abdominal breathing

This is controlled by the diaphragm. The peripheral muscle fibres of the diaphragm are more or less vertical and take origin from the lower six ribs. When the muscular fibres of the diaphragm contract, the diaphragm descends, increasing the vertical diameter of the thorax. As the central tendon descends, its vertical movement eventually arrests as it reaches the upper surface of the liver. The central tendon then behaves as an origin for the muscle fibres, which now elevate the lower six ribs in the final stages of inspiration. The combination of thoracic and abdominal breathing results in an increase in all diameters of the thorax. This in turn brings about an increase in the negative intrapleural pressure and expansion of the lung tissue occurs. Abdominal and thoracic breathing occur in quiet inspiration. In deep and in forced inspiration, additional muscles are used, i.e. the accessory muscles of respiration. These include sternocleidomastoid, the scalene muscles, pectoralis minor, pectoralis major and serratus anterior.

Expiration

Expiration is normally a passive process produced by the elastic recoil of the lungs and the tissues of the chest wall. However, forced expiration such as in coughing or playing a trumpet requires muscular activity. Such muscles include rectus abdominus, external oblique, internal oblique, transversus abdominus, latissimus dorsi.

STRUCTURE OF THE RESPIRATORY TREE

The basic structure of the lower respiratory tree is shown in Figure 11. 7. The respiratory tree is designed to transport humidified air into the distal airways and alveoli where exchange between CO_2 and oxygen takes place. The trachea is composed of C-shaped plates of cartilage with the curve of the C anteriorly; the ring is completed posteriorly with smooth muscle. The trachea contains mucous glands and is lined with ciliated epithelium. The trachea divides into bronchi and these contain discontinuous pieces of cartilage in their wall together with smooth muscle. They too are lined by columnar ciliated epithelium and contain mucous glands. The cilia beat rhythmically in a thin liquid layer and effectively transport the surface film of mucus and particles out of the lungs by way of the trachea.

The bronchi decrease in diameter and length with each successive branching. The cartilaginous support eventually disappears. In airways of about 1 mm the cartilage

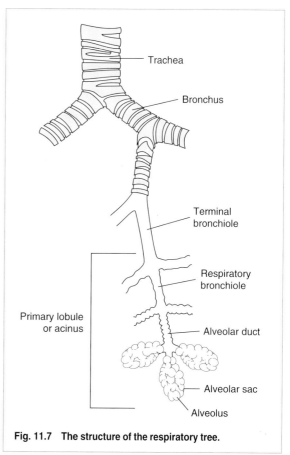

Fig. 11.7 **The structure of the respiratory tree.**

disappears completely. By convention all subsequent airways are called bronchioles. Bronchioles contain no cartilage or submucosal mucous glands. They contain cuboidal epithelium with ciliated cells as well as some additional cells which are thought to provide a watery secretion. The most distal air passages are the respiratory bronchioles, which are so called because the first alveoli open directly into them. Respiratory bronchioles end in several alveolar ducts, which are short channels which open into alveolar sacs which contain many alveoli. A single respiratory bronchiole, its alveoli and their blood supply are called a primary lobule or acinus. The alveoli are lined by flattened Type I pneumocytes together with some Type II pneumocytes. Type II cells secrete surfactant and replicate rapidly after injury to alveolar walls. These alveolar cells lie on a basement membrane together with an interstitial matrix including some elastin fibres which separate the air spaces from the pulmonary capillary walls. The structure of the alveolar–capillary membrane permits rapid and efficient diffusion of oxygen and carbon dioxide.

MEDIASTINUM

The mediastinum (Fig. 11.8) is the name given to the space between the two pleural cavities. It extends from the sternum in front to the thoracic vertebrae behind and from the thoracic inlet above to the diaphragm below.

For descriptive purposes it is divided into a superior and an inferior mediastinum, the latter being again subdivided into anterior, middle and posterior.

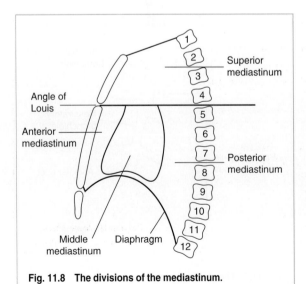

Fig. 11.8   The divisions of the mediastinum.

Superior mediastinum

This is bounded in front by the manubrium sterni and behind by the first four thoracic vertebrae. Above, it continues up to the root of the neck; below, it is continuous with the three divisions of the inferior mediastinum at a level of a line drawn horizontally through the angle of Louis. It contains the lower end of the trachea, the oesophagus, the thoracic duct, the arch of the aorta, the innominate artery, part of the carotid and subclavian arteries, the innominate veins, the upper part of the superior vena cava, the phrenic and vagus nerves, the left recurrent laryngeal nerve, the cardiac nerves, lymphatic glands, and the remnants of the thymus gland.

Anterior mediastinum

This is the space between the two pleural cavities in front of the pericardium and behind the sternum. In children part of the thymus gland may occupy this space, but in the adult it contains only the anterior mediastinal lymph glands.

Middle mediastinum

The middle mediastinum contains the pericardium itself with the heart and great vessels. The phrenic nerve and pericardiacophrenic vessels run down the lateral surface of the pericardium to reach the diaphragm.

Posterior mediastinum

This lies behind the pericardium and the diaphragm below. Anteriorly lie the pericardium and roots of the lungs, with the diaphragm lying anteriorly below. Posteriorly lies the vertebral column from the lower border of the 4th to the 12th thoracic vertebrae. Inferiorly lies the diaphragm and superiorly is a horizontal plane drawn through the angle of Louis. The posterior mediastinum contains the descending thoracic aorta, the oesophagus, the vagus and splanchnic nerves, the azygos and hemiazygos veins, the thoracic duct and the posterior mediastinal lymph glands.

Because of the arrangement of structures in the mediastinum, its appearance is different when viewed from the right and left hand sides. These differences and their relationships to the roots of the lungs are shown in Figures 11.9 and 11.10.

PHYSIOLOGY

CONTROL OF VENTILATION

The body succeeds in keeping arterial PO_2 and PCO_2 within remarkably narrow limits. This is made possible by highly developed negative feedback systems that consist of sensors, controllers and effectors.

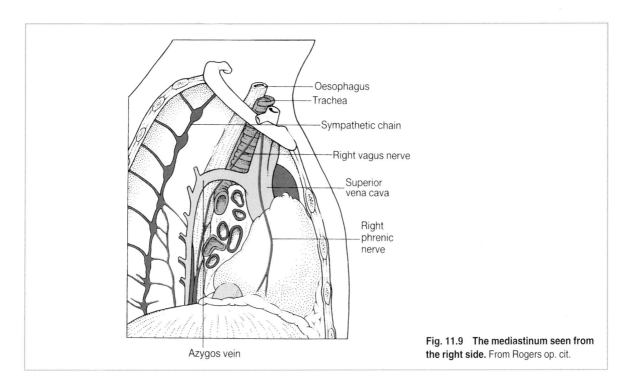

Fig. 11.9 The mediastinum seen from the right side. From Rogers op. cit.

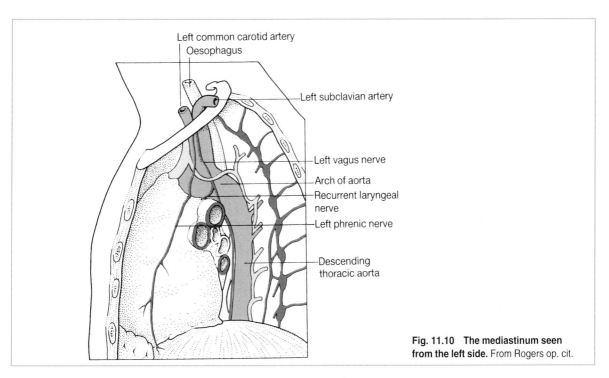

Fig. 11.10 The mediastinum seen from the left side. From Rogers op. cit.

Controllers

The controllers of ventilation are situated in the brain. Impulses from the brainstem effect normal automatic respiration, which can be overridden by the several mechanisms when voluntary control is warranted. The respiratory sensors are located in the pons and medulla. These can be thought of as three main groups of neurons, as follows.

1. Medullary respiratory centre. There are two groups of cells: one is associated with inspiration and one with expiration. These groups interact to produce the inherent rhythmicity of respiration.
2. Apneustic centre. This is located in the lower pons. If the brain of a cat is sectioned above this site inspiratory gasps develop. These are called apneuses and are interrupted transient expiratory efforts.
3. Pneumotaxic centre. This is found in the upper pons. This centre seems to inhibit inspiration after it has reached a certain point.

Other areas of importance include the cortex, which can override, to a large extent, the automatic, subconscious control of breathing. In affective states such as fear or extreme anger the limbic system and hypothalamus can influence respiration.

Effectors

These are the muscles of respiration. They are respectively the diaphragm, intercostals, abdominal wall muscles and accessory muscles (see anatomy section).

In order for respiration to be effective in extremes of demand these muscles must work in a fully coordinated way, under the auspices of the central control.

Sensors

These are the central chemoreceptors, peripheral chemoreceptors, and several others. In the lung, sensors include primary stretch receptors, irritant receptors and J receptors. In the nose and upper airway there are sensitive irritant receptors, while joints and muscles utilise the gamma stretch receptor and associated reflex. It should not be forgotten that the arterial baroreceptors may influence respiration (see later).

Central chemoreceptors

These are the most important receptors involved in day to day respiratory control. They are situated in the ventral surface of the medulla. Here the extracellular fluid (ECF) of the brain surrounds the central chemoreceptors. Changes in hydrogen ion concentration of the ECF cause these receptors to respond. As hydrogen ion concentra-

tion increases, so ventilation increases, and the opposite is true. The pH of the ECF is most affected by the cerebrospinal fluid (CSF) hydrogen ion content. CSF is separated from the circulation by the blood–brain barrier. Whilst ions such as hydrogen and bicarbonate do not easily cross the blood–brain barrier, CO_2 can cross readily. Thus as arterial PO_2 ($PaCO_2$) rises, CSF PCO_2 goes up, liberating hydrogen ions, which in turn lower the pH of the ECF. This stimulates central chemoreceptors to effect increased ventilation. Increased ventilation will decrease arterial $PaCO_2$. An increased $PaCO_2$ causes cerebral vasodilatation facilitating more rapid diffusion of CO_2 into the CSF.

A feature of CSF is that it has much lower buffering capacity than blood. Small changes in PCO_2 effect larger changes in CSF pH than in blood pH. However, bicarbonate can diffuse slowly across the blood–brain barrier, and so changes in pH of CSF are eventually compensated for by a rise or fall in bicarbonate. This process takes about 36 h to complete, so that if $PaCO_2$ is elevated for a prolonged period the chemoreceptors will 'reset', e.g. chronic lung disease, where patients may have an elevated $PaCO_2$ with a normal CSF pH and normal respiratory rates.

Peripheral chemoreceptors

As the name suggests these are located outside the CNS in the carotid bodies where the common carotid arteries bifurcate, and in the aortic arch. These bodies contain glomus cells, with a large dopamine content. Because of their location, they have a very high blood flow per unit weight. These receptors increase their firing rate in response to:

- decreased PaO_2
- decreased pH
- increased $PaCO_2$.

Curiously the response to a fall in PaO_2 begins at about 70 kPa, a state not likely to be encountered naturally. However, the sensitivity of the cells is much greater in the range below 13.5 kPa, when the firing rate increases dramatically.

These receptors are responsible for the increase in ventilation which occurs in hypoxaemia — a response easily abolished by small doses of morphine or anaesthetic agents. The response to hypoxaemia is the important one. The peripheral chemoreceptors have a much less important response than the central ones to changes in $PaCO_2$.

The response to a change in arterial pH is mediated only by the carotid bodies — hydrogen ions cannot readily cross the blood–brain barrier. A fall in pH will increase ventilation.

Receptors within the lung

Mechanical   Stretch receptors within the lungs discharge in response to distension of the lungs. Impulses are sent via the vagus nerve and result in a decreased respiratory rate. This is often referred to as the Hering-Breuer reflex. This may be important in newborn babies but is not useful for day to day control of respiration.

Chemical

1. J receptors. 'J' stands for juxta capillary, i.e. in juxtaposition to the capillaries, but in the alveolar wall. This is based on the observation that injection of chemicals into the pulmonary circulation produces almost instantaneous rapid shallow breathing, even apnoea. The function of these receptors is unclear.
2. Irritant receptors. These respond to noxious gases, smoke, cold air, etc. They probably lie in airway epithelial cells and their impulses are sent via the vagus nerve, resulting in bronchospasm and hyperpnoea.

Receptors outside the lung

Chemical   Receptors found in the nose and upper airway which respond to chemical stimulation, resulting in coughing and sneezing, and laryngeal spasm, which occurs during choking or sometimes during anaesthesia.

Mechanical   Joint and muscle receptors stimulate respiration at the start of exercise, whilst the respiratory muscle contains sensors which relay information on muscle length and help control the force of contraction and possibly the sensation of dyspnoea.

Finally, stimulation of aortic and carotid sinus baroreceptors following increased blood pressure results in hypoventilation or even apnoea, whilst a decrease in blood pressure can cause hyperventilation.

How do these mechanisms combine to control ventilation?

Consider the three main chemical factors which affect respiration:

1. arterial CO_2
2. arterial O_2
3. arterial pH.

Arterial CO₂

Under normal conditions the most important determinant of ventilation control is the $PaCO_2$. The mechanism is sufficiently sensitive to keep the variation in arterial level of CO_2 within about 0.4 kPa. Sedation, alcohol and sleep will all tend to increase $PaCO_2$.

If subjects are given CO_2 to breathe then their rate and depth of respiration increase so that for each 0.1 kPa increase in $PaCO_2$ an increase in minute volume of about 1.5 L occurs. If the subject becomes hypoxic the rate of increase in minute volume increases. If the amount of CO_2 inspired is allowed to increase to very high levels (15%) then no further increase in minute volume occurs and the subject may become drowsy and exhibit depressed ventilation. Conversely, if $PaCO_2$ levels are allowed to fall (e.g. following hyperventilation), then ventilation becomes depressed. This can easily occur when mechanically ventilating patients.

Arterial O₂

Arterial oxygen tensions do not control respiration on a minute to minute basis in the same way as $PaCO_2$. Indeed lowering PaO_2 by breathing hypoxic mixtures produces no effect until PaO_2 = 6.5 kPa. These are very low levels of arterial O_2 and they are not seen in day to day life. They may occur in illness (e.g. pneumonia) or on ascent to high altitude. However, when $PaCO_2$ is raised, the effects of a low PaO_2 are seen at levels approaching 13 kPa.

In severe, longstanding, lung disease, patients may exhibit a persistent $PaCO_2$ elevation with a low PaO_2. These patients may rely on hypoxaemia to provide an adequate respiratory drive. If oxygen is administered to these patients it may well result in depression of ventilation. This is a relatively rare event and should not prevent the prescription of oxygen in adequate amounts to patients who remain tachypnoeic. It can be predicted by taking arterial blood for baseline gas analysis and then administering oxygen in increasing percentages. If the patient has a ventilatory drive dependent on hypoxaemia then the minute volume will decrease as oxygen is administered, and arterial carbon dioxide will increase. (NB: the response to hypoxaemia is mediated by peripheral chemoreceptors — it has no effect on central chemoreceptors except when hypoxia in the brain directly depresses output from the CNS.)

Arterial pH

As might be expected a decrease in arterial pH gives rise to increased ventilation. pH will, of course, fall as $PaCO_2$ increases, so it is difficult to separate the two phenomena. However, patients who develop a metabolic acidosis exhibit a marked increase in minute volume. This is mediated by peripheral chemoreceptors (the blood–brain barrier is relatively impermeable to hydrogen ions).

Summary

In summary, a rise in $PaCO_2$ or H^+ stimulates respiration via the central and peripheral chemoreceptors. Hypoxia stimulates only the peripheral chemoreceptors. Stimulation of either sensor mechanism increases both rate and depth of respiration.

MECHANICS OF BREATHING

The major function of the lungs is the transport of gas in and out of the alveoli and the exchange of respiratory gases. This is achieved not just by the lungs, but by the surrounding tissues, bones and muscles.

Muscles of respiration

See the anatomy section.

Elastic properties of the lung

As the thoracic volume increases during inspiration the lung tissues become stretched; the greater the degree of chest expansion, the greater the degree of stretching of the lungs. However this relationship is not entirely linear. Figure 11.11 shows the relationship between the volume of the lung and the negative pressure surrounding it. As the negative pressure increases, so the lung volume increases, up to a point where further negative pressure does not increase lung volume. When the pressure around the lung decreases, the lung volume also decreases, but it

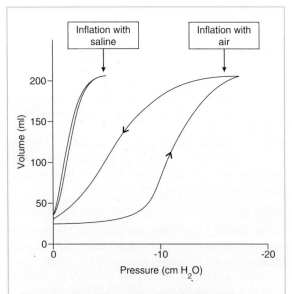

Fig. 11.11 Compliance and hysteresis. The graph illustrates the differences in compliance between the lungs inflated with air and the lungs inflated with saline. The saline-filled lungs have greater compliance and less hysteresis. The difference can be explained by the lack of surface tension in saline-filled lungs.

does not follow the same curve. This is called hysteresis. The lung volume at any given pressure during deflation is larger than that during inflation.

The slope of the volume pressure curve (the volume change per unit pressure) is known as the compliance. The usual compliance of the human lung is about 200 mL/cmH$_2$O pressure, but from the slope of the line it can be seen that compliance decreases at higher lung volumes as the lungs become stiffer. Lung compliance can also be reduced, for example, in pulmonary venous engorgement or in alveolar oedema. The compliance of the lung falls if the lung remains unventilated for a long period. This may occur, for example, following anaesthesia, resulting in atelectasis. Lung compliance is decreased by fibrosis of the lung and certain diseases. Age and emphysema increase it.

Because the change in lung volume per unit change in pressure will be larger in a large lung and smaller in a small lung, the compliance per unit volume of lung is often quoted. This is known as the specific compliance.

The elastic properties of the lung are in part due to the elastic tissue clearly visible in histological section. The arrangement of the elastin fibres is also important to the compliance of the tissue, and this has been likened to that of the filaments in nylon stocking.

For all its elastic properties the compliance of the lung would be greatly reduced without the presence of surfactant.

The following is a summary of the major factors affecting compliance:

- Increasing lung size increases the volume per unit pressure change.
- Compliance decreases on adopting a supine position.
- Small tidal volumes decrease compliance, probably due to changes in alveolar size.
- A decline in pulmonary blood flow will increase compliance. This will occur, for example, when a patient is put on a ventilator.
- Breathing 100% oxygen decreases compliance, probably because of alveolar collapse, as oxygen is rapidly absorbed in the alveoli with no nitrogen to maintain pressure.
- Age increases compliance.
- Emphysema increases compliance.
- Fibrosis and inflammation, and engorgement decrease compliance.

Surface tension

Surface tension is defined as the force acting along an imaginary line drawn on the surface of a liquid. This force exists because of the strong cohesive forces between molecules along the surface. Its importance in the lung can be demonstrated by comparing the pressure volume behaviour in isolated lungs inflated with either water or air. Lungs inflated with air have a much greater compliance and so are easier to distend than lungs filled with water (Fig. 11.11).

Uninhibited, the surface tension within the alveoli would significantly decrease the compliance of the lungs, perhaps by as much as 50%. However, specialised cells within the alveolar epithelium secrete surfactant, a lecithin-rich, detergent like substance that significantly decreases surface tension. Although these cells are plentiful in adult life they are not productive until a late stage of fetal maturity. Premature babies are very prone to develop respiratory distress, characterised by stiff lungs, atelectasis and pulmonary oedema.

Surfactant promotes several important properties within the lung, as follows.

- Lower surface tension within the alveoli promotes increased stability and lessens atelectasis. It is important to note that alveoli are inherently unstable and smaller alveoli have a tendency to inflate larger alveoli — Laplace's law states that the pressure in a bubble is equal to twice the wall tension divided by the radius, i.e. smaller bubbles (alveoli) have greater pressures.
- Surfactant helps keep the alveoli dry and free from oedema. Surface tension forces within the alveoli tend to force liquid from the capillaries into the alveoli. This tendency is reduced by surfactant.
- Compliance of the lung is increased.
- Work of respiration is decreased.

Regional differences in ventilation

Ventilation of the lung does not occur uniformly. Indeed dependent regions of the lung are much better ventilated than non-dependent regions of the lung. There are two main reasons for this:

- the weight of the lung
- the shape of the compliance curve (Fig. 11.12). In the dependent regions of the lung, resting intrapleural pressure is lower than in the apical regions. The

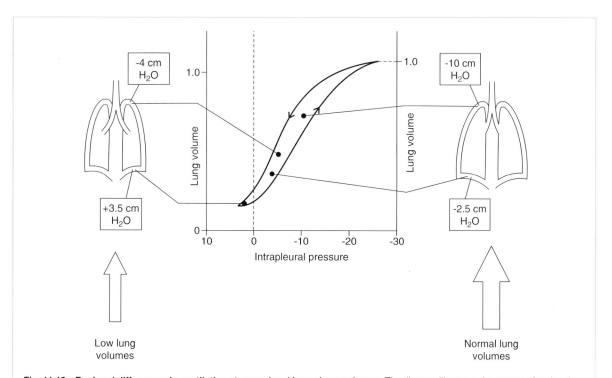

Fig. 11.12 Regional differences in ventilation at normal and lower lung volumes. The diagram illustrates the causes of regional differences in ventilation due to the weight of the lung. During normal breathing (right), the base of the lung is on a steeper part of the compliance curve and expands more per unit of negative pressure. The situation is reversed on the left, where, at lower lung volumes, the apex is on the steeper part of the curve.

dependent parts of the lung are on the steeper part of the compliance curve and are more easily distended. Thus ventilation is about 50% greater at the lung bases than at the apex.

This situation can be changed dramatically when the lung is ventilating at low volumes. Under these circumstances the lung tissue at the base becomes compressed after full expiration. The intrapleural pressures are now positive at the lung base and much less negative at the apex. When the lung expands, the non-dependent region is in the most advantageous part of the compliance curve, so that its volume will increase rapidly, whilst the dependent lung cannot increase its volume at all until the intrapleural pressures become subatmospheric. This situation can occur during anaesthesia in a spontaneously breathing patient.

Closure of small airways

There is another important effect, which can be observed at low lung volumes. As the volume of the lung decreases during expiration the intrapleural pressure in the dependent regions becomes positive. The small airways begin to close, trapping gas within the distal alveoli. In normal subjects this airway closure only occurs at very low lung volumes. However in patients whose lungs have lost elastic tissue (for example the elderly or those with emphysema), airway closure occurs at higher lung volumes. This airway closure can begin before the lung has reached its normal postexpiratory resting volume or functional residual capacity (FRC). The distal alveoli involved may be incompletely ventilated.

Elastic properties of the chest wall

Just as the lung has elastic properties which tend to make it collapse, the chest wall has elastic properties which tend to make it expand. When the two are in equilibrium the lung volume is said to be at functional residual capacity (FRC). The elastic recoil of the lung is balanced by the tendency of the chest to expand and the lung is at the end of a normal expiration. When the lung volume becomes smaller than FRC then intrapleural pressure must be positive.

Sites of airway resistance

As the airways penetrate toward the periphery of the lungs they become narrower, but more numerous. However, although the radii of these terminal bronchi are very small, they do not account for a great deal of resistance. The major site of resistance is in the medium-sized bronchi, and the very small bronchioles contribute very little. Most of the pressure drop across the airways occurs up to the

seventh generation of bronchi and less than 20% beyond this point.

Because the peripheral airways contribute so little to resistance, the detection of lung disease here is made much more difficult.

The major factors affecting airway resistance are the following.

- Lung volume — the bronchi are supported by elastic tissue of the lungs; thus, when the lungs expand, the bronchi are widened. Conversely at very low lung volume the airway calibre is reduced and airway resistance increased. Patients with significant chronic obstructive airways disease often breathe at high lung volumes in order to decrease airway resistance.
- Bronchial smooth muscle — contraction of bronchial smooth muscle decreases airway calibre, increasing airways resistance. The causes of bronchial smooth muscle contraction include irritant gases or allergens such as smoke or pollen. The nerve supply to bronchial smooth muscle is via the vagus nerve. The resting tone is under the control of the autonomic nervous system. Sympathetic stimulation causes bronchial dilatation, whilst parasympathetic stimulation causes bronchial constriction. Similarly adrenaline, isoprenaline and noradrenaline cause bronchodilatation. Acetylcholine causes bronchial constriction, which is reversed by atropine. The injection of microemboli or histamine into the pulmonary circulation results in the constriction of smooth muscle in the alveolar ducts. A fall in PCO_2 in alveolar gas increases airway resistance, for example in pulmonary embolism.
- The density and viscosity of inspired gas affects resistance within the airways. At high altitude the density of air is reduced, so that airway resistance is also reduced. Conversely, during deeper dives under the ocean, increased pressure increases the density of inspired gases so that airway resistance is increased. This is one reason why divers breathe mixtures of helium and oxygen.
- Dynamic compression of the airways. When a subject takes a maximal inspiration and then forcefully expires, not only are the lungs compressed but also the small airways. So significant is this effect that under these conditions flow becomes 'effort independent': no matter how forcefully the subject expires, the factor limiting expiratory flow rate will always be the compression of the small airways (Fig. 11.13).
- Anaesthesia, for a variety of reasons, increases resistance: e.g. narrowed endotracheal tube; release of bronchial constrictors, e.g. histamine-releasing drugs.

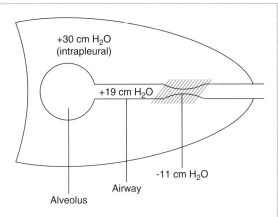

Fig. 11.13 A schematic diagram to represent forced expiration through the lungs. At high positive intrapleural pressures airways collapse and the flow becomes 'effort independent'.

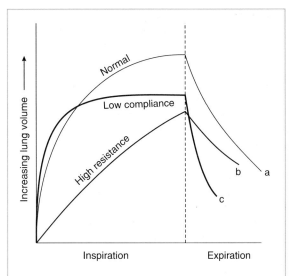

Fig. 11.14 Uneven ventilation. The diagram shows how the variation in resistance and compliance between lung units can cause uneven ventilation. Normal units (a) fill and empty quickly. Units with increased resistance fill and empty slowly and incompletely. Units with low compliance fill and empty rapidly but incompletely. These last two types of unit cause uneven ventilation (see text).

Tissue resistance

Just as gas transport within the airways contributes to resistance, so do the frictional forces between tissues. The tissue resistance accounts for about 20% of the total in a fit and healthy adult. The sum of tissue and airway resistance is sometimes called pulmonary resistance to distinguish it from airway resistance.

Uneven ventilation within the lungs

Until now we have assumed that compliance and resistance within the lung were uniform. In practice this is not so and there is uneven ventilation of lung units (Fig. 11.12). Figure 11.14 shows firstly a normal lung unit (a). Here the volume change in inspiration is both large and rapid, so it is completely filled before expiration begins. Lung unit (b) has stiff walls of low compliance; its volume change is rapid but small, although it is complete before expiration begins. Lung unit (c) has increased airway resistance, so that filling is slow and therefore incomplete before expiration begins. Units (b) and (c) contribute to uneven ventilation, but the pattern of inequality will depend on the depth and frequency of respiration.

Differences in compliance and resistance are not the only mechanism of uneven ventilation within the lungs. Another mechanism is incomplete diffusion beyond the fifteenth generation of airways. Beyond this point the airways constitute the respiratory zone where distances are so short that diffusion of gas is the dominant mechanism of transport. The rate of diffusion of gas molecules is so rapid that differences in concentration are abolished within 1 s, despite the very low velocity of gas within this region. However, in the diseased lung the terminal airways may be dilated. Under these circumstances the distances within this region will be greatly increased and diffusion ceases to be an adequate mechanism for gas transport.

WORK OF BREATHING

This is the work required to move the lung and chest wall. Since work is equal to pressure multiplied by volume, a pressure–volume diagram describes the work done (Fig. 11.15). As the respiratory rate increases, flow rates become faster and the viscous work becomes larger. When tidal volumes increase, the elastic work area increases. Expiration is normally passive and so the energy used is stored in the area 0ABCD0. In patients with reduced compliance, for example in fibrotic lung disease, breaths tend to be rapid and small. Patients with chronic obstructive lung disease tend to take slower, deeper breaths. These breathing patterns are optimised for decreasing respiratory work.

Interestingly, at rest a healthy individual is using about 5% of his resting oxygen consumption to breathe. In disease states this figure becomes much higher. Five

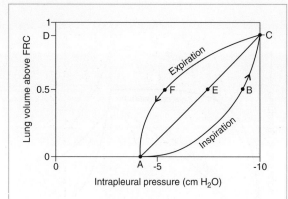

Fig. 11.15 The work of breathing. During inspiration the lung follows the line A,B,C. The work done is the area 0ABCD. 0ACED0 is the work required to overcome elastic forces. ABCEA is the work required to overcome airway and tissue resistance. During expiration, area AECFA is the work required to overcome airway and tissue resistance. If airways resistance increases, the curve ABC increases towards the right.

Table 11.1 Table of normal values

Volume	Value	Units
Tidal volume	500	mL
Minute volume	7500	mL
Total lung volume	5000–6500	mL
Anatomical dead space	150	mL
Functional residual capacity	2300–2600	mL
Alveolar gas volume	3000	mL
Pulmonary capillary blood volume	70	mL
Pulmonary blood flow	5000	mL/min
Tension		
Arterial PO_2	10.6–13.3	kPa
Arterial PCO_2	4.6–5.3	kPa
Mixed venous PO_2	5.3	kPa
Mixed venous PCO_2	6.1	kPa

percent is also the efficiency of breathing (as defined by useful work/energy expended). In some patients, where oxygen delivery is critically impaired, paralysing and ventilating the patient can make useful savings in oxygen consumption.

RESPIRATORY FUNCTION TESTS

Respiratory function tests are simply the practical application of respiratory physiology. They range from complicated laboratory techniques to simple procedures which can be performed at the bedside or in the doctor's office. These tests can be a useful adjunct to assessing the patient's fitness for surgery. It should be noted that respiratory function tests alone rarely provide a diagnosis or a definitive judgement on a patient's fitness to undergo surgery.

Respiratory function tests can be classified according to what they measure: ventilation and lung volumes, compliance, control of ventilation, and diffusion. There are some tests which take into account many aspects of respiratory physiology, e.g. arterial blood gases. Normal values are shown in Table 11.1.

VENTILATION

Normal adult lung values are shown in Figure 11.16. Although most lung volumes can be measured by a simple spirometer, the FRC can only be measured by helium dilution, body plethysmography, or by a nitrogen wash-out technique. These techniques are not applicable at the bedside.

Nitrogen washout is frequently performed in the clinical setting by the anaesthetist, not to measure lung volumes, but to replace all nitrogen in the lungs with oxygen so that, once asleep, a paralysed patient will remain well oxygenated if there is any difficulty in intubation or ventilation. (With nearly 2 L of oxygen left in the lungs it will require several minutes of apnoea for a patient to become hypoxic.)

The simplest (and most useful) bedside test of lung function is the single forced expiration. This involves measurement of lung volume using a simple vitalograph (Fig. 11.17).

The usual measurement is the volume forcefully expired over 1 s after a maximum inspiration: the FEV_1. This is compared with the total volume expired after a maximal inspiration: the FVC. The ratio of FEV_1/FVC is normally about 80% but is altered in disease states. Two patterns of disease emerge, though frequently these patterns overlap.

Restrictive lung disease comprises small, stiff lungs with low compliance: for example, pulmonary fibrosis. Both the FEV_1 and the FVC are reduced, so that the ratio FEV_1/FVC is normal or even increased. Obstructive lung disease implies a reduction in FEV_1, with a normal FVC giving a low FEV_1/FVC ratio. An alternative bedside measurement to FEV_1 is the maximum mid-expiratory flow (MMEF).

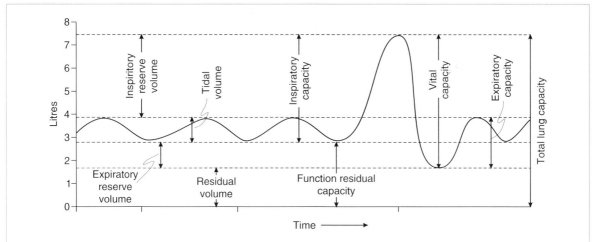

Fig. 11.16 Normal adult lung values. Tidal volume (TV) = 7 mL/kg. Vital capacity (VC) = 4.5 L. Total lung capacity (TLC) = 7.5 L. Functional residual capacity (FRC) = amount of gas in the lungs after a normal breath (2.8 L).

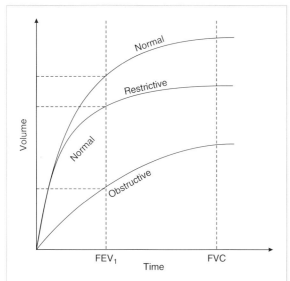

Fig. 11.17 FEV₁/FVC ratios. Normal FEV_1/FVC = 4 L/5 L = 80%. Obstructive FEV_1/FVC = 1.2/3 = 40%. Restrictive FEV_1/FVC = 2.9/3.2 = 93%.

ANATOMICAL DEAD SPACE

This is defined as the volume of the conducting airways down to a level where rapid mixture of inspired gas (with gas that is already in the lung) occurs. The gas in this part of the respiratory tree does not take part in the exchange of respiratory gases. This volume is normally about 150 mL but increases with inspiration due to elastic forces on the bronchial tubes.

Anatomical dead space is measured by Fowler's method. The patient breathes from a tube connected to a rapid nitrogen analyser. After a single intake of pure oxygen, the subject breathes out. Initially nitrogen concentration increases as dead space gas is washed out by alveolar gas. Towards the end of expiration the subject is expiring pure alveolar gas, giving rise to a 'plateau phase'. The expired volume is also recorded and the dead space found by plotting nitrogen concentration against expired volume (Fig. 11.18). The dead space is the volume expired up to a point where a line intersects the curve such that areas x and y on Figure 11.18 are equal.

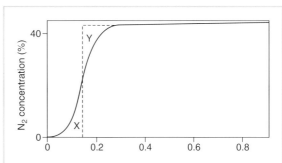

Fig. 11.18 Measurement of anatomical dead space using Fowler's method (see text).

PHYSIOLOGICAL DEAD SPACE

This is defined as the lung volume which does not take part in gas exchange. It includes the anatomical dead space and also the alveoli that are not ventilated (the alveolar dead space).

It is important to be clear on the differences between physiological and anatomical dead space. Anatomical dead space represents the volume of gas which is undiluted by that which is already in the lungs. The physiological dead space is the total volume of gas that has not taken part in gas exchange. This is a subtle but important difference, because the physiological dead space will include any gas from the alveoli which have not been perfused (the alveolar dead space).

In normal circumstances these anatomical and physiological dead spaces are the same, but if inequalities develop in blood flow and ventilation then physiological dead space will increase.

Major factors increasing anatomical dead space are:

- increasing size of subject
- assuming a standing position
- increased lung volume
- adrenaline, isoprenaline and noradrenaline, all of which cause bronchodilatation.

Factors increasing alveolar dead space are:

- hypotension, which decreases apical perfusion; this leads to some alveoli being underperfused (but still ventilated)
- hypoventilation, which decreases apical perfusion, again resulting in poor perfusion of some apical lung units
- emphysema and pulmonary embolism
- positive pressure ventilation, which decreases the capillary flow through lung units with low perfusion pressure, typically the upper zone. Such units will make a reduced contribution to gas exchange.

COMPLIANCE

The volume change in the lung per unit pressure change is measured in the spontaneously breathing patient by comparing the intrapleural pressure with the lung volume. In practice the intrapleural pressure is assumed to be equal to midoesophageal pressure in an erect subject. The subject breathes in and out of a spirometer in small steps, relaxing completely between breaths. A graph is plotted of pressure against volume (see Fig. 11.11).

Unfortunately this method is only useful in healthy lungs. In patients with airway disease, increased resis-

tance in some lung units means that movement of gas is still going on within the lung even if not through the upper airways. Units of low resistance are now gradually filling those of greater resistance until pressures equalise.

CLOSING CAPACITY

This is the volume of the lungs at which small airways start to close. This volume rises with age. As gas leaves the lungs some airways will close before expiration has finished, trapping gas in the alveoli. These alveoli do not play a full part in the exchange of respiratory gases. Small airways disease is especially difficult to detect until it is quite advanced. One method is to measure the amount of air trapped in the alveoli after expiration. The subject takes a full (TLC, total lung capacity) breath of 100% helium and then breathes out. The helium concentration of expired gas is measured and four discrete phases can be recognised:

1. Pure dead space is exhaled.
2. Mixed alveolar and dead space are exhaled.
3. Pure alveolar gas is exhaled (plateau phase).
4. There is preferential emptying of the apex of the lungs, which have a relatively high concentration of helium. This indicates closure of small airways at the base of the lung. There is more helium in the apex of the lungs because, as we have seen, this region expands less, and nitrogen is less diluted here (Fig. 11.19).

Alveoli that are closed off before end-expiration do not fully contribute to gas exchange and constitute 'alveolar

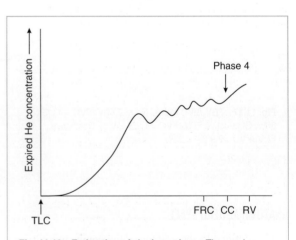

Fig. 11.19 Estimation of closing volume. The graph shows the expired helium concentration following a maximum single inspiration of 100% helium (see text for details).

dead space'. The closing volume is normally about 10% of vital capacity in a young, healthy subject, but by age 65 it has reached 40% of vital capacity. The closing capacity is increased by airway disease.

Major factors affecting closing capacity are as follows.

- It increases with age.
- Posture: in the supine position lung volume declines and closing capacity reaches FRC at 40 years old. At 60 closing capacity reaches FRC in the erect position.
- Anaesthesia: the decline in lung volumes during anaesthesia contributes to an increase in closing capacity, which exceeds FRC even in the youngest patients.

There are many more very complicated tests of respiratory function. For the attending doctor in a hospital setting, the single most useful tests are the FEV_1 and the FVC, followed by arterial blood gas analysis.

BLOOD GAS ANALYSIS

Modern technology has resulted in the development of portable gas analysers, which can easily measure $PaCO_2$, PaO_2 and pH, in a side room on the ward. Arterial blood should be taken from the radial, brachial, or femoral artery either with a single needle stab or from an indwelling cannula. The dead space of the syringe should be filled with dilute heparin and the blood should be analysed promptly. If there is to be any delay, the sample should be kept cool in iced water, otherwise the natural metabolism of the blood will result in significant errors.

Arterial pH is usually measured with a glass electrode at the same time as PaO_2 and $PaCO_2$. The pH of the blood is closely linked to $PaCO_2$ via the equation:

$$pH = pK + \log (HCO_3^-) /0.004 \times PaCO_2$$

where pK is the pH at which bicarbonate is 50% dissociated (normally 6.1), HCO_3^- is the plasma bicarbonate concentration in millimoles per litre, and $PaCO_2$ = arterial carbon dioxide tension in kPa.

The following brief descriptions of acid–base abnormalities can be more clearly understood by reference to Figure 11.20.

Acidosis

Acidosis means an increase in the arterial hydrogen ion concentration. It may be caused by respiratory or metabolic abnormalities or more frequently both.

Respiratory acidosis

Respiratory acidosis signifies a failure of the respiratory system to eliminate CO_2. There are two mechanisms by

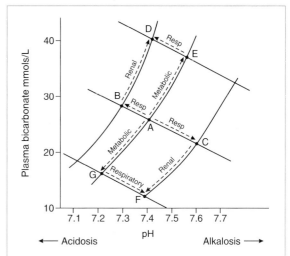

Fig. 11.20 Davenport diagram. The graph shows the relationship between the plasma bicarbonate and pH in various metabolic and respiratory states (see text for details).

which this can occur: hypoventilation and ventilation perfusion ratio inequalities. There are two forms of respiratory CO_2 retention: acute and chronic. A patient who has been overdosed with morphine is likely to develop acute respiratory acidosis as a result of depressed ventilation, whereas the chronic form of CO_2 retention is seen in chronic obstructive airway disease.

In acute respiratory acidosis, there is little time for bicarbonate to increase as a consequence of raised arterial CO_2. The pH falls rapidly as $PaCO_2$ increases (point B on Fig. 11.20).

In chronic CO_2 retention, although CO_2 levels may be high the pH is not so depressed. This is because the kidneys compensate by retaining bicarbonate in response to increased $PaCO_2$. This is termed partially compensated respiratory acidosis (point D).

Metabolic acidosis

This is a relative lack of bicarbonate, the best example being diabetic ketoacidosis (point G). In practice the fall in arterial pH stimulates the peripheral chemoreceptors, increasing ventilation and lowering $PaCO_2$ (point F). Lactic acidosis may occur following severe acute respiratory failure, as a consequence of prolonged tissue hypoxia.

Alkalosis

There are two forms of alkalosis: respiratory and metabolic.

Respiratory alkalosis

Acute respiratory alkalosis is seen in acute hysterical hyperventilation where the pH rises as a consequence of a fall in PaCO$_2$. A chronic form is seen in ascent to high altitude, where hyperventilation occurs as a result of hypoxaemia (point C). Under these circumstances the pH is returned to normal as the kidney excretes more bicarbonate (point F again). This is termed compensated respiratory alkalosis.

Metabolic alkalosis

Metabolic alkalosis is most often seen following prolonged vomiting, for example in pyloric stenosis. The plasma bicarbonate concentration rises, increasing plasma pH and causing a slight respiratory depression. Metabolic alkalosis may also occur if a patient with chronic obstructive airway disease is ventilated too enthusiastically so that the PaCO$_2$ is brought down to normal. Following the successful treatment of ventilatory failure, metabolic alkalosis and associated potassium chloride deficiency may occur.

Arterial PO$_2$

Any interpretation of the value of arterial oxygen tension must be based upon a full understanding of the oxyhaemoglobin dissociation curve (Fig. 11.21). Most importantly it must be realised that above 60 mmHg (8 kPa) the oxyhaemoglobin curve is flat, so that hypoxaemia is almost impossible to detect without the aid of a pulse oximeter. Normal arterial oxygen tension is about 13.3 kPa, which corresponds to a saturation of 97%. Mixed venous blood has a tension of about 5.3 kPa, giving a saturation of 75%. The oxyhaemoglobin dissociation curve is shifted to the right in exercising muscle; where temperature increases; PaCO$_2$ rises; and pH falls. An increase in 2,3 DPG inside the red cells also shifts the curve to the right, enabling haemoglobin to more readily give up oxygen. Levels of 2,3 DPG are low in stored blood but often raised in chronic obstructive airway disease.

There are five primary causes of hypoxaemia:

1. hypoventilation
2. impaired diffusion
3. shunt
4. ventilation and perfusion inequality
5. reduction in inspired oxygen tension.

Reduction in inspired oxygen tension

This may occur on ascent to high altitude and to a small degree in the cabin of a modern jet airliner. It may occur during the course of an anaesthetic or diving accident.

Hypoventilation

This is simply a reduction in the volume of fresh gas going into the alveoli per unit time. This will inevitably result in hypoxaemia unless the basal metabolic rate is also reduced. The most common causes of hypoventila-

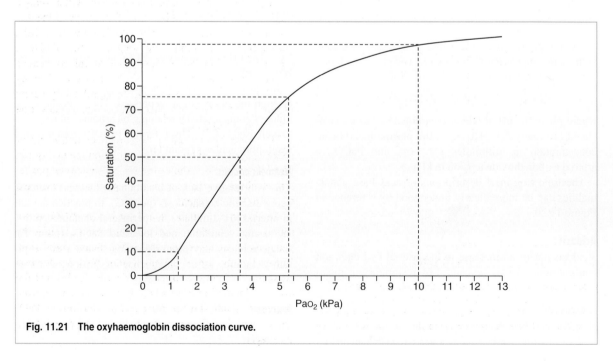

Fig. 11.21   The oxyhaemoglobin dissociation curve.

tion are drugs which affect the mechanics or control of ventilation, e.g. barbiturate or morphine overdose, or anaesthesia. Trauma, haemorrhage or abnormalities of the nervous system, e.g. a high cervical transection, polio or myasthenia gravis will decrease ventilation as will an obstruction to the upper airway. A particularly interesting example occurs in the morbidly obese, where a characteristic picture of hypoventilation is called Pickwickian syndrome.

The relationships between hypoventilation and $PaCO_2$ and PaO_2 are fundamentally different. This is shown in Figure 11.22. Hypoventilation is always associated with an increase in $PaCO_2$ and a decrease in PaO_2. However, the magnitude of the increase in $PaCO_2$ is much greater than the decrease in PaO_2. If the alveolar ventilation is halved, the $PaCO_2$ is doubled. The hypoxaemia caused by hypoventilation can *always* be decreased by administration of oxygen. Reference to the diagram will show that arterial oxygen tension cannot fall to a very low level simply because of hypoventilation: *hypoxaemia is not the dominant feature of hypoventilation*.

Impairment of diffusion

Impairment of diffusion implies that equilibration does not occur between oxygen tension in the alveolar gas and that within the capillaries. In a normal alveolar capillary unit under resting conditions the capillary blood oxygen tension has reached that of alveolar gas by the time it has traversed one-third distance along the capillary. Even in extreme exercise, as the cardiac output rises, there is sufficient reserve for equilibration to be complete before the blood has left the capillary. In some diseases the blood gas barrier (the alveolar membrane) is thickened, slowing diffusion and rendering equilibration incomplete, especially during exercise.

Diseases that may cause impaired diffusion include asbestosis, sarcoidosis and diffuse interstitial fibrosis.

Since diffusion across a membrane is proportional to the concentration gradient of the gas diffusing across that membrane, hypoxaemia which is caused by diffusion impairment can be corrected by the administration of oxygen.

Diffusion is also dependent upon the solubility of the gas in question. For this reason, CO_2 elimination is probably unaffected by impaired diffusion.

Shunt

Shunting describes the passage of blood through the lungs without coming into contact with ventilated alveoli, e.g. the bronchial circulation and Thebesian veins. This is greatly increased in patients with atrial or ventricular septal defects or PDA. In pneumonia the passage of blood through a consolidated lobe will also constitute a shunt.

This kind of hypoxaemia cannot be greatly improved by the administration of oxygen. The reason for this is the flat top of the oxyhaemoglobin dissociation curve. If the patient is given 100% oxygen to breathe, capillary blood coming into contact with ventilated alveoli will develop a high oxygen tension, but because of the shape of the dissociation curve the oxygen content will only rise a little. On the other hand, blood traversing unventilated alveoli will have an oxygen tension equal to mixed venous blood. When the two pools of blood mix on leaving the alveoli, oxygen tensions will be significantly below normal because well-oxygenated blood contributes little extra oxygen content.

The hypoxaemia resulting from hypoventilation, diffusion impairment and ventilation perfusion inequality can all be improved by administration of oxygen. Hypoxaemia resulting from a shunt is not significantly corrected by giving extra oxygen.

Another characteristic of a shunt is that $PaCO_2$ is not raised. Any potential rise in $PaCO_2$ is kept in check by the peripheral chemoreceptors that will increase ventilation. Because of the top of the oxyhaemoglobin dissociation curve this will not increase PaO_2. Figure 11.23 shows the effect of increasing inspired oxygen tension on differing degrees of shunt. If the inspired oxygen tension and PaO_2 are known, then the percentage shunt can be read from the graph.

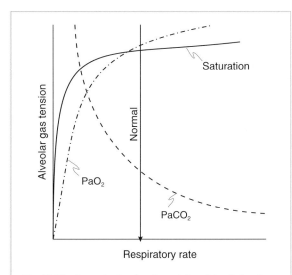

Fig. 11.22 A graph showing the relationship of alveolar ventilation to PaO₂, PaCO₂ and saturation. Note that very low levels of ventilation are required to significantly decrease PaO₂ but that PaO₂ increases very quickly.

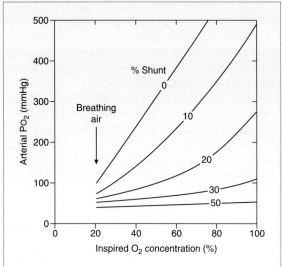

Fig. 11.23 **Oxygen shunt diagram showing arterial oxygen tensions achieved by increasing inspired oxygen.** Note that for shunts of 50%, no useful increase in arterial PO_2 occurs, but for smaller shunts very high concentrations of oxygen can be effective.

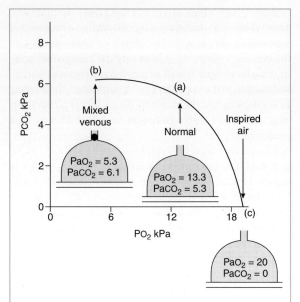

Fig. 11.24 **Relationships between ventilation and perfusion.** The ventilation–perfusion ratio line (b)–(a)–(c) shows the possible ratios for all lung units when breathing air.

Ventilation–perfusion inequality

Simply put, this means that ventilation (V_A) and blood flow (V_Q) are mismatched. The result is that all gas exchange becomes inefficient. This mechanism is responsible for most of the hypoxaemia seen in chronic lung disease, e.g. COAD and pulmonary embolism. Although it is the most common cause of hypoxaemia it is also the most difficult to detect. Inequality of ventilation and perfusion is the norm as we have seen. In the upright lung the apices are poorly perfused compared with the bases. The apices are poorly ventilated compared with the bases, but the difference is much smaller than for perfusion, with the result that the ventilation perfusion ratio increases from base to apex. In disease states this relationship is severely disturbed.

If we consider three different types of lung unit (Fig. 11.24), it is possible to illustrate the effects of uneven ventilation and perfusion. (a) Shows a normal lung unit and the gas tensions within it. (b) Shows the gas tensions in a unit which is completely unventilated but normally perfused. In an unventilated unit the gas tensions become equal to those of mixed venous blood. (c) Shows a unit which has no perfusion but which is normally ventilated. There will be no blood leaving this unit to mix with arterial blood, and the gas tensions within this unit will be equal to those of inspired air.

Here (a) represents the norm, (b) represents the extreme of decreased V_A:V_Q ratio, (c) shows the most extreme example of an increased V_A:V_Q ratio. Since (b) and (c) represent the extremes of ventilation–perfusion abnormalities and (a) represents the norm, all units ventilated and perfused must lie along the line as drawn in Figure 11.24.

It is obvious that if the lung consisted solely of units that were uniformly ventilated and perfused then gas exchange would be much more efficient. Those lung units that are ventilated but not perfused will be a waste of ventilation, whereas those lung units that are perfused but not ventilated constitute a waste of perfusion. Because of the flat top of the oxyhaemoglobin dissociation curve, those units which are ventilated but have poor perfusion will contribute little increase in oxygen content to arterial blood. Interestingly, these units can still eliminate carbon dioxide reasonably since the CO_2 dissociation curve is a straight line with no flat top in this region.

In normal patients, ventilation–perfusion inequalities within the lung result in only a small depression in arterial PO_2, from what might be expected in the ideally ventilated lung, where alveolar and arterial PO_2 would be equal. In practice there is about a 0.5 kPa difference in oxygen tension between alveoli and artery. This is known as the alveolar–arterial difference for PO_2, or A–a difference.

Just as ventilation–perfusion inequality results in a depression of PaO_2 these same inequalities must also result in some decrease in output of carbon dioxide. However, elevation of arterial CO_2 is unusual, because stimulation of the chemoreceptors would result in hyperventilation. Patients with increased ventilation–perfusion inequalities tend to have greater minute volumes, and this increase is often termed wasted ventilation. The flat top of the oxyhaemoglobin dissociation curve means that there is no significant increase in PaO_2. Lung units with high ventilation:perfusion ratios constitute alveolar dead space.

In practice most hypoxaemia (low arterial oxygen tension) results not from a single cause but from a mixture of the four main causes of hypoxaemia. An inadequate supply of oxygen to the tissues from all causes is collectively called hypoxia. A low PaO_2 is only one cause. Anaemia and carbon monoxide poisoning, a reduction in cardiac output, or a toxin that prevents cells from using oxygen (e.g. cyanide) will all result in tissue hypoxia. These types of hypoxia are called anaemic hypoxia, circulatory hypoxia and histotoxic hypoxia, respectively.

Arterial PCO_2

$PaCO_2$ is measured with a modified pH electrode, which is surrounded by a bicarbonate buffer but separated from blood by a thin membrane. Carbon dioxide diffuses into the buffer, decreasing the pH, from which the tension of carbon dioxide can be gauged.

There are two major causes of CO_2 retention: hypoventilation and ventilation–perfusion inequality. We have already seen that hypoventilation must cause CO_2 retention and hypoxaemia, but the effect on CO_2 is much greater.

We have also seen that ventilation–perfusion inequality is frequently accompanied by a normal $PaCO_2$ because of stimulation of the chemoreceptors and resulting hyperventilation. Patients who cannot hyperventilate, possibly because the increased work of breathing is beyond them, will have an elevated $PaCO_2$.

Blood gas exchange

Oxygen uptake

We have seen how gas gets into the alveoli and then diffuses across the alveolar membrane along the concentration gradient. The vast bulk of respiratory gases are transported in the red cells, and the distance from the capillary membrane to the red cell is greater than the thickness of this membrane. Patently a significant component of diffusion resistance is to be found within the

capillary. The story is made more complex by the finite rate of reaction of oxygen with haemoglobin.

Although the rate of combination of oxygen with haemoglobin is fast (less than a fifth of a second), oxygenation is so rapid within the pulmonary capillary that this forms a significant delay in the uptake of oxygen into the red cell. Thus the diffusion capacity of the lung D_L is made up of two components: the diffusion capacity of the membrane, D_M, and diffusion through plasma and the red cell, and the chemical reaction between gas and haemoglobin. This can be thought of as the diffusion capacity, θ, for the volume of capillary blood (V_C):

$$D_L = D_M + \theta\, V_C$$

where θ is the rate of reaction of oxygen with haemoglobin in mL/min/mm Hg/mL blood.

From this equation it can be seen that the diffusion capacity for any gas in the lungs must depend in part upon the volume of blood in the capillaries. Many diseases affect the volume of capillary blood. For this reason the term *transfer factor* is a better clinical description of the diffusion capacity of the lung.

Oxygen carriage

Once in the blood, oxygen is carried in two forms: that which is dissolved and that which is combined with haemoglobin.

Oxygen carried by haemoglobin Haemoglobin consists of four polypeptide chains, joined to an iron porphyrin compound. In normal adult haemoglobin (haemoglobin A), the polypeptide chains are of two distinct types: alpha and beta. A variety of amino acid substitutions give rise to various abnormal forms of haemoglobin. HbS (sickle) has an abnormal beta chain that results in a shift of the dissociation curve to the right. More importantly, when the molecule becomes deoxygenated then it becomes relatively insoluble, forming crystals within the red cell. The name derives from the crescent-shaped cell seen on a blood film when this happens.

Just as oxygen can react with haemoglobin so can various drugs. Most commonly these result in hyperoxidation of the ferrous ion to the ferric form, causing the formation of methaemoglobin, e.g. sulphonamides, prilocaine and nitrates. Methaemoglobin is not useful for oxygen carriage. There are two forms of haemoglobin in the blood: oxyhaemoglobin and haemoglobin. The two molecules are in equilibration, with an easily reversible reaction:

$$O_2 + Hb \rightleftharpoons HbO_2$$

The amount of oxygen in the blood can easily be measured in vitro, giving the oxyhaemoglobin dissociation curve (Fig. 11.21).

There are many features of this curve which are fundamental to understanding respiratory physiology. The importance of the flat top has already been mentioned, but most obviously it means that increasing the oxygen tension in the alveoli will have proportionately little effect on the amount of oxygen carried in the blood. Conversely, if the oxygen tension in alveolar gas falls, oxygen tension will be little affected in the capillaries until relatively low levels. The steep slope of the curve in the range of uptake means that a large concentration gradient exists when most oxygen is being transferred. This speeds up the diffusion process. pH, PCO_2, temperature and 2,3 DPG (2,3 diphosphoglycerate — a chemical found in red cells) alter the position of the oxyhaemoglobin dissociation curve. A rise in temperature or a fall in pH or PCO_2 shifts the curve to the right. This will increase unloading of oxygen, for example in capillaries in exercising muscle. Increased 2,3 DPG also shifts the curve to the right, for example in prolonged hypoxia of chronic lung disease. The introduction of carbon monoxide into the alveoli severely decreases oxygen transport because it combines with haemoglobin to form carboxyhaemoglobin. The affinity of haemoglobin for carbon monoxide is much greater than for oxygen. Very small concentrations of carbon monoxide will occupy large amounts of haemoglobin, making it unavailable for oxygen transport. The presence of carbon monoxide also shifts the curve to the left, which decreases the unloading of oxygen in the tissues.

The degree of shift of the curve can be gauged from the value of oxygen tension for a 50% saturation. This is known as the P50 and is normally about 3.5 kPa. The presence of carbon monoxide also shifts the curve to the left, which decreases the unloading of oxygen in the tissues.

Haemoglobin that is carrying the maximum amount of oxygen is said to be 100% saturated. The maximum amount of oxygen that 1 g of haemoglobin can combine with is about 1.34 mL oxygen. If normal blood has a haemoglobin concentration of 15 g/100 mL, then:

$$1.34 \times 15 = 20.1 \text{ mL } O_2/100 \text{ mL blood}$$

To this figure of 20.1 mL oxygen per 100 mL blood can be added the oxygen dissolved in the plasma.

Dissolved oxygen   Dissolved oxygen is carried in small amounts in the plasma in equilibrium with the partial pressure in the alveoli (Henry's law). The partial pressure of oxygen in arterial blood is 13.3 kPa; since plasma will contain 0.0225 mL O_2/100 mL blood/kPa,

then 100 mL plasma will only contain 0.3 mL oxygen. This is nowhere near enough to provide adequate oxygenation of the tissues. We can assume that the contribution made by the plasma to oxygen transport is normally small. However, if a patient is given 100% oxygen to breathe the partial pressure in the alveoli rises to about 93.3 kPa, enough to provide seven times as much oxygen in 100 mL of plasma — enough to provide for an increased chance of survival in patients with severe anaemia.

Under normal circumstances and with PaO_2 of 13.3 kPa, haemoglobin is 97.5% saturated. The oxygen tension in mixed venous blood is about 40 mmHg, corresponding to 75% saturation. Reduced haemoglobin is purple in colour, and sufficient circulating concentration will result in cyanosis. In practice this requires at least 4 g haemoglobin per 100 mL blood, and so is easy to detect in polycythaemia but difficult to see in anaemia.

Carbon dioxide

We have noted that the solubility of carbon dioxide is much greater than that of oxygen. Hence the rate of diffusion of CO_2 through the alveolar membrane is about 20 times faster than that of oxygen. However, the reaction of carbon dioxide with blood is complex, so that small degrees of impaired CO_2 elimination can occur if the alveolar membrane is very thickened.

Carbon dioxide is found in three forms in the blood: dissolved, bicarbonate and combined with proteins.

Dissolved carbon dioxide   Carbon dioxide is 20 times more soluble than oxygen, so that about 5% of CO_2 is carried in this form in venous blood.

Bicarbonate   Carbon dioxide combines with water under the influence of the enzyme carbonic anhydrase, and then dissociates into hydrogen ions and bicarbonate ions:

$$CO_2 + H_2O \rightleftharpoons H_2CO_3 \rightleftharpoons H^+ + HCO_3^-$$

This enzyme is found in the red cells only. As the concentrations of hydrogen ions and bicarbonate ions increase, there is a tendency for both to leave the red cell, down their respective concentration gradients. However, the cell membrane is relatively impermeable to hydrogen ions, so that only bicarbonate diffuses out, whilst chloride ions diffuse in to maintain electrochemical neutrality. This is called the *chloride shift*.

Some of the hydrogen ions are 'mopped up' by oxygenated haemoglobin, helping the unloading of oxygen, but also helping with the uptake of carbon dioxide. Hence, deoxygenated blood helps to transport CO_2. This is called the *Haldane effect*.

In venous blood 90% of CO_2 is carried as bicarbonate.

Carbon dioxide combined with proteins Carbon dioxide combines with blood proteins to form carbamino compounds. The bulk of CO_2 combines with haemoglobin to form carbamino haemoglobin. Reduced haemoglobin can carry more CO_2 than oxygenated haemoglobin.

The carbon dioxide dissociation curve is virtually a straight line over the physiological range. Because the carbon dioxide content is greater as haemoglobin becomes desaturated, the slight curve in the line is straightened out. This is due to the *Haldane effect.*

Blood gas exchange in the tissues

Just as oxygen and CO_2 move across the alveoli, so these gases must move between the blood and the tissues. The same process of simple diffusion through the capillary membrane accomplishes this. Once again, the elimination of CO_2 is much easier than the uptake of oxygen, because of its greater solubility, and hence faster diffusion. As the distance from a capillary increases, so the concentration of oxygen falls until, if the distance is great enough, anaerobic metabolism and lactic acidosis will occur. The diffusion distance between capillaries decreases during exercise as more capillaries open up.

RESPIRATORY FAILURE

Respiratory failure occurs if the lungs fail to adequately oxygenate arterial blood or to prevent CO_2 retention. There are no absolute arterial oxygen or carbon dioxide tensions that indicate respiratory failure since individual adaptation occurs. In practice, hypoxia, hypercapnoea and acidosis occur to varying degrees.

Hypoxaemia

The five causes of hypoxaemia (lack of oxygen in the blood) have been discussed. Clinical signs of hypoxaemia are cyanosis, tachycardia and confusion. With the advent of pulse oximetry, detection is now much easier. If the oxygen demands of the tissues are not met, then tissue hypoxia will develop. Delivery of O_2 to the tissues is given by the equation:

$$\text{arterial } O_2 \text{ content} \times \text{cardiac output} = O_2 \text{ delivery}$$
$$\text{(or flux)}$$
$$\{[(Hb \times \text{saturation} \times 1.34) + 0.3]/100\} \times 5000 =$$
$$1000 \text{ mL } O_2/\text{min}$$

Some tissues are especially robust in their ability to cope with hypoxia. However, the brain and heart are especially vulnerable. If oxygen supply to the cerebral cortex ceases, consciousness is rapidly lost and irreversible changes follow after about three minutes. In less sensitive tissues,

aerobic metabolism ceases and is replaced with anaerobic glycolysis. This is much less efficient and results in lactic acidosis.

As tissue oxidation drops, the only initial clinical abnormalities are a slight deterioration in mental performance and visual acuity. When arterial PO_2 drops further, the patient may develop headache or confusion. Severe hypoxaemia causes convulsions, retinal haemorrhages and permanent brain damage. The heart rate and blood pressure increase due to the release of adrenaline, but if hypoxaemia persists cardiac failure supervenes. Eventually renal function declines and sodium retention occurs.

Hypercapnia

The two causes of CO_2 retention have been discussed: hypoventilation and V_A:V_Q inequality. In respiratory failure, hypoventilation can be exacerbated by inappropriate use of oxygen therapy. Patients with severe, longstanding chronic obstructive airways disease may develop severe hypoxaemia and CO_2 retention. These patients can lead a reasonable existence despite their blood gases. However, persistently high arterial CO_2 tensions may mean that much of the patient's ventilatory drive is derived from stimulation of the peripheral chemoreceptors in response to hypoxaemia. Although $PaCO_2$ is raised, arterial pH will be near normal because of the renal retention of bicarbonate.

If this patient is given oxygen therapy, hypoxaemia may be significantly decreased, resulting in a decreased ventilatory drive. Ventilation may become severely depressed, leading to high levels of arterial carbon dioxide. Sudden discontinuation of oxygen at this point may be extremely dangerous. This does not mean that a severely tachypnoeic patient should be deprived of high concentrations of oxygen. The oxygen given to patients with severe COAD may have a secondary effect. Units in the lung that were poorly perfused due to hypoxic vasoconstriction may now become well perfused but remain poorly ventilated, resulting in a further rise in $PaCO_2$. This effect is probably of much less importance. Typically these patients suffer from chronic bronchitis and emphysema, and often asthma. Their disease is longstanding, and they are usually incapable of sustained physical activity. Arterial blood gas analysis, when these patients are at their best, often reveals depressed PaO_2 (about 6.5 kPa) and elevated $PaCO_2$ (greater than 6.5 kPa). In an acute infective episode, these patients develop 'acute on chronic lung disease'. This requires careful management with moderate oxygen enrichment (24–28%) and regular blood gas analysis. Antibiotics, bronchodilators and diuretics may be necessary. If exhaustion occurs a period of mechanical ventilation may be required.

Hypercapnia results in increased cerebral blood flow causing raised CSF pressure, headache and eventually papilloedema, and clouding of consciousness. It is usually accompanied by hypoxaemia resulting in confusion, slurred speech and flapping tremor. The degree of acidosis depends upon the rate of rise of $PaCO_2$. If it is prolonged, then renal compensation will occur. Sudden rises in $PaCO_2$ produce a profound degree of acidosis.

AIRWAYS OBSTRUCTION

Patients with longstanding lung disease are especially at risk from an increase in bronchial tone. Infections, irritants, or allergens may result in a life-threatening situation. The work of breathing is increased further until the patient may not be able to cope, resulting in CO_2 retention, hypoxaemia and respiratory acidosis. Treatment should include bronchodilators such as aminophylline, salbutamol, steroids, and anticholinergic drugs such as ipatropium bromide. Physiotherapy to encourage coughing, humidification of inspired gases, and adequate hydration are essential.

MECHANICAL VENTILATION

If oxygen therapy and general supportive measures, outlined above, fail then a further option is mechanical ventilation. Some early machines devised for this purpose did not involve positive pressure to the airway, but rather negative pressure to the thorax — the 'iron lung'. Modern hospital ventilation involves intubation or tracheostomy with a cuffed tube to provide an airtight seal. Patients who are not unconscious are frequently heavily sedated and no longer able to cough. The nasal passages are bypassed and hence humidification is reduced. Without expert nursing, secretions will become copious, thick and retained. Humidification must be provided, usually by a heated water system, whilst secretions must be removed via suction catheters at regular intervals. Endotracheal tubes are prone to kinking and obstruction, so that sophisticated monitoring and alarm systems must be in place, together with one to one nursing. Overinflation of the endotracheal tube cuff may cause severe damage to the mucosa of the trachea, resulting in fibrosis of the underlying cartilage and subsequent stenosis. All materials used must be inert.

Intermittent positive pressure ventilation (IPPV)

The lung is inflated by the application of increased airway pressure (20–30 cmH$_2$O) to about 10 mL/kg body weight, and allowed to deflate passively. The pattern of ventilation can be adjusted so that the tidal volume, rate, time for expiration and inspiration, and inspired oxygen concentration can be optimised. As we have seen, the pressure inside the thorax is normally negative on inspiration. The application of positive pressure tends to decrease venous return and compress the heart, leading to a decline in cardiac output especially at high ventilation pressures. It is important to maintain the patient's circulatory volume. Positive pressure ventilation also increases dead space. This is because the lung volume is raised and blood is diverted away from the ventilated regions by the higher airways pressure. This occurs most readily in the uppermost units of the lung, where hydrostatic pressure is lowest. If alveolar pressure rises to greater than capillary pressure then perfusion may be abolished in these units.

It is very important to avoid hyperventilation; this will not only result in hypocapnia but, if this follows a period of hypoventilation, it may result in a low serum potassium.

High concentrations of oxygen are extremely damaging to lung tissues, resulting in alveolar oedema, inflammation and eventually permanent fibrotic changes.

Positive end expiratory pressure (PEEP)

If a small positive pressure (5–10 cmH$_2$O) is maintained at the end of expiration a significant improvement in the patient's arterial oxygen tension may occur. Application of PEEP will result in an increase in FRC. This will tend to decrease the airway closure that occurs at low lung volumes, recruiting previously underventilated alveoli. In addition, alveolar oedema will decrease as fluid is 'pushed' back into the capillaries.

PEEP is not without hazards. The effects of IPPV are exaggerated and the individual response unpredictable. Venous return to the thorax is further decreased, especially if the circulatory volume is low. For this reason it is often necessary to measure cardiac output and calculate total oxygen delivery. Inotropic support may be necessary. The increased pressure in the lungs may result in barotrauma, most seriously in pneumothorax. High levels of PEEP especially depress venous return. There have been recent reports of bronchiectasis with prolonged PEEP.

Continuous positive airways pressure (CPAP) is the term applied to spontaneous respiration with a continuously raised airway pressure. It provides benefit in exactly the same way as PEEP, but is useful for weaning patients from a ventilator.

Intermittent mandatory ventilation (IMV)

This is the name given to IPPV, but with large tidal volumes given at a low rate, to a patient who is otherwise breathing spontaneously. It may be combined with PEEP or CPAP and is useful for weaning patients from ventilators.

SIMV (synchronised IMV) is a variant of this. Here the patient can breathe spontaneously during IPPV, but a spontaneous breath will delay the next positive pressure cycle.

Extended mandatory minute volume (EMMV)

The patient is allowed to breathe spontaneously, but is 'topped up' to a preset minute volume. It is synchronised as in SIMV (above).

Triggering

Triggering is a technique that allows patients to take a breath by decreasing airway pressure, initiating a positive pressure cycle.

Inspiratory assist

With this technique the patient's inspiratory efforts are assisted with positive pressure by the ventilator, decreasing the work of respiration.

High frequency ventilation

High frequency ventilation, i.e. cycles greater than 20 per second, with very small tidal volumes can maintain blood gases. This method has yet to find its clinical application, but is useful in the management of bronchopleural fistula.

ADULT RESPIRATORY DISTRESS SYNDROME

This is the name given to a specific disease of the lung characterised by hypoxaemia, alveolar inflammation and oedema and, later, pulmonary fibrosis. It follows a variety of insults, and these are further described in the pathology section and in Chapter 7. Typically the syndrome is recognised some hours or even days after the initial insult.

Early histological change shows both interstitial and alveolar oedema. The alveoli can be seen to contain cell debris, proteinaceous fluid, hyaline membrane and haemorrhage. Signs of chronic inflammation usually follow these signs of acute inflammation; organisation and fibrosis occur. By this stage, damage will be permanent.

Typically the patient has an increased respiratory rate, cyanosis, and, on arterial blood gas analysis, hypercapnia. Chest x-ray shows patchy white clouding. The compliance of the lung is severely reduced, so that the work of breathing is beyond the patient's capability. The patient soon requires ventilation, with high inspiratory pressures. The increased stiffness of the lungs is due to alveolar collapse and oedema.

Because the alveoli are filled with exudate and oedema,

a large percentage of pulmonary blood flow goes through unventilated units, giving rise to severe inequality of ventilation and perfusion. Treatment includes oxygen enrichment, often up to 100%, to correct hypoxaemia. PEEP often improves oxygenation by decreasing pulmonary oedema and recruiting underventilated alveoli.

A similar condition occurs in infants — infant respiratory distress syndrome. Pathological features are similar and there is profound hypoxaemia. Treatment is similar to that of adults, but the addition of synthetic surfactant to inspired oxygen helps correct the underlying defect, i.e. the inability of the premature fetal lung to produce sufficient surfactant.

OXYGEN THERAPY

Although inhalation of 100% oxygen can increase the arterial oxygen tension to more than 80 kPa, the carriage of oxygen is not increased ten-fold, because of the shape of the oxyhaemoglobin dissociation curve. The alveolar oxygen tension is given by the equation:

$$PaO_2 = P_B - PaH_2O - PaCO_2$$
$$= 100 - 4.9 - 5.3$$
$$= 89.8 \text{ kPa}$$

where P_B = barometric pressure, PaH_2O = alveolar water saturated vapour pressure, and $PaCO_2$ = alveolar pressure of carbon dioxide. (Note that the alveolar oxygen tension will always be higher than arterial oxygen tension because of shunt and ventilation–perfusion inequality.) Although the dissociation curve has a flat top, considerable increases in dissolved oxygen within the plasma occur when patients breathe 100% oxygen. When breathing air, about 0.3 mL O_2/100 mL blood are carried. On 100% oxygen this increases to 1.8 mL O_2/100 mL blood. When one considers that the normal arterial–venous difference in oxygen content is 5 mL/100 mL blood, this is a useful amount.

Some types of respiratory impairment respond much more to treatment with oxygen than others. For example, hypoxaemia due to hypoventilation is readily corrected by only small increases in inspired oxygen concentration. Similarly hypoxaemia due to impaired diffusion is readily corrected. The reason for this is simply that the rate of diffusion is proportional to the concentration difference across the alveolar membrane.

Hypoxaemia due to ventilation–perfusion inequality is not so readily corrected. Some lung units may be so poorly ventilated that it may take many minutes for nitrogen washout to be complete. The presence of oxygen in these units may lead to the abolition of hypoxic vasoconstriction and also absorption atalectasis, as these units are inherently unstable. Some lung units will be so poorly perfused that they will contribute little to improved arterial oxygenation. Finally, increased inspired oxygen may result in the development of unventilated areas. The clinical effect will depend on the pattern of $V_A:V_Q$ inequality. Arterial oxygen tension will rise but often not as high as necessary.

Administration of 100% oxygen would not significantly correct hypoxaemia due to shunt. In this case venous blood bypasses the ventilated lung units, so that no improvement in oxygenation occurs. That venous blood which is exposed to higher alveolar oxygen concentrations can only contribute a small increase in oxygen carriage, because of the flat top of the oxyhaemoglobin dissociation curve. However, carriage by dissolved oxygen will also increase, so that small but useful gains can be made by the administration of high concentrations of oxygen. It is possible to calculate the degree of shunt from the arterial oxygen tension and the inspired oxygen concentration (Fig. 11.23).

Delivering oxygen to the patient

Several systems exist for increasing inspired oxygen concentration in spontaneously breathing patients. They can be divided into two sorts: those which provide a known inspired oxygen concentration (fixed performance systems) and those which provide a variable degree of oxygen enrichment (variable performance systems).

Simple oxygen masks and nasal cannulae increase the patient's inspired oxygen, but the increase depends upon the respiratory pattern, the rate and depth of breathing, and most importantly the patient's peak inspiratory flow. If this significantly exceeds the rate of oxygen flowing into the mask, then there will be significant dilution with air. If the inspired oxygen tension is not known then arterial blood gas analysis has little meaning. Hence simple oxygen masks and nasal cannulae are variable performance systems.

Oxygen masks utilising the Venturi principle can provide accurate concentrations of oxygen of up to 60%, which will exceed the patient's peak inspiratory flow. These devices rely on using a high flow, low pressure principle generated by passing oxygen through a narrow orifice into a special mask. Because fast moving gas has a low pressure, surrounding air enters the mask at a rate determined by the flow rate of oxygen and the size of special perforations in the mask. Since both these two factors can be varied, a range of concentrations is available. These masks are especially appropriate for treating patients who may be dependent upon hypoxaemia to

supply their respiratory drive. Venturi masks are fixed performance systems. It is difficult to give spontaneously-breathing patients 100% oxygen without using an endotracheal tube and a special anaesthetic circuit. In practice this is probably no bad thing, because oxygen, like any other drug, has side effects.

Harmful effects of oxygen

We have already seen how increasing the patient's inspired oxygen concentration can result in depression of ventilation. Oxygen can also be directly toxic to the tissues. Since the lungs are exposed to the highest oxygen concentrations, it is not surprising that the toxic manifestations of oxygen are most often seen in the alveoli. Exposing alveoli to 100% oxygen for more than a few hours will result in normal subjects complaining of discomfort and difficulty in breathing. This is because, in the absence of nitrogen, alveoli tend to collapse as oxygen is rapidly removed. Further prolonged exposure to oxygen results in a progressive fall in arterial oxygen tensions, as the capillaries become increasingly permeable, leading to interstitial oedema,. After about 48 h, organisation and fibrosis occur in a similar fashion to ARDS. Thus patients treated for ventilatory failure with high concentrations of oxygen, enter a vicious circle, where ever-increasing oxygen enrichment is required to compensate for the deterioration in lung function caused by oxygen. The development of this syndrome requires exposure to high concentrations with time. It is much less likely to occur if inspired oxygen concentration is kept below 60%.

In the newborn infant treated with high inspired oxygen concentrations, a condition called retrolental fibroplasia may develop, with permanent blindness resulting.

PNEUMOTHORAX

Under normal conditions, the pressure in the intrapleural space is less than atmospheric, as a result of the opposing elastic forces of the lung and chest wall. If air is allowed to enter the intrapleural space then the lung will collapse as the chest wall moves outward. This is called a pneumothorax, and these features can readily be seen on an erect chest x-ray. It can be classified as spontaneous or traumatic.

Spontaneous pneumothorax

Most pneumothoraces are spontaneous, because the pressure within the alveoli is always greater than intrapleural pressure. If a weakened alveolus ruptures, then air will pass from the lung into the intrapleural until space pressures equalise. The chest wall does not usually expand as much as the elastic forces would suggest; probably splinting occurs due to pain. The decrease negative pressure in the chest causes depression of the diaphragm and shift of the mediastinum away from the affected side. PaO_2 tends to fall due to areas of decreased ventilation–perfusion in the collapsed lung. When the source of the pneumothorax is sealed, re-expansion takes place at about 1.25% of the volume of the hemithorax per day. This reabsorption takes place because the total gas tension in venous blood is less than that in arterial blood (94 kPa and 101 kPa, respectively). This difference can be increased by increasing inspired oxygen, hastening reabsorption.

A primary spontaneous pneumothorax occurs in an otherwise healthy patient. A secondary spontaneous pneumothorax arises as a complication of disease. The former usually occurs in tall young men, in whom the negative pressure in the pleural space at the apex of the lung is greater than normal. Rupture of a small bulla in this area is the usual cause.

Secondary spontaneous pneumothorax usually occurs in patients over 30, and is almost always associated with pulmonary disease.

The symptoms of pneumothorax are pleuritic pain on the affected side, and dyspnoea. Signs of a pneumothorax may be absent if it is small. Larger pneumothoraces cause a tachycardia, and an expanded chest wall on the affected side. There are reduced chest movements and breath sounds, and the percussion note is more resonant on the side with the pneumothorax.

A small pneumothorax (less than 20% of the hemithorax) in a patient with healthy lungs requires no treatment. A large pneumothorax or one causing significant dyspnoea requires a chest drain with an underwater seal.

Tension pneumothorax

A tension pneumothorax develops when the hole in the pleura remains unsealed, and a valve develops so that air can pass into the pleural space on inspiration but cannot escape during expiration. The pressure in the intrapleural space rises, so that the chest on the affected side becomes distended, the mediastinum is pushed away and the liver depressed. During inspiration the trachea moves away from the affected side. This does not occur following a simple pneumothorax. There is rarely time for a chest x-ray. The patient rapidly deteriorates due to reduced venous return, and hypoxaemia caused by shunting through the compressed lung. Life-saving treatment is necessary and provided by rapid insertion of a hollow needle into the affected side of the chest.

A tension pneumothorax may occur during IPPV of a patient with high pressures or with PEEP. Because of the positive pressure applied to the lungs the tension may develop with startling rapidity and catastrophic consequences if immediate treatment is not provided.

Traumatic pneumothorax

Severe injuries to the chest wall may be complicated by a pneumothorax. Usually there are associated rib fractures, but the pneumothorax can occur as a result of compression of the lung causing rupture of the alveoli. Interstitial emphysema develops and can clearly be seen on x-ray.

An open pneumothorax is caused by a penetrating wound of the chest that allows air from the outside world to communicate with the intrapleural space. If the communication is greater in size than the cross-sectional area of the larynx, there will be a mediastinum shift to the opposite side. The wound must be sealed immediately, followed by surgical closure and a chest drain.

PULMONARY OEDEMA

Pulmonary oedema is the abnormal accumulation fluid in the tissues of the lung. It may occur from a variety of causes and can be life threatening.

The epithelium of the capillaries is very permeable to water, small molecules and ions. Large molecules such as proteins have a restricted capacity to diffuse across the cells. The alveolar epithelium is permeable to water, but not to small molecules or even ions. Hydrostatic forces tend to push forward out of the circulation, while osmotic forces tend to keep fluid in. The rate of flow of fluid from the circulation can be predicted from Starling's equation:

$$Q = K \left[(P_c - P_i) - \theta(\pi_c - \pi_i) \right]$$

where Q is the net flow out of the capillary, K is the filtration coefficient, P_c is the hydrostatic pressure in the capillary space, P_i is the hydrostatic pressure in the interstitial space, π_c is the colloid osmotic pressure in the capillary space, π_i is the osmotic pressure in the interstitial space, θ is the reflection coefficient — an indication of the usefulness of the membrane in preventing the passage of protein.

In practice the equation is of little use, since only the colloid osmotic pressure in the capillary is known. This is usually about 28 mmHg. Whatever the other pressures, it is known that there is a net pressure excess causing a lymph flow of 20 mL/h.

If excess fluid moves out of the circulation it will cause, first, interstitial oedema. This has little effect on primary function but can be seen on x-ray. If fluid continues to move into the lungs it will overwhelm the lymphatics, resulting in alveolar oedema. The alveoli become filled with fluid which increases surface tension forces, causing them to shrink. Ventilation of these units ceases, and, while they remain perfused, hypoxaemia results. If the passage of fluid continues it will fill the small and then large airways as frothy sputum, which may be tinged pink from red blood cells.

There are several causes of pulmonary oedema, not all of which are fully understood. The commonest cause is raised capillary hydrostatic pressure, usually seen after acute myocardial infarction, left ventricular failure, or transfusion overload. The left atrial pressure rises and there is an increase in pulmonary venous and pulmonary capillary pressures. If the pressure rise is slow and gradual, then remarkably high pressures may occur without alveolar oedema, although x-ray often reveals marked interstitial oedema. Sudden rises in capillary pressure will result in alveolar oedema.

The permeability of the capillaries may also rise, causing fluid to accumulate in the alveoli. This occurs from a variety of causes including endotoxic shock, exposure to irritant gases such as chlorine or nitric oxide, and as part of ARDS.

If the lymphatic drainage of the lung becomes impaired, for example because of obstruction by tumour cells, then pulmonary oedema will result.

From the Starling equation it can be seen that colloid osmotic pressure has a major effect on diffusion of fluid through the capillaries. However, although decreased colloid osmotic pressure rarely results in pulmonary oedema, it may exaggerate existing oedema, for example in overtransfusion with saline.

Pulmonary oedema can also occur during rapid ascent to high altitude. The aetiology is unclear, and pulmonary capillary wedge pressure is normal. Pulmonary artery pressure is raised, probably because of hypoxic vasoconstriction, and the condition is relieved by oxygen therapy or descent to a lower altitude.

Neurogenic pulmonary oedema may occur following insult to the central nervous system, usually severe head injury. It is probably caused by massive overactivity of the sympathetic nervous system.

Whatever the cause the clinical features of pulmonary oedema are usually: dyspnoea, also orthopnoea, paroxysmal nocturnal dyspnoea, cough and cyanosis. Breathing is rapid and shallow, driven by arterial hypoxaemia and an effort to minimise the increased work of breathing. On auscultation fine inspiratory crepitations are heard at the lung bases. A chest x-ray reveals an enlarged heart with prominent pulmonary vessels. Interstitial oedema causes short, linear horizontal lines near the pleural surface in the lower zones — the Kerley B lines.

The physiological effects of pulmonary oedema are widespread. The compliance of the lung decreases as surface tension causes alveolar collapse. Airway resistance increases, partly because of the smaller lung volume and partly because the larger airways may be partially blocked by oedema. Reflex bronchoconstriction also increases resistance. Although interstitial oedema has little effect on pulmonary gas exchange, alveolar oedema has dramatic, and often fatal, effects. Those alveoli filled with fluid no longer take part in gas exchange, but instead collapse. They continue to be perfused, causing massive $V_A:V_Q$ mismatch. Some lung units will have minimal ventilation and normal perfusion. These units are especially likely to collapse during oxygen therapy. Rapid ventilation by the patient usually maintains $PaCO_2$ at normal or even reduced levels. Pulmonary vascular resistance is increased because of hypoxic vasoconstriction and external pressure on the vessels due to interstitial oedema. There is often diversion of blood to the upper zones.

The treatment of pulmonary oedema includes the administration of high concentrations of oxygen, vasodilators, diuretics, and ultimately IPPV and PEEP. The application of raised end expiratory pressure decreases oedema in the larger airways and decreases the shunt.

PULMONARY EMBOLUS

Thrombus formation in the great veins of the legs may result in blood clots breaking off and lodging in the pulmonary arteries. A large clot may completely obstruct the pulmonary outflow, resulting in death. Smaller clots may block a single large artery or break up and block several small vessels. The lower regions of the lung have the greatest blood flow and so are most often affected. If the patient survives the initial insult, then there may either be distal infarction or haemorrhage into the affected segment.

With small pulmonary emboli, the patient complains of dyspnoea and pleuritic pain. There may be a raised temperature and a productive cough with bloodstained sputum. There may be a tachycardia, and auscultation may reveal a pleural rub. X-ray rarely reveals an abnormality, so that diagnosis depends on specialised techniques such as a ventilation–perfusion scan, which will reveal areas of normal ventilation but reduced perfusion. Treatment is with antithrombolytics, anticoagulation and supplementary oxygen if required.

Larger emboli produce shock, central chest pain, sudden collapse and sometimes distended neck veins. Rapid surgical intervention may be life-saving.

The physiological effects of pulmonary emboli range from minimal to massive. The pulmonary artery resistance is only increased with large pulmonary emboli, since there is considerable reserve and capillary recruitment. If pulmonary artery pressure rises significantly, then the right ventricle may fail. Occlusion of the pulmonary artery in humans has shown that ventilation to the affected area is reduced, probably due to a reduction in alveolar PCO_2, causing bronchoconstriction in the small airways. The effect is weak and short-lived. It can be abolished by adding carbon dioxide to inspired air. Physiological dead space and shunt are increased. Hypoxaemia occurs without a corresponding rise in $PaCO_2$, because alveolar ventilation increases.

PLEURAL EFFUSION

The presence of fluid in the pleural cavity is called a pleural effusion. Small effusions do not cause symptoms. Larger effusions may cause dyspnoea and pleuritic pain. There will be reduced movements on the affected side of the chest, decreased breath sounds, and dullness on percussion.

The fluid that accumulates is either an exudate or a transudate. An exudate has a high protein content and is usually associated with infection or malignancy. A transudate is usually the result of capillary hypertension, for example from left ventricular failure. The physiological effects are similar to those seen in a small simple pneumothorax.

If the fluid in the pleural space is blood, from a haemorrhage, it is called a haemothorax. The physiological effects will be the same, but there may be associated haemorrhagic shock. Low blood pressure will result in decreased perfusion of alveoli, which will add to alveolar dead space and will lower arterial PO_2.

ENDOTRACHEAL INTUBATION

The insertion of an endotracheal tube is necessary for a variety of reasons, both in anaesthesia and resuscitation.

During anaesthesia an endotracheal tube provides a clear airway, and is useful where the patient is in an unusual position, and where the surgical field is shared with the anaesthetist. It is also necessary in order to facilitate IPPV during procedures that require muscle relaxation.

It is vital to remember that during the acute phase of resuscitation, endotracheal intubation is not necessary for the patient's survival, rather it is the delivery of oxygen to the alveoli which is essential. This can usually be achieved with a 'bag and mask' system, facilitated with either a laryngeal mask or Guedel airway until successful intubation can be performed.

A detailed description of the process of intubation is beyond the scope of this chapter, and the interested reader is encouraged to visit one of the many comprehensive anaesthetic textbooks on this matter.

Endotracheal intubation has several important effects:

1. Normal processes of humidification are bypassed.
2. There is a reduction in anatomical dead space.
3. There is an increase in airway resistance — this is most marked in children, where the radius of the tube is small.
4. The insertion of a laryngoscope blade into the vallecula and subsequent traction on the tissues causes profound reflex stimulation, tachycardia and increased blood pressure. In patients with pre-existing heart failure or ischaemic heart disease, this may be sufficient to provoke myocardial infarction or left ventricular failure. This response may be abolished by a variety of pharmacological means, including the use of high dose intravenous opiates. This is neither necessary nor advisable during resuscitation but is important during the conduct of anaesthesia.

A prolonged attempt at intubation may result in the patient becoming hypoxic. This can be avoided by pre-oxygenation with 100% oxygen as described earlier.

PATHOLOGY
RIB FRACTURES

A rib fracture is the most common chest injury. This may vary from a simple fracture with no complications to severe multiple fractures with flail chest and underlying lung contusion. Rib fractures usually occur as a result of direct violence. Rib fractures may occur as a result of strenuous coughing, but this is unusual if the rib is normal. Rib fractures caused by spontaneous coughing are usually pathological fractures and may be associated with such conditions as osteoporosis or secondary deposits in the ribs. Because of the associated pain on breathing, fractured ribs may cause hypoventilation, sputum retention, atelectasis and pneumonia, especially in the elderly.

If a number of ribs are broken in two places this creates a flail chest, the segment involved moving independently of the chest wall and moving paradoxically, i.e. inwards on inspiration and outwards on expiration. The underlying lung therefore does not expand. Often there is an associated underlying haemothorax, pneumothorax, or lung contusion. If ventilation becomes inadequate, atelectasis, hypoxia, hypercapnia, and accumulation of secretions will occur. Endotracheal intubation and positive pressure ventilation is often required.

PNEUMOTHORAX

Pneumothorax is air in the pleural cavity.

Aetiology

- Primary spontaneous (idiopathic). This most commonly occurs in young males aged 15–40 and is occasionally bilateral and recurrent. There is usually no evidence of underlying pulmonary disease, and the cause is unknown.
- Secondary spontaneous. Occurs in patients with evidence of underlying lung disease, e.g. emphysema, asthma, cystic fibrosis.
- Traumatic following penetrating injuries of the chest.
- Tension. Occurs where there is a valve-like mechanism at the site of communication between air and pleural cavity allowing air to enter the pleural cavity on inspiration but not to escape on expiration. The rise of pressure in the pleural cavity causes collapse of the lung and mediastinal shift to the opposite side, with both respiratory and circulatory embarrassment.
- Iatrogenic. This results from the inadvertent introduction of air into the pleural space during a therapeutic procedure. It may occur following intercostal nerve block, percutaneous placement of a subclavian catheter, thoracocentesis, or brachial plexus block. Inadvertent lung rupture may occur with ventilatory support.

PLEURAL CONDITIONS

Pleural effusions

These may occur from a variety of causes and may involve blood, a transudate (low protein fluid), an exudate (high protein fluid), pus and chyle. Haemothorax is blood in the pleural space. It is usually the result of trauma or a ruptured thoracic aortic aneurysm. Hydrothorax is due to either a transudate (liver, renal, or cardiac failure) or an exudate (tumour, infection, inflammation). Chylothorax is usually due to neoplastic infiltration of thoracic lymphatics or may rarely follow trauma. Pyothorax (empyema) results from pus secondary to infected lesions within the lung.

Mesothelioma

This is associated with exposure to asbestos. The interval between exposure and development of the disease may be as long as 30 years. The tumour develops as nodules on the pleura which coalesce to form a sheet extending into the lung fissures. Invasion of the chest wall and involvement of the intercostal nerves occurs, causing severe chest wall pain. Lymphatic spread occurs to the hilar nodes. There is no treatment, the disease progressing with dyspnoea and chest pain, and death occurring usually within 2 years of diagnosis.

LUNG INFECTIONS

Only those with which surgeons should be familiar are described here. Respiratory infections are common after surgery. This may be due to:

- loss or suppression of the cough reflex, e.g. anaesthesia or after surgery
- suppression of ciliary action by anaesthesia
- plugging of the respiratory passages with mucus
- smoking, which causes inhibition of macrophage function
- hypoxia
- pulmonary oedema.

There may be predisposing conditions to respiratory infection after surgery. These include chronic obstructive airways disease, mucus disorders, e.g. cystic fibrosis, immunosuppressive disorders, immunosuppressive drugs.

Pneumonia

This is usually due to infection of the distal airways, especially the alveoli. Primary pneumonia occurs in otherwise healthy persons. Secondary pneumonia occurs in a patient where defence mechanisms are lowered, e.g. the immunocompromised. There are two types of pneumonia: bronchopneumonia and lobar pneumonia.

Bronchopneumonia

This occurs chiefly in old age and infancy and in patients with debilitating disease e.g. cancer, cardiac failure, or renal failure. Other predisposing factors include chronic obstructive airways disease and cystic fibrosis. Bronchopneumonia also occurs in the early postoperative period due to failure to remove respiratory tract secretions. Causative organisms include *Streptococcus pneumoniae* and *Haemophilus influenzae*. Rarer causes include *Staph. aureus* and coliforms. *Staph. aureus* pneumonia is seen in hospital patients, after influenza, and as a severe secondary bacterial pneumonia in intravenous drug abusers.

It is also seen in the immunocompromised. It may be fulminating and rapidly fatal. Coliform organisms are a rare cause of bronchopneumonia. They are encountered as a cause of pneumonia in hospital patients, the immunocompromised and those on ventilatory support on ITUs.

Bronchopneumonia is of characteristic patchy distribution and tends to be basal and bilateral. Histological examination reveals inflammatory cells in the bronchi and bronchioles, with the alveoli filled with an inflammatory exudate. With appropriate treatment the areas of inflammation either resolve or heal by scarring.

Lobar pneumonia

This is seen more rarely in surgical patients. However, it may result in referred pain to the abdomen, particularly right lower lobar pneumonia may enter into the differential diagnosis of appendicitis, the intercostal nerves being irritated and pain being referred to the right iliac fossa. It is commonly caused by *Streptococcus pneumoniae* and may be seen as part of postsplenectomy sepsis. It is relatively uncommon in infancy and old age.

Clinical features   These include cough, fever, and 'rusty' sputum. Rigors may occur. Acute pleuritic chest pain occurs. Consolidation of the lobe or part of a lobe results. Classically, four stages of the disease are recognised pathologically, as follows.

1. Congestion. This lasts about 24 h and is due to a protein rich exudate filling the alveoli, with venous congestion.
2. Red 'hepatisation'. This stage lasts a few days, with inflammatory cells and red cells in the alveolus spaces. There is a fibrinous exudate on the pleura. The lung is red, solid and airless and bears a resemblance to the cut surface of fresh liver.
3. Grey 'hepatisation'. There is accumulation of fibrin with destruction of white cells and red cells. The lung appears grey and solid.
4. Resolution. This occurs in 8–10 days. The inflammatory cells and fibrin are reabsorbed, and the underlying lung architecture is preserved.

This is the classical pattern of lobar pneumonia. Most cases resolve as above, although the pattern may be modified by early and appropriate antibiotic therapy.

Aspiration pneumonia

This occurs when upper gastrointestinal contents are aspirated into the lung, resulting in consolidation and inflammation. Clinical situations in which this may occur include induction of anaesthesia, recovery from anaesthesia, sedation, coma, and severe debility. The parts of the lung affected depend on the patient's posture. Lung

abscess and empyema may result. Causative organisms are usually commensals of the upper respiratory tract, principally *Streptococcus pneumoniae,* although anaerobes are also involved in the majority of cases. Anaerobes are rarely isolated from sputum. Where necessary, samples should be obtained from a fine catheter passed down a bronchoscope or by transthoracic needle aspiration.

Atypical pneumonia

The main causative organisms are: *Mycoplasma pneumoniae, Coxiella burneti, Chlamydia psittaci, Chlamydia pneumoniae. Mycoplasma pneumoniae* is responsible for most cases of primary atypical pneumonia. School age children and young adults are the group most affected. It is spread by droplet infection. Effective drugs include tetracycline and erythromycin.

Legionnaire's disease

This is caused by *Legionella pneumophila.* Patients are typically middle aged smokers, often in poor general health. It may also affect patients who were previously healthy. The spread is by water droplets from contaminated air humidifiers or water storage tanks. Symptoms are initially those of a flu-like illness which progresses to a severe pneumonia and respiratory failure. Other features include headache, mental confusion, myalgia, nausea, vomiting, diarrhoea and acute renal failure. About 10–20% of cases are fatal. Treatment is usually with erythromycin but, in those failing to respond, rifampicin and ciprofloxacin either singly or in combination are effective drugs.

Chest infections in the immunocompromised

The lungs are prone to infection by unusual organisms that are non-pathogenic in non-immunocompromised individuals, i.e. opportunistic infections. Common opportunistic organisms include: protozoa, e.g. *Pneumocystis carinii*; fungi, e.g. *Candida, Aspergillus fumigatus*; and viruses, e.g. cytomegalovirus. Infections with opportunistic organisms are characterised by fever, cough and shortness of breath, with pulmonary infiltrates on chest x-ray.

Pneumocystis carinii   This is a result of reactivation of latent infection. It is common in patients with AIDS and transplant recipients. Diagnosis depends on the demonstration of characteristic organisms in bronchial aspirates, bronchial lavage, or lung biopsy. Treatment is with intravenous co-trimoxazole.

Fungi   Both *Candida* and *Aspergillus* can cause widespread areas of necrosis. Microabscesses containing characteristic fungal filaments may occur in the lungs. Treatment requires intravenous amphotericin B alone or in combination with 5-fluorocytosine. Oral administration of new imidazoles, e.g. fluconazole, may also be effective.

Viruses Cytomegalovirus causes diffuse alveolar damage. Characteristic intranuclear inclusions are seen with CMV infections. Treatment is with intravenous ganciclovir.

ADULT RESPIRATORY DISTRESS SYNDROME

(See also the physiology section.) Adult respiratory distress syndrome is a serious condition characterised by a reduction in pulmonary compliance, arterial hypoxaemia refractory to oxygen therapy, associated with ventilation–perfusion inequality. It is associated with many different clinical conditions:

- shock, e.g. hypovolaemic, cardiogenic, septic, anaphylactic
- trauma, e.g. direct lung trauma or multisystem trauma
- infection, e.g. septicaemia, pneumonia
- embolism, e.g. fat, air, amniotic fluid
- inhalation, e.g. smoke, vomit, water, high oxygen concentrations, chlorine, ammonia
- drugs, e.g. opiates (especially drug abuse), barbiturates
- cerebral, e.g. head injury, cerebral haemorrhage
- others, e.g. pancreatitis, DIC, blood transfusion, cardiopulmonary bypass.

All the situations referred to above result in diffuse alveolar damage with hyaline membranes. The precise pathogenesis is unknown. Contributing factors include endothelial cell damage, loss of surfactant, alveolar oedema, and free radical production. Polymorphs may be involved in the release of enzymes and activation of complement. About 50% of cases die despite intensive therapy. Of the survivors the majority make a full recovery with restoration of normal alveolar architecture, but in a small number of cases pulmonary fibrosis results.

PULMONARY EMBOLUS

(See also Ch. 9.) This may be caused by thrombus, fat, air, amniotic fluid, or tumour fragments. The commonest cause by far is venous thromboembolism.

Thromboembolism

A piece of thrombus becomes detached from the leg veins or pelvic veins, is carried in the venous circulation to the right side of the heart, where it becomes lodged in a pulmonary artery. The clinical sequelae depend on the size of the embolus. A saddle embolus at the bifurcation of the pulmonary arteries usually causes sudden death. Occlusion of one of the main pulmonary arteries also frequently leads to death, although occasionally there is severe chest pain and shock and the patient may survive with appropriate treatment. Occlusion of a lobar or segmental artery causes sudden onset of chest pain and leads to a wedge-shaped infarct of the peripheral lung tissue. Multiple small emboli may occur. These result initially in occlusion of the arterioles but slowly occlude the larger vessels in the pulmonary arterial tree, resulting in pulmonary arterial hypertension.

BRONCHIECTASIS

Bronchiectasis is a condition in which there is permanent dilatation of the bronchi and bronchioles. Recurrent infection and inflammation lead to further airway damage and destruction of lung tissue. The condition results from bronchial obstruction with distal infection or severe infection alone. There is destruction of the alveolar walls, especially interstitial elastin, and fibrosis of the lung parenchyma. Clinical features include a cough productive of large amounts of foul-smelling sputum, together with dyspnoea.

Complications include pneumonia, lung abscess, empyema, septicaemia, amyloid formation, pulmonary fibrosis, and cor pulmonale. Remote abscesses, e.g. cerebral abscesses and meningitis, may also occur.

The condition may be congenital or acquired. The chief congenital cause is cystic fibrosis, although it is also seen in immunodeficiency syndromes. Acquired causes include whooping cough and measles in childhood, tuberculous mediastinal lymph nodes, and bronchial tumours.

LUNG ABSCESS

There may be a single lung abscess or the condition may be multiple. They occur usually in patients who are malnourished, cachectic, or immunocompromised. Causes include aspiration pneumonia, bronchiectasis, carcinoma, inhaled foreign bodies, infected pulmonary infarcts following pulmonary embolus, and intravenous drug abuse. Organisms include *Streptococcus pneumoniae, Haemophilus influenzae, Staphylococcus aureus, Klebsiella,* and *Entamoeba histolytica,* the latter spreading from the liver via the diaphragm.

LUNG TUMOURS

These are common and may be either primary or secondary.

Primary carcinoma of the lung

This is the most common primary malignant tumour in the United Kingdom. The prognosis is extremely poor, the overall survival being 5% at 5 years. Only about 15% of cases are operable at diagnosis. The disease usually presents between 40 and 70 years of age. It accounts for about one-third of all cancers in males, and its incidence in females is increasing, being second only to breast cancer.

Aetiology

The major risk factors are cigarette smoking, occupational hazards, e.g. asbestosis or radioactive gases, and pulmonary fibrosis.

Cigarette smoking The association between cigarette smoking and lung cancer is well established. Progressive changes occur in the bronchial mucosa, associated with smoking. Initially squamous metaplasia occurs, and this is followed by dysplasia.

Occupational hazards Occupational exposure to asbestos results in a significant increase in the risk of lung cancer. A latent period of approximately 20 years is usual between exposure and the development of cancer. Radioactive gases may also predispose to lung cancer. There is also an increased risk in workers who are exposed to nickel, arsenic, chromium, or coal tar distillates. Some peripheral tumours may arise in areas of scarring, e.g. old tuberculous foci or infarcts. There is also a significant increase in adenocarcinoma in patients with pulmonary fibrosis.

Clinical features

Cough, haemoptysis and weight loss are the commonest presenting factors. With intrathoracic spread, dyspnoea and chest pain occur. Patients may present with symptoms related to metastases or as a result of hormonal symptoms: e.g. ADH or ACTH for small cell carcinomas, and PTH for squamous cell carcinoma. Clubbing and hypertrophic pulmonary osteoarthropathy may occur. Meta-stases occur to regional lymph nodes, liver, bone, brain, and occasionally to adrenal glands.

Morphology

Most tumours arise from bronchi close to the hilum. Some arise peripherally, and it is these small peripheral adenocarcinomas which are amenable to surgery if detected prior to metastatic spread. Four histological types are recognised: (i) squamous cell carcinoma; (ii) small cell carcinoma (oat cell carcinoma); (iii) adeno-carcinoma; and (iv) large cell undifferentiated carcinoma.

Squamous cell carcinoma This type of cancer is most closely associated with smoking. The tumour occurs in the hilar regions usually in areas of squamous metaplasia and dysplasia. Spread to hilar nodes is common but distant metastases occur late.

Small cell carcinoma (oat cell carcinoma) This type of cancer usually arises in the hilar region. They meta-stasise early, often producing large secondary deposits; in some cases the primary tumour remains very small.

Adenocarcinoma These are usually peripheral. They are associated with pulmonary fibrosis, honeycomb lung and asbestosis.

Large cell undifferentiated carcinoma These are usually centrally placed and are highly aggressive tumours associated with necrosis and haemorrhage.

Other lung tumours

These are rare and include benign bronchial gland adenomas and mesenchymal tumours. Sarcomas and lymphomas occur but are also rare.

Secondary lung tumours

These are extremely common, being more common than primary lung cancers. They arise by either blood or lymphatic spread. Discrete nodules may be scattered throughout the lung fields, or the lymphatics may be diffusely involved, a condition known as lymphangitis carcinomatosa. Secondary deposits are most common from breast, kidney, gastrointestinal tract, sarcoma and lymphomas.

12

Locomotor system

Richard L M Newell

In each part of this chapter, the main text is preceded by short sections giving an overview of the content and outlining key concepts and learning objectives.

ANATOMY

OVERVIEW OF CONTENT

The anatomy will be described on a mainly regional basis, dealing with the vertebral column, girdles and limbs. Transitional zones between these and other major anatomical regions will be included. For each anatomical subsection the organisational pattern will be the same:

- osteology
- arthrology
- areas between the joints
- related transitional zones
- neural patterns and relationships, stressing sites at which nerves are particularly vulnerable
- diagnostic clinical anatomy.

KEY CONCEPTS AND LEARNING OBJECTIVES

Anatomy should be learned in a clinically useful and retrievable way. Base your learning on the common loco-motor disorders presenting in a typical busy Accident and Emergency department: think in terms particularly of trauma and of infection. For each bone, joint, or region being learned, ask yourself two questions:

1. How do common injuries affect the local anatomy? It is a good anatomical exercise also to ask the reverse question: how are common patterns of injury — and their complications — determined by the local anatomy?
2. How could this bone/joint/region safely be approached surgically? The reverse exercise here is to ask: Which features of the local anatomy determine the possible complications of the operation?

In the limbs, build your anatomical knowledge around the major joints.

As for the regions which lie anatomically between the joints, learn them in terms of osteofascial compartments and important fascial planes. Such a three-dimensional approach is clinically more useful than trying to memorise lists of apparently unrelated facts such as the details of individual muscle attachments.

The old concept of anatomical 'relations' should not be neglected. Whether managing a soft-tissue wound or a fracture, or planning a surgical approach, you will need to know the exact relationships of the important structures at any given point or region of the body. This observation does not apply only to the locomotor system. It is much more relevant and clinically useful to be able to visualise the exact relative position of a nerve or artery at the site of pathology than it is to be able to recite from memory the anatomical 'course' of such a structure from beginning to end. You will also need to be aware of the commoner variations in the neurovascular patterns, especially those of the major arteries.

VERTEBRAL COLUMN

The column may be considered as a longitudinal series of bones, linkages and 'holes'. The bones are the individual vertebrae, the linkages are the joints (including the inter-vertebral discs), ligaments, muscles and fasciae, and the 'holes' are the foramina, vertebral and intervertebral. The serially linked vertebral foramina constitute the vertebral canal. The intervertebral discs constitute about a quarter of the length of the adult column.

The vertebral column as a whole is a protective seg-mented duct for neural and vascular tissue, which acts as a 'mast' guyed and supported by muscles, ligaments and fasciae, as a weight-bearing supportive strut, and which behaves mechanically as a cantilever or as an arch. Viewed from its lateral aspect the column has a series of curves. The primary curves, thoracic and pelvic, are present throughout development, and are both convex posteriorly (kyphoses). The curvature is due chiefly to the shape of the component vertebrae. The secondary curves, cervical and lumbar, are lordoses (convex anteriorly), and appear as the column starts to bear the weight of the head (cervical) and of the trunk and limbs (lumbar). In these regions the intervertebral discs contribute to the curve, being thicker anteriorly than posteriorly. The presence of these curves increases the ability of the column to withstand axial compression. The line of weight in the standing position intersects the curves at the cervicothoracic, thoracolumbar and lumbosacral junctions, then passes through the centre of gravity of the body at about the level of the second sacral vertebra. The varying curvature of the vertebral column determines the changing cross-sectional profile of the trunk. At a lordosis, as in the lumbar region, the anteroposterior diameter of the body cavity decreases markedly.

From the functional standpoint, the occipito-atlantoaxial region may be considered separately from the remainder of the mobile vertebral column (C3–L5). The majority of cervical rotation occurs at atlantoaxial level, while nodding movements and fine positioning (tilting) of the head on the neck occur mainly between atlas and occiput. In the rest of the mobile column, the final range of movement results from the summation of small movements at individual intervertebral levels ('motion segments'). The regions with the most movement, and hence the least stability, are the junctions of the more 'fixed'

levels (thoracic and sacral) with the more mobile levels (cervical and lumbar). The commonest forms of the unstable spinal injury occur at these junctional regions. At mid- and lower cervical levels and in the lumbar region the configuration of the facet joints, the arrangement of the muscles and the topography of the neighbouring soft tissues allow (forward) flexion, extension and lateral flexion (side-bending) movements which are largely prevented at thoracic level by the presence of the rib-cage. Axial rotation (about the vertical axis of the column) occurs maximally at thoracic level.

Osteology

Parts of a typical vertebra

A typical vertebra (Fig. 12.1) consists of an anteriorly placed body and a group of less substantial bony structures lying behind the vertebral canal and known as the posterior elements. These structures are connected to the body by a pair of pedicles, and comprise an arch or lamina from which project muscular and articular processes. The body bears the major part of the weight transmitted by the vertebra, while the posterior elements protect neural and vascular tissue and give attachment to muscles in such a way as to maximise their efficiency of action.

The internal bony architecture of the vertebral body is adapted to resist compressive forces. There are interlocking plates of cancellous bone, the trabeculae being

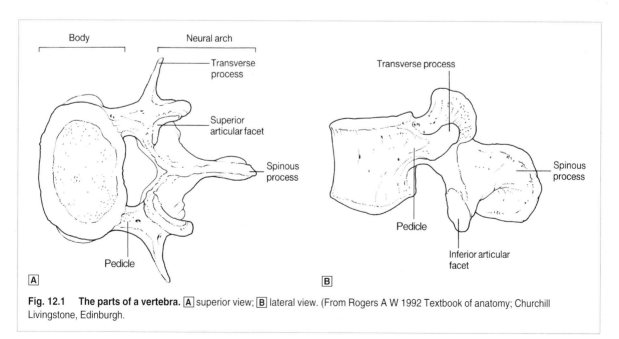

Fig. 12.1 **The parts of a vertebra.** A superior view; B lateral view. (From Rogers A W 1992 Textbook of anatomy; Churchill Livingstone, Edinburgh.

arranged mainly at right-angles to each other. The interstices between the trabeculae contain red marrow: erythropoiesis continues throughout life in the axial skeleton. The posterior elements consist largely of compact bone. The vertebral bodies articulate by means of symphyses — the intervertebral discs — while the posterior elements articulate separately by means of pairs of synovial joints, the zygoapophyseal or facet joints. The facets of these joints are borne on the pairs of articular processes, superior and inferior, projecting from each neural arch. The muscular processes are the midline spinous process, projecting posteriorly from the apex of the arch, and the paired transverse processes, which project laterally. In the cervical and sacral regions the costal elements lie anterior to the foramina transversaria and thus to the pedicles. These elements also lie anterolaterally in the sacrum, forming the ventral parts of the alae. In both cervical and sacral regions the costal, transverse and articular processes are often grouped descriptively as the 'lateral masses' of the vertebrae.

Special additional features at specific vertebral levels

Cervical All cervical vertebrae have a pair of foramina transversaria, through which pass the vertebral vessels (the artery missing out the seventh pair). These foramina lie between the costal and 'true' transverse process elements of the lateral masses. The first two cervical vertebrae are very atypical in form, as together with the occipital condyles of the skull they form a specialised functional region of the spine to allow nodding movements and rotation of the head on the neck. The atlas (C1) has an anterior arch but no vertebral body and no spinous process, while the lateral masses are large and anteriorly placed so that the first and second cervical nerves emerge posterior to them. In the axis (C2) the dens or odontoid process projects superiorly from the vertebral body, and bears an anterior facet for its synovial articulation with the anterior arch of the atlas. The foramina transversaria run superiorly and laterally within the lateral masses. The spinous process is strong and bifid. The size and orientation of the articular facets also differ markedly in the atlas and in the superior part of the axis from the conditions seen in the typical cervical vertebrae C3–C7. The inferior part of the axis resembles a typical cervical vertebra.

The typical cervical vertebra (C3–C6) has a bifid spine and a small oval body which is smaller than the vertebral foramen. The body has lateral lips on its superior surface which articulate with the bevelled lateral edges of the inferior surface of the body above, often by synovial joints (of Luschka). The articular surfaces of the zygoapophyseal (facet) joints lie obliquely, approaching the

horizontal plane more nearly than at any other vertebral level and thus predisposing to instability.

The seventh cervical vertebra is very variable in the shape and size of its lateral masses. The costal element of the 'transverse process' is often thin and slight, and the foramina transversia vary greatly in size and shape both between individuals and between sides in a single individual. The costal elements may be prolonged to form a cervical rib. The spine is large but not bifid.

Thoracic The typical thoracic vertebra (T2–T10) is characterised by its long, obliquely sloping spine and by the presence of the articular facets of its synovial joints with the ribs. The facets for the tubercles of the ribs lie on the anterosuperior surfaces of the transverse processes, facing more superiorly in the lower vertebrae. The heads of the ribs articulate with small posterolaterally placed demi-facets on the vertebral bodies, each typical rib articulating with two demi-facets.

The first, eleventh and twelfth thoracic vertebrae are atypical. The body of the first is very like that of the seventh cervical, and its transverse processes are large. There are complete (circular) facets posterolaterally on each side of the body, for the heads of the first pair of ribs, which articulate only with this vertebra. The eleventh and twelfth thoracic vertebrae also bear single rib-head facets, which are large, complete and may extend posteriorly onto the pedicle. The transverse processes are small and bear no facets. The twelfth (sometimes the eleventh) is the transitional vertebra between thoracic and lumbar: its superior articular facets are flat and lie mainly in the coronal plane, while the inferior facets are curved and face more laterally.

Lumbar Lumbar vertebrae have large, strong bodies with relatively small vertebral foramina. Psoas and the crura of the diaphragm attach anteriorly. The transverse processes vary in length, those of L3 usually being the longest. In L5 the body is somewhat longer anteriorly than posteriorly, and the pedicles are short and thick. If a lumbar vertebra is inspected from behind, the tips of its four articular processes form a rectangle. This rectangle is longer in its vertical axis in the upper lumbar vertebrae and longer in its horizontal access in the lower.

Sacral and coccygeal There are ususally five fused vertebrae in the sacrum, but segmentation anomalies are not unusual, giving four or six sacral vertebrae. The coccyx typically consists of four fused vertebrae, but the demarcation may be difficult to see. The fused lateral masses of the upper sacral vertebrae are massive, those of S1 forming the alae. The vertebral foramina of the fused vertebrae form the sacral canal, whose inferior opening is the sacral hiatus, flanked by the cornua.

Arthrology

The mobile vertebral column can be considered functionally as a series of linked pairs of vertebrae. Each pair of vertebrae and the linkages between its members constitute a motion segment. These linkages include joints, ligaments and muscles.

The joints are the interbody joints and the zygoapophyseal ('facet') joints. The major interbody joints are symphyses or secondary cartilaginous joints, occurring, as do all such joints, in the midline of the skeleton. In the cervical region the vertebral bodies also articulate peripherally on each side by means of the small joints of Luschka, which may be synovial. The posterior elements of the motion segment articulate at the superior and inferior pairs of facet joints. These joints are synovial, including all the anatomical features and subject to all the pathological conditions of this type of joint, e.g. osteoarthritis, rheumatoid arthritis, ankylosing spondylitis. All joints of a motion segment function as an integrated unit: malfunction of one member of the unit leads to dysfunction of the others.

The major interbody joints are symphyses: the bones of the vertebral bodies are linked by two layers of hyaline cartilage (the end-plates) between which lie the fibro-cartilaginous intervertebral discs (Fig. 12.2). The outer part of the disc, the annulus fibrosus, consists of concentric laminae of fibrous tissue, the more peripheral laminae being the least fibrocartilaginous. The collagen bundles of each lamina run obliquely, crossing those of the adjacent laminae at an angle. The most peripheral laminae are adherent to the anterior and posterior longitudinal ligaments. The central portion of the disc, the nucleus pulposus, is in early life gelatinous and semi-fluid, but is gradually replaced by fibrocartilage. The nucleus pulposus is situated nearer the posterior than the anterior margin of the disc, and lies in contact with the hyaline cartilage of the vertebral end-plates superiorly and inferiorly.

Sometimes this end-plate is breached, allowing the nuclear tissue to penetrate the bone of the vertebral body as a Schmorl's node. After early childhood the intervertebral disc is avascular, obtaining its nutrition entirely by diffusion from the vertebral bodies and from surface vessels around the periphery of the disc.

Other direct static linkages between vertebrae are mainly ligamentous. The vertebral bodies are linked by the anterior and posterior longitudinal ligaments. The former is a strong band extending from the basi-occiput to the upper sacrum, attached firmly to the upper and lower margins

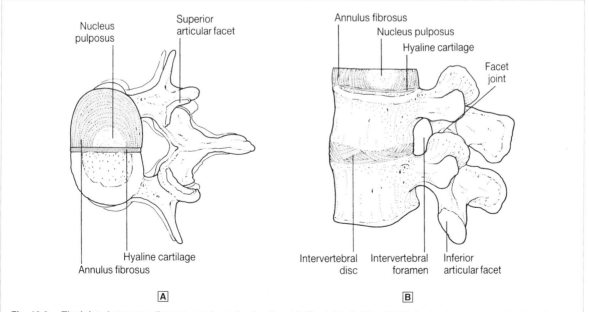

Fig. 12.2   The joints between adjacent vertebrae: lumbar 3 and 4. The left half of the L2–L3 disc has been cut away to show the plate of hyaline cartilage at the upper surface of L3. This, also, has been cut away to the left of the midline, exposing the upper surface of L3. A Superior view. B Lateral view. From Rogers op. cit.

of the vertebral bodies and to the intervertebral discs, and loosely to the intermediate anterior surfaces of the bodies. The latter is less strong, extending on the anterior wall of the vertebral canal from axis to sacrum, again attached to discs and vertebral margins but separated from the backs of the vertebral bodies by the basivertebral veins. The laminae are linked by the ligamenta flava, containing elastic tissue, and the spines are linked by interspinous ligaments thickened posteriorly to form a supraspinous ligament. The supraspinous and interspinous ligaments in the neck are replaced by the fibroelastic ligamentum nuchae. There are also flimsy intertransverse ligaments at most levels.

Note the ways in which the vertebral column is linked to the limb girdles, and to the thoracic cage, of which it forms the posterior 'strut'. There are no direct joint linkages to the pectoral girdle, though muscles such as trapezius, scalenes and rhomboids help suspend the girdle from the axial skeleton. The sacrum of the vertebral column is 'stepped' into the pelvic girdle like a mast into a deck, and linked to it directly by the massive weight-bearing sacroiliac joints and their powerful ligaments. The thoracic column is linked to the rib-cage both by the numerous costovertebral synovial joint complexes and by the small spinal muscles.

The rôle of the muscles in forming both direct and indirect dynamic links between the vertebrae must not be forgotten. There are small intersegmental muscles which run between adjacent vertebrae, but much more common and far more important are the larger, polysegmental muscles which cross a number of vertebrae in their course. These are discussed in the next section.

Summary
Joints (Fig. 12.2)
- Interbody: symphysis (secondary cartilaginous). There is no interbody joint at atlantoaxial level, but there is a plane synovial joint between the odontoid and the anterior arch of the atlas.
- Facet (zygoapophyseal): plane synovial. These occur at all mobile levels. (The atlanto-occipital joints are specialised facet joints.)

Movements and muscles (See also next section.) Large movements involve the bigger muscles, more distant from the vertebral column; finer movements involve muscles acting on few segments. Gravity plays a very important rôle in spinal movements: apparent antagonists to the movement often contract eccentrically as antigravity muscles, e.g the spinal extensors 'pay out rope' to control trunk flexion from the standing position.

- Flexion ('bending forward'): bilateral action of all muscles running anterior to the spinal segment(s) involved, e.g. longus colli, sternocleidomastoid, psoas, rectus abdominis.
- Extension ('bending backward'): bilateral action of all muscles running posterior to the involved segments, e.g. semispinalis capitis, splenius, trapezius, erector spinae, multifidus.
- Lateral flexion ('bending sideways'): balanced unilateral action of the long flexors and extensors; oblique abdominal muscles on the side of flexion.
- Rotation: contralateral sternocleidomastoid; ipsilateral splenius; oblique abdominals; rotatores.

Major anatomical relations These are best appreciated by the examination of axial (transverse) sections of the body at serial levels. The list below is not comprehensive, and excludes many muscles.

- Posterior and posterolateral: spinal dural sheath (theca) in the vertebral canal; spinal nerves (loosely called the 'nerve roots') and their accompanying vessels in the intervertebral foramina; internal vertebral venous plexus.
- Anterior and lateral: pharynx; oesophagus; thoracic duct; major longitudinal vessels at all levels (e.g. vertebral, descending aorta, azygos; inferior vena cava); crura of diaphragm, psoas muscles; sympathetic trunk.

Fasciae and muscles
All fasciae in the body are essentially in continuity, as they represent the mesenchymal framework within which the striated musculature later differentiates during development. Try and imagine in three dimensions the fascial 'skeleton' of the region of the body which you are studying. In the axial and paraxial regions of the body the important fascial constituents include the prevertebral fascia (Fig. 12.3), the endothoracic and retroperitoneal fasciae, the thoracolumbar fascia and the central (sacral) components of the pelvic fascia. The thoracolumbar fascia links anteriorly with the musculature of the abdominal wall to form a very important hydraulic mechanism which augments the weight-bearing capacity of the lumbar spine.

The muscles which are immediately evident beneath the skin of the back are not the 'true' back muscles: trapezius and latissimus dorsi are both developmentally 'immigrant' muscles from neck and upper limb, respectively, as indicated by their nerve supplies. The 'true' posterior and local back muscles are those lying anterior to the posterior leaf of the thoracolumbar fascia — the erector spinae group, which cross many segments in their action, and the more medially placed multifidus, whose separate fibres cross only two or three segments. These true, epaxial back muscles are characterised by their innervation from the posterior primary rami of the spinal nerves. All other muscles acting on the spine, locally or at a distance, are hypaxial in origin and are thus innervated by anterior primary rami.

Fine detail of the neck muscles need not be learned. Anteriorly lie the long flexors: sternocleidomastoid, the scalenes and the prevertebral (longus) group. Posteriorly are the long extensors, overlaid by trapezius and innervated by posterior primary rami: note particularly the two easily palpable 'columns' largely formed by semispinalis capitis. Deep to the long extensors in the upper part of the neck lie the suboccipital muscles. These lie almost in the horizontal plane, and control rotation and fine positioning of the head on the neck.

The actions of the major muscles have already been summarised (p. 318).

Study of a transverse section of the trunk shows that many muscles acting locally on the vertebral column are enclosed within osteofascial compartments limited by layers or 'leaves' of the thoracolumbar fascia. A few cases of 'compartment syndrome' causing low back pain have been documented.

Transitional zones
With the increasing use of anterior approaches to the vertebral column at all levels, the anterior relations of the column are becoming more surgically relevant. The interface between the musculoskeletal axial structures and the viscera anterior to them is a good example of an anatomical 'transitional zone'. Such areas tend to be neglected, both by anatomists and by clinicians.

In the neck, the interface is demarcated by the prevertebral fascia: the visceral 'column' of the neck moves actively and passively on the musculoskeletal 'column' in the plane of this fascia. The fascial anatomy of the neck is of great surgical importance, and is best seen in transverse (axial) sections (Fig. 12.3). The prevertebral fascia of the neck extends inferiorly as the endothoracic fascia and subsequently the retroperitoneal fascia of the abdomen.

Revise in sequence all structures related directly to the anterior and anterolateral aspects of the vertebral bodies, starting at the atlas and ending at the coccyx. You will be surprised how much anatomy will be covered in such an exercise.

Neurovascular patterns and relationships: the 'holes' and what they contain
The 'holes' are the serial vertebral foramina (together constituting the vertebral canal), the intervertebral foramina, and in the cervical spine the foramina transversaria. The vertebral canal contains the spinal cord and cauda equina in their meningeal coverings, an incomplete epidural layer of fat containing the internal venous plexus, and some tenuous connective tissue connecting the dural tube or theca with the posterior longitudinal ligament. The most lateral parts of the canal contain the roots of the spinal nerves in their dural sheaths, within which each pair of dorsal and ventral roots joins, immediately lateral to the dorsal root ganglion. The epidural

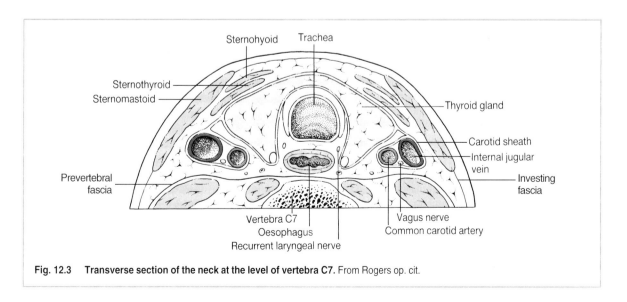

Fig. 12.3   Transverse section of the neck at the level of vertebra C7. From Rogers op. cit.

'space' is only 'potential' until defined by air or liquid let into it as a result of pathology or medical intervention (e.g. epidural injection, epidural anaesthesia, laminectomy). The cross-sectional size and shape of the vertebral canal varies with vertebral level, as does the proportion of its cross-sectional area occupied by the spinal cord and its coverings. The normal canal is large in the upper cervical and lower lumbar regions, and smallest in the midthoracic region.

The arterial supply of the cord is longitudinal via anterior and posterior spinal arteries lying on its surface. These arteries branch from the vertebrals, with segmental reinforcement at many levels via radicular arteries entering through the intervertebral foramina. The most important and largest of these radicular arteries, the *arteria radicularis magna*, usually occurs in the thoracolumbar junctional region on the left and may itself be responsible for the supply of a large part of the lower cord. The veins of the cord also run longitudinally on its surface, and communicate with each other and with the cerebellar veins and cranial venous sinuses. Each typical intervertebral foramen (Fig. 12.2) is bounded superiorly and inferiorly by the pedicles, anteriorly mainly by the intervertebral disc and posteriorly mainly by the facet joint. The foramen contains the foraminal segment of the exiting 'nerve root' (spinal nerve), together with the radicular vessels and fine recurrent meningeal (sinuvertebral) nerves. Owing to the varying obliquity and length of the nerve roots, which run increasingly distally as the spine is descended, the dorsal root ganglia may lie in the lateral zone of the vertebral canal or in the intervertebral foramen. The foramina transversaria in the lateral masses of the cervical vertebrae contain the vertebral vessels and a plexus of sympathetic nerves. The foramina of the seventh vertebra do not contain vertebral arteries. The arterial supply of the vertebrae themselves is segmental. Paired arteries arise from the deep arteries of the posterior neck, from the aorta and from the internal iliac arteries. The radicular arteries arise from these segmental arteries to the vertebrae. The venous drainage from the vertebrae is mainly via large basivertebral veins into venous plexuses. In addition to the internal venous plexus described above, there is an external plexus, best developed in the cervical region. These valveless plexuses communicate freely with each other and with the caval systems, and constitute important routes for the spread of infection and malignancy.

The main clinically relevant variations in the neurovascular patterns concern the effect of vertebral segmentation anomalies on the number and position of nerve roots (spinal nerves) exiting the vertebral column. Such segmentation anomalies are not uncommon, and chiefly affect the lumbosacral region. The lumbar spine may be shortened to four vertebrae ('sacralised L5'), or lengthened to six ('lumbarised S1'), with accompanying rearrangement of the nerve roots leading to possible confusion in the clinical assessment of neurological signs in the lower limbs.

In spinal injuries, the spinal cord, the nerve roots and the spinal nerves may be involved separately or together. The site of injury may be within the vertebral canal or in the intervertebral foramen and 'root canal'. Both cord and roots may be involved at any level above L1, where the cord stops in an adult. Below L1 only the roots of the cauda equina or the spinal nerves can be affected. The motor signs in spinal injury may be those of an upper motor neuron lesion, a lower motor neuron lesion, or a mixed picture may be seen. The whole spectrum of severity of nerve injury is possible, including the effects of acute or chronic nerve compression. The injury may be open (rarely) or closed, and the cause may be spinal fracture-dislocation, disc prolapse, or bony compresssion (spinal stenosis, which can occur at one or several spinal levels and which may affect the whole vertebral canal or only its lateral recesses). Clinical examination should include testing for both motor and sensory signs of root lesions: familiarity with dermatomes and muscle 'root values' is essential.

Diagnostic clinical anatomy

This includes the ability accurately to examine the range of spinal movements at all vertebral levels, to test the action of the muscle groups which produce these movements, and to conduct an efficient screening neurological examination of the limbs and trunk. You must also be able to identify all easily visible and palpable spinal and pelvic landmarks. You should be able to identify the major features of plain radiographs of the spine, and to recognise normal soft tissue structures and patterns on magnetic resonance imaging (MRI) and computerised tomographic (CT) scans. Interventional investigations of a basic nature requiring anatomical understanding include lumbar puncture and caudal epidural injection.

You should also know the anatomical principles underlying the planning of surgical access to the spine, particularly in the midcervical and lumbosacral regions where intervention is common.

The management of spinal injuries is largely based upon the anatomical principles informing the concept of stability. Holdsworth's pioneering idea of the prime rôle of the intact posterior vertebral elements and their linkages, bony and ligamentous, for stability has been developed by Denis to incorporate consideration of the 'three columns' of the spine as viewed in the lateral projection. These columns, anterior, middle and posterior, may be damaged individually or together, at single or multiple spinal levels. The posterior column includes the pedicles and all structures posterior to them, the middle column includes the posterior longitudinal ligament and the posterior halves of the vertebral bodies and discs, and the anterior column comprises the anterior halves of body and disc together with the anterior longitudinal ligament. Denis accords prime importance to integrity of the middle column in the maintenance of stability after injury.

PECTORAL GIRDLE

Though the term 'girdle' implies a complete, circumferential structure, the human pectoral girdle is usually described as consisting of two bones rather than four. Each separate 'hemi-girdle' comprises the scapula posteriorly and the clavicle anteriorly, and articulates with the axial skeleton by a single synovial joint, the sternoclavicular joint. Unlike the pelvic girdle, the pectoral girdle articulates neither with the vertebral column nor with its own contralateral fellow. Each pectoral girdle can therefore move independently of the other and of the vertebral column, thus giving the prehensile upper limb a versatile fixation platform. The clavicle also functions as a prop, maintaining the necessary relative separation of the limb from the trunk.

Osteology

Clavicle

This is one of the most frequently fractured bones, and has important muscle and ligament attachments and soft-tissue relations. It is subcutaneous throughout its length, but the overlying skin is very mobile, and open fracture is uncommon. The lateral half of the bone is concave forwards and flattened, with prominent anterior and posterior borders, while the medial half is convex forwards and almost cylindrical. The inferior surface is roughened laterally for the attachment of the coracoclavicular ligament and medially for that of the costoclavicular ligament (Fig. 12.4). These ligaments are very strong: the bone always fractures between their attachments, in the segment on the inferior surface of which the subclavius muscle is attached. Deltoid and pectoralis major are attached to the anterior surface, while trapezius attaches posterolaterally. The clavicular head of sternocleidomastoid attaches superomedially. The most important soft-tissue relations lie posteriorly, particularly at the medial end where the subclavian and brachiocephalic vessels are near. The divisions of the brachial plexus lie behind the medial two-thirds of the bone, separated from it by an often surprisingly large suprascapular vein. The clavicle is crossed anteriorly and subcutaneously by the palpable supraclavicular nerves from the cervical plexus.

The clavicle ossifies mainly in membrane, and is the first bone in the body to ossify.

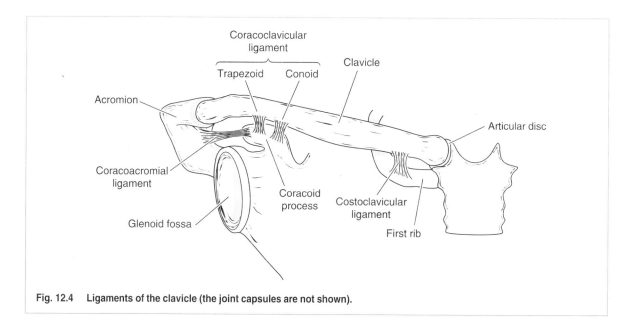

Fig. 12.4   Ligaments of the clavicle (the joint capsules are not shown).

Scapula

The scapula lies posterolaterally over the 2nd to 7th ribs. It consists of a flat, thin triangular body whose lateral border is thickened for force transmission and to act as a lever for the action of the attached teres muscles. A notch at the lateral end of the superior border transmits the suprascapular nerve, which may become entrapped here, and demarcates the bases of the coracoid process and 'neck' of the scapula from the remainder of the bone. The coracoid process projects mainly anteriorly in the anatomical position, and gives attachment to three muscles (coracobrachialis, short head of biceps and pectoralis minor) and three ligaments (coracoclavicular, coracoacromial and coracohumeral). The thick, cylindrical neck, to which the suprascapular nerve and vessels are very closely related posteriorly, bears the shallow articular surface for the humerus, the glenoid cavity. A tubercle immediately above the glenoid gives attachment to the long head of biceps, while the long head of triceps attaches in the corresponding position below. The spine of the scapula projects from its posterior surface, and ends laterally in the flattened acromion process. The spine is a lever for muscle attachment, with trapezius superiorly and deltoid inferiorly. The posterior surface of the body gives origin to the supraspinatus and infraspinatus muscles, both of which are tightly bound down by thick fascia. Subscapularis fills the concavity of the body anteriorly, 'padding' the bone against the chest wall and its covering muscles. Serratus anterior, 'slinging' the scapula from the upper eight ribs, attaches to the inner aspect of the medial border of the scapula. The edge of the medial border gives attachment to the rhomboids and levator scapulae, which together with trapezius connect the pectoral girdle, and thus the upper limb, with the axial skeleton. Intra-articular fractures involving the glenoid may require internal fixation, but fractures of the body of the scapula displace little and unite well, owing to the close coverage, firm fascial binding to bone, and excellent blood supply of the overlying muscles.

Arthrology

The 'shoulder joint' is not the 'shoulder' joint. When a patient is asked to move the shoulder, or complains of pain in the shoulder, he or she is not concerned only with the glenohumeral joint. The shoulder complex — the mechanism by which the upper limb is positioned and fixed in space — includes all the joints of the pectoral girdle as well as the important ligaments and muscles which link the limb to the trunk. The pectoral girdle as a whole is very mobile, movements of the 'shoulder complex' conferring wide versatility of function on the upper limb. The limb skeleton is linked to the trunk by a chain of synovial joints: this comprises the glenohumeral joint (see p. 329), the acromioclavicular joint and the sternoclavicular joint. The pectoral girdle is 'slung from' the trunk and the vertebral axis by the numerous muscles attaching to scapula and clavicle and mentioned above, while the limb is in turn connected to the girdle by a further series of muscles attaching mainly to the scapula but including pectoralis major and deltoid, attached also to the clavicle. Both pectoralis major and a further large, 'migrant' limb muscle, latissimus dorsi, attach the limb directly to the trunk. Note that both these muscles can act as accessory muscles of respiration if their attachment to the limb is fixed.

Neither the sternoclavicular nor the acromioclavicular joint have inherent bony stability, though both contain fibrous intra-articular discs which aid congruity. Both these synovial joints rely on their capsules and on strong, closely adjacent ligaments to provide the stability necessary for effective action of the limb (Fig. 12.4). The capsule of the sternoclavicular joint is strong, with anterior and posterior thickenings. The fibrous disc, passing obliquely across the joint from the clavicle superiorly to the sternum inferiorly, acts as an intra-articular ligament. The accessory ligaments of the sternoclavicular joint are the very strong costoclavicular (rhomboid) ligament, passing to the first rib and its cartilage, and the weaker interclavicular ligament passing between the medial ends of the clavicles. The capsule of the acromioclavicular joint is weaker, though it is strengthened superiorly by the acromioclavicular ligament. The strongest ligament is the bipartite coracoclavicular. The coracoacromial ligament, connecting the tips of the bony processes, lies at some distance from the joint. It may be considered 'accessory' both to the acromioclavicular and to the glenohumeral joints.

Summary

Joints (Fig. 12.4)
- sternoclavicular
- acromioclavicular.

Both are synovial, with articular surfaces of fibrocartilage, and each has an intra-articular fibrous disc (incomplete in the acromioclavicular joint).

Movements and muscles
- elevation: levator scapulae, trapezius
- depression: gravity, pectoralis muscles, serratus anterior
- protraction: serratus anterior, pectoralis minor
- retraction: rhomboids, trapezius

- rotation of scapula in the plane of its body: trapezius, serratus anterior.

Note also that the clavicle must move with the scapula during all of these movements, and that it also rotates on its own longitudinal axis during many of them.

Major anatomical relations   The brachiocephalic veins begin behind the sternoclavicular joints.

Transitional zones

Area enclosed by the pectoral girdle(s)
The thoracic spine, the axioscapular muscles (rhomboids and trapezii), the scapulae, clavicles and manubrium sternae form a 'ring' which may be considered as the complete pectoral 'girdle'. This outer ring encompasses an inner ring made by the first ribs and their cartilages, the thoracic inlet. Thus in addition to including the major anatomical transitional zone between the neck and the thorax, this outer ring also encloses structures on their way between the root of the neck and the upper limbs (brachial plexus, subclavian vessels). There are also several surgically important named fasciae related and attached to the girdle(s) and to the boundaries of these inner and outer rings. The apices of the lungs lie beneath the suprapleural membranes (Sibson's fascia) which attach around the medial borders of the first ribs. The clavipectoral fascia runs inferiorly from the clavicle, from which it suspends the concave fascial 'floor' of the axilla, splitting to enclose both subclavius and pectoralis minor muscles and forming part of the anterior axillary 'wall' during its course. The investing layer of the deep cervical fascia (Fig. 12.3) attaches to the clavicle, as does the fascial sling from the intermediate tendon of the omo-hyoid muscle. The prevertebral fascia (Fig. 12.3) overlies the roots of the brachial plexus then runs posterolaterally between inner and outer rings and becomes the axillary sheath around the axillary vessels. Both the prevertebral and the pretracheal fasciae of the neck pass inferiorly through the inlet into the superior mediastinum. The patterns and attachments of these fasciae, as well as acting as surgical guides and landmarks, may determine the direction and extent of spread of infection and haemorrhage. Note also that the anatomy of the inner ring — the thoracic inlet — may be compromised in the presence of a complete or partial cervical rib or band.

Between girdle and limb — the axilla
The next major anatomical region through which longitudinally running structures pass in continuity to and from the area of the pectoral girdle thus becomes the axilla. The main structures to consider are the brachial plexus

and the axillary vessels. It is tempting to imagine the brachial plexus as a flat, two-dimensional 'railway junction' structure, as usually illustrated in diagrams. Before it is disssected, however, the infraclavicular part of the plexus is closely grouped around and parallel with the axillary artery. The relationship of the cords of the plexus to the second part of the artery gives them their names. The distinction between supraclavicular and infraclavicular parts of the plexus is infrequently made in anatomical texts, but is very useful in the clinical approach to disorders and injuries of the plexus. The roots of the plexus emerge into the neck between the scalene muscles, the trunks lie in the posterior triangle, the divisions behind the clavicle, and the cords group around the axillary artery to reach their definitive lateral, medial and posterior positions behind pectoralis minor.

Nerves
The morphological pattern of the brachial plexus is subject to great individual variation. Such variations are common, and may cause confusion during cadaveric dissection and at operation. The pattern to be described is the standard version found in most texts.

The plexus (Fig. 12.5) is formed from the anterior primary rami of spinal nerves C5 to T1, with common

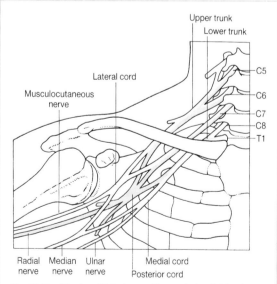

Fig. 12.5   The brachial plexus. The posterior division has been shaded to distinguish it from the anterior division. From Rogers op. cit.

(10%) variation of origin each way: C4–C8 (pre-fixed) or C6–T2 (post-fixed). The two superior roots of the plexus — usually C5 and C6 — emerge between scalenus anterior and scalenus medius and unite to form the upper trunk in the posterior triangle of the neck. The C7 root proceeds alone as the middle trunk, while C8 unites with T1, which has ascended out of the thoracic inlet across the neck of the first rib, to form the lower trunk which lies behind the subclavian artery. Each trunk then divides behind the clavicle into anterior and posterior divisions which pass into the apex of the axilla. The anterior divisions supply the flexor aspect and muscle compartments of the limb; the posterior divisions supply their extensor equivalents. The cords form from the divisions and come to lie closely grouped around the second part of the axillary artery behind pectoralis minor. The lateral and medial cords both form entirely from anterior divisions, the lateral from those of the upper and middle trunks and the medial from that of the lower trunk. All three posterior divisions join to form the posterior trunk. Branches from the plexus pass from the roots, from the upper trunk, and from the cords. There are no branches from the middle and lower trunk or from the divisions.

The more proximal ('higher') the branch, the more proximal in neck, trunk or limb its area of supply. Thus the motor branches from the roots supply the scalene muscles (C5–C8), the rhomboids (C5), and serratus anterior (C5–C7 via the long thoracic nerve, passing behind the plexus onto the upper chest wall). Those from the upper trunk supply supraspinatus and infraspinatus (suprascapular nerve, C5 and C6) and subclavius (C5,6). Proximal motor branches from the posterior cord supply subscapularis (upper and lower subscapular nerves C5,6) and latissimus dorsi (thoracodorsal nerve, C6–C8). The lower subscapular nerve also supplies teres major. From the lateral cord, a proximal branch supplies the pectoral muscles (lateral pectoral nerve, C5–C7); a similar branch from the medial cord (medial pectoral nerve, C8,T1) also supplies both pectorals. The remainder of the posterior cord divides to supply the extensor component of the limb via the axillary (C5,6) and radial (C5–T1) nerves: both are mixed nerves. The lateral cord supplies part of the flexor component, including all the flexors in the upper arm, via the musculocutaneous (C5–C7) and the median (lateral root, C5–C7) nerves. The median nerve supplies nothing above the elbow. The medial cord also contributes to the median nerve via its medial root (C8,T1), and goes on to form the ulnar nerve (C7–T1). All of the above are mixed nerves. The medial cord also gives off two sensory nerves, the medial cutaneous nerves of the arm and forearm (C8,T1).

Note that the plexus also has an autonomic component. This is entirely sympathetic. All cervical ventral rami receive grey rami communicantes from the cervical sympathetic ganglia. The first and second thoracic ventral rami send white rami communicantes to the sympathetic chain; these white rami contain the sympathetic outflow to the head and neck. Thus sympathetic autonomic deficit is an important component of brachial plexus injuries at all levels.

Brachial plexus injuries are not uncommon. The plexus and its branches may be injured supraclavicularly or infraclavicularly; it is rarely involved in clavicular fractures. The supraclavicular plexus is usually affected by closed traction injury, whereas the infraclavicular part may be stretched over the displaced humeral head in antero-inferior shoulder dislocation. Open injury of the plexus may occur at any level. The site of injury may be localised clinically, using knowledge of the points of branching. For example, sparing of serratus anterior would indicate a lesion distal to the roots, while if the spinati muscles were also spared the lesion could be placed more distally. The extent of the injury can also be assessed by careful clinical examination: complete paralysis of both heads of pectoralis major would indicate damage to all roots. Traction lesions of the upper roots (C5,6) produce the well-known Erb's palsy (paralysis) with signs throughout the limb proximal to the wrist.

- *Erb's palsy.* The muscles primarily supplied by C5 and C6 are affected. The shoulder is adducted because of paralysis of deltoid and supraspinatus, and medially rotated because of that of infraspinatus, teres minor and the posterior fibres of deltoid. Paralysis of the elbow flexors biceps, brachialis and brachioradialis leaves the elbow fully extended, and that of biceps and supinator leave the forearm pronated.

  Lesions of the lower roots (C8,T1) produce the less common Klumpke's palsy.

- *Klumpke's palsy.* This mainly affects the small muscles of the hand, particularly the intrinsics (interossei and lumbricals) which are almost entirely supplied by T1. The wrist flexors may also be weakened. Thus the hand is flattened, extended at the metacarpophalangeal (MCP) joints because the active long extensors are unopposed by the intrinsics, and possibly extended at the wrist. The interphalangeal (IP) joints are in flexion, as the long finger flexors remain active. Damage to T1 may also cause a Horner's syndrome.

In both types of injury it is important not to forget the sensory component: there will be numbness in the dermatomal distribution of the affected roots. Compression lesions of the lower plexus may occur in the 'thoracic inlet syndrome' in the presence of a normal plexus and an incompletely ossifed cervical rib. Associated vascular compression or stenosis may predispose to thrombosis at the subclavian–axillary transition. Complete cervical ribs may be associated with a pre-fixed plexus, and thus cause no neurological problem.

Another site of possible nerve entrapment in the pectoral girdle involves the suprascapular nerve, as it passes beneath the transverse scapular ligament into the suprascapular notch. A lesion here may present with weakness and wasting of both supraspinatus and infraspinatus muscles. Non-traumatic lesions of the brachial plexus include tumours of the plexus itself such as neurofibromata, which may present as a supraclavicular mass or as more distal neurological impairment in the limb, as well as malignant lesions which may involve the plexus by local spread. An example of the latter is the Pancoast syndrome, in which an apical carcinoma of the lung involves the lower root(s) of the plexus and produces a neural deficit similar to that described in Klumpke's palsy. Remember that autonomic (sympathetic) deficit may also be present and clinically detectable in the assessment of brachial plexus lesions.

Diagnostic clinical anatomy

In the pectoral girdle region this involves the assessment of brachial plexus and axillary vascular lesions as described above, together with that of the very common fractures and dislocations which occur in this area. It is here that the anatomical relations of the clavicle and of its joints become particularly relevant. The surface anatomy of the bony points and individual muscles must be known, as must the anatomical principles of testing the movements and motors of all joints of the 'shoulder complex'. Consult a dermatome 'map' and note that the cutaneous sensory supply of most of the pectoral girdle region comes from the cervical plexus rather than from the brachial. Complete radiological assessment of injuries in this area may require angiography and myelography in addition to the use of plain films and magnetic resonance imaging (MRI).

UPPER LIMB

The anatomy of the upper limb will be dealt with according to the given general framework, with a separate subsection on the anatomy of the hand.

Osteology

The anatomy of the bones of the limbs should be learned in a way relevant to the pattern and complications of common fractures and joint injuries, to the planning of surgical access, and to the understanding of the pathology and management of bone and joint infection. Close detail of individual muscle attachments is unnecessary. Detail of joint capsular, fascial and ligamentous attachment to bone, and of the way in which these attachments relate to the growth plates and to the blood supply of the long bones, are much more surgically relevant. The major named features and processes of each bone should be known, together with detail of the points or areas at which major nerves or vessels are directly related to the bone. You should also be familiar with the general principles of the blood supply and of the growth and development of the long bones. Each long bone consists of a shaft, or diaphysis, and two expanded ends (epiphyses) each of which typically forms part of a joint (Fig. 12.6). The epiphyses of the immature bone are separated from the shaft by the growth plates (strictly the *physes* or epiphyseal plates, though often loosely called the epiphyses). The widened

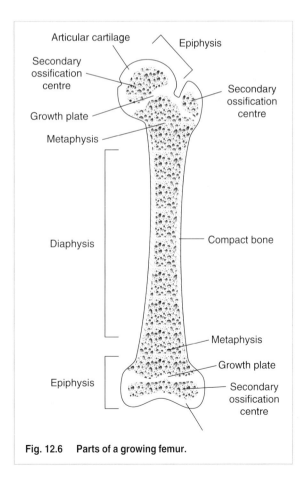

Fig. 12.6   Parts of a growing femur.

parts of the shaft immediately adjacent to the growth plates are the metaphyses. A typical long bone (e.g. femur, humerus) ossifies endochondrally from a hyaline cartilage precursor. Primary ossification commences in the centre of the diaphysis and continues proximally and distally into the metaphyses before birth. Around the time of birth in a few cases (distal femur, proximal tibia) or during childhood, secondary centres of ossification appear in the still-cartilaginous epiphyses at the ends of the bone. These centres remain separated by the growth plates from the ossified diaphysis until growth in length is complete and the centres fuse. The temporal pattern of secondary ossification varies between upper and lower limbs. In the upper limb the majority of growth in length takes place at the shoulder and wrist, while in the lower limb growth is maximal around the knee. Thus older adolescents and young adults up to the age of 20, regularly involved in often high violence injuries, still have open growth plates in these areas. Bones grow in thickness by appositional subperiosteal osssification. Where a medullary cavity is present, associated endosteal bone removal takes place. All growing bones remodel to retain the basic shape defined for each by its cartilaginous precursor.

Humerus

The proximal expanded end of the humerus has three major components: the head and the two tuberosities or tubercles. The head, covered with articular cartilage, lies immediately above the anatomical neck. The greater tuberosity, less obviously the larger of the two when viewed from the front, lies lateral and posterior to the head. The lesser tuberosity lies anteriorly, and is separated from the greater by the bicipital (intertubercular) groove in which runs the tendon of the long head of biceps. The tendon lies in a synovial sheath which is continuous with the synovium of the glenohumeral joint. The proximal metaphysis of the humerus, below the head and tuberosities, is commonly fractured and is known as the 'surgical neck' of the bone. The tuberosities are processes for the attachment of the muscles of the rotator cuff, a very important group of four short muscles whose function as stabilisers of the shoulder joint overrides their function as motors of the limb. All four pass across the joint from scapula to humerus; only one lies anteriorly, and is thus a medial rotator of the humerus. This is subscapularis, attaching to the lesser tuberosity and reinforcing the anterior aspect of the joint. The other three attach to the greater tuberosity: supraspinatus, an abductor, lies above the joint and reinforces the superior capsule, while infraspinatus and teres minor lie posteriorly, are external rotators, and reinforce the posterior part of the capsule. Three other muscles pass anterior to the sagittal axis of the shoulder and are thus medial rotators; all attach to the anterior aspect of the upper shaft in the region of the bicipital groove. Pectoralis major crosses the groove to its lateral lip, latissimus dorsi attaches in the floor of the groove, and teres major to its medial lip. The line of attachment of the joint capsule excludes the tuberosities but includes the medial metaphysis, crossing the growth plate and making its medial end intracapsular. The axillary nerve lies just medial to this point, just below the capsule. The circumflex humeral arteries lie in close circumferential relationship with the bone at the surgical neck. The first important feature of the shaft of the humerus is the spiral groove, in which the radial nerve and the profunda brachii vessels run between the lateral and medial heads of triceps and in direct contact with bone. The other main feature is the tubercle for the attachment of the deltoid muscle, almost half way down the lateral border of the bone. The triangular shape of deltoid gives it its name: its broad base lies proximally on the pectoral girdle, so that it has fibres running anteriorly, superiorly and posteriorly to the shoulder joint. It can thus flex and extend the joint, in addition to its main function as an abductor. The motor supply of deltoid is the axillary nerve (C5,6), vulnerable just below the joint capsule at the surgical neck. The distal half of the front of the shaft is covered anteriorly by the attachment of brachialis and posteriorly by that of the medial head of triceps. Coracobrachialis attaches medially opposite the deltoid attachment.

The distal expanded end of the humerus is formed by the two condyles, medial and lateral. The complex articular surface comprises elements of both condyles: the lateral condyle includes the rounded capitulum, which articulates with the radius, and the lateral part of the pulley-like trochlea which articulates with the ulna. The medial part of the trochlea belongs to the medial condyle. The peripheral projections on each condyle are the epicondyles, medial and lateral. The ulnar nerve is directly related to bone behind the medial epicondyle, and anconeus muscle attaches behind the lateral. The cross-sectional profile of the shaft changes from tubular to flattened from front to back at the distal metaphysis. This is the supracondylar region, where fracture is common in childhood. All three major nerves of the arm and forearm lie on or close to bone here, the ulnar posteromedially, the radial anterolaterally and the median anteriorly with the brachial artery. The sharp medial and lateral borders of the metaphysis are the supracondylar ridges, to which pronator teres and extensor carpi radialis longus (ECRL) attach respectively. The main group of forearm flexors attaches to the medial epicondyle (common flexor origin), and the extensors to the lateral (common extensor origin). Brachioradialis attaches to the lateral and distal shaft just proximal to ECRL; the radial nerve appears in the anterior compartment between brachioradialis and brachialis at this level.

The humerus is connected to the deep fascia of the arm by the medial and lateral intermuscular septa. The medial septum extends distally from the teres major attachment to the medial epicondyle, and the lateral similarly from the deltoid attachment to the lateral epicondyle. These septa divide the upper arm into flexor and extensor osteofascial compartments.

The line of capsular attachment for the elbow includes the trochlea and capitulum but excludes both epicondyles. There are two definitive growth plates for the distal humerus: that for the medial epicondyle is entirely extracapsular, while that for the trochlea and lateral condyle crosses the capsular attachment and is extracapsular only posterolaterally.

Radius

The radius has two expanded ends of which the distal is by far the larger. The cylindrical proximal end or head forms part both of the elbow joint and of the superior radioulnar joint, its articular surfaces for both these joints being in continuity. Immediately distal to the circumferential radioulnar articular surface of the head is the narrower neck of the bone. The annular ligament runs around this articular surface of the head, not around the neck. The main muscles attaching to the proximal radius are the biceps medially, to the bicipital tuberosity, and the supinator laterally, wrapping around the neck and proximal shaft.

The shaft of the radius is convex laterally; it is narrow and cylindrical in its proximal part, and has a sharp medial border to which attaches the interosseous membrane. Muscles attaching to the shaft anteriorly include flexor digitorum superficialis proximally, flexor pollicis longus over most of the middle third, and pronator teres in the distal third. Posteriorly, the lateral attachments of abductor pollicis longus and extensor pollicis brevis occupy the middle third, while pronator teres attaches posterolaterally at midshaft level.

The distal expanded end is smooth and concave anteriorly but grooved and convex posteriorly (dorsally). It is prolonged laterally into the radial styloid process, and its concave distal surface articulates with the scaphoid and lunate bones of the proximal carpus. The dorsal grooves bear the extensor tendons in their sheaths, most importantly that of extensor pollicis longus lying just medial to

the dorsal tubercle (of Lister). Attrition rupture of this tendon can occur here when the wrist is immobilised in a cast. The lateral surface of the distal end is grooved by the tendons of abductor pollicis longus and extensor pollicis brevis in their sheaths, while the medial surface is concave and bears an articular surface for the inferior radioulnar joint. The distal growth plate of the radius lies entirely outside the capsule of the wrist joint. The interosseous membrane between radius and ulna divides the forearm into its flexor and extensor osteofascial compartments.

The posterior interosseous nerve (the deep branch of the radial) is vulnerable where it winds around the neck of the radius within the supinator muscle. The cutaneous terminal portion of the radial nerve runs quite close to the lateral aspect of the distal radius, in the favoured site for insertion of intravenous cannulae and crossing the common distal radial fracture lines.

Ulna

In the ulna the proximal expanded end is far larger than the distal. The proximal end terminates in the olecranon, the bony process for attachment of the triceps tendon. Anteriorly lies the trochlear notch, for articulation with the humerus, and just distal to this the coronoid process, to which brachialis attaches anteriorly, flexor digitorum superficialis and pronator teres medially, and supinator laterally. Anconeus attaches to the posterior surface of the olecranon and of the proximal metaphysis. The lateral side of the metaphysis bears the concave articular surface of the superior radioulnar joint (radial notch), which is in continuity with that of the trochlear notch. The annular ligament is attached anteriorly and posteriorly to the radial notch. The proximal growth plate of the ulna lies outside the capsular attachment of the elbow joint. The shaft of the ulna 'mirrors' in shape and cross-sectional profile that of the radius, with a sharp lateral border for the attachment of the interosseous membrane. The ulnar shaft is cylindrical and narrower distally, and is slightly convex medially. Flexor digitorum profundus attaches widely to its middle two fourths, and pronator quadratus to the distal fourth. Flexor digitorum profundus also shares an aponeurotic attachment to the posterior border of the ulna with flexor and extensor carpi ulnaris. This posterior border is subcutaneous throughout its length. Distal and medial to this aponeurosis, abductor pollicis longus, extensor pollicis longus and extensor indicis attach to the medial part of the posterior surface of the shaft. The distal expanded end of the ulna is prolonged medially as the ulnar styloid process, and bears a groove dorsally for extensor carpi ulnaris tendon. There is an articular surface laterally for the inferior radioulnar joint, and distally for the triangular cartilage whose distal surface is part of the wrist joint. The ulna does not articulate directly with any carpal bone. The distal growth plate of the ulna lies outside the line of attachment of the wrist joint capsule.

The ulnar nerve lies close to the medial aspect of the olecranon as it enters the forearm within flexor carpi ulnaris. Its dorsal branch runs closely around the distal shaft about 4 cm proximal to the styloid process.

Wrist

The carpal bones (Fig. 12.7) are arranged in two rows. The proximal row, from radial (lateral) to ulnar (medial) side, comprises scaphoid, lunate and triquetral, with the pisiform, a sesamoid bone in the tendon of flexor carpi ulnaris, located anteromedially. Some features of the scaphoid, the most commonly fractured carpal bone, should be recognised, in particular the waist of the bone and the way in which the blood supply enters mainly from the distal end, making avascular necrosis of the proximal end likely after a displaced waist fracture. The distal row, again from radial to ulnar, is made up of the trapezium, trapezoid, capitate and hamate bones. The carpal bones form a shallow arch, convex dorsally. The height of this arch is increased by ventral (palmar) bony processes, the hook of the hamate, the ridge of the trapezium and the tubercle of the scaphoid, and by the pisiform

medially. These 'pillars' of the arch give attachment to the flexor retinaculum so that the concavity of the arch forms the carpal tunnel.

Metacarpals and phalanges

These are structurally 'mini' long bones. Individual muscle attachments will not be dealt with here, but you should know those of the major flexors and extensors of the wrist and the digits.

Arthrology

The glenohumeral joint is the site of several very common clinical problems, both in trauma (dislocation) and in non-emergency work (painful and stiff shoulders). You need to know its anatomy in more detail than that of the elbow or wrist. The small joints of the hand are commonly injured or arthritic, and may become infected as a complication of trauma.

For each major limb joint the descriptive order will be as follows:

* shape of articular surfaces
* linking structures: capsule, ligaments
* synovium: reflections, extra-articular extensions, bursae
* menisci or other structures included within the joint; these often form important arthroscopic landmarks
* muscles crossing the joint, and therefore acting on it; these will be summarised for each joint

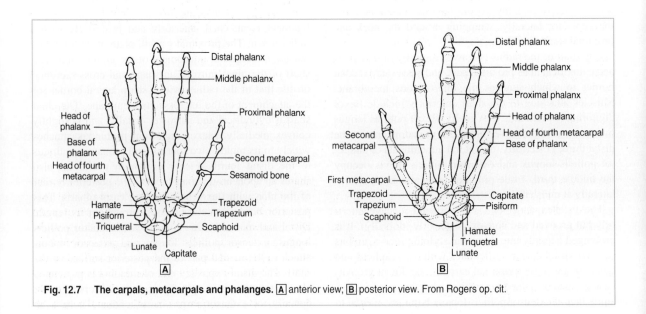

Fig. 12.7   The carpals, metacarpals and phalanges. [A] anterior view; [B] posterior view. From Rogers op. cit.

- nerve supply — remember Hilton's Law: the same nerves whose branches supply the muscles moving a joint supply the skin over the insertions of the same muscles and also the joint itself
- arterial supply: periarticular anastomoses occur around all major limb joints, and may form important collateral vascular pathways to the distal limb
- position of maximal stability (when the capsule is at its 'tightest')
- applied anatomy: access for aspiration and surgery; imaging methods.

Glenohumeral joint

This is a ball-and-socket joint, the relative shape and size of whose articular surfaces make it totally reliant on soft tissue structures for static and dynamic stability (Fig. 12.8). The capsule is attached around the margin of the glenoid cavity of the scapula, extending onto the base of the coracoid superiorly to include the biceps attachment. The glenoid labrum, deepening the concavity of the glenoid fossa, is entirely intracapsular. On the humerus, the capsule is attached around the anatomical neck except where it passes onto the medial metaphysis inferiorly. The latter attachment brings the inferior capsule into close relation with the axillary nerve, rendering the nerve vulnerable in anteroinferior dislocations. It also means that a metaphyseal osteomyelitic lesion of the proximal humerus may be intracapsular, leading to the possibility of septic arthritis as a sequel. The capsule is reinforced by the tendons of the rotator cuff muscles, which blend with it everywhere except inferiorly, and additionally by the coracohumeral ligament superiorly. There are also variable thickenings in the capsule anteriorly: these are the glenohumeral ligaments, whose detailed anatomy is of importance to the shoulder arthroscopist. The capsule is lax inferiorly, allowing wide abduction of the joint. The tendon of the long head of biceps passes through the joint over the head of the humerus, within its synovial sheath: it is intracapsular but extrasynovial (cf. the cruciate ligaments of the knee) and is a major arthroscopic landmark. The synovial sheath extends distally beneath the transverse ligament of the humerus into the bicipital groove. The two major bursae associated with the joint are the subacromial/subdeltoid bursa superiorly and the subscapular bursa anteriorly. The former lies between the 'layers' of the abductor mechanism of the shoulder (the acromion, with the attached deltoid muscle and coracoacromial ligament, and supraspinatus attaching to the greater tuberosity). It does not normally communicate with the synovial cavity of the glenohumeral joint. The latter is an extension of the glenohumeral synovium passing between the gleno-

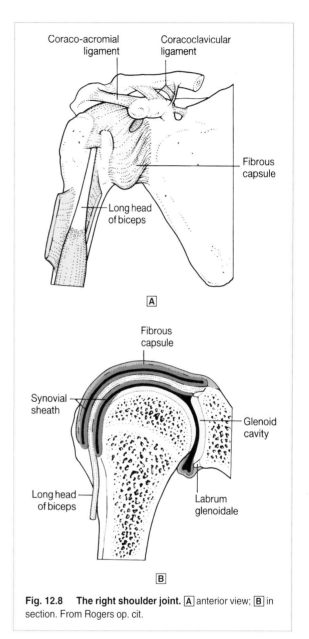

Fig. 12.8   The right shoulder joint. [A] anterior view; [B] in section. From Rogers op. cit.

humeral ligaments and deep to subscapularis muscle. The muscles crossing the glenohumeral joint and their actions upon it are summarised below. The joint is innervated by the nerves which supply those muscles, mainly by the axillary and suprascapular. The suprascapular artery, from the subclavian, and the subscapular and circumflex humeral arteries, from the axillary, are the main participants in the anastomosis around the scapula and the head of the humerus. The glenohumeral capsule is said to be at its tightest when the joint is abducted and externally rotated, though this position is often that which produces antero-inferior dislocation. The joint may be aspirated or injected anteriorly or posteriorly, the posterior subacromial approach being somewhat easier and also being that usually used for arthroscopy. Diagnostic arthrography of the shoulder has been largely superseded by magnetic resonance imaging. The common approach for open shoulder surgery is anterior, passing between deltoid and pectoralis major. The muscles attaching to the coracoid are displaced medially, protecting axillary neurovascular structures, and the capsule is entered after dividing subscapularis.

Summary Glenohumeral joint (Fig. 12.8) synovial, ball-and-socket.

- Movements and muscles
  - flexion: anterior part of deltoid, pectoralis major, biceps brachii, coracobrachialis
  - extension: posterior deltoid, teres major, latissimus dorsi
  - abduction: mid-part of deltoid, supraspinatus
  - adduction: pectoralis major, latissimus dorsi, teres major, coracobrachialis, [gravity]
  - medial rotation: subscapularis, anterior deltoid, latissimus dorsi, teres major
  - lateral rotation: posterior deltoid, infraspinatus, teres minor
  - circumduction: all of the above.
- Major anatomical relations
  - anterior: brachial plexus; axillary vessels

  - inferior: axillary nerve; circumflex humeral vessels
  - posterior: suprascapular nerve and vessels (on the neck of the scapula medial to the capsular attachment).

The tendons of the rotator cuff muscles merge with the capsule anteriorly, superiorly and posteriorly.

Elbow joint

This is a modified hinge joint between the humerus and the forearm bones (Fig. 12.9). The main part of the joint is the humero-ulnar, between the trochlea of the humerus and the trochlear notch of the ulna. The trochlear diameter is greater medially than laterally, thus creating the valgus 'carrying angle' of the elbow. The trochlear articular surface of the humerus is continuous laterally with that of the rounded capitulum, which is confined to the anterior aspect of the bone and which articulates with the concavity of the head of the radius. The trochlear articular surface of the ulna continues laterally and distally over the radial notch, which articulates with the circumferential part of the radial articular surface. The superior radio-ulnar joint is thus continuous with the elbow joint, sharing a synovial 'cavity'. The humeral attachment of the capsule of the elbow joint leaves the articular margins of trochlea and capitulum anteriorly and posteriorly to include the coronoid, radial and olecranon fossae. The capsule is thin anteriorly and posteriorly but thicker medially and laterally where reinforced by the collateral ligaments. It attaches distally to the articular margins of the trochlear notch, then passes onto the superior border

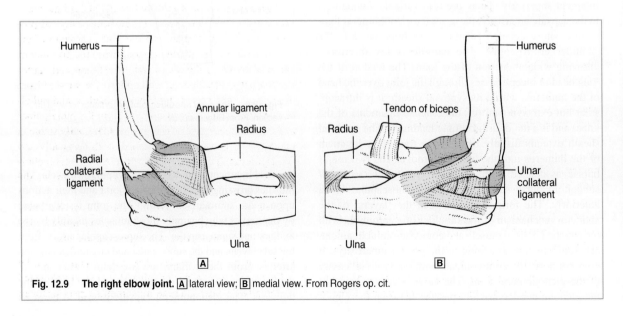

Fig. 12.9   The right elbow joint. [A] lateral view; [B] medial view. From Rogers op. cit.

of the annular ligament, with which it becomes continuous. The collateral ligaments of the elbow differ in shape: the radial is fan shaped, radiating onto the annular ligament from the lateral humeral epicondyle, while the ulnar has three bands constituting a triangle betwen the medial epicondyle and the lateral sides of the coronoid and olecranon processes (Fig. 12.9). The synovium of the elbow, lining the capsule, is continuous with that of the superior radio-ulnar joint, and extends distally a little way below the annular ligament. The synovium is separated from the capsule anteriorly and posteriorly by fat pads, whose displacement can be used in the radiological diagnosis of small effusions or haemarthroses of the elbow. Muscles crossing, and thus acting upon, the joint are summarised below. The nerves to the elbow derive, by Hilton's Law, from all three major nerves of the limb. The arterial anastomosis around the elbow is made up of branches from the brachial, radial and ulnar vessels. The elbow is maximally stable in full extension, when the anterior capsule is tense. A swollen elbow is best aspirated from the lateral side, where no important neurovascular structures cross the joint. A posterior approach, lateral to the main body of the triceps tendon, may also be used. Open surgical approaches are mainly lateral or posterior, depending upon the size of exposure required.

Summary Elbow joint (Fig. 12.9): synovial, hinge.

- Movements and muscles
  — flexion: brachialis, biceps brachii, brachioradialis, pronator teres
  — extension: triceps brachii, anconeus.
- Major anatomical relations
  — anterior: median nerve; brachial artery
  — anterolateral: radial nerve
  — posteromedial: ulnar nerve.

Radio-ulnar joints

The shafts of radius and ulna are strongly linked in all positions of the forearm by the interosseous membrane, whose fibres pass distally and medially, transmitting force from radius to ulna. The proximal ends of the bones articulate at the superior radio-ulnar joint, described above with the elbow, with which it is structurally continuous. The distal ends articulate at the inferior radio-ulnar joint, between the cylindrical ulna and the concave ulnar notch of the radius. The capsule of this joint is weak, but the joint is strengthened by a triangular intra-articular fibrocartilage passing betwen the ulnar styloid and the distal margin of the ulnar notch of the radius. If intact, this fibrocartilage separates the synovial lining of the inferior radio-ulnar joint from that of the wrist joint. The radio-ulnar joints move together during forearm rotation into pronation and supination, the axis passing from the centre of the radial head to the ulnar styloid.

Summary

- Joints
  — superior (proximal) radio-ulnar (Fig. 12.9): synovial, pivot, in synovial continuity with elbow joint
  — inferior (distal) radio-ulnar: synovial, pivot, with fibrous intra-articular disc. The interosseous membrane and oblique ligament constitute an intermediate, fibrous joint.
- Movements and muscles
  — supination: biceps brachii (especially when elbow flexed), supinator
  — pronation: pronator teres (especially when elbow flexed), pronator quadratus.
- Major anatomical relations
  — superior radio-ulnar joint: the posterior interosseous nerve runs in supinator close to the distal capsular attachment
  — inferior radio-ulnar joint: the dorsal branch of the ulnar nerve passes close to the joint posteriorly.

Wrist joint

In strict terms the 'wrist' joint is the radiocarpal joint, that between the distal radius (and the distal surface of the triangular fibrocartilage) and the proximal row of carpal bones. There are also the intercarpal joints, between the individual carpal bones, and the midcarpal joint, between the two rows of carpal bones. The capsule of the radiocarpal joint is attached distal to the (distal) growth plates of radius and ulna, and is stronger in its palmar than in its dorsal component. There are two collateral ligaments, radial and ulnar, attaching to the respective styloid processes and fusing with the capsule. The synovium of the radiocarpal joint is usually separate from the continuous synovial lining of the intercarpal, midcarpal and carpometacarpal joints. The nerve supply to the wrist is from the interosseous nerves (branches of median and radial) and there is an arterial anastomosis from the radial, ulnar and interosseous vessels. The wrist is maximally stable in extension. It is usually approached, both surgically and for aspiration, from the dorsal aspect. Note that, on clinical examination, most of the carpus lies *distal* to the distal wrist crease, i.e. 'in the hand'.

Summary Wrist joint (strictly radiocarpal, but intercarpal and midcarpal included in clinical usage), synovial, ellipsoid with plane and sellar components.

- Movements and muscles. The wrist complex can be flexed, extended, adducted (ulnar deviated) and abducted (radially deviated). These movements rarely occur in isolation. A combination of all four produces circumduction. In the working wrist, extension usually occurs with radial deviation, against gravity, while flexion and ulnar deviation occur together as gravity-assisted movements. Flexion and radial deviation both take place mainly at the midcarpal joint, extension and ulnar deviation at the radiocarpal. Translational and rotational movements also occur in the carpus. The movements are produced by all the named flexors and extensors of wrist and digits. Radial and ulnar deviation are produced by the respective flexors and extensors of the wrist working together.

- Major anatomical relations
  — anterior: median nerve; ulnar nerve and vessels; radial vessels
  — lateral: radial vessels; radial cutaneous nerve.

(For tendons and sheaths crossing the wrist, see Fig. 12.13.)

Joints of the hand

The carpometacarpal joints move little, with the exception of the carpometacarpal joint of the thumb. This is a very mobile saddle-shaped joint, giving the thumb much of its versatility and precision of movement. The metacarpophalangeal (MCP) and interphalangeal (IP) joints each have a pair of obliquely running collateral ligaments reinforcing the capsule. The IP joints are hinge joints, while the MCP joints also allow abduction, adduction and a little rotation. Note that the palmar skin crease at the base of each finger does *not* overlie the MCP joint: the joint is situated much more proximally in the palm. Make a fist and check this.

Between the joints: fasciae and compartments; nerves

The muscles of the limb are ensheathed in a continuous 'tube' of deep fascia: this is not as conspicuous or as thick as the deep fascia of the lower limb, and is more easily defined in the forearm than in the upper arm. It is locally thickened to form subcutaneous extensor retinacula at the wrist; the corresponding flexor retinaculum is more deeply placed. The intermuscular septa attach to the inner surface of this fascial sleeve, limiting the osteofascial compartments. In the proximal segment of the limb, the anatomical 'arm', there are two such compartments, separated by the humerus and the medial and lateral intermuscular septa. The flexor compartment contains the elbow flexors, innervated by the musculocutaneous nerve (Fig. 12.10) and with a functional root value of C5,6. The extensor compartment contains triceps (and anconeus), innervated by the radial (Fig. 12.11), root value C7,8. Its main artery is the profunda brachii. The median nerve

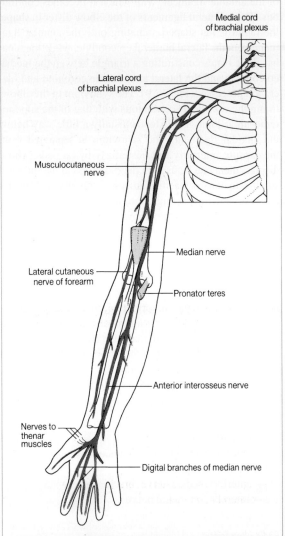

Fig. 12.10 The course and distribution of the median and musculocutaneous nerves. From Rogers op. cit.

(Fig. 12.10) and the brachial artery remain in the flexor compartment. The ulnar nerve (Fig. 12.12) lies in the flexor compartment proximally but passes into the extensor compartment before crossing the elbow. The radial nerve does exactly the reverse, lying anterolaterally at the elbow.

In the distal segment, the forearm, there are two flexor osteofascial compartments and one extensor, separated and defined by the bones and the interosseous membrane. The superficial flexor compartment contains flexores carpi radialis and ulnaris, flexor digitorum superficialis, palmaris longus (if present) and, proximally, pronator

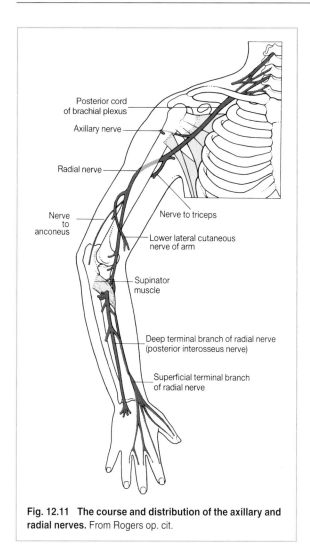

Fig. 12.11 The course and distribution of the axillary and radial nerves. From Rogers op. cit.

Posterior cord
of brachial plexus

Axillary nerve

Radial nerve

Nerve
to
anconeus

Nerve to triceps

Lower lateral cutaneous
nerve of arm

Supinator
muscle

Deep terminal branch of radial nerve
(posterior interosseus nerve)

Superficial terminal branch
of radial nerve

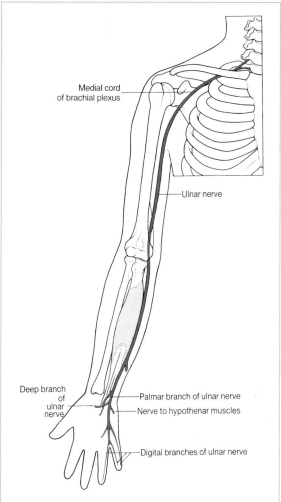

Fig. 12.12 The course and distribution of the ulnar nerve. From Rogers op. cit.

Medial cord
of brachial plexus

Ulnar nerve

Deep branch
of
ulnar
nerve

Palmar branch of ulnar nerve

Nerve to hypothenar muscles

Digital branches of ulnar nerve

teres. The deep compartment contains flexor digitorum profundus, flexor pollicis longus and, distally, pronator quadratus. The extensor compartment contains all the wrist and finger extensors, with, at a deeper level, supinator proximally and the group of muscles passing to the extensor aspect of thumb and index distally. This group includes extensors pollicis longus and brevis, abductor pollicis longus and extensor indicis (proprius). The brachioradialis muscle is unusual in that, although most of it lies in the forearm, it does not cross the wrist. It lies along the radial side of the forearm, and, like extensor carpi radialis longus, is supplied by the radial nerve before it divides. It is thus part of the extensor group, though its position allows it to function as an elbow flexor and as a

rotator of the forearm. The nerves of the flexor compartments are median and ulnar superficially and anterior interosseous (of median) deeply. The nerve of the posterior compartment is the posterior interosseous branch of the radial, and its artery the posterior interosseous branch of the ulnar (usually via the common interosseous). The sensory cutaneous branch of the radial lies superficially.

Transitional zones

The axilla has been dealt with above. The wrist could also be considered as a small transitional zone: the anatomy and three-dimensional relationship of the many structures crossing it in continuity and superficially are particularly important in this commonly injured region (see the wrist joint 'summary' above). This includes especially the anatomy of the carpal tunnel and its contents, and of the those structures which border and constitute the 'anatomical snuff-box' on the radial side of the wrist.

Hand

The clinical importance of the hand is such that its anatomy must be well understood even at a junior level of postgraduate training. Both trauma and infection are particularly common in the hand, and cannot be managed effectively without a firm understanding of its anatomy.

You must know in detail the areas of cutaneous supply of the spinal nerves (dermatomes) and those of the peripheral nerves, as these are constantly used in clinical diagnosis. The anatomy of the carpal tunnel, of the flexor tendons and of their sheaths, and the relationship of these structures to the digital nerves and vessels must be carefully learned. You should also understand the functional anatomy of the extensor mechanism of the fingers. Knowing the arrangement and functional distribution of the small muscles of the hand is more important than detailed knowledge of their individual attachments. A three-dimensional grasp of the relationships of these muscles will also help you understand the concept of the palmar 'spaces' and their proximal and distal extensions (see p. 369). The anatomy of the muscles and fasciae in the hand may be built up, initially on the palmar side and then on the dorsum, around that of the bones and of the long tendons. Knowing the branching pattern of the major nerves and the anastomotic patterns of the major arteries, these structures may then be superimposed upon and integrated with the musculoskeletal framework. On the palmar side note first the anatomy of the carpal tunnel. Its boundaries have been described in the osteology section above. Note its surface marking: the proximal edge of the flexor retinaculum underlies the distal wrist crease, so that the tunnel lies effectively in the palm. Running through the tunnel are the eight long finger flexor tendons, lying in a common synovial sheath which is incomplete radially. This common sheath extends distally into the palm (Fig. 12.13). The superficialis tendons run in two pairs, those to the middle and ring fingers lying nearer the retinaculum. The profundus tendons run more dorsally in a single row of four, that to the index being separate from the medial three. The tendon of flexor pollicis longus (FPL) runs through the tunnel radial to the finger flexors, in its own synovial sheath. The median nerve lies just beneath the retinaculum, radial to its midpoint. Also related to the retinaculum are the ulnar nerve and vessels and the tendon of flexor carpi

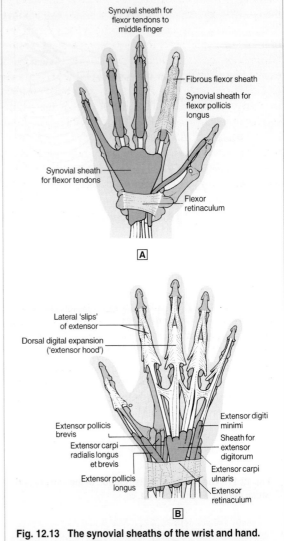

Fig. 12.13 The synovial sheaths of the wrist and hand. Ⓐ anterior view; Ⓑ posterior view. From Rogers op. cit.

radialis (FCR). The ulnar nerve and vessels run superficial to the retinaculum just radial to the pisiform, while the FCR tendon lies in its own osseofascial compartment in the tunnel superficial and radial to the FPL. The retinaculum is also crossed superficially near its midpoint by the palmar cutaneous branch of the median nerve. The muscles of the thenar and hypothenar eminences attach proximally to the radial and ulnar sides of the palmar surface of the retinaculum. The thenar eminence contains abductor pollicis brevis superficially, with flexor pollicis brevis (FPB) and opponens pollicis lying more deeply. All are usually supplied by the motor branch of the median nerve, given off as that nerve leaves the carpal tunnel, though FPB and opponens may be supplied by the ulnar. The hypothenar eminence contains a similarly named trio of muscles: abductor, flexor and opponens digiti minimi. All are supplied by the ulnar nerve. In both eminences, all except the opponens muscles attach distally to the base of the proximal phalanx. The opponentes attach to their respective metacarpals. The central part of the palmar surface of the flexor retinaculum is overlaid by the proximal 'apex' of the triangular palmar fascia: the tendon of palmaris longus attaches to this apex. Thin expansions from the radial and ulnar sides of the palmar fascia cover the thenar and hypothenar muscles. A septum from the dorsal surface of the fascia passes to the shaft of the third (middle) metacarpal, dividing the potential space deep (dorsal) to the common flexor synovial sheath into two compartments. These are the palmar spaces: the mid-palmar medially and the thenar laterally (see p. 369 and Fig. 12.28). The triangular adductor pollicis muscle lies deep to the thenar space, its base attaching, like the fascial septum, to the third metacarpal shaft, and its apex to the proximal phalanx of the thumb. Attached to the radial sides of the deep finger flexor tendons as they lie in the common sheath in the palm are the lumbrical muscles, each running distally to attach to a digital extensor expansion. These little muscles control the relative tension in the long finger flexors, and help the interossei in flexing the MCP joints. Deeper still lie the interosseous muscles,

attached as shown in Figure 12.14. From the level of the MCP joints distally into the digits, the flexors for each digit share a fibrous sheath which surrounds the synovial sheath. This fibrous sheath is subdivided into thick bands or 'pulleys' opposite the phalangeal shafts, and thinner, flexible areas opposite the joints. On the dorsal side the only muscle belly easily palpable is that of the first dorsal interosseous. This, with adductor pollicis, forms the bulk of the web between thumb and index. As both muscles are innervated by the ulnar nerve, weakness and wasting here are important diagnostic signs. The tendons of the digital extensors pass in their own synovial sheaths beneath the extensor retinaculum on the dorsum of the wrist (Fig. 12.13). Note that the extensors and long abductor of the thumb bound the 'anatomical snuff-box', in whose base lies the scaphoid bone crossed by the radial artery. Each finger extensor inserts into an arrowhead-shaped fibrous 'hood', which wraps around the dorsum of the finger (Fig. 12.13). The thumb extensors insert more directly into bone. The intrinsic muscles of the digits (lumbricals and interossei) insert into the digital extensor hoods from the flexor side (Fig. 12.14), so that as they contract together they tighten the hood around the proximal phalanx and thus flex the MCP joint. The main body of the extensor tendon attaches to the base of the middle phalanx, while its lateral extensions come together to attach to the distal phalanx (Fig. 12.14).

The median nerve branches as it leaves the carpal

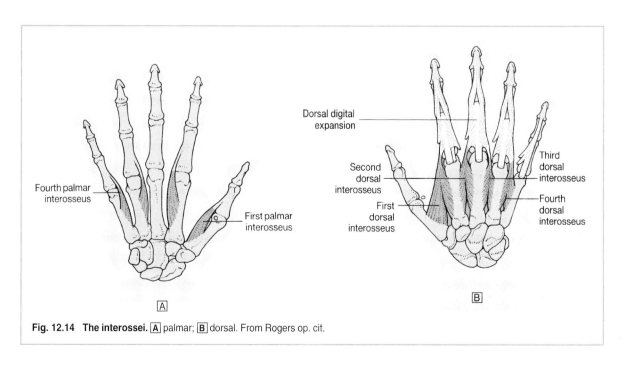

Fourth palmar interosseus

First palmar interosseus

Dorsal digital expansion

Second dorsal interosseus

First dorsal interosseus

Third dorsal interosseus

Fourth dorsal interosseus

A

B

Fig. 12.14 The interossei. A palmar; B dorsal. From Rogers op. cit.

335

tunnel, giving sensory branches to the digits and a motor branch to the thenar eminence (Fig. 12.10). The ulnar nerve branches where it lies just radial to the pisiform bone (Fig. 12.12). Its deep branch supplies the interossei, adductor pollicis and the ulnar lumbricals. The branching pattern of the radial nerve on the dorsum of the hand is shown in Figure 12.11. The ulnar nerve supplies an area of the dorsum which exactly matches its area on the palmar side. The median nerve supplies the dorsum of the distal phalanges of thumb and of the radial two-and-a-half fingers. The digital nerves and arteries run together along the sides of the digits, either side of the fibrous flexor sheaths. Their surface marking in a digit is given by joining the posterior ends of the interphalangeal skin flexor creases.

Nerves of the upper limb: where liable to injury and compression

The axillary nerve is vulnerable at the surgical neck of the humerus (Fig. 12.11). A lesion here will denervate the deltoid muscle and give an area of numbness over the lateral aspect of the upper arm in the 'badge' area. In a patient with an injured shoulder it is easier and kinder to test for the sensory rather than for the motor deficit.

The radial nerve (Fig. 12.11) may be damaged by compression or by a fracture as it runs in the spiral groove. A lesion at this level will denervate the wrist extensors and those of the digits, resulting in 'wrist drop' and there will be sensory loss on the back of the radial side of the hand. The deep branch of the radial nerve (posterior interosseous) is at risk where it passes around the neck of the radius within the supinator muscle. A lesion here will have purely motor effects, as the sensory component of the radial nerve leaves the main trunk as it enters supinator. Some wrist extension will also be retained, as extensor carpi radialis longus is innervated from the main trunk. The extensors of the fingers and the extensors and long abductor of the thumb will be paralysed. At the wrist the sensory component of the radial nerve is immediately subcutaneous as it lies on the radial side of the distal radius near the cephalic vein. Damage here in lacerations, incisions or while siting an intravenous line causes dysaesthesia on the dorsum of the hand.

The ulnar nerve (Fig. 12.12) is particularly vulnerable behind the medial epicondyle, where it may be involved in closed or open injury. An ulnar lesion at this level will not cause a typical 'claw hand', as the deep ulnar finger flexors will be paralysed as well as the majority of the small muscles of the hand (all except the thenar muscles and the first and second lumbricals, which are supplied by the median nerve). There will also be sensory loss in the ulnar distribution in the hand — medial one-and-a half digits and corresponding areas of palm and dorsum.

The median nerve (Fig. 12.10) is less vulnerable at elbow level, but may be damaged in a supracondylar humeral fracture. A median lesion here will denervate most of the contents of the flexor compartments of the forearm (all except flexor carpi ulnaris and the ulnar 'half' of flexor digitorum profundus), in addition to the median-supplied muscles in the hand (see below). Sensory loss in the hand involves the palmar aspects of the lateral three-and-a-half digits, the dorsal aspects of their distal phalanges, and the corresponding area of the palm.

Neither the ulnar nor the median nerve supplies any skin in the forearm. Both nerves are vulnerable at the wrist, though the ulnar has some protection from the overlying tendon of flexor carpi ulnaris, and the median, more distally, from the flexor retinaculum. Damage here is usually from open injury: nerve involvement must be excluded in every patient with a volar wrist laceration. An ulnar lesion at the wrist will not denervate the 'ulnar half' of flexor digitorum profundus, so the ring and little fingers will be more flexed at the IP joints, but extended at the MCP joints due to intrinsic muscle paralysis — the typical 'claw hand' position. There may also be retention of some ulnar sensation on the dorsum of the hand, if the lesion is distal to origin of the dorsal cutaneous branch. A median nerve lesion at the wrist will give the sensory loss described above for the 'high' lesion, with possibly some sparing of central palmar skin if the palmar cutaneous branch has been given off proximal to the lesion. The muscles supplied in the hand include all those of the thenar eminence, together with the lateral two lumbricals. Most importantly, the power of opposition of the thumb will be lost. The most significant deficit from a median lesion at the wrist is the loss of sensation in the pulps of the thumb and index finger.

The digital nerves to the thumb lie just beneath the skin as they cross the palmar aspect of the MCP joint, and all digital nerves proper are vulnerable throughout their course. The radial digital nerve to the index and the ulnar digital nerve to the little finger are especially liable to injury.

The commonest sites of nerve entrapment and compression are the carpal tunnel (median nerve) and the medial epicondyle (ulnar). The effects are as described above for acute lesions at those levels, but in longstanding nerve entrapment both may in addition present with wasting of muscles in the hand in the appropriate distribution. Both interosseous nerves may be entrapped in the forearm, the posterior (radial) within supinator and the anterior (median) as it passes through and distal to pronator teres. The former gives the clinical picture already described for a posterior interosseous nerve lesion, while the latter gives a purely motor lesion paralysing flexor pollicis longus and the deep flexors of the index and middle fingers.

Diagnostic clinical anatomy

The great importance of the neurological clinical examination of the hand has already been emphasised. The neurological examination of the whole of the upper limb is an essential component of the assessment of patients with neck and shoulder pain. You must understand the anatomical basis of the assessment of muscle function throughout the limb, including that of the commonly examined stretch reflexes. This assessment is closely linked with that of joint function, including the major joints of the limb and the small joints of the hand. Radiological assessment of the limbs now makes great use of MRI, so that an appreciation of cross-sectional anatomy assumes a new importance here as in the trunk. Plain films are still extensively used in the management of fractures and dislocations; it is a good anatomical exercise to try and explain the pattern and degree of displacement seen in such injuries in terms of the muscles producing the displacement.

PELVIC GIRDLE

With the pelvic as with the pectoral girdle, the term 'girdle' is rather confusing. Strictly anatomically, the pelvic girdle is a unilateral structure and the sacrum is part of the vertebral column. Each girdle primitively consists of three separate bones: ilium, ischium and pubis. However, as each pelvic girdle is strongly linked both to its fellow and to the sacrum, making it virtually incapable of independent movement, it is functionally more helpful to think of the pelvic girdle as a completely circumferential structure comprising both innominate ('hip') bones and the sacrum. This girdle is then seen as a weight-bearing protective structure, to which both limb and trunk muscles gain attachment. It also forms the skeletal framework of the birth canal: note the sexual differences in the pelvis in this respect.

Osteology

Always consider the pelvis in its anatomical position. In the standing subject, the symphysis pubis and the anterior superior iliac spine lie in the same coronal plane, and the ischial spine and upper border of the symphysis lie in the same transverse plane. The acetabulum thus

faces laterally, as well as a little inferiorly and anteriorly. All palpable bony landmarks of the pelvis are important clinically, in the management of patients with conditions as wide-ranging as pregnancy, hip and pelvic injury, scoliosis and hernia. These points include the iliac crest with its paired anterior and posterior spines, the pubic tubercle and rami, and the ischial tuberosities.

There are several important differences between the typically male and the typically female pelvis: intermediate, less typical forms commonly occur. The male pelvis is narrower and more funnel-shaped, both the pelvic inlet (bounded by the pelvic brim) and the pelvic outlet (bounded by the ischial tuberosities, the pubic symphysis and the coccyx) being smaller than in the female. In the female pelvic inlet the transverse diameter exceeds the anteroposterior. Both the pubic arch (beneath the symphysis) and the greater sciatic notch are more acutely angled in the male, with more prominent muscle markings on the inferior (ischiopubic) rami.

The ilium consists anterosuperiorly of a broad thin blade for muscle attachment and visceral protection, and posteroinferiorly of a thick weight-transmitting bar with an articular surface (for sacrum and head of femur) at either end. This bar also forms part of the pelvic brim. The posterior border of the ilium curves inferiorly between the sacroiliac joint and the ischial spine, forming the greater sciatic notch. The gluteal and tensor fasciae latae muscles attach to the outer aspect of the blade, and iliacus to its inner aspect with obturator internus below the pelvic brim. The three layered abdominal wall muscles attach to the anterior two thirds of the crest, with latissimus dorsi and erector spinae posteriorly and sartorius and the inguinal ligament attaching anteriorly. Rectus femoris, the only component of the quadriceps to cross (and thus act upon) the hip joint, attaches anteriorly above the acetabulum.

The ischium is a J-shaped bone, with a massive body posteriorly bearing the ischial component of the acetabulum. Inferiorly is the tuberosity, which bears the weight of the sitting trunk. Anteriorly is the ramus, uniting with the pubis. The posterior border of the body bears the ischial spine, separating the greater sciatic notch superiorly from the lesser inferiorly. The tuberosity and the spine are linked to the sacrum by the sacrotuberous and sacrospinous ligaments (Fig. 12.15), which convert the sciatic notches into foramina. The hamstrings and the short hip rotators (except piriformis) attach to the outer aspect of the tuberosity and lower body. Obturator internus attaches to the internal surface of the body and ramus anteromedially, while obturator externus and adductor magnus attach to the ramus externally. The ischium and

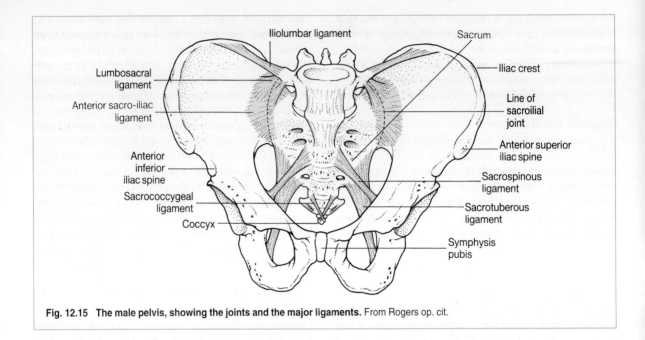

Fig. 12.15 The male pelvis, showing the joints and the major ligaments. From Rogers op. cit.

pubis together form the circumference of the obturator foramen.

The pubis is shaped like a rotated L. Its longer, horizontal, superior ramus connects the acetabular and symphyseal articular surfaces of the pubis. The inferior ramus extends downwards from the tubercle to its point of fusion with the ischium. Rectus abdominis and pectineus attach to the superior ramus, and the inguinal ligament attaches to the tubercle. The adductors and the perineal muscles and membrane attach to the inferior ramus.

The mature acetabulum consists of about one-fifth pubis and two-fifths each of ilium and ischium. Its articular surface is in the shape of a horseshoe open anteriorly, the gap being bridged by the transverse ligament. The ligament of the head of the femur attaches to the thin, medially placed floor.

Arthrology

The joints which involve the pelvic girdle are the sacroiliacs, the pubic symphysis, and the hip joints. The hip will be considered with the lower limb.

The large and very stable sacroiliac joints connect the girdle proper to the axial skeleton. The joints change in character with age: in the very young, they are synovial, with almost plane surfaces, while in the elderly they are almost entirely fibrous, with very irregular surfaces. They rely largely for stability on numerous and powerful ligaments (Fig. 12.15). The tendency for downward and backward displacement of the sacrum between the innominate (hip) bones is opposed by the anterior and posterior sacroiliac ligaments, the latter being widely attached to the dorsal surface of the sacrum, and by the iliolumbar ligaments attaching the transverse processes of L5 to the iliac crests. The tendency for downward rotation of the sacrum in the sagittal plane is additionally opposed by the sacrotuberous and sacrospinous ligaments attaching the sacrum to the ischium.

The symphysis pubis, like all symphyses, lies in the median plane and comprises a disc of fibrocartilage firmly fixed between two articular surfaces of hyaline cartilage. A non-synovial cavity often appears in this disc in adult life. The joint is strengthened anteriorly by decussating bands of collagen, and inferiorly by the arcuate pubic ligament.

Summary
- Joints (Fig. 12.15)
  - sacroiliac: irregular plane synovial, becoming fibrous with age
  - pubic symphysis: secondary cartilaginous (symphysis).
- Movements. Apart from very slight rotation in the sagittal plane there is virtually no sacroiliac movement in the normal adult male. There is a little more movement during pregnancy and childbirth as the ligaments relax slightly. At the pubic symphysis there is normally

little or no movement, except during pregnancy and childbirth when some stretching may occur.

- Major anatomical relations
  - sacroiliac joints: the internal iliac vessels pass anteriorly
  - pubic symphysis: the urethra and the deep dorsal vein of the penis or clitoris pass inferiorly.

Transitional zones

Area enclosed by the pelvic girdle(s)

The pelvic brim or inlet is bounded by the arcuate and pectineal lines of the innominate bones on either side, the sacral promontory posteriorly and the pubic crests and symphysis anteriorly. The true pelvis lies below this brim, with its outlet bounded by the ischial bones, the pubic arch and the coccyx. The obturator foramina in its lateral walls are 'filled in' by the obturator membranes with the obturator muscles on either side, allowing only the obturator nerve and vessels to pass through their canals superolaterally. Obturator internus extends back to the greater sciatic notch and almost meets the belly of piriformis, which fills in the concavity of the sacrum and leaves the pelvis through that notch. The muscles which form the pelvic floor or diaphragm, levator ani and coccygeus, are attached along the inner wall of the true pelvis. Levator ani attaches laterally from the back of the pubis, across the obturator fascia lining obturator internus, to the ischial spine. Medially it attaches to its fellow to complete the 'floor', except where the gastrointestinal and urogenital tracts pass through to their respective outlets. Coccygeus, which is the pelvic aspect of the sacrospinous ligament, completes the 'floor' posteriorly. Above this floor lies the 'cavity' of the pelvis, below it the anatomical perineum (which includes the ischiorectal fossa). Thus the greater sciatic notch (foramen) connects pelvis and buttock (gluteal region), while the lesser connects buttock and perineum. The continuous layer of fascia covering the superior surface of levator ani, coccygeus and the pelvic wall (superior) parts of obturator internus and piriformis is the parietal pelvic fascia. Note that the emerging sacral anterior primary rami lie deep to this fascia, while the internal iliac vessels lie superficial to it. The parietal fascia merges medially with the visceral pelvic fascia surrounding the pelvic organs and their nerves and vessels. Thickenings in this merged fascia of the pelvic floor pass to the pelvic walls and help support the viscera: such fascial supports are often termed 'ligaments'. Above the pelvic brim the extraperitoneal parietal layer of fascia covers iliacus and psoas. The entire muscles are ensheathed in fascia in such a way that

collections of fluid (pus, blood) within the sheaths can pass beneath the inguinal ligament into the upper thigh and may present as masses in the 'groin'. The iliacus fascia joins the tranversalis fascia of the lower abdominal wall to form the femoral sheath. The anterior part of the pelvic outlet forms the urogenital triangle of the perineum, and is bridged by the perineal membrane to which are attached the genital erectile structures and their overlying muscles.

Between girdle and limb

There are three important transitional zones between the area enclosed by the 'girdles' and the lower limb. All are common sites of pathology, traversed by major nerves and vessels in continuity. Anteriorly lie the pelvicrural and obturator areas, and posteriorly the sciatic foramina connecting the gluteal region with pelvis and perineum.

The pelvicrural junction is really part of the 'groin', and includes all those structures which pass between the inguinal ligament and the bony pelvis. The femoral vessels in their sheath, the femoral nerve, the femoral canal, muscles (psoas, iliacus and pectineus), and cutaneous nerves (genitofemoral and lateral femoral) all traverse this region. Anteromedially the obturator nerve and vessels emerge from the obturator canal into the thigh deep to obturator externus, and immediately divide into their anterior and posterior branches.

The courses of two muscles are the keys to the posterior transitional zones (Fig. 12.16). The greater sciatic foramen, connecting pelvis and buttock, is traversed by piriformis, and the lesser sciatic foramen, between perineum and buttock, by obturator internus. Obturator internus lies both in the lateral wall of the pelvis, above the levator ani, and in that of the perineum below it. Structures leaving the pelvis with piriformis include the superior gluteal nerve and vessels above the muscle, and the sciatic nerve, inferior gluteal nerve and vessels, and the pudendal nerve and vessels below it. The last named nerve and vessels immediately cross the ischial spine and enter the lesser sciatic foramen above obturator internus to reach the pudendal canal on the lateral wall of the ischiorectal fossa.

Nerves

Several major nerves related to the pelvic girdle may be involved in injuries and disease of the bones of the pelvis and its contained viscera. These include the lumbosacral plexus and its major branches.

The nerves of the lower limb derive from the anterior (ventral) primary rami making up the lumbosacral plexus, and thus must cross all or part of the pelvis early in their

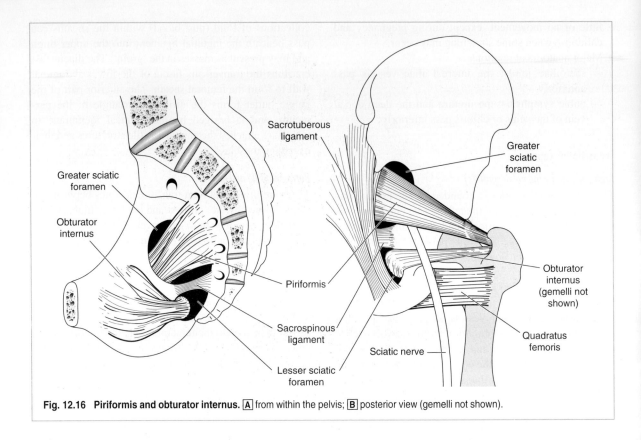

Fig. 12.16 **Piriformis and obturator internus.** [A] from within the pelvis; [B] posterior view (gemelli not shown).

course (Fig. 12.17). As in the brachial plexus, some of the rami are destined to supply muscles and dermatomes of the flexor and adductor components of the limb, and some to supply those of the extensor component. As a result of rotation during development, the extensor component of the lower limb distal to the hip lies anteriorly, with the flexor component posterior. This rotation means that the distribution of dermatomes is not quite so straightforward as in the upper limb. The lumbosacral plexus and its branches lie extraperitoneally and deep to the parietal pelvic fascia, and are thus closely related to the musculoskeletal structures of the body wall and pelvic girdle. All three major limb nerves lie on or near bone in the proximal part of their course, making each vulnerable in pelvic and in lower spinal trauma.

The lumbar and sacral components of the plexus are shown in Figures 12.18 and 12.19. The lumbar plexus receives input from all the lumbar ventral rami and from that of T12, and the sacral plexus from the upper four sacral and the lower two lumbar rami. The key to the lumbar plexus is the psoas muscle: the rami lie within it, and the major limb nerves from the plexus emerge and run either side of it. The femoral nerve is lateral, while

the obturator nerve and the lumbosacral trunk (on its way to the sciatic nerve) are medial to the muscle. The lumbosacral trunk is vulnerable where it lies on bone and on the sacroiliac joint as it crosses the pelvic brim. The femoral nerve is close to bone where it crosses the pubis between psoas and iliacus, and is thus vulnerable in anterior pelvic injury. The obturator nerve crosses the pelvic brim posteriorly behind the common iliac vessels, then runs in close relation to the lateral pelvic wall to reach its canal in the superolateral angle of the obturator foramen. It is thus liable to involvement in anterior and posterior pelvic injuries. The key to the sacral plexus is the piriformis muscle, on which the plexus lies and above and below which its major branches leave the pelvis. The plexus is vulnerable in injuries of the sacrum and of the posterior pelvis. The nerve to the flexor component of the lower limb is the tibial part of the sciatic. The other main branches of the sacral plexus to the limb (common peroneal, gluteal nerves) supply the extensor component. The sacral plexus also supplies the perineum, via the pudendal nerve: this fact is of great importance in the clinical assessment of spinal injuries.

The autonomic input to the lumbosacral plexus is

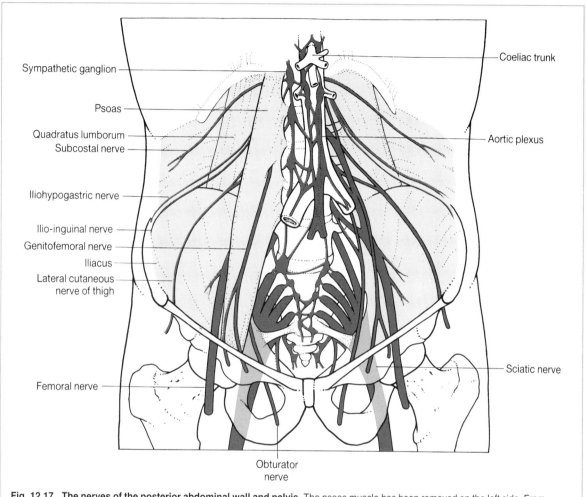

Fig. 12.17 The nerves of the posterior abdominal wall and pelvis. The psoas muscle has been removed on the left side. From Rogers op. cit.

perhaps even more important than that to the brachial plexus, as, in the former, both major components of the autonomic system are involved. All lumbar and sacral ventral rami receive grey rami communicantes from the corresponding sympathetic ganglia. The upper two lumbar ventral rami, with all the thoracic, send white rami communicantes to the sympathetic chain. The second to fourth sacral ventral rami convey the sacral parasympathetic outflow to the pelvic splanchnic nerves, supplying the pelvic viscera. Remember that the body wall and limbs have no parasympathetic supply.

Diagnostic clinical anatomy

This includes the assessment of patients with spinal injuries, pelvic fractures and hip injuries. Familiarity

with the clinical anatomy of the lumbosacral plexus is also essential in the assessment and management of patients with low back and leg pain. MRI and CT reconstruction have revolutionised the clarification of disturbed anatomy in complex pelvic fractures.

LOWER LIMB

There are major differences in functional anatomy between the upper and lower limbs, explained by the differing rôles of the limbs. The upper limb moves and fixes the hand in space, while the lower limb is mainly a strong weight-bearing structure whose distal end, the foot, is usually in contact with the ground. The joints of the upper limb are versatile, and their muscles are precisely

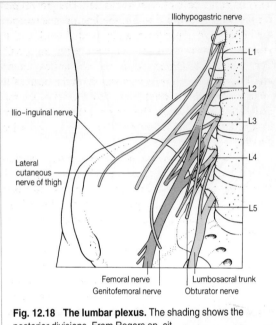

Iliohypogastric nerve

Ilio-inguinal nerve

Lateral cutaneous nerve of thigh

L1
L2
L3
L4
L5

Femoral nerve
Genitofemoral nerve
Lumbosacral trunk
Obturator nerve

Fig. 12.18 The lumbar plexus. The shading shows the posterior divisions. From Rogers op. cit.

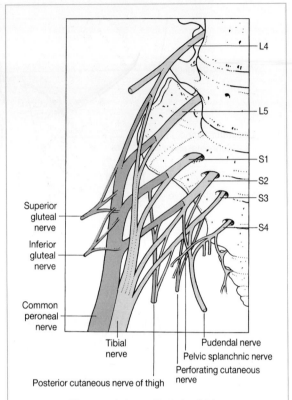

L4
L5
S1
S2
S3
S4

Superior gluteal nerve
Inferior gluteal nerve
Common peroneal nerve

Tibial nerve
Pudendal nerve
Pelvic splanchnic nerve
Perforating cutaneous nerve
Posterior cutaneous nerve of thigh

Fig. 12.19 The sacral plexus. Posterior divisions are shaded darker to distinguish them from the anterior divisions. From Rogers op cit.

attached. These muscles almost always work from their proximal attachments (origins) to their distal (insertions), as the distal end of the limb is free and mobile. Muscles in the lower limb mainly have large, diffuse attachments, and work largely from their distal attachments to 'stand up' the trunk and proximal lower limb on the feet, then to stabilise these structures during standing and locomotion. It is the distal ends of lower limb muscles which are usually the fixed ends: the foot does not act like a 'surrogate hand'. In addition to the fact that most muscles spend most of their time 'acting in reverse', there are many muscles in the lower limb which cross, and can therefore act upon, more than one major joint. They usually have important rôles both as stabilisers and motors of the joints which they cross.

Osteology

Femur

The proximal end of the femur has three major components: the head and the two trochanters. The head is borne on a relatively long neck, which forms an angle both with the shaft and with the transcondylar axis (coronal plane) of the bone. The neck is angled medially on the shaft, the open neck-shaft angle being about 130°. It is also normally angled forward (anteverted) from the coronal plane by about 15° in the adult. These angles are

important in the consideration of proximal femoral fractures and in the insertion of proximal femoral prostheses. Their presence also determines the line of action of muscles acting about the hip. The head is more than half a sphere, and is completely covered with articular cartilage except in the base of the central pit or fovea for the attachment of the ligament of the head of the femur (ligamentum teres). The neck is narrower proximally than distally, and is demarcated from the shaft by the intertrochanteric crest posteriorly and line anteriorly. Subcapital femoral fractures occur through the narrow more proximal neck, and (per)trochanteric fractures pass through the intertrochanteric region. The line of capsular attachment from the hip joint passes distal to the line of subcapital fractures but proximal to that of trochanteric fractures (Fig 12.20). Almost the entire blood supply of the adult femoral head reaches it from vessels entering the neck at or distal to the capsular attachment. Thus subcapital fractures can lead to avascular necrosis of the femoral head whereas trochanteric fractures do not.

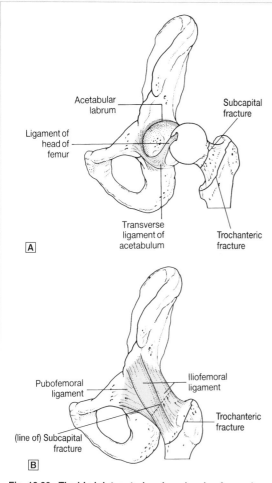

Fig. 12.20 The hip joint: anterior view showing femoral nerve fracture-line. A the head of the femur has been separated from the acetabulum to show the labrum and ligament of the head of the femur; B external view. From Rogers op. cit.

(Figure labels, panel A:) Acetabular labrum; Subcapital fracture; Ligament of head of femur; Transverse ligament of acetabulum; Trochanteric fracture

(Figure labels, panel B:) Pubofemoral ligament; Iliofemoral ligament; (line of) Subcapital fracture; Trochanteric fracture

The greater trochanter is mainly an attachment for the abductors and short rotators of the hip, but vastus lateralis encroaches upon it anteriorly. Gluteus medius attaches superiorly, gluteus minimus more anteriorly, and the short rotator (obturators and piriformis) attachments are grouped around the trochanteric fossa medially. That of quadratus femoris has its own tubercle posteriorly. The lessser trochanter lies posteromedially at the base of the neck. Psoas attaches to its tip, with iliacus and pectineus inferiorly and posteriorly. Vastus medialis attachment extends anterior to the lesser trochanter. There are three growth plates in the proximal femur, one at the junction of the capital or 'upper femoral' epiphysis with the neck,

and one at the base of each trochanter. The growth plate for the head is entirely within the line of attachment of the hip capsule. Apart from a tiny medial portion of the greater, the trochanteric growth plates are extracapsular. The arterial anastomosis from the circumflex femoral arteries, from which the blood supply to the head of the femur derives, lies close to bone at the level of the mid- and distal femoral neck. The posterior surface of the neck is separated only by the short rotators from the sciatic nerve.

The shaft of the femur is a very strong, anteriorly bowed tube of compact bone, expanding distally into the metaphyseal supracondylar region. Its main feature is the posteriorly placed linea aspera, a raised and roughened muscle attachment. This line splits superiorly, continuing laterally into the raised area for the femoral attachment of gluteus maximus. It also splits inferiorly as the shaft expands, giving the two supracondylar lines and ridges which border the popliteal surface of the bone. The three named adductors of the femur attach to the linea aspera, together with the short head of biceps femoris, the vasti and the intermuscular septa. Vastus intermedius also attaches to the proximal two-thirds of the anterior aspect of the shaft. The shaft of the femur is attached to the stocking-like fascia lata by the medial and lateral inter-muscular septa, dividing the thigh into anterior extensor and posterior flexor osteofascial compartments. The septa attach along the whole of the linea aspera and its distal prolongations. The perforating arteries, branches of the profunda femoris, pass very close to the shaft as they run from the extensor into the flexor compartment. Thus they are very vulnerable in fractures of the femoral shaft, their damage often contributing to the significant blood loss from such injuries.

The distal expanded end of the femur includes the metaphysis and popliteal surface and the two condyles. The extra-articular parts of the condyles are the epicondyles. The adductor tubercle, the distal attachment of adductor magnus, lies just proximal to the medial epicondyle. Adductor magnus has a very long femoral attachment extending from just below the lesser trochanter down the whole of the linea aspera and medial supracondylar line to the adductor tubercle. The femoral vessels become the popliteal as they pass through a hiatus in the lower part of this attachment, and are thereafter closely related to the popliteal surface of the femur, the artery lying on the bone and consequently being very liable to injury in supracondylar fractures of the femur. The medial head of gastrocnemius attaches to the medial 'corner' of the popliteal surface, while the lateral head attaches to the back and lateral side of the lateral condyle above the attachment of the lateral collateral ligament of the knee. Below and behind the ligament lie the attachment and groove for popliteus. The medial collateral ligament attaches to the medial epicondyle. The horseshoe-shaped articular surface for the tibia is prolonged anteriorly into that for the patella, which extends further forward laterally than medially. Between the condyles is the intercondylar notch, whose surface is intracapsular but extrasynovial. The lateral wall of the notch is part of the lateral condyle and gives attachment to the anterior cruciate ligament, while its medial wall, from the medial condyle, bears the attachment of the posterior cruciate.

The growth plate of the distal femur runs almost horizontally at the level of the adductor tubercle, and is extracapsular except for a small central segment anteriorly.

Patella

The patella, the largest sesamoid bone, develops in the tendon of quadriceps femoris. From its lower pole the patellar tendon (ligamentum patellae) runs to the tibial tubercle, and the bulk of the quadriceps tendon inserts into its upper (proximal) surface. The quadriceps expansions, aponeurotic attachments from the vasti, join its medial and lateral borders. Its anterior, non-articular surface is subcutaneous, with the prepatellar bursa intervening. Its posterior surface articulates with the femur, and is divided by a longitudinal ridge into a smaller medial and a larger lateral facet for the respective femoral condyles. Viewed from behind, the patella lies in a circumferential cushion or pad of fat, which articulates in extension with a similar pad on the anterior surface of the femoral metaphysis.

Tibia

The proximal expanded end of the tibia consists of the two condyles separated by the intercondylar eminence and area, to which the cruciate ligaments and the horns of the menisci are attached (Fig. 12.21). Its superior surface or plateau articulates with the femur and menisci: the fibula articulates with the inferior surface of the lateral condyle. The medial condyle has a posterior transverse groove for the attachment of semimembranosus, and the smaller, more circular, lateral condyle has a flattened area anterolaterally for the attachment of the iliotibial tract of fascia lata. Anteriorly in the midline is the prominent tibial tubercle, to which attaches the patellar tendon (ligament). In the intercondylar region the central eminence divides the anterior from the posterior non-articular areas. The anterior cruciate ligament attaches to the centre of the anterior area, with the anterior meniscal attachments anteromedially and posterolaterally. The posterior cruciate attaches to the posterior lip of the posterior non-articular area, with both the meniscal attachments anterior to it. The articular facet for the fibula lies posteriorly beneath the lateral condyle; just above it is a groove in which lies the popliteus tendon where it interrupts the capsular attachment. The capsule of the knee joint attaches at the margins of the articular surface except anteriorly, where it extends almost down to the tibial tubercle. The proximal growth plate of the tibia lies entirely outside the capsule, and has an anterodistal projection to include the tibial tubercle.

On the medial side of the proximal metaphysis lie the attachments for the superficial part of the medial collateral ligament and for the *pes anserinus*, the flattened common tendon of sartorius, gracilis and semitendinosus. Popliteus attaches to the posterior metaphyseal surface above the oblique linear attachment of soleus, lying between the popliteal artery and the bone.

The shaft of the tibia is triangular in section. The anterior border and medial surface are subcutaneous throughout their length, making the tibia particularly liable to open fracture. No muscles attach to this surface. The lateral surface, lateral to the anterior border, is covered proximally by the attachment of tibialis anterior. The interosseous membrane attaches to the lateral border of the shaft. Posteriorly, distal to the linear soleal attachment, tibialis posterior attaches laterally and flexor digitorum longus medially. The distal third of the shaft is devoid of muscle attachments, the consequent reduced vascularity adversely affecting fracture healing in this area.

The distal expanded end continues distally and medially into the medial malleolus, grooved posteriorly by the tendon of tibialis posterior. On the lateral surface at the same level lies the notch for articulation with the fibula. The inferior surface bears the articular surface for the talus, and is wider anteriorly than posteriorly. The capsule of the ankle joint attaches around the margins of the articular surface: the distal growth plate of the tibia, like the proximal, is entirely extracapsular.

Fibula

The proximal expanded end of the fibula is the head, bearing the styloid process laterally for attachment of the lateral collateral ligament of the knee, and the facet for the tibia medially. Biceps femoris attaches to the head around the base of the styloid process, and the common peroneal nerve is vulnerable where it crosses the neck of the bone just below the head. The attachments of the muscles to the upper shaft extend proximally onto the head anteriorly and posteriorly. The growth plate for the head lies entirely outside the capsules of the knee and superior tibiofibular joints.

The shaft has a very narrow anterior surface, to which extensores hallucis longus and digitorum longus and peroneus tertius are attached, a wider posterior surface to which soleus and flexor hallucis longus attach, and a spiral lateral surface to which peronei longus and brevis are attached. The interosseous membrane attaches between the anterior and posterior surfaces. The superficial peroneal nerve runs close to bone at midshaft level.

The distal expanded end forms the lateral malleolus, the talar articular surface lying medially. Proximal to this surface lies the area of attachment for the interosseous ligament. There is a groove posteriorly for the peroneus brevis tendon. Both ends of the fibula are easily palpable subcutaneously.

The distal growth plate lies outside the capsule of the ankle joint, which attaches to the articular margins.

Tarsal bones

These seven bones comprise the large calcaneum (calcaneus, os calcis) and talus posteriorly, the navicular medially and the cuboid laterally in the midfoot, with the three wedge-like cuneiforms anterior (distal) to the navicular and medial to the cuboid. Only the talus articulates with the tibia and fibula, while the cuneiforms and cuboid articulate with the metatarsals. The talus is the key bone

of the foot: it is the apex of the longitudinal arch, and is the sole direct bearer and distributor of the weight of the standing body. Detailed knowledge of individual bones is not required, though the way in which the talus articulates with the calcaneum and navicular should be noted, as the important movements of eversion and inversion occur at this joint complex. Some muscle attachments are particularly important, such as those of the tendo Achillis to the calcaneum, tibialis posterior to the navicular tuberosity, and the 'matching' attachments of tibialis anterior and peroneus longus to the medial cuneiform and first metatarsal. The talus is unusual for a bone of its size in that it has no muscle attachments. Like the scaphoid, its blood supply is asymmetrical and somewhat tenuous. The body of the bone is supplied by vessels entering it distally, rendering it liable to avascular necrosis when a fracture occurs across the 'neck'. On the plantar aspect of the foot, flexor hallucis longus grooves the sustentaculum tali of the calcaneum, and peroneus longus grooves the cuboid.

Metatarsals and phalanges

Like the metacarpals these are 'mini' long bones. Apart from the first, the metatarsals are slender and narrower from side to side than metacarpals.

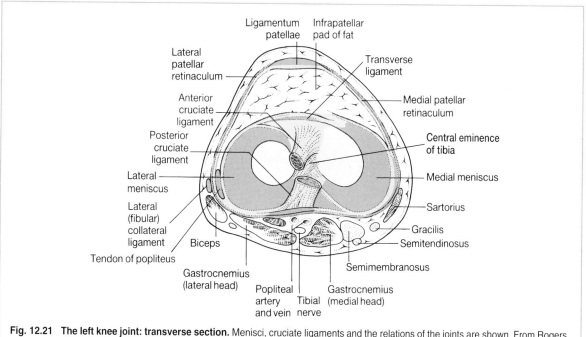

Fig. 12.21 The left knee joint: transverse section. Menisci, cruciate ligaments and the relations of the joints are shown. From Rogers op. cit.

Arthrology

The joints of the lower limb will be described according to the framework used for those of the upper limb. The anatomy of the large, weight-bearing joints of the lower limb is very important: these joints are very commonly involved in trauma and in degenerative joint disease. Some knowledge of the topography of the tarsal joints is required in order to understand the biomechanics and movements of the foot, especially with regard to the maintenance of the arches of the foot and the action of the foot as a whole in gait and propulsion. The small joints of the forefoot are commonly injured and deformed as a result of arthritis, degenerative and inflammatory.

Hip joint

This is a ball-and-socket joint in which the ball, the femoral head, forms more than two-thirds of a sphere and is held very firmly in the socket, the acetabulum. The acetabulum is deepened by an intra-articular fibrocartilaginous labrum, and the ligament of the head of the femur (ligamentum teres) attaches the head to the floor of the acetabular notch (Fig. 12.20). The circumference of the acetabulum is completed anteriorly by the transverse ligament, running in continuity with the labrum. Other named ligaments are capsular thickenings. The capsule attaches proximally to the margins of the acetabulum outside the labrum, and to the transverse ligament. It attaches distally to the base of the femoral neck anteriorly, inferiorly and superiorly. Posteriorly its fibres pass medial to the intertrochanteric line: some traverse the neck without attachment to bone. The thickenings in the capsule spiral around the neck in such a way that the capsule is tightest, and the joint thus maximally stable, in extension, abduction and medial rotation — the position in which the limb is placed to reduce and internally fix a subcapital fracture of the femur. These capsular thickenings are the ischiofemoral ligament posteriorly, the pubofemoral anteroinferiorly, and most importantly the iliofemoral ligament anteriorly. This ligament, in the shape of an inverted Y, is extremely strong, as it resists the weight of the body which tends to extend the pelvis on the femora in the standing position. The synovial lining of the joint covers the intracapsular part of the femoral neck and the ligament of the head, and may communicate anteriorly with a bursa beneath the iliopsoas tendon. There is often a non-communicating bursa lying between gluteus maximus and the greater trochanter, and another beneath gluteus maximus overlying the ischial tuberosity.

The hip is a universal joint, moving in all three orthogonal planes. The actions of the various groups of muscles related to the joint may be deduced from their positions. Lying anteriorly are the flexors. Lying laterally are the abductors, medially are the adductors, and posteriorly lie the short external rotators and the extensors. Obturator externus lies inferiorly. The muscles producing rotation vary with the position of the hip and also with the weight-bearing status of the limb. Following Hilton's Law, all the nerves supplying these muscles will also supply the joint. The sciatic nerve lies on the short rotators posteriorly, and the medial circumflex femoral vessels pass immediately inferior to the capsule. The joint is best aspirated from an anterior approach, keeping well (about 3 cm) lateral to the femoral artery. The hip may be approached surgically from all four sides, but approaches immediately anterior to gluteus medius, those splitting the gluteus medius-vastus lateralis 'hood', and posterior approaches dividing the short rotators are most often favoured for adult reconstructive surgery.

Summary Hip joint (Fig. 12.20): synovial, ball-and-socket.

- Movements and muscles (movements described are those of the femur on the pelvis, as in the non-weight-bearing limb)
  — flexion: iliopsoas, pectineus, sartorius and rectus femoris
  — extension: gluteus maximus and the hamstrings
  — adduction: named adductors, gracilis, pectineus
  — abduction: gluteus medius and minimus, tensor fasciae latae
  — external (lateral) rotation: piriformis, obturator internus, quadratus femoris
  — internal (medial) rotation: anterior parts of gluteus medius and minimus, tensor fasciae latae.
- Major anatomical relations
  — anterior: femoral vessels; femoral nerve
  — posterior: sciatic nerve.

Knee

The knee is a very common presenting site both of trauma and of degenerative conditions. Its functional anatomy must be well understood by the junior surgeon. This understanding should be based on a sound grasp of the anatomy of the constituent bones and in particular of the attachments of the fibrous structures on which the knee relies entirely for its static stability. These include the capsule of the joint with its medial and posterior thickenings, the cruciate and collateral ligaments, the iliotibial tract, the fibrous attachments of the patella, and the intra-articular menisci. Figures 12.21, 12.22 and 12.23 show many of these attachments, together with important soft-tissue relations of the knee.

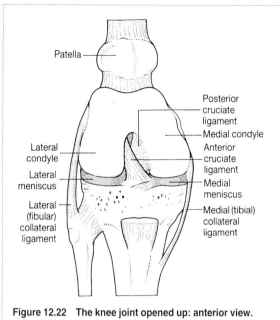

Figure 12.22 The knee joint opened up: anterior view.
From Rogers op. cit.

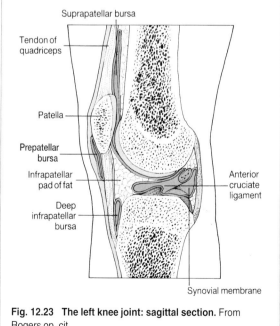

Fig. 12.23 The left knee joint: sagittal section. From Rogers op. cit.

Note especially that the knee also has important dynamic stabilisers: all those muscles which cross it and act upon it. There is no intrinsic bony stability.

The 'knee' joint has two major components: the tibio-femoral and the patellofemoral articulations. Though these joints share a synovial lining, their functional anatomy, like their clinical disorders, can be considered separately. The tibiofemoral joint has two compartments, medial and lateral, separated by the intercondylar region where the cruciates and menisci are attached. The femoral condyles differ in size and in radius of curvature, the lateral being the larger. The radii of curvature are themselves variable, the articular surfaces for the tibia being flattened centrally. The tibial condyles are also asymmetrical, and the reciprocity of the articulating surfaces is improved by the presence of the menisci. The capsular attachment on the femur follows the articular margin distal to the growth plate posteriorly and laterally, but crosses the plate anteriorly to extend up onto the anterior femoral surface. Here the attachment is deficient superiorly where the suprapatellar bursa communicates with the joint. On the tibia, the capsular attachment largely follows the articular margin, but is deficient pos-terolaterally where popliteus tendon enters the joint. The capsule is thickest posteriorly, where it is reinforced by the oblique popliteal ligament. Like the biceps tendon in the shoulder, the cruciate ligaments and the popliteal tendon are intra-articular but extrasynovial, being 'invagi-nated' into the synovium from behind (Fig. 12.23). The anterior cruciate runs from lateral femoral to medial tibial condyle, crossing anterior to the posterior cruciate. The latter runs from the medial femoral condyle to reach the posterior lip of the tibia almost in the midline. Stand with your right leg crossed over your left: your legs now indi-cate the relative positions and attachments of the cruciate ligaments of the right knee. The medial fibrocartilagi-nous meniscus attaches by its horns to the intercondylar region of the tibia, and peripherally via the capsule to the circumference of the medial tibial condyle. The central part of this capsular attachment includes the deep part of the medial collateral ligament. The lateral meniscus, more nearly circular than the medial and covering more of the tibial articular surface, has similar attachments to the tibia except posterolaterally, where its capsular attachment is interrupted by the tendon of popliteus. In addition to its tibial attachments, the lateral meniscus attaches both to popliteus tendon and to the femur either side of the posterior cruciate ligament. It does not attach to the lateral collateral ligament. The collateral ligaments of the knee differ markedly in size and shape. The tibial collateral or medial ligament has two layers. A wide, long and flat superficial part runs from the medial femoral epicondyle obliquely forwards to merge with the periosteum of the tibia beneath the attachments of sartorius, gracilis and semitendinosus. Its free anterior margin is separated from the capsule by a bursa, but its posterior margin blends with the capsule. The deep part of the ligament is a thickening in the capsule of the joint, attached to the central part of the periphery of the medial meniscus. The fibular collateral or lateral ligament is a rounded fibrous cord running from the lateral epicondyle of the femur obliquely backwards to the head of the fibula. It is entirely separate from the capsule and underlying lateral meniscus.

The patellofemoral joint and the soft-tissue attachments to the patella constitute the extensor mechanism of the knee. The superior attachment is the rectus femoris insertion, while the patellar tendon (ligamentum patellae) is attached inferiorly. Both are continuous with the aponeurotic quadriceps expansions which attach to the remainder of the patellar cirumference. The oblique line of pull of the quadriceps on the patella (revise the attachments of rectus femoris) forms an angle with that of the patellar tendon, which lies in the midline of the limb. This angle is greater in females, whose pelvis is wider, so that the horizontal component of the resultant force exerted by the quadriceps is increased. This explains the fact that patellar dislocation is both commoner in females and almost invariably lateral in direction.

The synovial lining of the knee joint extends well proximal to the patella, forming the suprapatellar bursa (Fig. 12.23) in which effusions of the knee are best observed. The synovium also commonly extends posteromedially as a bursa between the attachments of semimembranosus and gastrocnemius, and posterolaterally along the tendon of popliteus.

The line of weight bearing runs anterior to the centre of the knee, putting the thickened posterior capsule under tension in the standing position. The knee is maximally stable in full extension, when all four major ligaments are taut. The knee is not a simple hinge: its active movement incorporates an element of rotation, and its axis varies in flexion and extension owing to the differing geometry of the two femoral condyles. In the weight-bearing knee the femur rotates medially on the tibia in the later part of extension, 'screwing home' into the maximally stable position. As flexion begins, the femur 'unscrews' into lateral rotation by the action of popliteus. Owing to their capsular attachments, the menisci move with the tibia rather than with the femur. The recognition that rotational movement occurs at the knee is vital to the understanding of cruciate ligament action. In very simple terms, the cruciate ligaments control stability of the joint in the sagittal plane (anteroposterior glide) while the collaterals control coronal stability, preventing abduction and adduction. In fact all four ligaments work together, and the anterior in particular is more concerned with rotational than with purely sagittal stability. In considering the stabilising function of ligaments, note that their rôle may be exceeded or even usurped by that of the muscles (especially the quadriceps) in the mobile patient.

As with all joints the knee receives its nerve supply from those nerves supplying the muscles which act upon it. Note however that the nerve supply to the skin overlying the knee also includes, medially, an important contribution from the obturator nerve. Thus all three major nerves which supply the hip joint also supply the knee.

Summary Knee joint (Figs 12.21, 12.22, 12.23): synovial, modified hinge with intra-articular menisci (femorotibial) and gliding patellofemoral component.

- Movements (of tibia on femur) and muscles
  — flexion: biceps femoris, semimembranosus, semitendinosus, sartorius, gracilis, popliteus
  — extension: quadriceps femoris, tensor fasciae latae
  — medial rotation with knee flexed: semimembranosus, semitendinosus, sartorius and gracilis, popliteus
  — lateral rotation with knee flexed: biceps femoris.
  Note that when the knee is extended and weight bearing, popliteus 'unlocks' the joint by laterally rotating the femur on the tibia, and gastrocnemius helps in flexion.
- Major anatomical relations
  — posterior: popliteal artery on the capsule (with popliteal vein and tibial nerve only a little further away)
  — posterolateral: common peroneal nerve
  — medially and laterally: the inferior genicular arteries (from the popliteal)
  — medial: saphenous nerve emerging through the deep fascia to run with the great saphenous vein.

Tibiofibular joints

The shafts of tibia and fibula are strongly linked by the interosseous membrane, whose fibres run distally and laterally. Proximal to the membrane and just distal to the synovial superior tibiofibular joint is an aperture through which the anterior tibial vessels pass: here the arteries of the leg are very vulnerable in proximal tibial fractures and surgery. The membrane is continuous distally with the interosseous ligament of the fibrous inferior tibiofibular joint. There are also anterior and posterior ligaments of this joint: some or all of these ligaments may be disrupted in severe ankle injuries. There is very little movement at the tibiofibular joints, though some rotation occurs during ankle movements.

Ankle joint

This very commonly injured, major weight-bearing joint is surprisingly rarely the site of troublesome osteoarthritis. It is a hinge joint with some variation of its transmalleolar axis during movement. The 'mortise' is formed by the adjacent articular surfaces of tibia and fibula, deepened posteriorly by the inferior tibiofibular ligament. The 'tenon' is the trochlea of the talus, with its continuous articular surface superiorly, laterally and medially. The joint is wider anteriorly, so that the position of maximal stability is in full dorsiflexion when the 'fit' is tightest. The capsule attaches around the articular margins of tibia and fibula, and around that of the talus except anteriorly where it extends onto the neck of the bone. This capsule is thinnest anteriorly, and is strengthened medially and laterally by the collateral ligaments. The stronger medial or deltoid ligament (Fig. 12.24) is a uniform triangular structure attached by its apex to the medial malleolus and by its base to the medial side of the skeleton of the foot from calcaneum to navicular. The lateral ligament is a weaker, tripartite structure. The central band runs from the lateral malleolus to the calcaneum, while anterior and posterior bands attach the malleolus to the talus either side of it. The anterior talofibular band is the most commonly injured in an ankle sprain. The synovium lines the capsule and extends proximally a short way between tibia and fibula just below the fibrous inferior tibiofibular joint. Active, useful movements of the ankle joint are confined to flexion (plantar flexion) and extension (dorsiflexion). All muscles passing anterior to the transmalleolar axis produce dorsiflexion, and all passing posterior to the axis produce plantarflexion. The nerve supply to the joint is derived from the nerves to these muscles. The extensor tendons cross the joint anteriorly in their synovial sheaths beneath the extensor retinacula. The flexors pass behind the medial malleolus in their sheaths beneath the flexor retinaculum, while the larger two peronei pass similarly behind the lateral malleolus. The (posterior) tibial neurovascular bundle runs medially across the deltoid ligament, while the anterior tibial artery and deep peroneal nerve are closely related to the capsule anteriorly (Fig. 12.25). The ankle is best aspirated anteriorly between the tendons of tibialis anterior and extensor hallucis longus. Surgical approaches, usually for the internal fixation of fractures, are determined by the fracture pattern.

Summary Ankle joint (Fig. 12.24): synovial, hinge.

- Movements and muscles
  — dorsiflexion (extension): tibialis anterior, extensor digitorum longus, extensor hallucis longus, peroneus tertius
  — plantar flexion (flexion): gastrocnemius, soleus, tibialis posterior, flexor hallucis longus, flexor digitorum longus, peronei longus et brevis.

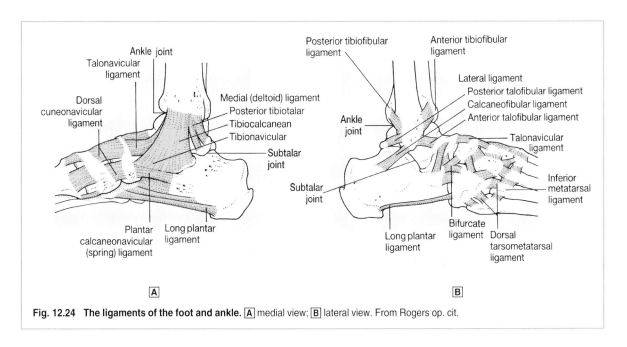

Fig. 12.24 The ligaments of the foot and ankle. A medial view; B lateral view. From Rogers op. cit.

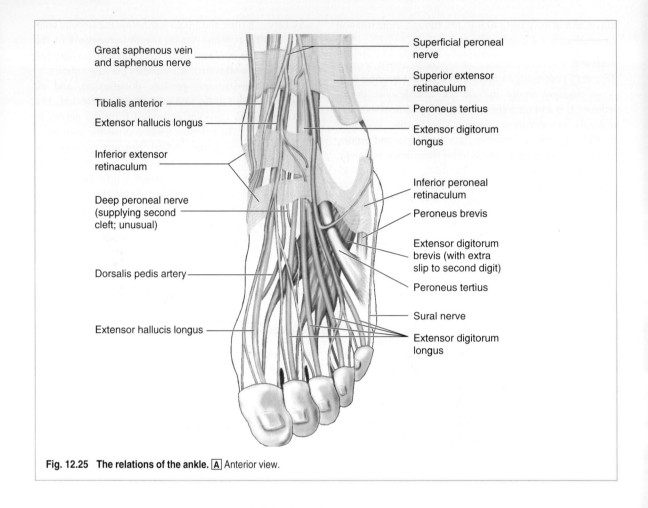

Great saphenous vein and saphenous nerve

Tibialis anterior

Extensor hallucis longus

Inferior extensor retinaculum

Deep peroneal nerve (supplying second cleft; unusual)

Dorsalis pedis artery

Extensor hallucis longus

Superficial peroneal nerve

Superior extensor retinaculum

Peroneus tertius

Extensor digitorum longus

Inferior peroneal retinaculum

Peroneus brevis

Extensor digitorum brevis (with extra slip to second digit)

Peroneus tertius

Sural nerve

Extensor digitorum longus

Fig. 12.25 The relations of the ankle. [A] Anterior view.

- Major anatomical relations (Fig. 12.25A,B,C)
  - medial: behind medial malleolus: tibialis posterior, (posterior) tibial neurovascular bundle, flexor digitorum longus, flexor hallucis longus; in front of medial malleolus: great saphenous vein and saphenous nerve
  - lateral (all behind lateral malleolus): peroneus longus and brevis, small saphenous vein and sural nerve
  - anterior (medial to lateral): tibialis anterior, extensor hallucis longus, anterior tibial vessels and deep peroneal nerve, extensor digitorum longus, peroneus tertius   *TEA DEP*
  - posterior: tendo calcaneus, flexor hallucis longus.

Joints of the foot

Those joints proximal to the tarsometarsals are difficult to understand, and some of the terminology is confusing, with differences between anatomical and clinical usage. In simple terms, there are two interlinked joint complexes, the subtalar and the midtarsal. The subtalar complex includes the (posterior) talocalcaneal joint ('subtalar joint proper') and the talocalcaneonavicular joint. The midtarsal complex includes the latter and the calcaneocuboid joint. The movements occurring at the subtalar complex are eversion and inversion of the foot on the talus. The midtarsal joint allows some pronation and supination, and a little dorsiflexion and plantarflexion, of the forefoot on the hindfoot. All muscles whose line of action crosses medial to the axis of the subtalar joints will invert — pull up the medial border of the foot, make the sole face medially and bring the lateral border of the foot into contact with the ground. Those muscles whose line of action crosses lateral to the axis will do the opposite — evert.

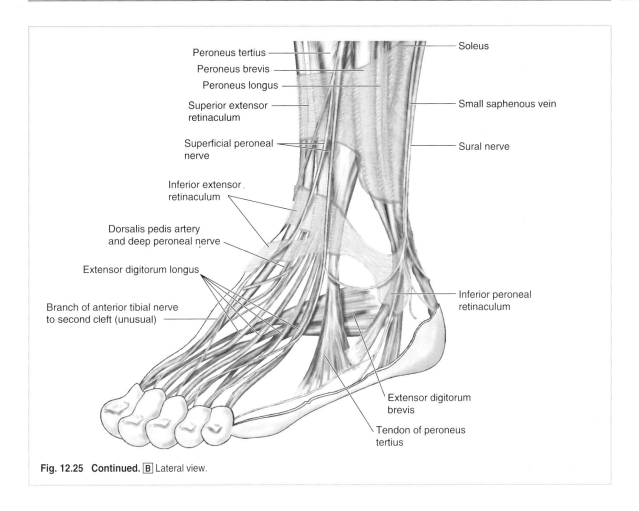

Peroneus tertius

Peroneus brevis

Peroneus longus

Superior extensor retinaculum

Superficial peroneal nerve

Inferior extensor retinaculum

Dorsalis pedis artery and deep peroneal nerve

Extensor digitorum longus

Branch of anterior tibial nerve to second cleft (unusual)

Soleus

Small saphenous vein

Sural nerve

Inferior peroneal retinaculum

Extensor digitorum brevis

Tendon of peroneus tertius

Fig. 12.25 Continued. B Lateral view.

The axis of inversion and eversion is oblique, so that eversion of the free (non-weight-bearing) foot includes some dorsiflexion and abduction while inversion includes the opposite movements. When the foot is bearing weight, movements at the subtalar complex are modified by pronation or supination at the midtarsal joints, in order to keep the sole plantigrade. In crossed-leg and in wide-abduction standing, or in walking across a slope, the feet are simultaneously everted/inverted and plantigrade. All joints are synovial, with capsules strengthened by many interosseous ligaments. The talocalcaneonavicular joint is functionally a ball-and-socket, the socket being completed by the cartilage-lined plantar calcaneonavicular or 'spring' ligament which plays a crucial part in the maintenance of the longitudinal arch of the foot.

Summary

- Joints (Fig. 12.24)
  - subtalar complex: posterior component of talocal-caneal joint: synovial, ellipsoid; talocalcaneonavic-ular joint: synovial, 'ball-and-socket'
  - midtarsal: talocalcaneonavicular, plus calcaneo-cuboid: synovial, plane.
- Movements and muscles
  - inversion (with supination): tibialis posterior, tibialis anterior
  - eversion (with pronation): peroneus longus, brevis and tertius, pulling up the lateral border of the foot and producing eversion and pronation.

There is very little movement at any of the tarso-metatarsal joints. The structure and movements at the metatarsophalangeal (MTP) and interphalangeal (IP) joints resemble those in the hand, and as in the hand the IP joints are hinge joints, while the MTP joints also allow abduction and adduction. The function of the foot as an elastic prop and its propelling role in locomotion require it to be more than a flat, weight-bearing platform. The

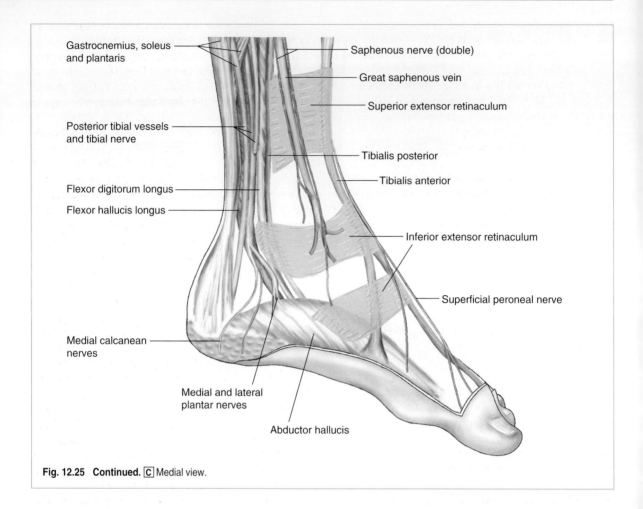

Gastrocnemius, soleus and plantaris

Saphenous nerve (double)

Great saphenous vein

Superior extensor retinaculum

Posterior tibial vessels and tibial nerve

Tibialis posterior

Tibialis anterior

Flexor digitorum longus

Flexor hallucis longus

Inferior extensor retinaculum

Superficial peroneal nerve

Medial calcanean nerves

Medial and lateral plantar nerves

Abductor hallucis

Fig. 12.25 Continued. C Medial view.

shape of the bony foot incorporates a series of resilient arches, which are maintained by balanced soft-tissue elements. These comprise static, passive structures — ligaments and fasciae — and dynamic, active structures — short muscles and the tendons of long muscles. The elastic, propellant side of the foot is the medial, whose longitudinal bony arch includes the calcaneus, talus, navicular, the three cuneiforms and the three medial metatarsals. The supportive lateral side of the foot has a much lower, less mobile arch comprising the calcaneus, cuboid and lateral two metatarsals. In addition, there is a transverse arch, made by the articulating cuneiforms and cuboid and their associated metatarsals. The integrity of the longitudinal arches is maintained by a layered pattern of ligaments, muscles and fasciae in the sole of the foot, together with the suspensory action of the long tendons from the leg. The ligaments include the plantar calcaneonavicular or 'spring' ligament which forms part of the

talocalcaneonavicular 'socket', overlying which are the short and long plantar ligaments (Fig. 12.24), the flexor digitorum brevis and the plantar fascia (aponeurosis). In walking, when the toes are dorsiflexed and the heel is off the ground, tension in the aponeurosis heightens the arch by the 'Spanish windlass' effect. The dynamic action of tibialis posterior with its multiple bony attachments radiating from the navicular combines with that of tibialis anterior to elevate the medial arch. The corresponding action of peroneus longus, whose tendon obliquely crosses the sole, acts chiefly to close up the transverse arch.

Between the joints: fasciae and compartments; nerves

The fascial 'stocking' enclosing the lower limb is much more complete and well developed than is that of the upper limb. This stocking improves the efficiency of action of the muscles, both as motors of the joints and as agents of venous return. The stocking of the thigh, the

Hamstrings :- Sciatic Nerve - L5, S1
↳ Medial side - Tibial division
↳ Short head - Common Peroneal division
↳ Obturator - Adductors + Gracilis. (L2, 3)

LOCOMOTOR SYSTEM 12

fascia lata, splits proximally and laterally to enclose its muscle, the tensor fasciae latae, has the saphenous opening proximally and anteriorly, and is thickened laterally to form a band, the iliotibial tract, extending from iliac crest to anterolateral tibia. In the (lower) leg, thickenings at the ankle form the retinacula, extensor, flexor and peroneal. The intermuscular septa attach to the inner surface of the 'stocking', defining the osteofascial compartments. In the thigh there are three compartments but only two septa, medial and lateral, both attaching to the linea aspera of the femur. The adductors are separated from the flexors by adductor magnus, which belongs functionally to both groups. Anteriorly, the extensor compartment contains the extensors of the knee (quadriceps) and sartorius, a flexor of the knee though innervated by the nerve of the extensor compartment, the femoral. The root value of knee extension, and hence of the knee jerk reflex, is L3,4. Posteriorly, the flexor compartment contains the hamstring muscles, innervated by the sciatic nerve (L5,S1). The medial hams and the long head of biceps are innervated by the tibial division of the nerve, while the short head is innervated by the common peroneal division. The smaller named adductors and gracilis are innervated by the obturator (L2,3) while adductor magnus has a dual nerve supply from obturator and tibial sciatic.

In the distal segment, the anatomical 'leg', there are three main osteofascial compartments, of which one is further subdivided. The anterior and posterior intermuscular septa attach the inside of the fascial stocking laterally to the fibula, enclosing between them the lateral or peroneal compartment. The interosseous membrane and the bones separate the anterior and posterior compartments. The posterior compartment is further subdivided by the deep transverse fascia into deep and superficial components. The anterior compartment contains the dorsiflexors of the foot and the extensors of the toes; its nerve is the deep peroneal and its artery the anterior tibial. The root value of dorsiflexion is L4,5 and of toe extension L5,S1. The lateral compartment contains peroneus longus and brevis. Its nerve is the superficial peroneal, root value L5,S1 (the root value of eversion), and its artery the peroneal. The superficial posterior compartment contains the muscles which form the Achilles tendon, gastrocnemius and soleus, with plantaris if present. These are all supplied by the tibial nerve, root value mainly S1 (the root tested by the ankle jerk reflex). Gastrocnemius crosses the knee joint, whereas soleus can act only on the ankle. The deep posterior compartment contains tibialis posterior and the long toe flexors, with popliteus more proximally. Its nerve is the tibial, which traverses the compartment with its artery, the posterior

tibial. The root value for tibialis posterior (and thus for inversion) is L4,5, and that of toe flexion S1,2.

There is a single muscle on the dorsum of the foot, the extensor digitorum brevis, which usually runs to all except the little toe. It is best considered with the muscles of the anterior compartment of the leg, as it belongs to their functional group and shares their innervation.

The muscles of the sole of the foot are traditionally described in a series of layers, but will here be considered, like the muscles elsewhere in the limb, in terms of functional groups and osteofascial compartments. It has recently been accepted that there is an important 'muscle pump' for venous return in the foot as well as in the calf, dependent upon the efficient working of the muscles of the foot within their fascial compartments. The arrangement of the deep fascia within the foot is complex, but its outermost layer can usefully be regarded as the continuation of the fascial 'stocking' of the limb. The dorsal fascia is thin, with transverse thickenings for the extensor retinacula. The 'sole' of the fascial stocking is the plantar fascia, which, as in the hand, is connected to bone by a series of septa. Within the fascial framework so created lie the groups of muscles. The medial group comprises the intrinsic muscles of the hallux (great toe), abductor hallucis and flexor hallucis brevis, and corresponds to the thenar eminence in the hand. The lateral group corresponds to the hypothenar muscles of the hand and includes the abductor and short flexor of the little toe. The central group includes the short toe flexor and the muscles attached to the long toe flexor (lumbricals and flexor accessorius). The deeper-lying adductor hallucis and the interossei lie dorsal to this central group. The muscles of the medial group are innervated by the medial plantar nerve, which corresponds to the median in its motor and sensory distribution. All other muscles are supplied by the lateral plantar, which in terms of its distribution is the 'ulnar nerve of the foot'. These nerves are accompanied by the vessels of the same name.

Transitional zones

The zones of transition from the trunk into the limb have been dealt with above. There are two regions in the limb whose clinical importance merits their separate consideration as small transitional zones: the popliteal fossa and the ankle. The popliteal fossa lies behind the knee, and with the knee extended is a diamond-shaped recess whose 'floor' consists largely of the posterior surface of the distal femur. The floor extends, distal to its transverse axis, to include the central part of the posterior capsule of the knee, then narrows off to include part of the fascia overlying popliteus muscle. The fossa is bounded proximally by the diverging hamstrings, and distally by the heads of gastrocnemius which lie in contact unless dissected apart. It is 'roofed over' by the fascia lata, through which passes the short saphenous vein on its way to the popliteal vein. Within the fossa, passing down the longitudinal axis of the 'diamond', is the major neurovascular bundle. Most superficially and vertically lies the tibial nerve (the direct continuation of the sciatic), and deepest, running more obliquely and very vulnerably against the bone of the femur and the capsule of the knee, lies the popliteal artery. The popliteal vein runs between the nerve and the artery throughout. The common peroneal nerve runs down the lateral border of the fossa immediately medial to the tendon of biceps femoris, with which it may easily be confused. The tibial and common peroneal nerves give off the sural and sural communicating nerves, respectively. The tibial nerve gives genicular and muscular branches. The popliteal artery gives off important genicular branches to form the periarticular anastomosis of the knee, and the popliteal vein receives the corresponding tributaries. The remainder of the fossa is filled with fat in which are found the popliteal lymph nodes.

Like the wrist, the ankle region is a small transitional zone where many important structures run superficially in continuity across a major joint and are vulnerable in closed and open trauma (Fig. 12.25).

Nerves of the lower limb: where liable to injury and compression

All three major nerves are vulnerable where they enter the limb from the pelvis. The sciatic and the femoral are at risk in injuries and surgery involving the hip joint. The sciatic in the buttock may be damaged by misplaced intramuscular injection, so the surface marking of the nerve is of major importance. The nerve lies mainly in the lower and inner quadrant of the buttock, running in a curved course between the midpoint of a line joining the posterior superior iliac spine with the ischial tuberosity and the midpoint of a second line joining the ischial tuberosity with the greater trochanter. The course of the nerve then runs vertically down the midline of the thigh posteriorly. The safe area for intramuscular injection lies in the upper outer quadrant of the whole buttock when the iliac crest is exposed; the injection is made into the hip abductors rather than into gluteus maximus. The lateral femoral cutaneous nerve may become entrapped as it passes through or beneath the lateral end of the inguinal ligament, giving dysaesthesia of the lateral thigh (meralgia paraesthetica). The sciatic nerve and its major branches are vulnerable in the popliteal fossa, with the common

peroneal becoming almost subcutaneous and particularly liable to pressure from without (bedrest, casts), and to open injury, at the neck of the fibula. A complete sciatic lesion is quickly distinguished clinically from a common peroneal lesion by the fact that in the former there is no movement below the knee, i.e. both plantar flexion and dorsiflexion are absent. In a full sciatic lesion all sensation is lost below the knee apart from that mediated by the saphenous nerve from the femoral: an area of skin extending down the medial side of the leg onto the medial surface of the foot. A common peroneal lesion is characterised by 'foot drop' (loss of ankle dorsiflexion), loss of eversion and loss of sensation over the dorsum and lateral side of the foot. The clinical picture of a common peroneal lesion does not localise the lesion to the region of the knee; trauma in the buttock sometimes spares the tibial component of the sciatic, particularly if the major division of the sciatic occurs at the level of pyriformis. Any of the major nerves of the true leg (below the knee) may be involved in compartment syndromes in that segment of the limb, with the deep peroneal in the anterior compartment being most commonly implicated. Cutaneous sensory loss from a deep peroneal lesion is limited to the cleft between the hallux and second toe; the motor component innervates the ankle and toe extensors (dorsiflexors). The superficial peroneal runs close to the fibula, innervating the two main peroneus muscles before merging through the deep fascia laterally at midcalf level to supply the skin of the anterolateral lower leg and dorsum of the foot. Tarsal tunnel entrapment syndrome affects the tibial nerve and its branches as it passes beneath the flexor retinaculum at the ankle. A lesion at this level causes pain and dysaesthesia in most of the plantar surface of the mid- and forefoot, with paralysis of the small muscles of the foot. The purely sensory saphenous nerve, the only branch of the femoral to cross the knee, accompanies the great saphenous vein and is vulnerable when this vein is excised or ligated.

Diagnostic clinical anatomy

Find this heading in the section on the upper limb (p. 337). Much of what is written there applies equally to the lower limb. In particular, you must understand the anatomical basis of the examination of the major joints and of the muscles which act upon them. The neurological examination of the lower limb is an essential component of the assessment of patients with low back pain. Knowledge of the vascular patterns, arterial and venous, is of even more importance and clinical value in the lower limb, owing to the prevalence of vascular disorders therein.

PHYSIOLOGY

OVERVIEW OF CONTENT

The section will deal with four aspects of musculoskeletal physiology: neuromuscular transmission, the physiology of skeletal muscle, the structural physiology of bone, and locomotion.

The physiology of skeletal muscle is dealt with at intracellular, tissue and organ level, incorporating important clinical principles of muscle action.

Certain areas of the physiology of bone are dealt with elsewhere (see below); here more attention will be given to the physiological aspects of the structural maintenance of bone mass.

KEY CONCEPTS AND LEARNING OBJECTIVES

Learn the physiology in a clinically relevant way, so that disorders of function can be accurately diagnosed and interpreted.

Locomotor physiology is largely applied neurophysiology. In forming an overall view of the subject, central aspects of motor function and its coordination should not be neglected in favour of peripheral neuromuscular detail. The sensory side of locomotor physiology, from proprioception to the locomotor responses to pain, must not be forgotten.

NEUROMUSCULAR TRANSMISSION

The sequence of events by which a signal is transmitted from nerve to striated muscle is the pivotal process in the physiology of the locomotor system. The basic mechanisms involved are the same as those utilised in synaptic transmission in general. The neuromuscular junction or motor end-plate is a chemical synapse between the motor axon and the skeletal muscle fibre. The myelinated axon of the alpha motor neuron is the 'final common pathway' in the neurophysiology of motor activity. Each skeletal muscle has its own particular set of innervating motor neurons, called the motor neuron pool, whose cell bodies lie in lamina IX of the ventral horn of the spinal cord or in the cranial nerve motor nuclei. Each muscle cell (a fibre is an elongated cell) has only one neuromuscular junction, but each alpha motor neuronal axon innervates a number of fibres. The alpha motor neuron and the fibres it innervates constitute the motor unit.

Just proximal to the neuromuscular junction the axon loses its myelin sheath and divides to form the axon terminals. Each axon terminal lies in a synaptic trough on the surface of its target muscle cell (fibre), separated from the postjunctional membrane of the muscle cell by the synaptic cleft. The passage of an action potential down the axon leads to depolarisation of the presynaptic terminal membrane. This depolarisation opens voltage-gated calcium (Ca) channels, allowing extracellular Ca to flow down its electrochemical gradient into the axon terminal. The increase in intracellular Ca concentration stimulates synaptic vesicles, containing acetylcholine (ACh), to fuse with the presynaptic membrane and release 'quanta' of ACh into the synaptic cleft. The ACh is synthesised in the motor neuron from acetyl CoA produced in the neuron and choline taken up actively by the neuron from the extracellular fluid. This choline is largely recycled from metabolised ACh. The ACh diffuses across the cleft and combines chemically with the receptor proteins in the postjunctional membrane. These proteins are integral parts of the membrane, constituting nicotinic cholinergic receptors. As a result of this chemical combination, ligand-gated ion channels open so that there is transiently increased permeability both to Na and K. The net inward ionic current leads to a transient local depolarisation of the postjunctional membrane, the end-plate potential (EPP). This itself is non-propagating, but sets up local electrotonic depolarising currents in the adjacent muscle cell membrane (sarcolemma). When these currents reach threshold, an action potential (AP) propagates along the muscle fibre and initiates muscle contraction via the excitation-contraction coupling mechanism to be described below. The size of an AP in nerve and in muscle, cannot vary (all-or-nothing principle), but its frequency can, leading to summation and subsequently to a tetanic response. The number of motor units recruited can also vary. The released ACh is constantly being hydrolysed in the synaptic cleft into acetate and choline: the process is catalysed by the enzyme acetylcholinesterase, which occurs in high concentration at the normal post-junctional membrane. Small spontaneous releases of ACh also occur, without axonal stimulation, causing miniature depolarisations of the postjunctional membrane (miniature end-plate potentials, MEPP).

It is important to understand the way in which this process can be modified, both pharmacologically and by disease. Transmission can be altered in a number of ways. Non-depolarising drugs such as curare, a plant alphatoxin, work by binding to the receptor protein and blocking transmission. This causes longer-term paralysis than do the depolarisers, such as succinylcholine, which bind to the receptor and cause temporary depolarisation. These different forms of action are utilised in anaesthesia. The action of such drugs can be reversed by neostigmine, which blocks the action of acetylcholinesterase and thus promotes transmission. In the disease myasthenia gravis, circulating antibodies to the cholinergic receptor proteins are present.

SKELETAL MUSCLE PHYSIOLOGY

A skeletal muscle may be considered as a specialised organ for the conversion of the chemical energy held in adenosine triphosphate (ATP) into mechanical work. Its physiology can be approached at several levels of structural organisation, from molecular through cell and tissue to 'organ' level. Recent and exciting major advances in the understanding of muscle function at molecular and cell level have tended to obscure the clinical importance of the 'macrophysiology' of skeletal muscles as the organs of locomotion. A further 'supra-organ' level, that of neurological motor control, will be considered in the section on the physiology of locomotion.

Molecular and intracellular level

Only an overview can be given here. The critical process is that of excitation–contraction coupling, the mechanism by which electrical changes at the muscle cell membrane (sarcolemma) are coupled to the activation of the intracellular contraction apparatus. This apparatus consists of highly organised regular lattices of protein filaments which interdigitate in such a way that the filaments can move past each other — the sliding-filament model. In terms of connective tissue architecture, each muscle has an almost fractal structure, in that each level of magnitude replicates the next (Fig. 12.26). The whole muscle consists of numerous bundles (fasciculi) of fibres. The fibres are bound together by endomysium and the fasciculi by perimysium. The whole muscle is enclosed in a sheath of epimysium. Each fibre is an elongated multinucleate cell bounded by a limiting membrane, the sarcolemma. Within each cell lie further 'bundled' structures, the myofibrils, which contain the interdigitating contractile elements actin ('thin filaments') and myosin ('thick filaments'). These lie within the cytoplasm of the cell, and are organised into serially repeating units or sarcomeres, giving the familiar striped or striated appearance on light microscopy. The transverse components of the sarcomeres are cytoskeletal elements, anchoring the contractile proteins and connecting them to the sarcolemma to enable contraction of the whole fibre. The bundles of myofibrils are separated by the complex membranous network of the sarcoplasmic reticulum and by other intracellular organelles, notably mitochondria. Calcium is specifically stored within the reticulum; muscle cells are

too large to rely on the diffusion of calcium from the extracellular pool. The membrane of the reticulum is in structural continuity with the sarcolemma via a system of membranous T-tubules. Thus the whole of the sarcolemma and reticulum can become electrically activated as the AP is propagated. Calcium stored within the reticulum acts as the second messenger in the process of excitation–contraction coupling. When the AP reaches and depolarises the T-tubular membrane, voltage-gated Ca channels are opened in the contiguous reticulum, releasing Ca into the cytoplasm surrounding the myofibrils. This calcium binds to troponin, a protein bound to the actin, causing it to change its molecular conformation, displace a second actin-bound protein (tropomyosin) and expose binding sites on the actin for the attachment of the adjacent myosin filaments. Conformational change in the myosin, once bound to the actin, produces the sliding movement which is magnified into contraction of the fibre and thus of the muscle.

The cycle of changes in the binding region of the myosin filament which produces the change of shape is called the cross-bridge cycle. The process is powered by the hydrolysis of ATP to ADP, and is cyclical because of the alternating and differing levels of affinity for myosin of ATP and ADP. The ADP is rephosphorylated to form more ATP as the cycle progresses. There are three possible biochemical pathways for this phosphorylation, in muscle as in all other cells. These pathways are oxidative phosphorylation, glycolysis, and direct phosphorylation. The first of these relies on the oxidation of imported substrates such as carbohydrates and fatty acids, occurs in the mitochondria, and requires the presence of a copious capillary blood supply and an oxygen-binding protein (myoglobin). The second, a much more rapid process, is anaerobic and involves the breakdown of locally stored glycogen via the pyruvate cycle, with lactate as the main 'waste' product. The third process, direct phosphorylation of ADP, utilises locally-stored creatine phosphate; it is not directly synthetic, and serves as a rapid and quickly available 'holding mechanism' until one or both of the other, synthetic, processes come into play.

Tissue level: fibre type and metabolism

Skeletal muscle contains two main cell (fibre) types, each specialised for a particular work rate and power output. The difference between types is determined by the rate at which ATP is used, this in turn being decided by the type of myosin isoenzyme present in the cell. Those which work more slowly and are adapted for sustained (low fatigue), lower power contraction utilise mainly

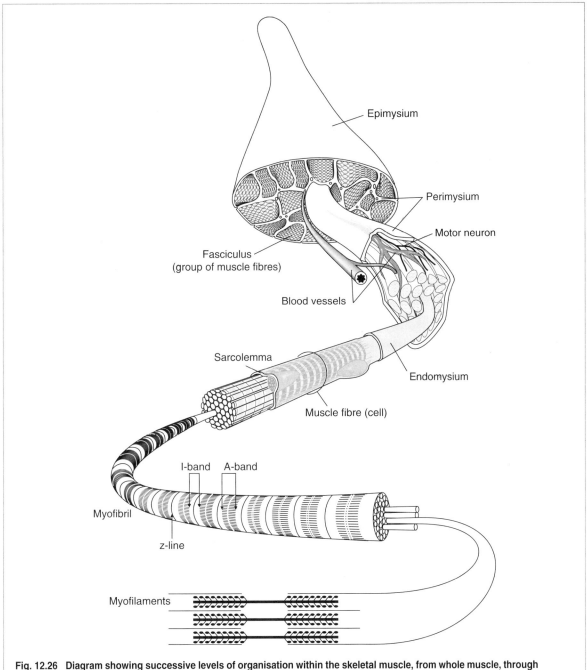

Fig. 12.26 Diagram showing successive levels of organisation within the skeletal muscle, from whole muscle, through fasciculi, fibres, myofibrils and myofilaments.

oxidative phosphorylation, and so are well vascularised and contain much myoglobin, accounting for their 'red' colour. Those which work fastest, and are adapted for rapid and high powered work, rely on anaerobic glyco-

lysis, have fewer capillaries and less myoglobin, and are thus 'white' fibres. They fatigue quickly as the intra-muscular glycogen is used up and lactate concentration rises. Slow, red, oxidative fibres are of Type I; fast, white, anaerobic glycolytic fibres are of Type IIB. There is also an intermediate group of fibres, which utilise oxidative glycolysis (Type IIA). Humans have a good balance of these fibre types; cats have mainly fast fibres, dogs mainly slow. Fibre types are never mixed within motor units. Each unit contains either slow or fast fibres. Slow units have small motor neurons and few fibres. The axons are slower conducting but the neurons are relatively more excitable, and are recruited first and act frequently. Fast units have large, fast conducting axons but less excitable cell bodies, and contain many muscle fibres. They are recruited in maximal efforts of short duration (rapid fatiguability). Controlled variation in the number and type of motor unit recruited, and in the frequency of stimulation, allows gradation of the power of contraction over a wide range. Exercise and training do not cause motor units to change in type nor to increase in number, though individual fibres increase in size and strength as more contractile filaments are synthesised. Disuse and denervation both lead to muscle atrophy. The regeneration pattern in terms of unit type is determined by the level of recruitment (frequency of activation).

Patterns of motor unit activity can be assessed clinically using electromyography (EMG). Diagnostic EMG is most efficiently carried out using fine needles inserted into the muscle; surface electrodes may be used for large superficial muscles. It measures electrical activity, recording action potentials from contracting fibres. It does not involve electrical stimulation (contrast nerve conduction studies). Recordings are made in four stages. Firstly, the potentials are recorded during and immediately after insertion of the needle (insertional activity). Secondly, a recording is made with the muscle at rest. Thirdly, the patient is asked to make a minimal contraction of the muscle. Lastly, a maximal voluntary contraction is made (this gives the so-called interference pattern record). The traces for all stages are compared with known normal patterns in order to make the diagnosis. Characteristic patterns occur in disease and in denervation, and vary with the age and severity of the lesion. For example, in a denervated muscle there is no activity on minimal or maximal contraction. If the denervation is due to recoverable nerve damage (neurapraxia) the recordings at insertion are normal, and there is the normal electrical 'silence' at rest. If there is severance of the axons (axonotmesis) or of the nerve (neurotmesis), there is increased insertional activity, with fibrillations present at rest. Patterns also alter with time from injury or onset of disease, as the extent of degenerative and regenerative change in nerve and muscle varies.

The subjective sense of 'fatigue' (tiredness) is not co-extensive with local, biochemical muscle fatigue. Central and systemic factors are also involved in tiredness.

Organ level

This covers the organisation of fibres within muscles (muscle architecture) and the action of muscles both as single entities and in groups. Fibres and fascicles tend to be aligned according to function. These differences of alignment may occur within a single muscle (e.g. deltoid, obliquus internus abdominis) or between muscles (compare sartorius and gluteus maximus). The architecture of the muscle also changes as it approaches its attachment to bone, often with a gradual transition into the structure of the tendon. Maximal force production relates directly to the cross-sectional area of the muscle concerned.

Muscles may contract in two functionally different ways: isotonically and isometrically. Isotonic contraction involves change in muscle length with constant load. This change in length does not have to be a decrease: when the external force exceeds that generated by the muscle, the muscle may lengthen as it contracts. In molecular terms, the stretched cross-bridges are unable to change their conformation to produce shortening. Bonds are broken and reform, almost in ratchet fashion. This type of contraction — eccentric contraction — has great potential for muscle injury. A common example of eccentric contraction is the simply tested action of biceps brachii during controlled active elbow extension with gravity: biceps is 'paying out rope' to prevent a sudden extension of the elbow. Triceps, the prime elbow extensor, remains flaccid. More commonly, muscle shortens as it contracts, tension being proportional to load: this is concentric contraction. A muscle may also contract isometrically, developing tension without changing its length: this happens if a load is applied which is greater than the muscle can lift. Muscles cannot generate force at the limits of their length: this fact supports the sliding-filament theory of muscle action. As in any machine, the energy cost of muscle action can be expressed in terms of its efficiency of action. This is the ratio of the mechanical work performed to the (chemical) energy produced by the hydrolysis of ATP. The maximal efficiency of this process occurs in partially loaded muscle and is about 45%, but loss of energy as heat and in other energy-consuming reactions within the muscle reduces the overall efficiency to 20–25%.

Muscles tend to work in groups rather than as individuals; in the limbs these functional groups are organised anatomically into separate osteofascial compartments. Muscles and groups may act together, when they are said to be synergists. Groups combining to produce an action may be widely separated anatomically: if your calf muscles did not act when you throw a ball, you would fall over. The main muscles producing the action are the prime movers. Muscles which act to oppose the prime movers are acting as antagonists; prime movers and antagonists may act together when muscles act as fixators, as in the stabilisation of the shoulder during precise action of the unsupported hand. In general, proximal limb muscles and trunk muscles tend to act in groups for stabilisation, while distal limb muscles act more precisely when the hand or foot is free-moving. The central neurological representation and control of these different groups reflect their functional differences. It should be emphasised again that the terms 'origin' and 'insertion' can be misleading in considering muscle function. All muscles act from their fixed end to their mobile end: the latter need not always be distal to the former. Think of the actions of the lower limb muscles when the foot is bearing weight, or of the pectoralis major and latissimus dorsi when the arms are fixed and the chest is moving. Such 'reverse action' explains the utility of many muscles as accessory muscles of respiration. Finally, in analysing muscle movements, never forget the action of gravity. The body is very economical: if gravity can supply the force necessary for a movement, then the muscles will let it do so. Feel the flaccidity of your abdominal muscles ('trunk flexors') as you bend forward.

BONE — STRUCTURAL PHYSIOLOGY

Bone looks as if it stays the same for decades, but in fact it is constantly changing. Stages and events in the life of a bone include its development and growth, its response to physical stress, its changes with age from maturity to senility, and its response to injury both macroscopic and microscopic. New bone must be formed throughout life: the process and sequence of events are always the same, involving both the laying down and the removal of bone. These processes must be coupled and coordinated. Development and growth entail the modelling of bone — morphogenesis and ossification — as well as remodelling to maintain its overall shape, proportion and soft-tissue relationships as it grows. All other events in bone involve structural remodelling. Thus the circumstances of remodelling are physiological, adaptive, age-related and reparative.

Bone has three main functional rôles:

1. mechanical
2. biochemical
3. haemopoietic.

Change occurring as part of the first is integral to the development and maintenance of the form of bone, both macroscopic and microscopic, and will be the subject of this section. Change as part of the second, the rôle of bone as an ion reserve, particularly with respect to calcium and phosphate, is dealt with elsewhere, especially in Chapter 14. Change as part of the third, the rôle of bone in haemopoiesis, is discussed in Chapter 10. All three groups of changes are inextricably linked, as all ultimately involve change in the structure of bone and in overall bone mass by the normally coupled mechanisms of bone formation and resorption. Physiological remodelling occurs during biochemical homeostasis and during haemopoiesis, as well as during the constant process of micro-repair and damage limitation which accompanies the normal response of bone to loading. Adaptive changes occur as loading promotes bone formation or unloading its resorption. Reparative remodelling occurs on both a microscopic and a macroscopic scale during the process of fracture healing. During ageing the coupling of bone formation and resorption is often disturbed.

The concept of bone mass is an important one, linking the anatomy, physiology and pathology of bone, especially as the latter relates to metabolic bone disease. Total bone mass, including organic and inorganic constituents, increases during development and growth to a maximum reached at 20–30 years of age. There is then normally a steady state for about 20 years, but even during this period, turnover of about 15% of the total bone mass occurs every year. In later life, bone mass decreases, hormonal influences such as that of oestrogen withdrawal being particularly important.

Bone formation and resorption

There are four main mechanisms by which bone mass can alter physiologically or pathologically: formation may be stimulated and/or resorption inhibited, resulting in an increase in bone mass; stimulation of resorption and/or inhibition of formation will have the opposite effect. The process of bone formation, and the nature of the final product — mature bone, cortical and cancellous — is generally consistent, though there are two distinct mechanisms of ossification distinguished by the local tissue environment in which the process occurs (see below). Bone, as a connective tissue, has a cellular component and an extracellular matrix. The matrix is mineralised.

Mechanisms of structural development and maintenance at cellular level are well recognised; the final common pathway at molecular level by which these mechanisms are translated into structural change has yet to be determined. The cellular agents of bone formation and bone resorption are the osteoblasts and osteoclasts, respectively. The osteoblasts belong to a mesenchymal lineage which includes both the surface lining cells of bone and the osteocytes in their lacunae. Osteoclasts develop from extraskeletal blood-borne precursors, sharing their stem cells with circulating monocytes and macrophages. Active osteoblasts produce the organic matrix of bone, based on Type I collagen and osteocalcin, to form a framework of osteoid on which mineralisation later occurs in the presence of normal plasma calcium and phosphate concentrations. Osteoclasts resorb bone as a whole, releasing the inorganic ions and breaking down the matrix proteins. The coupling mechanism must require communication between cells of the osteoblast and osteoclast lineages, the chemical basis of which remains to be elucidated. It is now thought that initial determinant factors act upon cells of the osteoblast series in all cases, and that osteoclast activity is thus under secondary control. The coupling process is thus facilitated, enabling the body mass to be 'defended' when threatened by physiological stress or by pathological change. Major regulating agents include hormones such as parathyroid hormone and the active metabolite of vitamin D, together with local autocrine and paracrine agents such as growth factors and other cytokines. In addition, bone both produces and transmits electrical signals, usually as a result of loading-related microdeformation. The structurally linked osteocytes, communicating via processes in canaliculi in the bone, are probably involved in transduction of mechanical stimuli. It is also important to remember that there are nerves in bone. The endothelial cells lining the copious blood vessels of bone are increasingly implicated in cellular processes of remodelling and of fracture healing. The extracellular matrix is also now being seen to have a rôle which exceeds that of passive support: it may also be involved in the sensation and transduction of mechanical stimuli. Morphogenesis and growth of bone also involve the increasingly frequently recognised process of 'programmed cell death' or apoptosis. It is very likely that it has a part to play in physiological remodelling.

The two mechanisms of ossification are termed intramembranous and endochondral. The former is a direct mechanism in which bone develops in vascularised mesenchyme without an intermediary stage. In the latter, bone develops on the template of a cartilage model: the developing bone replaces the pre-existing cartilage. Intramembranous ossification occurs in the formation of the 'membrane bones' — the vault of the skull, the face and mandible, and most of the clavicle. The remainder of the skeleton ossifies in cartilage, but not exclusively so, as all subperiosteal deposition of new bone (by which

bones grow in thickness) is intramembranous. Note that in growing tubular bones this deposition must be accompanied by coupled endosteal resorption to maintain the relative size of the medullary cavity.

Intramembranous ossification begins in an area of mesenchymal cell condensation vascularised by capillaries. The mesenchymal cells differentiate into osteogenic precursors and subsequently into osteoblasts which lay down the organic matrix which subsequently becomes mineralised. A network of mineralised bony trabeculae is thus formed, and by subsequent appositional growth, resorption by blood-borne osteoclasts, and remodelling, fully differentiated bone is produced. Endochondral ossification during development also begins with mesenchymal cell condensation, but here the mesenchymal cells first differentiate into chondroblasts. These produce a hyaline cartilage 'model' in the general shape of the future bone, limited by a fibrous perichondrium. As this model grows, the matrix of its central region becomes calcified but remains avascular. The perichondrium then becomes vascularised, and its inner layer forms bone intramembranously, becoming a periosteum. Capillaries from the periosteum then invade the calcified cartilage, bringing osteoprogenitor cells which become osteoblasts and form bone, initially on the framework of calcified cartilage. The original cartilage is eventually fully removed and replaced by mature bone. This area of the developing bone is the primary ossification centre. In growing long bones, the ends of the bones (epiphyses) remain cartilaginous until secondary centres appear. Endochondral ossification then continues in the growth plates until skeletal maturity is reached. Even after maturity it forms part of the fracture-healing process.

LOCOMOTION

The physiology of locomotion is a large area, involving both the coordinative neurophysiology of locomotor control and the physiology of joint movement. It is very easy to regard the locomotor system purely as a series of effectors, and to forget the essential part played by the afferent side of the system. A brief overview of locomotor control will be followed by a summary of joint physiology and some special considerations regarding posture, gait and the use of the upper limbs.

Locomotor control

The basic unit of motor control is the spinal reflex. The main spinal reflexes are the stretch and inverse myotatic (Golgi tendon organ) reflexes and the flexion withdrawal reflex. The first two are negative feedback loops, each with a different controlled variable. In the stretch ('tendon jerk') reflex the variable is muscle length and the sensor is the muscle spindle, lying functionally in parallel with the muscle. In the inverse myotatic reflex the variable is muscle tension, the sensor is the Golgi tendon organ which is found in extensor muscles and is functionally in series with the muscle. The stretch reflex is monosynaptic and excitatory to the prime mover and synergists, with associated inhibition of antagonists via Renshaw interneurons. The disynaptic inverse myotatic reflex is inhibitory to the prime mover. Such reciprocal innervation provides for coordination during rhythmic movements and during fixation of a joint. Postural control also involves brainstem reflexes whose receptors are in the vestibular apparatus and in the neck.

Modulation of these primitive reflexes is initially a property of the palaeocerebellum, with higher connections both cortical and subcortical. Injury of the spinal cord may damage these higher connections, so that the spinal reflexes become hyperactive. The archicerebellum is concerned with the control of posture and gait. Proximal and distal muscle activity in the limbs are under mainly separate systems of descending control, both pyramidal (from the cerebral cortex) and extrapyramidal (from the basal ganglia). Proximal muscles, together with trunk muscles, are involved mainly in posture, balance and locomotion, and are controlled by the more medially placed descending pathways. These pathways do not cross the midline in their entirety, so that both sides of the body can be controlled by them (trunk muscles often act bilaterally). Distal limb muscles, involved in more precise, manipulative movements, are controlled by the lateral descending pathways, which control only the contralateral side of the body. This descending motor activity is modulated by input from the neocerebellum and basal ganglia on the basis of afferent information from the moving structures. Locomotion and other rhythmic activities (e.g. chewing, respiration) are neurologically 'programmed' centrally, in specialised biological oscillators called pattern generators.

Joint movement

Normal function of synovial joints relies upon the presence of normal articular cartilage. This cartilage absorbs and transmits load, functions mediated by the water-imbibing and releasing properties of the proteoglycan component of the extracellular matrix. The proteoglycans are held within a complex network of collagen; the matrix is heterogeneous, varying at differing depths and areas within the articular surface of the joint. The subchondral bone, immediately beneath the articular cartilage, also has an increasingly recognised rôle in normal joint physiology.

Considering the joint as a whole, on the afferent side the most important sensory modalities are pain and proprioception. Joints contain copious pain receptors, as well as mechanoceptors responding both to transient and sustained spatial deformation. Proprioception as a whole also utilises sensory input from muscles and from skin, and is mediated centrally by the dorsal columns of the spinal cord.

Regarding joint motion, it is important to understand the directions in which a particular joint can move, the motors producing the movements, and the constraints on movement which determine the range of motion at that joint. In practical clinical, as opposed to biomechanical, terms, think of the movements of the joint in the three orthogonal axes ('x, y and z'). The axes of movement of many joints vary during movement: the knee, radio-ulnar and subtalar joints are examples.

Constraints to movement include the joint capsule, ligaments intra- and extra-articular, bone shape, and local soft tissues especially muscles. Every joint is a functional compromise between stability and mobility, the level of compromise being determined by the physiological requirements of the joint.

Special considerations — posture, gait and upper limb function

Muscles can act as movers, as fixators or as both. Many more muscles are involved even in apparently simple movements than would be suspected from superficial inspection. A 'whole body approach' to muscle action is advocated, particularly during the clinical diagnosis of sports injuries. To use Apley's well-known invocation, just 'look, feel and move' for yourself. The antigravity muscles may not be those initially apparent in a particular motor activity: remember eccentric muscular contraction (see above). There are other paradoxes in the physiology of posture. Few if any muscles are active during normal stance at rest: you stand on your ligaments and joint capsules. Only if the line of weight-bearing of the body sways 'out of true' do muscles come into play. It has already been pointed out that muscles in the lower limb usually act from their fixed distal attachments to their more mobile proximal ones as they change the position of the weight-bearing body (e.g. from sitting to standing) or support the trunk over the feet in adjustments of position during standing and walking.

Human gait is a cyclical, patterned movement which is maximally efficient when the centre of gravity of the body moves least from its position during standing, just anterior to the body of the second sacral vertebra. There are two main varieties of gait: walking, in which one foot is always on the ground, and running, in which there is a period when both feet are off the ground. In walking, each limb has a stance phase, when its foot is on the ground, and a swing phase when it is not. Stance phase constitutes about 60% of the cycle, and extends from heel strike through foot flat to toe off. In swing phase the limb accelerates to the mid-swing point, then decelerates to the next heel strike. Both concentric and eccentric muscle action occur during the gait cycle, the latter allowing more controlled joint movement. It is during this eccentric action (contraction while lengthening) in the running cycle that many sports injuries of muscle occur. The normal gait pattern is often characteristic for a particular individual, and is controlled by a pattern generator under modulation from higher neural centres. Abnormalities of gait pattern can be diagnostic in a variety of orthopaedic and neurological disorders.

Muscles of the upper limb usually act from their fixed proximal attachment to their mobile distal one. The more proximal groups frequently act as fixators, stabilising the shoulder complex while the hand is in use. Distal groups are capable of fine and precise movements as well as more powerful actions. These varieties of movement characterise the types of grip. The power grip, as when using a tool such as a hammer, requires the concerted action of normal wrist extensors together with the digital flexors. The precision grip, as in picking up a pin, uses thumb and index and requires the presence of normal median-nerve sensation as well as finely controlled muscle action. Other, intermediate types of grip include the key grip, involving strong adduction of the thumb against the radial side of the index finger, and the 'chuck' grip, in which all the digits are employed like the blades of a drill-chuck, as in picking up a ball. Modified forms of these grips can be learned by patients with arthritis of the hand and wrist, or with neurological deficits involving the small muscles of the hand.

PATHOLOGY
OVERVIEW OF CONTENT

The pathology of selected commonly-presenting conditions and disorders is dealt with at a basic science level. Some key principles of the management of these conditions will be included where indicated. Neuropathology (central and peripheral) and pathology of skeletal muscle are not included. The pathology of the bone marrow is dealt with elsewhere (Chapter 10).

KEY CONCEPTS AND LEARNING OBJECTIVES

In the locomotor system as elsewhere, surgical pathology is often erroneously considered as synonymous with morbid anatomy and histopathology. It is vital that in your revision of the surgical pathology of any system you do not neglect the relevant microbiology, clinical biochemistry and immunohaematology. The molecular approach to pathology, which tends to unify these four 'classical subdivisions' of the discipline, is now used increasingly.

It is important to relate the principles of morbid anatomy to those of normal topographical anatomy. Fascial planes and compartments, tissue layers and 'spaces' all determine the spread of pathological fluids and the protection of normal structures from pathological processes. Patterns of fibrosis and contracture, scarring and 'walling-off' of infection are all based on the underlying patterns of normal soft-tissue anatomy.

The microbiology of the locomotor system is largely concerned with common bacterial pathogens of soft-tissue, bone and joint infection and with infection as a complication of trauma (accidental and surgical). More recently, other pathogens have assumed great significance, e.g. the management of orthopaedic problems in the patient infected with HIV.

Clinical biochemistry here mainly concerns the endocrine and metabolic disorders of bone, while examples of the advent of molecular surgical pathology may be found in the immunology of the arthritides and in the genetics of the many heritable locomotor disorders.

Finally, remember that a wide range of haematological, neurological and neuromuscular pathology may present primarily as a locomotor problem.

FRACTURES AND THEIR COMPLICATIONS

Revise the anatomy and relations of the commonly fractured bones; neurovascular and fascial relations are especially important here. Note how muscle and fascial attachments to bone determine displacement after fracture. The anatomy of osteofascial compartments is of particular significance in the leg, where compartment syndrome is not infrequently seen as a complication of fractures. Remember the systemic physiological effects of major musculoskeletal trauma, and how disordered physiology can lead to systemic complications in circumstances of haemorrhage and shock (see Ch. 9).

In considering the basic pathology of fractures, the following questions need to be answered.

1. Why do bones break?
2. How do bones break?

3. How do bones heal?
4. How does the incidence of common fractures relate to the age of the patient?
5. What are the common complications of fractures?

Why bones break

Normal bones break when they are stressed beyond the load which they are 'designed' to bear. The pathological force leading to fracture is often sudden and large: physiological loading is cyclical. However, even cyclical loading of low magnitude can lead to fracture. Such fractures are known as stress or fatigue fractures, and occur mainly in the lower limb after excessive or unaccustomed exercise. If a bone breaks as a result of a force which should be within the physiological tolerance of that bone, then pre-existing abnormality of the bone should be suspected. The fracture is then said to be pathological. The bony abnormality does not have to be neoplastic: a wide variety of conditions, including infection and metabolic disease, can weaken bone.

How bones break

In children, bones commonly break intraperiosteally, often with only part of the cortical circumference involved. These are 'greenstick' fractures. In adults the pattern of fracture is decided by the magnitude and direction of the causative force. The size of the force determines whether the fracture is complete or incomplete, displaced or undisplaced, simple or comminuted, and open (involving a wound of the skin) or closed. The direction of the force applied determines the obliquity of the fracture, which may be transverse, oblique or (long) spiral. Most long-bone fractures are caused by a force which involves rotation. The direction of force must be diagnosed from clinical and radiological examination of the fracture, as it must be reversed during manipulative reduction.

How bones heal

Bone differs from other musculoskeletal tissues in that its healing involves tissue regeneration: bone heals by forming new bone. The process involved is considered below.

Age and fracture

Patterns of growth, development and ageing in certain bones combine with the prevalence of particular forms of injury to determine the relationship of common fractures with age. Elderly patients with reduced bone mass who fall frequently tend to fracture the proximal femur and the distal radius. Osteoporotic vertebral body fracture, strictly a form of pathological fracture, is also common in this age group. Only growing bones can sustain injuries of the growth plate.

Complications

These should always include both the complications of the fracture and the complications of its management. Complications of injury are traditionally and sensibly classified as general and local, the local being subdivided into 'early and late'.

Main general complications

- hypovolaemic shock
- adult respiratory distress syndrome
- systemic infection and septicaemic shock
- fat embolism.

Early local complications These chiefly reflect related soft-tissue involvement:

- infection
- nerve injury
- vascular injury
- injury to local viscera
- compartment syndromes
- associated local joint injury and infection.

Late local complications These are mainly complications which modify the healing process and which affect rehabilitation:

- delayed union
- malunion
- non-union
- joint stiffness and myositis ossificans
- ischaemic contractures
- algodystrophy (Südeck's atrophy)
- avascular necrosis of bone
- growth disturbance
- osteoarthritis.

Most of the above may also be complications of the treatment of the fracture. Particular complications of fracture management include those of splintage, such as compartment syndrome and nerve entrapment, and those of internal fixation, such as infection, delayed union, and wound problems.

Fracture healing

The process of fracture healing involves the recruitment of bone-forming cell precursors (osteoprogenitors) to the fracture site, the induction and activation of these precursors to differentiate into cartilage- and bone-forming cells (osteoinduction), and the presence of an osteoconductive surface or template on which this new bone can be produced (the various types of 'callus'). The process is best learned as a series of coordinated temporal stages whose progression is determined by numerous factors both local and systemic. The stages as classically described are based on light-microscopic histological appearances, but more recent approaches involve biochemical cascades, cell population kinetics and considerations of local strain environment. The process is regulated and coordinated, with a timescale which appears predetermined for each particular limb and bone.

The classical histological stages of fracture healing (Fig. 12.27) are:

- haematoma formation
- inflammation — the blood clot is organised to form granulation tissue
- callus formation:
  - primary, highly cellular soft callus formed mainly from uninjured periosteum a little distant from the fracture ends (where the bone is dead)
  - external bridging callus, formed mainly by locally induced osteoprogenitors in the 'fracture gap'
  - late medullary callus, formed mainly within the medullary cavity at the fracture
- conversion of callus to woven bone: bridging callus passes from granulation tissue through a cartilaginous or chondroid stage. The chondroid material is converted to woven bone by a process of endochondral ossification. Bone is also formed in the healing fracture by intramembranous ossification, both from the periosteum and in the medulla
- consolidation and remodelling of the woven bone ('osteoid') into lamellar bone

- reconstitution of the medullary canal and recovery of the shape of the bone.

These histological stages coincide biochemically with a series of changes in the predominant type of collagen produced as healing progresses from fibrous granulation tissue through 'chondroid' and osteoid to mature bone. The sources and sequence of appearance, proliferation, migration and differentiation of the various cell populations involved in the inflammatory and osteogenic stages remain controversial. Local and invading vascular endothelial cells and pericytes may be the prime source of osteoprogenitor cells.

Factors affecting fracture healing

The following can all be considered as aspects of the fracture environment.

General: the patient and local or systemic disease
- age — children heal faster than adults
- state of nutrition and general health
- the presence of infection at the fracture
- pre-existing abnormal bone at the fracture ('pathological fracture'). This may be genetically determined (e.g. osteogenesis imperfecta) or the result of acquired conditions (e.g. malignant disease, metabolic bone disease).

Local anatomical environment
- site — upper limb bones heal faster than lower
- blood supply — soft-tissue attachments

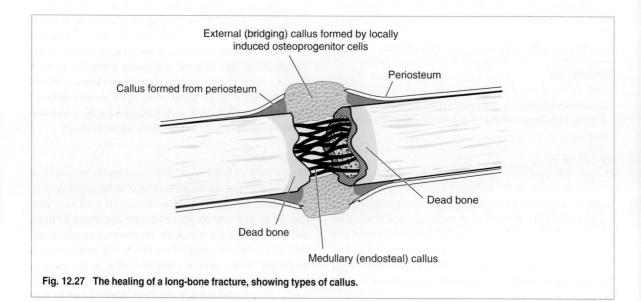

Fig. 12.27 The healing of a long-bone fracture, showing types of callus.

External (bridging) callus formed by locally induced osteoprogenitor cells

Periosteum

Callus formed from periosteum

Dead bone

Dead bone

Medullary (endosteal) callus

- the proximity of the bone ends — the amount of bone loss; soft-tissue interposition
- whether the fracture surfaces are intra-articular
- nerve supply.

Biomechanical environment   There is no doubt that the mechanical environment of the fracture has a great effect on the way in which it heals. There is an optimal compromise between desirable movement and stability of immobilisation. Healing bones need to be used: weight-bearing bones need to bear weight to heal soundly. Limited movement at the fracture site promotes external (bridging) callus formation. Fractures internally fixed with compression seem to omit the stage of external callus formation. Healing is said to be by primary bone union, in which groups of osteoclasts tunnel across the fracture line ('cutter heads') and are followed by osteoblasts so that lamellar bone is directly laid down. A special kind of callus forms between bone ends which are gradually distracted on external fixation devices as part of the surgical treatment of limb length inequality and of growth deformities.

How the mechanical signals are transduced is the subject of much current study in view of the possible therapeutic applications.

Electromagnetic environment   Stressed bone produces electrical currents. The rôle of such local currents and magnetic fields in the healing process is controversial. Some use has been made therapeutically of both direct and electromagnetically induced current.

Biochemical and pharmacological environment   The search for a pharmacological promoter of fracture healing has led to much recent work on local biochemical influences such as cytokines, growth factors, prostaglandins and changes in pH and oxygenation. Systemic biochemical factors such as circulating hormones also influence the rate and quality of healing. Humoral factors produced by the healing fracture may also circulate: there are measurable effects on the structure and biochemistry of distant bones as a result of single limb-bone fracture.

Many groups of prescribed drugs affect fracture healing, usually adversely (e.g. corticosteroids, NSAIDs). Certain herbal preparations, such as comfrey ('knitbone') have long been claimed to aid the process.

CONDITIONS OF TENDONS AND TENDON REPAIR

Again the local anatomy and the mechanical environment are of paramount importance. The relationship of the tendons to their sheaths, synovial and fibrous, and to their sources of blood supply, and the occurrence of specialised histological regions (e.g. fibrocartilage) within particular tendons should be borne in mind when considering their pathology. Conditions other than trauma which commonly affect tendons include pyogenic infections of their sheaths, and inflammatory disease both systemic and local. Rheumatoid arthritis often involves tendons, especially in the hands and feet. Synovial inflammation and proliferation may combine with local bony attrition to cause tendon rupture. Disproportion between flexor tendons and their fibrous sheaths in the hand leads to the 'triggering' phenomenon. Trauma to tendons may be open or closed, acute or chronic, single or repetitive. Overuse injury ('repetitive strain injury') falls into the latter category.

Open tendon injury is most commonly seen in the hand. The prognosis for successful function after repair of such injuries is affected by the anatomical 'zone' of the hand within which the injury occurs as well as by the quality of the surgical repair. Anatomical zones are described both for flexor and extensor tendons: their extent is largely determined by changes in the relationship of the tendon to its synovial and fibrous sheaths. Postoperative adhesions commonly cause poor results. Both early active and passive movement of the repaired tendon are advocated to improve the functional result. Such increase in mobility may, however, be obtained at the expense of strength of the repair. The process of tendon repair involves scar formation: the extent of this scar must be minimised. As in most wound healing, the process has inflammatory, proliferative and organisational stages. The cell populations involved, fibroblasts and macrophages, originate within the tendon itself. Synovial healing must also occur: sheaths must be accurately and separately repaired to ensure optimal return of function and tendon excursion. The same considerations apply when tendon grafts are inserted, though here the problem of vascularisation is greater than in primary repair. Tendon repairs are weakest a week or so after surgery. Though most of the strength is regained in 3–4 weeks, it is not maximal until 6 months after surgical repair.

INFECTION OF BONE AND JOINT

Anatomical factors largely determine the patterns of presentation and of spread of bone and joint infection. The anatomy of growing bone, particularly that of its blood supply and its relationship to the growth plate, explains the sites of predilection of acute haematogenous osteomyelitis. The varying susceptibility of synovial joints to infection is also related to their blood supply, to the anatomy of their capsular attachments and to their external vulnerability (e.g. the subcutaneous position of the knee joint or of the MCP joints).

Bone infection (osteomyelitis) and joint infection (septic arthritis) are usually pyogenic but may be granulomatous (e.g tuberculosis, syphilis). Pyogenic osteomyelitis may be acute, subacute, or chronic. The last-named may result from inappropriately treated acute infection, or from the presence of foreign material within the bone.

Osteomyelitis may follow penetrating injury of bone; surgical intervention must be included here (joint replacement, internal fixation of fractures). The usual pathogen in haematogenous osteomyelitis is *Staphylococcus aureus*, though haemophili and streptococci may occur in young children, and Gram negative organisms of urinary origin may cause spinal or pelvic osteomyelitis in the elderly. Subacute osteomyelitis is usually staphylococcal, resulting from untreated or unrecognised acute infection and often discovered radiologically in a patient with few local signs. Chronic osteomyelitis, including that seen around surgical implants, may involve varying pathogens, sometimes surprisingly difficult to isolate and eradicate. Surgical intervention, often radical, may be necessary.

Pyogenic joint infection may be haematogenous or may follow penetrating injury or surgery. The haematogenous kind is commonest in children, and may occur as a complication of the typically metaphyseal acute haematogenous osteomyelitis, especially if part or all of the affected metaphysis lies within the joint capsule. The anatomy of the proximal femoral growth plate and its relationship to the capsule of the hip joint is particularly relevant here. In adults septic arthritis may be seen in the immunologically compromised (HIV, drug abuse, or rheumatoid arthritis in which there may already be joint damage prior to infection) and after joint surgery. Tuberculous infection of bone and joint remains very common in the developing world, and its prevalence is increasing again elsewhere as HIV, social deprivation and anti-tuberculous drug resistance spread. A multiplicity of rarer pathogens, from fungi to anaerobes and protozoa, may also cause bone and joint infection, particularly in the immunocompromised subject. Viral infections of bone have been described: it has been suggested that the commonly-seen Paget's disease of bone (osteitis deformans) is caused by a slow virus.

The optimal management of all forms of bone and joint infection entails rapid and accurate microbiological diagnosis, efficient (usually intravenous) delivery of the appropriate antibiotic, and a low therapeutic threshold for surgical intervention when adequate conservative treatment has failed to produce rapid improvement.

ARTHRITIS

By far the most common forms of non-septic arthritis are osteoarthritis and rheumatoid. Forms of inflammatory arthritis other than rheumatoid include the spondylarthropathies (ankylosing spondylitis, Reiter's, and the enteropathic group), SLE, and the crystal deposition arthropathies (e.g. gout). Haemorrhagic and other non-inflammatory arthritides (e.g. neuropathic) also occur. Only osteoarthritis and rheumatoid will be considered further here.

Note the local anatomical effects of arthritis on the commonly affected joints, and, conversely, the way in which the anatomy of the particular joint can determine the clinical presentation of the arthritis (type of deformity, distribution of pain, detectability of effusion).

Osteoarthritis

Osteoarthritis is a manifestation of degenerative change: the prevalence of primary osteoarthritis increases with age. Secondary osteoarthritis occurs after pre-existing joint damage (e.g. following trauma or infection). The primary lesion in osteoarthritis is now thought to be failure of cartilage repair in stressed areas of the joint. Whether the initial failure lies in the chondrocytes or in the extracellular matrix, and, if the latter, whether in its proteoglycan/hyaluronan or in its collagenous component, is not yet established. Local enzyme dysfunction and abnormal cytokines have also been implicated. Subchondral bone changes are generally thought to be secondary to changes in the articular cartilage, but primacy of the bone changes has been proposed by some.

In summary, the main pathological features are:

- cartilage breakdown with failure of repair in stressed areas, giving the clinical appearance of fibrillation, loss of radiographic 'joint space' and leading ultimately to exposure of bone (eburnation)
- subchondral bone sclerosis with cyst formation
- proliferation and remodelling of cartilage and bone in unstressed areas, presenting as osteophyte formation
- capsular thickening and fibrosis, contributing to joint stiffness.

The pain of osteoarthritis probably arises from the capsule and from the exposed or damaged bone. Articular cartilage is not innervated.

Rheumatoid arthritis

This is a systemic disease, characterised by proliferative and destructive inflammation of synovium but with widespread extra-articular manifestations affecting serosa and blood vessels together with visceral, subcutaneous and ocular connective tissues. Joints tend to be involved symmetrically, the small joints of the hands and feet usually being affected first. More proximal joints, particularly the knees, shoulders and elbows, may also be involved. The cervical spine may be affected, leading to instability and neurological changes. In affected synovial joints, the proliferative synovium or pannus extends over and erodes the articular cartilage, with evidence both of acute and chronic inflammation. Genetic factors are involved in the pathogenesis of the disease, though the primary event is likely to be the activation of helper T (CD4+) cells by an as yet unknown microbial pathogen. These activated cells produce cytokines which activate and perpetuate the process of inflammation within the joint, and also activate the B cell system to produce rheumatoid factors. These are autoantibodies against IgG immunoglobulins in synovial fluid and in serum. Those in the synovial fluid form immune complexes which produce local tissue damage by a Type III hypersensitivity reaction. Secondary osteoarthritic changes may also occur.

BONE TUMOURS

Bones contain many different tissues, all of which may undergo neoplastic change (Box 12.1). Relate the pathology of tumours to the gross anatomy, noting how the blood supply of a bone and its fascial attachments may determine the site and spread of a tumour. The same factors also affect the design of ablative and reconstructive surgical procedures in the management of bone tumours.

The simplest general classification of bone tumours divides them first into benign and malignant groups, organised according to tissue of origin of the tumour. Malignant tumours are further divided into primary and secondary groups: note that secondary (metastatic) bone tumours are far commoner than primary tumours. Primary bone tumours are rare, and with certain well-defined exceptions tend to affect young patients. Older patients may present with chondrosarcoma, or with osteosarcoma as a late complication of Paget's disease or of radiation (secondary osteosarcoma). Metastatic bone tumours originate chiefly from primary lesions in prostate, breast, lung and kidney. Gastrointestinal and thyroid primaries are less common. The secondary tumour may be the first presentation of the disease; such a tumour may present as a pathological fracture. The secondary tumour may be destructive (osteolytic), new bone forming (osteoblastic), or both. Most are osteolytic, though prostate metastases are characteristically osteoblastic. Malignant conditions of haemopoietic origin may also present in bone and be confused with other primary or secondary lesions. Such conditions include leukaemias, lymphomas and multiple myeloma.

The classification of primary tumours according to tissue of origin is shown in Box 12.1.

The commonest primary malignancies are osteosarcoma, chondrosarcoma and Ewing's tumour. The first usually affects long-bone metaphyses (particularly around the knee) in adolescents, the second proximal long bones and girdles in middle-aged patients, and the third is unusual in that it often presents in mid-diaphysis (shaft) of the bone, typically in children and adolescents.

Malignant bone lesions are staged according to histological grade of differentiation, anatomical features (confinement or otherwise to bone and osteofascial compartments), and presence or absence of metastases.

Box 12.1   Classification of primary bone tumours

1. bone-forming tumours
   (a) benign: osteoma, osteoid osteoma, osteoblastoma
   (b) malignant: osteosarcoma

2. cartilage-forming tumours
   (a) benign: chondroma, osteochondroma, chondroblastoma
   (b) malignant: chondrosarcoma

3. tumours of fibrous origin
   (a) benign: fibroma, fibrous dysplasia (strictly a 'tumour-like' condition)
   (b) malignant: fibrosarcoma, malignant fibrous histiosarcoma

4. tumours of uncertain origin
   (a) 'benign' (may be locally aggressive): giant cell tumour of bone
   (b) malignant: Ewing's sarcoma

5. tumours of other tissues present in bone
   (a) benign: lipoma, neuroma, angioma
   (b) malignant: liposarcoma, neurosarcoma, angiosarcoma.

Mixed tumours occur, and there are many subclassifications of the above major groups.

HAND INJURIES AND INFECTIONS

It has been emphasised above that the effective management of hand injuries must be based on a sound knowledge of the anatomy of the hand and of the detailed relationships of its component structures. Read the section on the anatomy of the hand (p. 334) again. The discussion which follows also includes some principles of management.

General principles

The hand is unforgiving. Diagnosis of hand injuries and infections must be prompt and accurate, and effective management must start as early as possible. Failure results in stiffness, often irreversible and severely disabling. Injured hands are painful and tend to swell quickly. The cornerstones of management are elevation, correct splintage, and frequent clinical review for evidence of circulatory compromise. The hand is ideally splinted with the MCP joints flexed to a right-angle and the IP joints extended. The period of splintage should be the minimum consistent with safe healing and rehabilitation. Encircling bandages and plaster casts should be avoided if at all possible, and generously padded if essential. Even though the injury may be in the hand, remember that swelling may occur in the forearm and cause compartment syndromes.

Injuries of bone and joint

Common 'wrist' fractures usually affect the distal radius and ulna. Significant fractures of carpal bones other than the scaphoid are uncommon. Fractures of metacarpals and phalanges are 'mini' long-bone fractures: deforming forces, the pattern of fracture and directions of displacement, and the principles of management are the same as for the large long bones. Accurate reduction and adequate immobilisation are essential. Rotational malunion in particular causes great functional disability and ugly cosmetic deformity. Intra-articular fractures are common at all anatomical levels, and require exact reduction. Dislocations and subluxations of IP joints are often seen: damaged ligaments and joint capsules may require surgical repair. Open injuries of MP and IP joints may go unrecognised unless all lacerations over joints are carefully examined. Most of these joints are subcutaneous, especially when they form part of a clenched fist. Neglect of such injuries can lead to disabling septic arthritis.

Injuries of nerves and tendons

Assume that any laceration overlying a nerve or tendon has damaged that structure until proved otherwise. It is safest to consider all hand injuries 'guilty until proved innocent'. You must be totally familiar with the surface markings and exact anatomical distributions of all nerves and tendons in the wrist and hand. Clinical examination of the hand is incomplete until nerve and tendon function has been assessed. Remember the autonomic (sympathetic) component of the nerves: absence of sweating may be an important physical sign, especially in the uncommunicative patient.

In examining a hand for major tendon injury, look for three signs:

- the position of the digits at rest
- for the long flexors, test active individual interphalangeal movement: flexor superficialis flexes the PIP joint, flexor profundus the DIP joint (there is only one long flexor for the thumb)
- for the extensors, test extension of the digits at each joint (MCP, PIP and DIP).

Having excluded tendon injury, a good screening overview for the major nerves is obtained by examining:

- sensation in the pulps of index and middle finger (median)
- abduction and adduction of the little finger (ulnar)
- sensation on the dorsum of the first (thumb-index) web (radial).

For a more proximal injury (at or above the elbow) median and radial integrity can be quickly assessed by asking the patient actively to flex (FPL — median) then extend (EPL — deep radial) the IP joint of the thumb.

Any laceration over the course of a digital nerve demands careful testing of sensation distal to the lesion. Injuries of tendons are also dealt with above (p. 365).

Hand infections

Most acute hand infections are caused by *Staphylococcus aureus*, though a wide variety of pathogens may be present if the infection results from a bite or if it occurs in an immunocompromised patient. These include Gram negative and anaerobic bacteria, and viruses (e.g. herpes simplex). An infected hand commonly presents following a small and forgotten primary penetrating wound. As well as the local signs of infection in the hand, signs of systemic infection may also be present. Diabetics are particularly at risk. The importance of early diagnosis and prompt effective management has already been stressed. Hand infections must always be taken seriously. Parenteral antibiotics are usually required in all but the most minor cases, and the threshold for surgical intervention (incision and drainage) should be low. The infection may be confined to an anatomical compartment, though subcutaneous infection may occur anywhere. A subcuticular or subcutaneous abscess may communicate through a narrow 'neck' with a deeper, subfascial collection of pus ('collar-stud' abscess). Swelling may be confined to the dorsum of the hand, even when the infection is palmar or deep, as only in the dorsum is the skin loosely attached. The potential for proximal spread is great, especially when flexor tendon sheaths are involved. There may be evident lymphangiitis proximal to the wrist, with involvement of epitrochlear (elbow) and axillary lymph nodes. The main anatomical compartments to consider are:

- distal phalangeal infections: nailfolds (paronychia), pulp spaces (whitlow)
- flexor tendon sheaths and bursae
- palmar and web spaces.

Infection of the nailfold is very common, and frequently requires surgical drainage. The fat of the distal phalangeal pulp is subdivided into many small fascial compartments: the fascia is attached to the periosteum of the phalanx. Localised infection here presents as an acutely tender abscess; the blood supply to the phalanx may be compromised, leading to necrosis of the bone. Such infections usually remain distal to the termination of the digital flexor sheath if promptly treated, but the sheaths should always be examined for tenderness.

The anatomy of the synovial flexor sheaths is shown in Figure 12.13. The expanded sheath of the little finger is sometimes called the ulnar bursa, while that extending proximally from the thumb is the radial bursa; the bursae frequently communicate. Note how both bursae extend proximal to the flexor retinaculum. Flexor sheath infection usually results from penetrating injury, particularly if the wound lies over a joint crease, where the fibrous sheath is thin. The infected finger is held flexed, with pain on passive extension and marked tenderness along the line of the sheath. Established infection requires antibiotic irrigation of the sheath or open drainage.

The deep palmar spaces, thenar and midpalmar, lie dorsal to the flexor tendons. They are described on p. 335 above and shown in Figure 12.28. The web spaces lie between the bases of the digits; the anatomy of the first (betwen thumb and index) differs from that of the other three. The first 'space' lies betwen the skin and the fascia overlying the first dorsal interosseous and adductor pollicis muscles. The other spaces are bordered by the deep attachments of the palmar aponeurosis, and 'floored' by the deep transverse metacarpal ligaments linking the metacarpal heads. The web spaces communicate with the palmar spaces via the lumbrical canals, fine sheaths surrounding the lumbrical muscles as they run palmar to the deep transverse ligaments. Web spaces may be directly infected by penetrating injury, or by spread of a palmar space infection. Infection may involve the palmar spaces from direct penetrating injuries, or by spread from the webs or from the ulnar and radial bursae. Palmar space infections are now rarely seen.

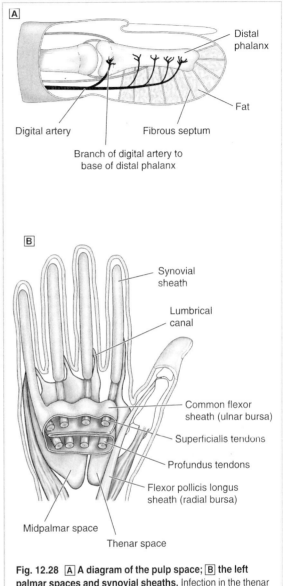

Fig. 12.28 Ⓐ **A diagram of the pulp space;** Ⓑ **the left palmar spaces and synovial sheaths.** Infection in the thenar or midpalmar spaces easily breaks through into the lumbrical canals (connective tissue sheath of the lumbrical muscles), so the canals are shown in continuity with the spaces. A segment of the ulnar bursa has been removed to indicate the disposition of the finger tendons embraced by it.

METABOLIC DISEASE OF BONE

Diseases of bone metabolism may affect both mineralisation and the non-mineralised component; they usually result in changes in bone mass. They are mainly, in the widest sense, disorders of calcium, phosphate and vitamin D metabolism, and may be endocrine, renal or gastroenterological in origin. Disorders of collagen formation may also affect bone (e.g. scurvy).

Metabolic bone diseases may also be classified fairly comprehensively into:

- those associated with hypercalcaemia: e.g. hyperparathyroidism
- those associated with hypocalcaemia: e.g rickets/ osteomalacia; renal osteodystrophy
- normocalcaemic disease with reduced bone mass: e.g. osteoporosis; scurvy
- normocalcaemic disease with increased bone mass: e.g. osteopetrosis; Paget's disease.

The main distinction to appreciate at this stage is that between the two major metabolic conditions which lead to reduced bone mass (osteopenia). These are:

- osteoporosis, which is a multifactorial disorder leading to an overall loss of bone mass and density but not affecting the mineralisation process
- osteomalacia, and its juvenile form, rickets, which are caused by defective bone mineralisation with increase in formation of non-mineralised bone. The underlying biochemical lesion is deficiency of vitamin D.

Osteoporosis

There is no single aetiological factor common to all forms of this condition. There are genetic factors determining maximal bone density, dietary factors related to calcium intake and possibly to vitamin D metabolism, mechanical factors involved in the control of bone remodelling throughout life, physiological age changes, and complex hormonal factors mainly involving deficiency of steroid hormones such as oestrogens. Smoking and excess alcohol consumption have also been incriminated.

Primary forms of osteoporosis occur postmenopausally in women, in the aged of both sexes, and rarely in younger age groups.

Conditions leading to secondary osteoporosis may be grouped, with examples, as follows:

- endocrine — hyperthyroidism, hypothyroidism, hyperparathyroidism, hypogonadism, Cushing's disease, Addison's disease, acromegaly
- gastrointestinal — malabsorption, malnutrition, gastric resections, liver disease
- malignant — multiple myeloma, carcinomatosis

- rheumatic — rheumatoid arthritis, ankylosing spondylitis
- drug-induced — anticonvulsants, alcohol, corticosteroids, anticoagulants
- respiratory — chronic obstructive airways disease, tuberculosis
- miscellaneous — disuse, scurvy, osteogenesis imperfecta.

The final common pathway leading to decreased bone mass is an uncoupling of bone formation from bone resorption, involving both a decrease in bone synthesis and an increase in bone loss. Note that the mineral content of the remaining bone is normal. The effects of osteoporosis are most evident in cancellous bone. Osteoporotic fractures are most commonly seen in bone which is predominantly cancellous, such as the vertebral bodies and the extremities of the long bones, particularly the proximal humerus and femur and the distal radius.

Osteomalacia and rickets

Defective mineralisation of mature bone as a result of disordered vitamin D metabolism leads to osteomalacia; if the bone is still growing, the condition is called rickets. The metabolically active form of the vitamin, 1,25-dihydroxycholecalciferol, acts in gut, bone and kidney in collaboration with parathyroid hormone (PTH) to maintain the serum calcium and phosphorus levels. About 80% of the normal vitamin D requirement is synthesised endogenously in the skin, with the aid of ultraviolet light; the remainder is obtained from the diet. Metabolism to give the biologically active form requires normal hepatic and renal function. The initial effect of a deficiency of vitamin D is a lowering of the serum calcium: compensation occurs as a result of increased PTH activity, but the resulting hypophosphataemia disturbs the $Ca \times P$ product and mineralisation is impaired. There is then an excess of osteoid, the unmineralised component of bone (contrast osteoporosis, in which the amount of osteoid is reduced). In growing bone the ordered sequence of changes at the growth plate is disrupted, with failure of mineralisation, overgrowth of uncalcified cartilage, and excess deposition of abnormal osteoid, resulting in the typical rachitic deformities and weakness of bone. In mature bone there is excess osteoid within the bone, often localised to give diagnostic radiological appearances, and weakness of bone leading to fatigue fracture.

13

Head and neck

Samuel Jacob

ANATOMY

MANDIBLE

The mandible, or the lower jaw, consists of a horizontal body bearing the alveolar process and the lower teeth, and a vertically oriented ramus. The junction between the body and the ramus is the angle of the mandible. The upper part of the ramus divides into an anterior coronoid process and a posterior condyloid process which bears the head and neck of the mandible (Fig. 13.1). The head articulates with the mandibular fossa at the base of the skull to form the temporomandibular joint. The neck has a depression, the pterygoid fovea, in its upper part for the insertion of the lateral pterygoid muscle. The coronoid process receives the attachment of the temporalis muscle.

Medial surface

On the medial aspect of the ramus is the mandibular foramen (Fig. 13.2). This is guarded anteriorly by a projecting process called the lingula to which the sphenomandibular ligament is attached. The inferior alveolar (dental) nerve enters the mandibular foramen and traverses the body within the mandibular canal. It divides into the mental nerve and the incisive nerve. The incisive nerve which supplies the incisors and canine teeth runs beyond the mental foramen within the body in the incisive canal. The trunk of the inferior alveolar nerve supplies the premolars and the molars.

A small groove runs inferiorly and forward from the mandibular foramen. This is the mylohyoid groove and is produced by the nerve to mylohyoid which supplies the mylohyoid and the anterior belly of the digastric muscles. Above the groove is a prominent ridge, the mylohyoid line for the attachment of the mylohyoid muscle. The muscle extends from the level of the last molar tooth to the midline. The two mylohyoids which form the floor of the mouth separate the oral cavity from the neck. The slight depression on the bone below the mylohyoid line is the submandibular fossa where the superficial part of

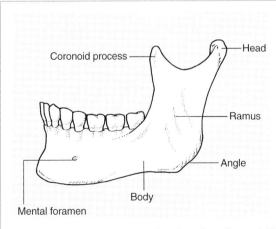

Fig. 13.1 **The mandible: external surface.** From Rogers A W 1992 Textbook of anatomy; Churchill Livingstone, Edinburgh.

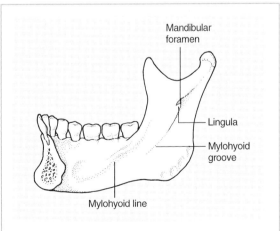

Fig. 13.2 **The mandible: internal surface.** From Rogers op. cit.

the submandibular gland is located. The deep part of the gland and the sublingual gland lie above the mylohyoid line in the oral cavity. This part of the mandible is lined by the mucous membrane of the mouth.

The rough area on the medial surface of the angle of the mandible is for the attachment of the medial pterygoid muscle.

Anteriorly in the midline are two pairs of irregular elevations: the genial tubercles or mental tubercles. The superior pair give attachments to the genioglossi and the inferior to the geniohyoids.

Lateral surface

The anterior border of the ramus extends forward on the body as the external oblique ridge. The buccinator muscle is attached to this ridge. The mental foramen lies halfway between the upper and lower border of the body of the mandible in the region of the apices of the premolar teeth. The mental nerve emerges through the mental foramen to supply the lower lip and the buccal and labial gingiva.

The lateral surface of the ramus gives attachment to the masseter which extends from the angle forward as far as the external oblique line and the second molar tooth.

TEMPOROMANDIBULAR JOINT

This is a synovial joint where the head of the mandible articulates with the mandibular fossa (glenoid fossa) and the articular eminence of the temporal bone. The articular surfaces of this joint are covered by fibrocartilage (not hyaline) and there is also a fibrocartilaginous articular disc dividing the joint cavity into upper and lower compartments.

The capsule of the joint is attached to the neck of the mandible around the head. Above it is attached just anterior to the articular eminence in front, and to the squamotympanic fissure posteriorly.

The articular disc is attached around its periphery to the joint capsule. Anteriorly it is attached to the lateral pterygoid muscle and posteriorly to the temporal bone. The posterior attachment is elastic, allowing forward movement of the disc with the mandible by the contraction of the lateral pterygoid during opening of the mouth.

The capsule of the joint is reinforced by a lateral temporomandibular ligament extending downwards and backwards from the tubercle of the zygoma to the posterior border of the neck of the mandible. The sphenomandibular ligament and the stylomandibular ligament act as accessory ligaments of the joint.

The temporomandibular joints allow depression, elevation, protrusion, retraction and side-to-side movements of the mandible.

MUSCLES OF MASTICATION

There are four pairs of muscles in this group attaching the mandible to the base of the skull:

- the masseter
- the temporalis
- the medial pterygoid
- the lateral pterygoid.

Masseter

The masseter extends from the zygomatic arch to the ramus of the mandible. It has a superficial and a deep part. The superficial fibres run downwards and backwards whereas the deep fibres are vertical. The superficial part elevates the mandible as well as assists in protrusion. When the jaw is protruded the superficial fibres become more vertical and the deep slightly oblique. The two sets of fibres thus allow the muscle to elevate the mandible in all positions of the mandible.

Temporalis

The temporalis takes origin from the temporal fossa and the temporal fascia covering the muscle and is inserted into the coronoid process. Its insertion extends into the retromolar fossa behind the last molar tooth. When lower dentures are fitted they should not extend into the retromolar fossa, to avoid soreness of the mucosa due to contraction of the temporalis muscle. The temporalis elevates the mandible. Its posterior fibres retract the mandible after protrusion.

Lateral pterygoid

The lateral pterygoid which originates from the lateral surface of the lateral pterygoid plate and from the infratemporal surface of the skull is inserted into the capsule of the temporomandibular joint, the articular disc, and also into the upper part of the neck of the mandible. Its contraction pulls the head of the mandible and the articular disc forward during protraction and during the act of opening the mouth. Unilateral contraction of the lateral pterygoid allows the mandible to move to the opposite side. The forward movement of the disc may help to pack the space between the incongruent articular surfaces of the condyle and the articular eminence, thus stabilising the joint.

Mouth opening, side to side movements.

Medial pterygoid

The medial pterygoid extends from the medial surface of the lateral pterygoid plate to the medial surface of the ramus of the mandible. It has a small superficial head of origin from the maxillary tuberosity. It is an elevator of the mandible. Unilateral contraction of the medial pterygoid is important in the side-to-side movement of the mandible, as it deviates the jaw to the opposite side.

The four muscles of mastication are supplied by the mandibular division of the trigeminal nerve. The actions of the muscles of mastication and movements of the mandible at the temporomandibular joint are:

- masseter
  — elevation
- temporalis
  — elevation
  — retrusion (posterior fibres)
- lateral pterygoid
  — depression (open mouth)
  — side-to-side movement (as in chewing)
- medial pterygoid
  — elevation
  — side-to-side movement.

Testing of the muscles of mastication

The muscles of mastication and their nerve supply are tested clinically by asking the patient:

- to clench the teeth; contractions of the masseter and temporalis can be felt
- to move the chin from side to side, testing activity in the pterygoid muscles.

Fractures of the mandible

Fractures of the mandible happen more often than those of the upper facial skeleton. In many cases they are bilateral. The condyle of the mandible can fracture as a result of a blow to the chin, and this may result in dislocation of the temporomandibular joint. Fractures of the angle can run downwards and forwards, or downwards and backwards. In the former case impaction of the two fragments prevents displacement. However, if the fracture line runs downwards and backwards, muscular contraction tends to displace the posterior fragment upwards.

Fractures of the body of the mandible are most common in the canine region, as the length of the root of the canine tooth weakens the bone in this position. A blow on the side of the face may fracture the body of the mandible on the side of impact and fracture the condylar process on the opposite side. Fractures of the body are always compound fractures lacerating the mucosa of the oral cavity.

Dislocation of the mandible

This most commonly occurs in a forward direction when the condyloid process of the mandible slides forward onto the articular eminence and then into the infratemporal fossa. This can be reduced by pressing down the mandible on the molar teeth to stretch the masseter and the temporalis which are in spasm and then pulling up the chin to lever the condyle back into the mandibular fossa.

If the dislocation is associated with a fracture of the neck of mandible, open reduction and wiring of the fractured fragments may be necessary.

ANATOMY OF THE NECK

A thorough knowledge of anatomy is required to treat surgical conditions affecting the neck. For descriptive purposes the neck is divided into various triangles (Fig. 13.3). The sternocleidomastoid (SCM) divides it into two large triangles: the anterior triangle between the SCM and the midline, and the posterior triangle between it and the trapezius.

Surface anatomy of the neck

The following can be felt in the midline from above downwards (Fig. 13.4):

- the mandible
- the hyoid bone — at the level of C3
- the thyroid cartilage — at the level of C4 C5
- the cricoid cartilage — level of C6
- the tracheal rings — the isthmus of the thyroid gland lies over the 2nd, 3rd rings
- the suprasternal notch.

The lower border of the cricoid is an important level in the neck and it corresponds to:

- the junction of larynx with the trachea
- the junction of pharynx with the oesophagus
- the site at which the carotid artery can be compressed against the carotid tubercle of the transverse process of C6 vertebra
- the site at which the needle insertion is made for blocking the brachial plexus (interscalene block) and the stellate ganglion
- the level at which the inferior thyroid artery and the middle thyroid vein enter the thyroid gland.

Each SCM can be tensed and tested by turning the head against resistance to the opposite side.

The pulsation of the common carotid artery can be felt at the anterior border of SCM at the lower border of the cricoid cartilage (C6 level). The common carotid artery

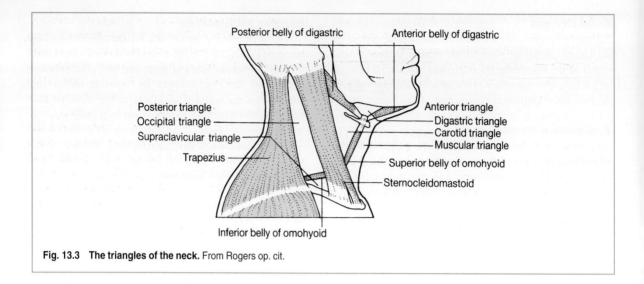

Fig. 13.3 The triangles of the neck. From Rogers op. cit.

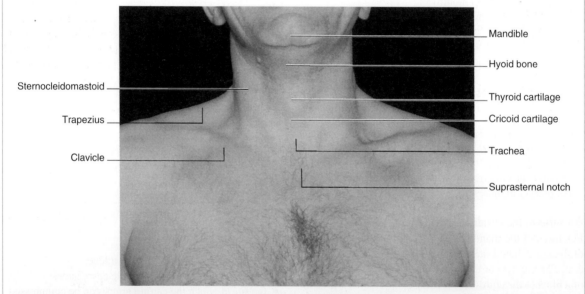

Fig. 13.4 Surface anatomy of the neck. From Jacob S 1996 Anatomy: a dissection manual and atlas; Churchill Livingstone, Edinburgh.

usually bifurcates at the upper border of the thyroid cartilage.

The lower end of the internal jugular vein is located in the gap between the sternal and the clavicular heads of the sternocleidomastoid muscle.

Skin and superficial structures

In the neck, skin incisions are made transversely following Langer's lines or crease lines. The superficial fascia contains the platysma, a striated muscle, which extends from the region of the clavicle, pectoralis major, and the deltoid to the mandible above. To prevent retraction of the severed muscle contributing to a broad scar, platysma is sutured with the skin when the neck wounds are sutured. The muscle has good vascularity. Hence, when skin flaps are raised, platysma is included to maintain good blood supply.

The cutaneous nerves and the superficial veins lie deep

to the platysma between it and the deep fascia. The anterior jugular veins course beneath the platysma on either side of the midline. Just above the suprasternal notch, the veins unite and then pass laterally beneath the SCM to drain into the external jugular vein. The external jugular vein will be described later.

Deep fascia of the neck

The neck has distinct fascial layers which facilitate block dissection in the treatment of metastatic tumours. The layers of the fascia form lines of cleavage during operative dissection and also to a certain extent limit the spread of pus during infection.

There are three distinct layers (Fig. 13.5):

- the investing layer of fascia
- the prevertebral fascia
- the pretracheal fascia.

The *investing layer* is the outer of the three, arising from the ligamentum nuchae and the spines of the cervical vertebrae to completely surround the neck. It splits to enclose the trapezius and the SCM and, between these two, forms the roof of the posterior triangle and also contributes to the fascial capsules of the parotid gland and the submandibular gland. Above, it is attached to the external occipital protuberance, mastoid process, and the zygomatic arch and the mandible. Below, it is attached to the manubrium sterni, the clavicle, the acromion and the spine of the scapula.

The *prevertebral fascia* is anterior to the vertebral column, the prevertebral muscles and the scalene muscles. It prolongs into the axilla as the axillary sheath enclosing the brachial plexus and the subclavian artery. In an axillary block of the brachial plexus the local anaesthetic is introduced into the axilliary sheath. In an interscalene block the plane deep to the fascia is infiltrated, as it contains the roots and trunks of the brachial plexus.

The *pretracheal fascia* splits into an anterior layer that encloses the infrahyoid (strap) muscles and a posterior layer which forms the fascial capsule of the thyroid gland. The fascia extends into the mediastinium and merges with the pericardium. Laterally it blends with the investing layer deep to the SCM. It also contributes to the carotid sheath.

ANTERIOR TRIANGLE

The anterior triangle is bounded by the anterior border of the SCM, the midline and inferior margin of the mandible. It is subdivided into four smaller triangles: submental, submandibular, carotid and muscular (Fig. 13.3). The anterior triangle contains among other structures the thyroid gland, the submandibular gland, the carotid sheath, the deep cervical group of lymph nodes, and the supra- and infrahyoid groups of muscles.

Muscles attached to the hyoid bone

These are in two groups:

- suprahyoids
- infrahyoids.

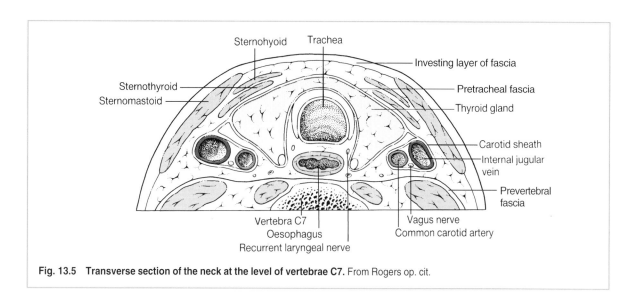

Fig. 13.5   Transverse section of the neck at the level of vertebrae C7. From Rogers op. cit.

The suprahyoids consist of:

- the stylohyoid
- the mylohyoid
- the digastric
- the geniohyoid.

The posterior belly of the digastric is closely related to the major blood vessels and nerves of the neck. The anterior and posterior bellies of the digastric bound the submandibular triangle, which contains the submandibular gland. The mylohyoid muscles of both sides fuse to form the floor of the mouth. The mylohyoid separates the deep part of the submandibular gland from its superficial portion.

The suprahyoids elevate the hyoid and pull it forward during swallowing. Both the supra- and infrahyoids are active in opening the mouth against resistance. The infrahyoids consist of:

- sternohyoid
- sternothyroid
- thyrohyoid
- omohyoid.

Deep to these lie the thyroid gland, the larynx, and the trachea. The infrahyoids or the strap muscles are supplied by the ansa cervicalis (C1, C2, C3), which is a nerve loop on the internal jugular vein (Fig. 13.6). The branches to the muscles enter in their lower half. During exposure of a large goitre the strap muscles are cut in their upper half to preserve the nerve supply from the ansa cervicalis.

Blood vessels in the anterior triangle

Carotid arteries

The right *common carotid artery* is a branch of the branchiocephalic trunk; the left common carotid is a branch of the arch of the aorta. The common carotid

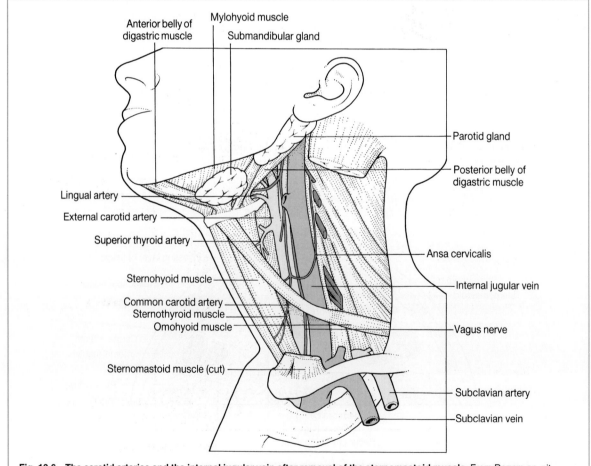

Fig. 13.6 The carotid arteries and the internal jugular vein after removal of the sternomastoid muscle. From Rogers op. cit.

artery divides into the external and the internal carotid arteries at the upper border of the thyroid cartilage. The bifurcation can be at a higher level, a point worth remembering to avoid ligation of the common carotid instead of the external carotid.

The common carotid artery is crossed at the level of the 6th cervical vertebra by the omohyoid muscle (Fig. 13.6). Above this level the artery is superficial and its pulsation can easily be felt, whereas, below, the artery is covered by the infrahyoid muscles and the SCM. The artery is enclosed in the carotid sheath with the internal jugular vein lateral to it and the vagus nerve between the artery and the vein at a deeper plane. The *internal carotid artery* passes vertically upwards as a continuation of the common carotid without giving any branches in the neck. The artery, which is also enclosed in the carotid sheath, is separated from the external carotid by (Fig. 13.7):

- the styloid process
- the stylopharyngeus muscle
- the glossopharyngeal nerve
- the pharyngeal branch of the vagus.

It is accompanied by a plexus of sympathetic nerves. At the base of the skull the artery enters the carotid canal. The intracranial part supplies the eye and the brain.

The *external carotid artery* extends from the point of bifurcation of the common carotid to a point midway between the angle of mandible and the mastoid process. The upper part of the artery enters the parotid gland, where it divides into its two terminal branches: the maxillary artery and the superficial temporal artery. At its commencement the artery is anteromedial to the internal and can be distinguished from the internal by the presence of branches (the internal carotid has no branches in the neck). The branches of the external carotid artery are (Fig. 13.8):

- the superior thyroid artery
- the lingual artery
- the facial artery
- the occipital artery
- the posterior auricular artery
- the ascending pharyngeal artery
- the maxillary artery
- the superficial temporal artery.

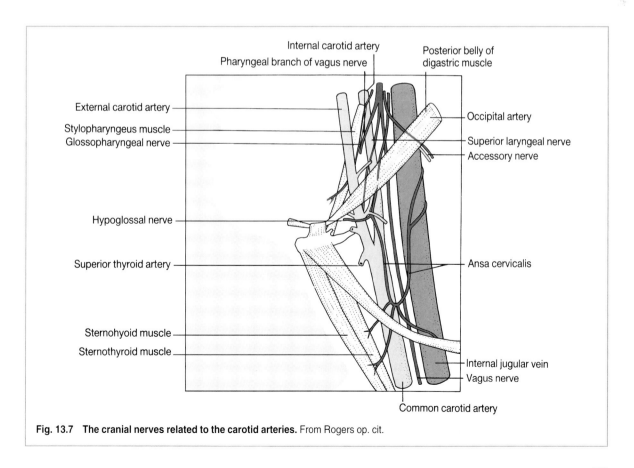

Fig. 13.7 The cranial nerves related to the carotid arteries. From Rogers op. cit.

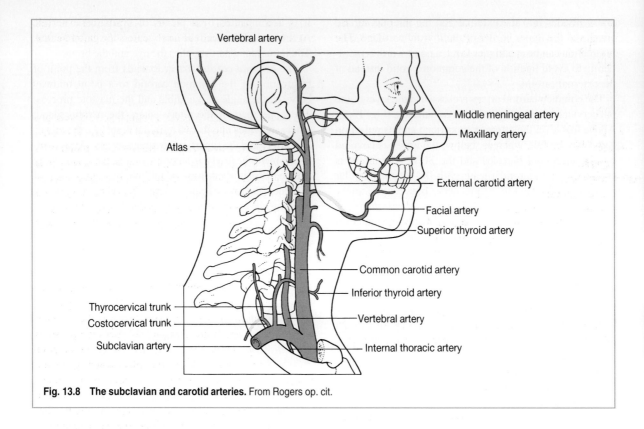

Fig. 13.8 The subclavian and carotid arteries. From Rogers op. cit.

The superior thyroid artery, arising at the commencement of the external carotid, is closely related to the external laryngeal nerve. The nerve should be identified and separated before ligating the artery during thyroid surgery.

The external carotid artery may have to be ligated to control bleeding from one of its inaccessible branches. However, ligation will not eliminate blood flow through it, because of the anastomoses of the branches of the arteries of the two sides.

Internal jugular vein

This is the largest vein in the neck and is formed in the jugular foramen as a continuation of the sigmoid sinus. At its commencement the vein lies behind the internal carotid artery. However, as it descends, the internal jugular vein occupies a position lateral to the internal carotid artery and the common carotid artery. The carotid sheath, in which the artery and the vein lie, is not thick over the vein, allowing the vein to distend. The deep cervical group of lymph nodes is found along the internal jugular vein within the carotid sheath. In a block dissection the internal jugular vein is removed to facilitate removal of the nodes.

In the root of the neck, the internal jugular vein lies behind the gap between the sternal and the clavicular heads of the SCM and ends by joining the subclavian vein to form the brachiocephalic vein. Just below the jugular foramen the inferior petrosal sinus joins the internal jugular vein. The pharyngeal veins, the common facial vein and the superior and middle thyroid veins also drain into the internal jugular vein. The middle thyroid vein or veins may vary in number. They are short and are thin walled. Undue traction during thyroid surgery can result in avulsion of these veins from the internal jugular. Gentle traction, double ligation and sectioning of these veins are important steps in mobilisation of the thyroid lobe.

Internal jugular vein cannulation

This can be done by using a high or low approach. Catheterisation is usually done on the right side, as the right vein is in a straight line with the right brachiocephalic vein and the superior vena cava. In the high approach the vein is palpated lateral to the common carotid artery pulsation deep to the anterior border of the sternocleidomastoid at the level of C6 vertebra, the vein is punctured and a cannula is introduced. In the low approach the needle is inserted near the apex of the triangular gap between the sternal and the clavicular heads of the sternocleidomastoid.

POSTERIOR TRIANGLE

The boundaries are:

- anterior — sternocleidomastoid
- posterior — trapezius
- apex — meeting points of upper attachments of the trapezius and SCM
- base — middle third of clavicle
- roof — investing layer of fascia extending between trapezius and SCM
- floor — splenius capitis, levator scapulae, scalenus medius, scalenus anterior, all covered by the prevertebra fascia.

The skin over the triangle has platysma only in its anterior part. Its absence and hence relatively lower vascularity makes development of skin flaps in the posterior part more difficult.

The posterior triangle contains the subclavian artery (3rd part), transverse cervical artery, suprascapular artery and the occipital artery.

The external jugular vein courses in the superficial fascia obliquely, pierces the deep fascia just above the clavicle and drains into the subclavian vein. Dissection of the lower part of the triangle may cause troublesome bleeding from this vein. The spinal accessory nerve is the most important structure in the posterior triangle. It exits from the jugular foramen, passes through the deep part of the sternocleidomastoid and enters the posterior triangle, where it lies fairly superficially embedded in the deep fascia along the roof. It then enters the undersurface of the trapezius. The nerve supplies the sternocleidomastoid and the trapezius. The accessory nerve can be damaged during biopsy of lymph nodes in the posterior triangle. This will paralyse the trapezius, resulting in inability to raise the arm above the level of the shoulder as well as inability to shrug the shoulder.

Surface marking of the accessory nerve

Draw a line connecting the junction between the upper third and the lower two-thirds of the posterior border of the stenocleidomastoid to a point two finger breadths (5 cm) above the clavicle on the anterior border of the trapezius. The nerve can be identified as it enters the deep surface of the SCM about 4 cm below the mastoid. It can also be found at Erb's point, just above where great auricular, transverse cervical and lesser occipital nerves (all branches of the cervical plexus) emerge from behind the SCM.

TONGUE

The tongue lies on the floor of the mouth and extends into the anterior wall of the oropharynx. It is a mass of striated muscles covered by mucous membrane. Its mobility is essential for mastication, swallowing and speech. It is derived from a variety of embryonic sources. The anterior two-thirds of the mucosa is developed from the first branchial arch, and the posterior third from the third. Both intrinsic and extrinsic muscles are from the occipital myotomes.

Mucosal surface

The dorsum of the tongue is divided into an anterior two-thirds and a posterior third by a V-shaped groove, the sulcus terminalis, the apex of which has the foramen caecum from which the thyroglossal duct giving rise to the thyroid gland develops. The mucosa of the anterior two-thirds carries the filiform papillae, which gives the tongue its rough feel. Slightly larger and reddish fungiform papillae are also present, scattered in between these papillae. Just in front of the sulcus terminalis and parallel to it is a row of even larger papillae, the vallate papillae, about 8–12 in number (Fig. 13.9). The vallate papillae carry taste buds.

The inferior surface of the tongue is smooth and shiny and in the midline has the frenulum of the tongue. On either side of the frenulum the deep vein of the tongue can be seen (Fig. 13.10).

The posterior third of the tongue faces the oropharynx and the laryngeal part of the pharynx. There are a number of elevations seen here which form the lingual tonsil, a lymphoid aggregation embedded in the musculature.

Muscles

The intrinsic muscles

A midline fibrous septum divides the tongue into right and left halves. Within these two compartments there are the four main groups of intrinsic muscles:

- superior longitudinal
- inferior longitudinal
- transverse
- vertical.

These muscles alter and control the shape of the tongue.

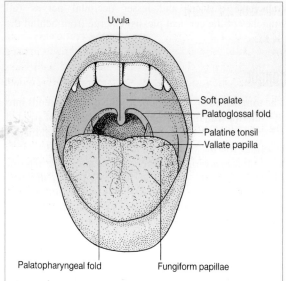

Fig. 13.9 The buccal cavity: the mouth and oropharynx. From Rogers op. cit.

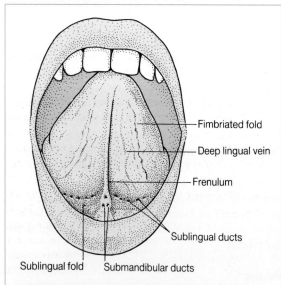

Fig. 13.10 The buccal cavity: the inferior surface of the tongue and the floor of the mouth. From Rogers op. cit.

The extrinsic muscles

There are four pairs (Fig. 13.11):

- the genioglossus
- the hyoglossus
- the styloglossus
- the palatoglossus.

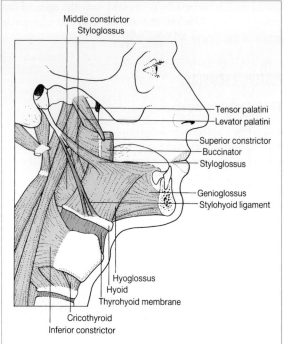

Fig. 13.11 The muscles of the tongue and pharynx. From Rogers op. cit.

These attach the tongue to the mandible, hyoid bone, styloid process and the soft palate, respectively. They alter the position of the tongue.

Nerve supply

The nerve supply of the tongue is based on its development. The lingual nerve which is a branch of the mandibular division of the trigeminal (nerve of the first branchial arch) carries common sensation from the anterior two-thirds. Taste is carried by the chorda tympani fibres with the lingual nerve. The sensory supply of the posterior third, including the vallate papillae, is by the glossopharyngeal nerve, which is the nerve of the third branchial arch. The intrinsic and extrinsic muscles are supplied by the hypoglossal nerve.

Blood supply

Arteries

The tongue is supplied by the lingual artery, a branch of the external carotid artery, the course of which is illustrated in Figure 13.12. The dorsal lingual arteries are branches which supply the mucous membrane as well as the palatine tonsil and the soft palate. The artery is accompanied by the deep lingual vein. At its commencement,

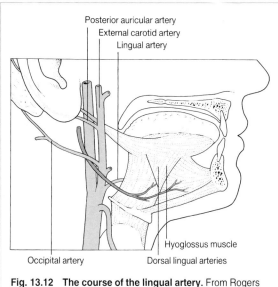

Posterior auricular artery
External carotid artery
Lingual artery

Hyoglossus muscle

Occipital artery   Dorsal lingual arteries

Fig. 13.12   The course of the lingual artery. From Rogers
op. cit.

the hypoglossal nerve and its companion vein crosses
superficial to the artery. At the posterior third, branches
from the tonsillar artery (branch of the facial) and ascending pharyngeal artery anastomose with those of the lingual artery. There is only a poor communication between
the two lingual arteries across the median septum.

Veins

The tongue has two main veins:

- the lingual vein accompanying the lingual artery
- the deep lingual vein, which is visible on the inferior
  surface and which drains the sublingual gland as well.

Lymphatic drainage

Lymphatic spread in cancer of the tongue is by tumour
emboli. The drainage is essentially to the deep cervical
nodes. In the anterior two-thirds there is only minimal
communication of lymphatics across the midline septum,
so that metastases from this portion tend to be ipsilateral.
Posterior third lymphatics form extrinsic networks and
facilitate early bilateral metastases.

Lymphatics from the tip of the tongue pass to the submental nodes and from there to the lower deep cervical
nodes. From the midportion, lymphatics pass to the submandibular nodes and then to the deep cervical from the
margin of the tongue ipsilaterally and the rest bilateral.
From the posterior third the drainage is to the upper deep
cervical of both sides.

FLOOR OF THE MOUTH

The floor of the mouth, separating the oral cavity from
the neck, is formed by the mylohyoid diaphragm formed
by the fusion of the mylohyoid muscles of both sides
along the midline raphe. Above the mylohyoid is the mouth
and below is the neck. The mylohyoids are reinforced
superiorly by the two geniohyoids. The anterior part of
the tongue rests on the mucosa covering the floor of the
mouth. In the midline, the frenulum of the tongue is seen
on the floor connecting the tongue to the mandible. On
either side of the frenulum is the sublingual papilla on
which the submandibular gland duct opens (Fig. 13.10).
Lateral to this is the sublingual fold produced by the
sublingual gland.

More posteriorly between the mylohyoid and the
tongue lies the hyoglossus muscle which, in fact, is the
side wall of the tongue. A number of important structures
in the floor of the mouth lie on the hyoglossus. These
from above downwards are:

- the lingual nerve
- the deep part of the submandibular gland and the
  submandibular duct
- the hypoglossal nerve.

The deep part of the submandibular gland and the
submandibular duct are described on page 384.

The lingual nerve, a branch of the mandibular division
of the trigeminal nerve, runs forward above the mylohyoid. It gives off a gingival branch which supplies the
whole of the lingual gingiva and the mucous membrane
of the floor of the mouth. The lingual nerve winds round
the submandibular duct (p. 385) before getting distributed
to the mucosa of the anterior two-thirds of the tongue.
The submandibular ganglion is suspended from the lingual nerve as it lies on the hyoglossus. The preganglionic
fibres in the chorda tympani synapse in this ganglion.
Before reaching the floor of the mouth the lingual nerve
lies against the periosteum of the alveolar process closely
related to the 3rd molar tooth. The nerve can be damaged
here during dental extraction.

The hypoglossal nerve descends between the internal
jugular vein and the internal carotid artery, giving branches
to thyrohyoid and geniohyoid muscles. It supplies the
superior limb of the ansa cervicalis (C1) to innervate the
infrahyoid muscles. It reaches the surface of the hyoglossus by passing deep to the posterior belly of the digastric.
On the hyoglossus it breaks up into branches to supply all
the muscles (both extrinsic and intrinsic) of the tongue
except the palatoglossus. Paralysis of the hypoglossal
nerve is manifested as fibrillation of the tongue as well as

wasting of the muscles. The latter will show the mucosa loose on the paralysed side.

SALIVARY GLANDS

Parotid gland

This serous salivary gland has a complex shape, irregular surfaces and important relations. An anatomy teacher told his students that during the Creation of Man the Creator poured 'liquid parotid tissue' into the area between the mastoid process and the ramus of the mandible, the liquid trickled into all the crevices in this region and solidified around a number of important structures. The story emphasises the complex configuration and relations of the gland which will no doubt be appreciated by a surgeon doing a total parotidectomy.

The parotid gland lies between the mastoid process and the SCM posteriorly, and the ramus of the mandible, which it clasps anteriorly (Fig. 13.13).

The upper pole of the gland has a small concave surface and it adheres to the cartilaginous part of the auditory tube and it is wedged between the latter and the capsule of the temporomandibular joint.

The lower pole extends below and behind the angle of the mandible into the neck on to the SCM and the posterior belly of the digastric.

The parotid gland is enclosed in a tough capsule

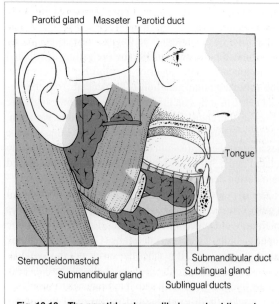

Parotid gland   Masseter   Parotid duct

Tongue

Sternocleidomastoid
Submandibular gland
Submandibular duct
Sublingual gland
Sublingual ducts

Fig. 13.13   The parotid, submandibular and sublingual glands. From Rogers op cit.

derived from the investing layer of the deep fascia. Inflammation of this gland produces pain as the gland swells within the unyielding capsule.

The parotid duct or Stensen's duct emerges from the anterior border of the gland, lies over the masseter, turns medially to pierce the buccinator to enter the oral cavity at the level of the upper second molar tooth. It lies between the muscle and mucous membrane for a short distance before piercing it, and the valvular flap thus produced prevents inflation of the gland when the intraoral pressure is raised. The duct is palpable over the masseter when the jaw is clenched. It lies along a line joining the tragus of the ear and the philtrum of the upper lip. Classical descriptions attribute three surfaces to the gland:

- the lateral or superficial surface
- the anteromedial or anterior surface
- the posteromedial or deep surface.

Superficial surface

There is natural plane of separation between the skin and the superficial surface. Platysma may be present between these two.

Anteromedial surface

This, in fact, is U-shaped extending from the lateral surface of the masseter to the medial surface of the medial pterygoid muscle winding round the posterior border of the mandibular ramus. Where this surface meets the superficial surface is the convex anterior border from which emerges the parotid duct and the five branches of the facial nerve. The stylomandibular ligament separates the deep aspect of this surface from the submandibular gland.

Posteromedial surface

This is very irregular and more complex. Part of it wraps around the mastoid process and the attached muscles, SCM laterally and the posterior belly of digastric medially. This part is also indented by these structures. The gland extends deep to the posterior belly of the digastric to be related to the styloid process and the stylo-hyoid muscle. The latter two separate the gland from the carotid sheath and its contents (internal carotid artery, internal jugular vein, and the last four cranial nerves).

Structures passing through the parotid gland

The external carotid artery, the retromandibular vein and the facial nerve pass through the parotid gland (Fig. 13.14).

The external carotid artery enters the posteromedial surface inferiorly and divides within the gland into its terminal branches, the maxillary and the superficial

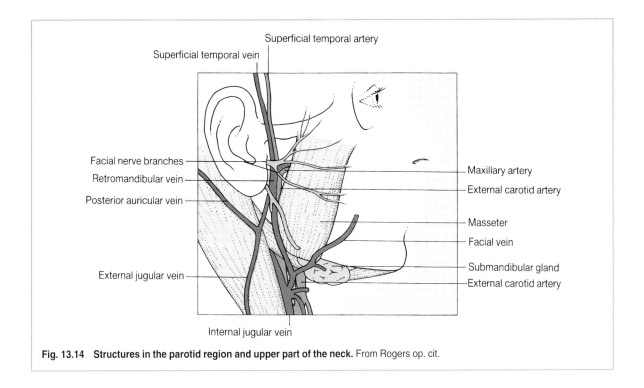

Fig. 13.14 Structures in the parotid region and upper part of the neck. From Rogers op. cit.

temporal arteries. The terminal branches leave the anteromedial surface. The retromandibular vein, which emerges from the posteromedial surface, is formed within the gland by the union of the maxillary and the superficial temporal veins which enter the gland on its anteromedial surface.

The facial nerve leaves the base of the skull through the stylomastoid foramen. The main trunk of the nerve is located in the triangle formed by the mastoid, the angle of the mandible and the cartilaginous part of the external auditory meatus. During parotidectomy, the trunk of the nerve is approached along a plane in front of the anterior margin of the cartilage. The cartilage in this region has a small projection pointing towards the nerve.

The stylomastoid branch of the posterior auricular artery is superficial to the nerve and is also a guide to its proximity.

Before entering the gland the following three branches are given off from the nerve:

- the posterior auricular branch
- a branch to the posterior belly of the digastric muscle
- a branch to the stylohyoid muscle.

The facial nerve enters the posteromedial surface of the parotid gland about 1 cm after emerging from the skull. It then passes forward in the gland as the most superficial of the three embedded structures. (The external carotid artery being the deepest.) Inside the gland the nerve usually divides into an upper temporofacial division having a vertical course and a cervicofacial division which is more horizontal. These two further divide to form the five terminal branches:

- temporal for the frontalis and the orbicularis oculi muscles
- zygomatic for the orbicularis oculi
- buccal supplying the buccinator and the upper lip muscles
- marginal mandibular supplying the lower lip muscles
- cervical for the supply of platysma.

There is considerable variation in the pattern of the branching inside the gland. There are also a number of communicating rami between the branches.

The concept of a superficial and deep lobes for the parotid, separated by the facial nerve, is controversial as these lobes are not well defined nor separated. The parotid is a common site for salivary gland tumours. Parotidectomy requires precise identification and dissection of the facial nerve, and hence a precise knowledge of anatomy of the gland is essential to avoid injury to the nerve.

Submandibular gland

The submandibular gland (Fig. 13.14) and the submandibular group of lymph nodes fill the submandibular triangle, which is bounded by the anterior and posterior bellies of the digastric muscle and the lower border of the mandible. The gland also extends upward deep to the mandible. Differentiating an enlargement of the gland from that of the lymph nodes can be difficult.

The superficial surface of the gland is covered by the skin, platysma and the investing layer of deep fascia, and is crossed by the facial vein, the cervical branch of the facial nerve, and also often by the marginal mandibular branch of the facial nerve. The marginal mandibular branch lies deep to the platysma and is one of the most important relations of the gland. This branch which supplies the depressor anguli oris and the depressor labii inferioris is liable to injury during surgery of the submandibular region. Injury of the nerve can result in facial asymmetry and occasional dribbling. Skin incisions in the submandibular region are made about 4 cm below the mandible to avoid injury to the marginal mandibular branch.

Each submandibular gland has a larger, superficial part and a smaller, deep part. The two are separated by the mylohyoid muscle. The two parts, however, are conti-nuous with each other posteriorly, and the concavity thus formed is occupied by the free posterior border of the mylohyoid muscle.

Superficial part

This part of the gland lying superficial to the mylohyoid muscle has a superficial surface facing inferiorly in the submandibular triangle. The upper part of this surface lies deep to the body of the mandible. Its deep surface is related to the digastric below, and above this to the mylohyoid anteriorly, and to the hyoglossus muscle posteriorly. The facial artery grooves the deep surface and emerges onto the face by passing between the gland and the mandible (Fig. 13.15). Several submandibular lymph nodes lie on the superficial surface.

Deep part

This lies in the floor of the mouth, superior (deep) to the mylohyoid and is covered by the mucosa of the oral cavity. Medially it lies on the hyoglossus and is related to the lingual nerve, the submandibular ganglion and the hypoglossal nerve.

Submandibular duct

The duct of the submandibular gland (Wharton's duct) starts in the superficial part, running posteriorly and

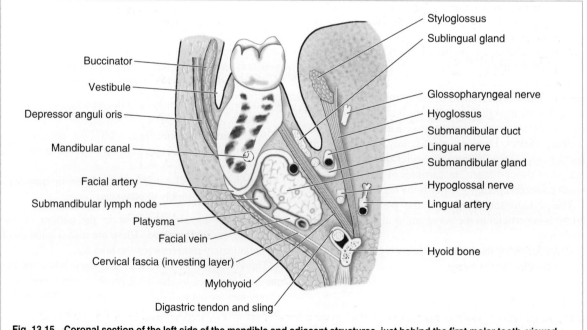

Fig. 13.15 Coronal section of the left side of the mandible and adjacent structures, just behind the first molar tooth, viewed from behind.

superiorly to reach the deep part. Here it turns forward and medially and emerges onto the surface of the hyoglossus muscle. It runs forward deep to the mucosa of the floor of the mouth between the mucosa and the sublingual gland and the geniohyoid muscle to open into the floor of the mouth on either side of the frenulum of the tongue. The duct, on the floor of the mouth is closely related to the lingual nerve. As it goes forward it crosses medial to the nerve to lie above the nerve and then crosses back, this time lateral to it to reach a position once again below the nerve (Fig. 13.16).

Sublingual gland

The sublingual gland lies in the floor of the mouth and raises the sublingual fold of the oral mucosa. The gland is related medially to the genioglossus muscle and laterally to the sublingual fossa of the mandible. Posteriorly it extends as far as the deep part of the submandibular gland. The submandibular duct runs along the medial side of the sublingual gland. Several small ducts emerge from the gland. The posterior ducts open directly into the mouth on the sublingual fold. The anterior part has a duct which drains into the submandibular duct.

Nerve supply of the salivary glands

The secretomotor supply to the parotid gland is from the glossopharyngeal nerve, the parasympathetic fibres synapsing in the otic ganglion. Postganglionic fibres reach the gland via the auriculotemporal nerve.

The parasympathetic supply of the submandibular and sublingual glands is from the facial nerve through its chorda tympani branch. The chorda tympani joins the lingual nerve, and the preganglionic fibres synapse in the submandibular ganglion. The postganglionic fibres rejoin the lingual nerve, to be distributed to the glands.

PHARYNX

The pharynx is a muscular tube attached above to the base of the skull and extends below as far as the sixth cervical

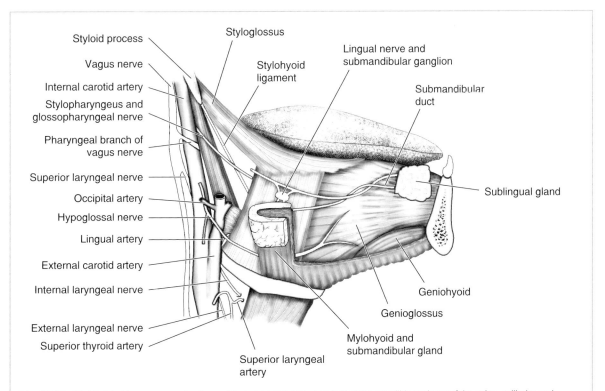

Fig. 13.16   Right styloid process and submandibular region. The right half of the mandible and part of the submandibular and sublingual glands have been removed. The glossopharyngeal nerve, styloid ligament and lingual artery pass deep to the posterior border of hyoglossus; the lingual nerve, submandibular duct of hypoglossal nerve are superficial to hyoglossus.

vertebra, where it continues down as the oesophagus. It has three parts:

- the nasopharynx opening anteriorly to the nasal cavities
- the oropharynx opening to the oral cavity
- the laryngopharynx or hypopharynx opening into the larynx and continuing downwards as the oesophagus.

Nasopharynx

The Eustachian tube (auditory or pharyngotympanic tube) which connects the pharynx to the middle ear opens into the nasopharynx. The cartilaginous end of the tube has a prominence at the posterosuperior part of the opening. This is the tubal elevation and is a guide to the opening during catheterisation. The area posterolateral to the tubal elevation is the pharyngeal recess. The roof and the posterior wall has lymphoid accumulation in the mucosa forming the adenoids. There is also lymphoid accumulation around the opening of the Eustachian tube.

Examination of the nasopharynx can be performed by placing a small angled mirror in the oropharynx. The following can be visualised:

- opening of the Eustachian tube
- the tubal elevation
- the pharyngeal recess
- adenoids — seen as vertical ridges separated by clefts
- the posterior choanae
- the posterior end of inferior concha or turbinate.

The nasopharyngeal tonsils are prominent in children, but like all lymphoid tissues, undergo atrophy after puberty. Infection from the nasopharynx can easily spread into the middle ear through the Eustachian tube.

Oropharynx and the anatomy of the tonsil

The most important structure in the oropharynx is the palatine tonsil, or the tonsil. It lies in the tonsillar fossa bounded by the anterior and posterior pillars of the fauces. The anterior pillar is the palatoglossal arch produced by the palatoglossus muscle, and the posterior pillar is the palatopharyngeal arch by the palatopharyngeus muscle. The superior constrictor forms the floor of the tonsillar fossa. Pharyngobasilar fascia lining the inner surface of the constrictor forms the capsule of the tonsil and lies between the tonsil and the muscle. The capsule is normally separated from the muscle by loose areolar tissue.

The tonsil is an accumulation of lymphoid tissue. Its oral surface is lined by mucous membrane having stratified squamous epithelium. Tonsillar crypts are clefts on the inner surface, and these too are lined by the mucosa

(these crypts are not present in adenoids, which are lined by ciliated columnar epithelium).

Blood supply

The main arterial supply is derived from the tonsillar branch of the facial artery which pierces the superior constrictor to enter the lower pole of the tonsil. There are additional branches from the lingual, ascending palatine and ascending pharyngeal arteries as well.

The venous drainage is to the pharyngeal plexus of veins. The troublesome paratonsillar vein which often bleeds during tonsillectomy extends from the soft palate to lie on the lateral surface of the tonsil before piercing the superior constrictor.

The lymphatic drainage is to the jugulodigastric lymph node situated behind the angle of the mandible. This node is often palpable in chronic tonsillitis.

The sensory nerve supply of the tonsillar fossa is through the glossopharyngeal nerve, with minor contribution from the lesser palatine nerve.

During tonsillectomy the tonsil and the underlying capsule are removed. The superior constrictor is not damaged, as it is separated from the capsule by areolar tissue.

Laryngopharynx

This part of the pharynx, which is also known as the hypopharynx, has the inlet of the larynx and the piriform fossa. The inlet of the larynx, which is vertical, is bounded by the epiglottis, aryepiglottic fold and the arytenoids. Anterolateral to the inlet is a recess known as the piriform fossa. It is a common site for lodging foreign bodies such as fish bones and also notorious for malignant tumours which may be silent in the early stages. The internal laryngeal nerve which supplies the laryngopharynx and most of the larynx is also found in the piriform fossa. As this part has a rich lymphatic drainage the tumour rapidly spreads into the deep cervical nodes.

Structure of the pharynx

The pharyngeal wall consists of the:

- mucosa
- submucosa
- pharyngobasilar fascia
- muscle
- buccopharyngeal fascia (areolar tissue).

The mucosa has pseudostratified columnar ciliated epithelium (respiratory epithelium) in the nasopharynx and stratified squamous epithelium in the rest of the pharynx.

The pharyngobasilar fascia lies deep to the mucosa and lines the muscles of the pharynx. It is thick in the upper part, and its attachment to the base of the skull gives firm anchorage to the pharynx. In the oropharynx the fascia contributes to the capsule of the tonsil.

Muscles of the pharynx

The main muscles of the pharynx are the three fan-shaped constrictor muscles:

- the superior constrictor
- the middle constrictor
- the inferior constrictor.

These are reinforced by much smaller longitudinal muscles:

- the stylopharyngeus
- the salpingopharyngeus
- the palatopharyngeus.

Each constrictor muscle starts from a limited origin anteriorly and broadens out laterally and posteriorly to insert into a posterior midline raphe — the pharyngeal raphe. Each constrictor overlaps the one above posteriorly. There are gaps laterally. The gap between the inferior and middle is occupied by the thyrohyoid ligament and associated structures. The stylopharyngeus muscle accompanied by the glossopharyngeal nerve enters the pharynx through the gap between the middle and superior constrictors. The gap between the upper border of the superior constrictor and the base of the skull is bridged by the thick pharyngobasilar fascia. The Eustachian tube enters the pharynx through this gap.

Anteriorly the superior constrictor is attached to the pterygomandibular raphe, and the middle constrictor to the greater horn of the hyoid bone. The inferior constrictor has two parts. The thyropharyngeus part of the inferior constrictor is fan shaped like the other constrictors and is attached to the lamina of the thyroid cartilage. The cricopharyngeus part of the inferior constrictor is circular and acts like a sphincter. The weakest area of the pharyngeal wall is the gap between the thyropharyngeus and the cricopharyngeus posteriorly in the midline. This is the Killian's dehiscence, a common site for pharyngeal diverticulum (pouch).

Innervation of the pharynx

Motor innervation

All the muscles of the pharynx except stylopharyngeus are supplied by the pharyngeal branch of the vagus, fibres coming from the nucleus ambiguus through the cranial part of the accessory nerve. Stylopharyngeus is supplied by the glossopharyngeal nerve.

Sensory innervation

- nasopharynx — maxillary division of trigeminal

- oropharynx — glossopharyngeal nerve
- laryngopharynx — internal laryngeal branch of the vagus.

LARYNX

The larynx is an integral part of the respiratory tract and is the organ of voice production. It also plays an essential role in the swallowing mechanism. It is held open by a series of cartilages on its wall.

Cartilages

There are five major cartilages:

- the cricoid cartilage
- the thyroid cartilage
- the epiglottis
- the paired arytenoid cartilages.

Cricoid cartilage

Shaped like a signet ring, the cricoid cartilage has a narrow arch anteriorly and a broad lamina at the back. The arch can be felt in the neck below the thyroid cartilage. The cricotracheal ligament connects the cricoid to the first tracheal ring.

Thyroid cartilage

The thyroid cartilage is the largest of the laryngeal cartilages and has two laminae meeting in the midline anteriorly. The oblique line on the lamina receives attachment of the infrahyoid muscles. This cartilage articulates inferiorly with the cricoid at the cricothyroid joints and is connected to the hyoid bone by the thyrohyoid ligament.

Epiglottis

This is a leaf-shaped cartilage forming the anterior wall of the inlet of the larynx. Its narrow lower end is attached to the thyroid cartilage by the thyroepiglottic ligament. The thyroepiglottic ligament tethers its anterior surface to the back of the hyoid bone in the midline.

Arytenoid cartilages

These are paired cartilages which are pyramidal in shape, articulating with the lamina of the cricoid. In its broader lower part the arytenoid has the vocal process projecting anteriorly and the muscular process laterally. The former receives attachment of the vocal ligament and the latter the abductors and adductors of the vocal cord.

There are two pairs of minor cartilages. The corniculate cartilage articulates with the apex of the arytenoid. The cuneiform cartilage is a nodule in the aryepiglottic fold. Though small, these are essential for complete approximation of the inlet of the larynx.

Intrinsic ligaments (membranes) of the larynx

Two broad fibroelastic membranes bridge the gaps between the cartilages and contribute to the walls of the larynx. These are as follows.

- The quadrangular membrane forms the upper part of the wall. Its upper free border forms the aryepiglottic fold, and the lower free border forms the core of the vestibular fold or the false vocal cord.
- The cricothyroid membrane (cricovocal membrane) is a tent-shaped membrane in the lower part of the larynx. It is attached below to the arch of the cricoid, above to the vocal process of the arytenoid posteriorly and the thyroid cartilage in the midline anteriorly. Between its thyroid and arytenoid attachment it has a free border, the vocal ligament, forming the core of the vocal fold or vocal cord. The part between the cricoid and the thyroid cartilage in the midline anteriorly is thickened to form the cricothyroid ligament. This is easily palpable, is relatively avascular, and is the site for laryngotomy (cricothyroid stab) in acute laryngeal obstruction.

Parts of the cavity

The cavity of the larynx is divided into different parts (Fig. 13.17):

- the inlet
- the vestibule
- the ventricle or the sinus
- the infraglottic part.

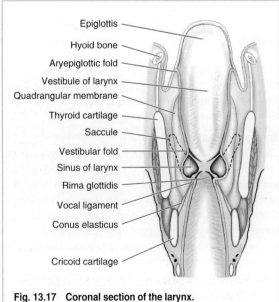

Fig. 13.17 Coronal section of the larynx.

Labels (top to bottom):
Epiglottis
Hyoid bone
Aryepiglottic fold
Vestibule of larynx
Quadrangular membrane
Thyroid cartilage
Saccule
Vestibular fold
Sinus of larynx
Rima glottidis
Vocal ligament
Conus elasticus
Cricoid cartilage

The laryngeal inlet, bounded by the epiglottis in front, the aryepiglottic folds on the side and the arytenoids and the corniculate cartilages at the back, opens into the laryngopharynx.

The vestibule of the larynx extends from the inlet to the vestibular fold.

The ventricle of the larynx is the short narrow space between the vestibular fold and the vocal fold. There is a small blind-ending diverticulum from the anterior end of the ventricle. This is the saccule. The ventricle, whose wall is not reinforced by thick membrane, is a potential site for laryngocele.

The space between the vocal cord, the rima glottidis, is the narrowest part of the upper airway.

The part of the larynx above the vocal cord is often referred to as the supraglottic region.

The infraglottic part lies below the vocal folds and widens to continue into the trachea.

The pre-epiglottic space lies anterior to the epiglottis, between it and the thyroid cartilage. It contains pre-epiglottic fat and is an area into which cancer can spread easily.

Mucous membrane

The mucosa in the supraglottic region is loosely bound to the underlying wall. It contains goblet cells and mucous glands. In laryngeal oedema fluid accumulates in the submucous space, and the mucosa swells up and obstructs the airway. The fluid cannot spread downwards, as at the vocal cord the mucosa is firmly adherent to the underlying structures without having a submucous space. The lack of a submucosal layer also makes the vocal cords relatively less vascular and hence they appear paler than the rest of the mucosa. There are no mucous glands in the vocal cords and only few in the subglottic region.

Intrinsic muscles of the larynx

One muscle abducts the vocal cord, two adduct it, one adjusts the length, and two adjust the tension.

Posterior cricoarytenoid muscle

This paired muscle abducts the cord. The muscle arises from the posterior surface of the lamina of the cricoid and is attached to the muscular process of the arytenoid. As it contracts, the arytenoid slides down on the slope of the cricoid, widening the rima glottidis.

Lateral cricoarytenoid muscle

This paired muscle arises from the lateral part of the arch of the cricoid and is attached to the muscular process. On contraction the muscular process is pulled anteriorly, and the vocal process moves medially, adducting the cord.

Transverse arytenoid (interarytenoid)

This unpaired muscle adducts the vocal cords by sliding the arytenoids towards each other. The muscle is attached to the posterior surfaces of the arytenoid cartilages.

Cricothyroid muscle

This arises from the oblique line on the lamina of the thyroid cartilage and is inserted into the anterior part of the arch of the cricoid. As it contracts, it approximates the cricoid and the thyroid cartilages anteriorly, increases the distance between the attachments of the cords and lengthens them.

Thyroarytenoid muscle

Lying in the cord, this muscle forms the main bulk of the vocal cord. On contraction it shortens the cord. However, the thyroarytenoid and its specialised free edge portion, the vocalis muscle, are important in adjusting the tension of the cord.

The *aryepiglottic muscle* and the *oblique arytenoid* muscle are small muscles, but are important in reducing the size of the laryngeal inlet, as in swallowing. The former lies in the aryepiglottic fold and the latter extends obliquely across from one arytenoid to the other.

Blood supply

The supraglottic region is supplied and drained by the superior laryngeal artery and vein, which enter the larynx through the thyrohyoid membrane. The region below the vocal cords is supplied and drained by the inferior laryngeal artery and vein. The artery is a branch of the inferior thyroid artery.

Nerve supply

- Motor innervation. All the muscles of the larynx are supplied by the recurrent laryngeal nerve except the cricothyroid, which is supplied by the external laryngeal nerve (branch of the superior laryngeal).
- Sensory innervation. The supraglottic part is supplied by the internal laryngeal nerve (branch of superior laryngeal). The infraglottic part is supplied by the recurrent laryngeal nerve.

Lymphatic drainage

The vocal cords have no lymphatic drainage, and hence this region acts as a lymphatic watershed. The supraglottic part drains to the upper deep cervical nodes through vessels piercing the thyrohyoid membrane. The subglottic part drains to the prelaryngeal and pretracheal nodes and also to the inferior deep cervical nodes. The ary-epiglottic fold and the vestibular fold have rich lymphatic supply, and hence malignancy in them metastasises rapidly.

THE NOSE, THE NASAL CAVITY AND THE PARANASAL SINUSES

The nose consists of the external nose and the nasal cavities. The two cavities are divided by a nasal septum which is often deviated to one side of the midline. Each cavity has an olfactory and a respiratory area covered by mucous membrane with the appropriate epithelium.

External nose

This is the most prominent part of the face, projecting as a pyramidal elevation. It has a bony and a cartilaginous part. The upper part is bony where the nasal bones form the bridge of the nose. Most laterally is the frontal process of the maxilla. The lower part has the following cartilages, which are shown in Figure 13.18:

- the upper lateral cartilage or the lateral cartilage
- the lower lateral cartilage or major alar cartilage
- the minimal cartilages — up to four of them reinforcing the fibrofatty tissue forming the ala of the nose
- the septal cartilage in the midline, which is the anterior part of the nasal septum.

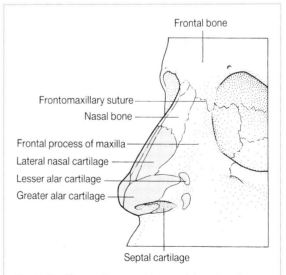

Fig. 13.18 The cartilages and bones of the external nose.
From Rogers op. cit.

Labels on figure:
Frontal bone
Frontomaxillary suture
Nasal bone
Frontal process of maxilla
Lateral nasal cartilage
Lesser alar cartilage
Greater alar cartilage
Septal cartilage

The cartilaginous part of the external nose is flexible. The delicate nasal bones can easily be fractured.

The external nose opens below by two nostrils separated by the midline septum. A number of small muscles which are compressors and dilators of the nostrils are present in the alar region. They are supplied by branches from the facial nerve.

The skin of the external nose is thin and adherent to the underlying bones and cartilages and has a number of sebaceous glands.

The arteries of the external nose are branches of the facial artery and the ophthalmic artery. The veins drain into the facial vein and the ophthalmic veins. There are connections between these veins and the cavernous sinus. Infections of the external nose can, if not treated, lead on to cavernous sinus thrombosis. The lymphatics drain to preauricular (parotid) nodes and to submandibular nodes.

Nasal cavities

Each nasal cavity continues upwards and backwards from the vestibule of the nose. The vestibule is the expanded part just above the nostrils and is lined by hair-containing skin reflected from the external surface. The skin finishes at the mucocutaneous junction where the nasal cavity starts. The two nasal cavities are partitioned by the nasal septum and they open posteriorly into the nasopharynx as the posterior nares or choanae. In coronal section, the nasal cavities are roughly triangular. The roof is narrow, the septum vertical and the lateral walls slope away laterally to give a wider floor. The walls of the nasal cavity are made of a number of bones. The only cartilage is on the septum in its anterior part.

Roof of the nasal cavity and its relations

The nasal cavity has a narrow roof where the septum is only 2 mm away from the lateral wall. The anterior third of the roof projects anteriorly and inferiorly and is related to the medial part of the frontal sinus. The middle third is horizontal and is formed by the cribriform plate of the ethmoid. This separates the nasal cavity from the cranial cavity (i.e. meninges, CSF, brain). Tumours from the nasal cavity, can easily spread into the cranial cavity, and fractures of the roof can produce CSF rhinorrhea. The posterior third of the roof slopes posteriorly and inferiorly and is related to the sphenoid sinus, into which the pituitary fossa projects. The transnasal route is a 'popular' approach to the hypophysis cerebri.

Floor of the nasal cavity

This is the roof of the oral cavity and is formed by the hard palate with a minimal contribution from the soft palate posteriorly.

Lateral wall

The lateral wall has the superior, middle and inferior conchae or turbinates. The superior concha is the smallest and the inferior the longest. The superior and middle conchae are parts of the medial wall of the ethmoid labyrinth (lateral mass of the ethmoid) whereas the inferior concha is a separate bone which articulates with the surface of the maxilla.

Below each concha lies the respective meatus, i.e. the superior, middle and inferior meatuses. The region above and posterior to the superior concha is the spheno-ethmoidal recess.

The superior meatus, the smallest of the meatuses, occupies the posterior third of the nasal cavity. The middle meatus occupies about two-thirds and the inferior the whole length of the nasal cavity. The inferior meatus is also the most expanded part, facilitating nasal intubations through this region.

The middle meatus presents a convex bulge beneath the concha. This is the ethmoidal bulla. Below the bulla is the hiatus semilunaris into which open the frontal, anterior ethmoidal and maxillary sinuses. The frontal sinus opens via the infundibulum. The anterior ethmoidal cells are few, and their openings may extend onto the wall of the infundibulum as well. The maxillary sinus may have more than one opening.

The nasolacrimal duct opens into the inferior meatus about 2 cm behind the nostril.

The sphenoid sinus opens on the roof of the nasal cavity into the spheno-ethmoidal recess posteriorly. The posterior ethmoidal sinuses drain into the superior meatus.

Lateral to the nasal cavity lie the ethmoidal sinuses which separate it from the orbit. The lower part of the lateral wall is related to the maxillary sinus. Further posteriorly lies the pterygopalatine fossa, which contains the maxillary nerve and sphenopalatine ganglion and maxillary artery. Branches from the maxillary artery and those from the sphenopalatine ganglion enter the nasal cavity through the sphenopalatine foramen.

Nasal septum

This is vertical but often may be deviated to one side. It consists of the vomer, perpendicular plate of the ethmoid and the septal cartilage. The latter occupies the wedge-shaped gap between the vomer and the perpendicular plate of the ethmoid and extends into the external nose to give it its shape and prominence.

The mucoperiosteum and mucoperichondrium (over the cartilaginous part) line the walls. Though it is firmly attached to the wall, it can be stripped off in submucous resection.

The mucosa over the inferior concha has large vascular spaces which act like erectile tissue which, along with mucus secretion from the goblet cells and mucous glands, produce nasal congestion.

The roof and upper part above the superior concha is the olfactory area containing the olfactory epithelium with receptors for smell. Axons of the olfactory neurons reach the olfactory bulb as the olfactory nerves through the cribiform plate of the ethmoid. Most of the nasal cavity contains respiratory mucosa with pseudostratified ciliated columnar epithelium containing goblet cells. The mucous secretion traps particles, and the cilia beat in such a way that the mucus is moved towards the naso-pharynx. The vestibule is lined by skin with hair follicles and glands.

Blood supply

Arterial supply   The arterial supply of the nasal cavity is derived from two sources. The main supply is through the maxillary branch of the external carotid artery via its sphenopalatine branch, which divides into inferior turbinate, middle turbinate and sphenopalatine branches. They run in the mucoperiosteum of the nasal cavity. The nasopalatine artery enters the nasal cavity from the pterygopalatine fossa through the sphenopalatine fora-men. It divides into two branches. The superior branch, which lies on the perpendicular plate of the ethmoid, remains in the nasal cavity. The inferior branch supplies the lower part of the septum and small branches to the palate through the incisive foramen. The second main source of arterial supply is the internal carotid artery through the anterior ethmoidal branch of the ophthalmic artery. The posterior ethmoidal artery is much smaller and is continued to the posterior part of the nasal cavity. The ethmoidal arteries enter the nasal cavity through the anterior and posterior ethmoidal foramina. The greater palatine artery, a branch of the maxillary artery, enters the nasal septum through the incisive foramen. The facial artery also contributes a branch to the nasal septum.

Venous drainage   The veins form a cavernous plexus beneath the mucous membrane and drain through the sphenopalatine and facial veins. Smaller ethmoidal veins drain to the ophthalmic veins and to the veins of the dura mater.

Lymphatic drainage

The anterior part of the nasal cavity drains to the subman-dibular and the upper deep cervical nodes whereas the posterior region drains to the inferior deep cervical nodes.

Nerve supply

The nerve supply of the nasal mucosa is extremely rich.

Olfactory nerves from the olfactory neurons emerge from the olfactory mucosa. They go through the cribi-form plate of the ethmoid to reach the olfactory bulb. The vestibular area is supplied by the nasal branches of the infraorbital nerve. The rest of the lateral wall (respiratory area) is innervated by four nerves:

- anterior ethmoidal nerve from the nasociliary branch of the ophthalmic
- anterior superior alveolar nerve
- lateral posterior superior nasal branches of the sphenopalatine ganglion
- nasal branches of the greater palatine nerve.

The septum is supplied by the following four nerves:

- olfactory nerve
- anterior ethmoidal nerve
- medial superior nasal nerves from the sphenopalatine ganglion
- nasopalatine nerve, also from the sphenopalatine ganglion.

Paranasal sinuses

A series of paranasal sinuses open into the nasal cavity on each side. They are effectively extensions of the nasal cavity. The sinuses are:

- the maxillary sinus, opening into the middle meatus
- the ethmoidal air cells (sinuses), which are variable in number and are in three groups: the anterior, middle and posterior. The anterior and middle cells open into the middle meatus. The posterior air cells open into the superior meatus
- the frontal sinus, opening into the middle meatus via the infundibulum
- the sphenoidal sinus, opening into the spheno-ethmoidal recess.

All the sinuses are lined by respiratory epithelium with goblet cells and cilia.

Maxillary sinus

This is the largest of the paranasal sinuses, with a mean volume of about 10 mL.

- The medial wall or base is composed of thin and deli-cate bones on the lateral wall of the nasal cavity. The opening of the sinus into the hiatus semilunaris lies high on the medial wall, just below the floor of the orbit. As the ostium is high on the wall, drainage depends on ciliary action and not gravity.
- The roof of the sinus is the floor of the orbit. The canal for the infraorbital nerve produces a ridge down into

the sinus from the roof. The roof is also of relatively thin bone.

- The posterior wall faces the pterygopalatine fossa and the infratemporal fossa.
- The anterior wall is comparatively thick and lies between the infraorbital margin and the premolar teeth.
- The floor is a narrow cleft between the posterior and anterior wall in the alveolar process of the maxilla overlying the second premolar and the first molar teeth. The canine and all the molars may be included in the floor, if the sinus is large. The roots of these teeth may produce projections into the sinus or occasionally perforate the bone. A tooth abscess may rupture into the sinus. The floor of the maxillary sinus is at a more inferior level than the floor of the nasal cavity.

At birth the maxillary sinus is rudimentary. During the period of secondary dentition it quickly expands to reach its adult size by the time of eruption of the third molar tooth.

For maxillary sinus wash-out a cannula is inserted into the sinus via the inferior meatus of the nasal cavity.

In the Caldwell–Luc operation for chronic maxillary sinusitis the anterior bony wall of the maxillary sinus is removed, the mucosa is stripped out and a permanent drainage hole is made into the nose through the inferior meatus.

Carcinoma of the maxillary sinus may invade the palate and cause dental problems. It may block the nasolacrimal duct, causing epiphora. Spread of the tumour into the orbit causes proptosis.

Nerve supply
The maxillary division of the trigeminal nerve supplies the sinus through its infraorbital and superior dental nerves. The pain due to sinusitis may often manifest itself as toothache.

Arterial supply
The maxillary sinus is supplied by branches of the maxillary artery.

Lymphatic drainage
The lymphatics of the maxillary sinus drain to the upper deep cervical lymph nodes.

Ethmoidal air cells
The ethmoidal air cells are small air cells which vary in size and number. They are thin-walled cavities in the ethmoidal labyrinth. They are relatively large at birth and grow slowly compared with other sinuses. The sinuses lie below the anterior cranial fossa. They are lateral to the nasal cavity, and lateral to them lies the orbit separated by the lamina papyracea (or paper-thin layer). The ethmoidal air cells are divided into anterior, middle and posterior groups of air cells. The anterior cells drain into the hiatus semilunaris, the middle (normally only one or two) on the bulla ethmoidalis and the posterior into the superior meatus.

Acute ethmoiditis in childhood can easily spread into the orbit through the lamina papyracea and cause proptosis, chemosis, ophthalmoplegia and periorbital oedema. The abscess may be drained through a small incision in the medial part of the orbit. Ethmoidal carcinoma may spread upwards, causing meningitis and CSF leakage, or it may spread laterally into the orbit, causing proptosis and diplopia.

Nerve supply
The sinuses are supplied by the ophthalmic division of the trigeminal nerve via the anterior and posterior ethmoidal nerves of the nasociliary branch.

Arterial supply
The arterial supply is from the anterior and posterior ethmoidal branches of the ophthalmic artery.

Frontal sinus
The frontal sinuses are not present at birth but start to appear in the second year of life. The frontal sinus is very variable in size and shape. It may be a single small air cell above the medial end of the orbit or a cluster of cells extending into the lateral end of the orbital roof and several centimetres up into the frontal bone. The sinuses of the two sides may be dissimilar in size and number. The anterior wall of the sinus is thick. The posterior wall facing the anterior cranial fossa is thin. The floor is also thin and it separates the sinus from the orbit.

The frontal sinus drains by the infundibulum or the frontonasal duct into the hiatus semilunaris of the middle meatus. Infection of the frontal sinus is often associated with infection of the maxillary sinus, as their openings are very close to each other.

Acute sinusitis can spread posteriorly into the anterior cranial fossa, causing extradural and subdural abscesses or meningitis. The pus in the sinus can be drained by washout through the nose or by a small incision on its wall just below the medial end of the eyebrow.

Nerve supply
The nerve supply is through the supratrochlear and supraorbital branches of the frontal division of the ophthalmic nerve, and the blood supply is via the corresponding branches of the ophthalmic artery.

Sphenoidal sinus

The sphenoidal sinus, like the maxillary sinus, is very small at birth. The size in the adult is variable and the right and left sinuses may not be symmetrical. It occupies the body of the sphenoid but may extend into its greater and lesser wings. The sphenoidal sinus opens into the sphenoethmoidal recess of the nasal cavity.

The floor of the sinus is in the roof of the nasal cavity and the nasopharynx. The roof of the sinus is thin. The pituitary fossa bulges into the roof in its posterior half, and anteriorly the roof separates the sinus from the optic chiasma and the optic nerves. The lateral wall also is thin and separates the sinus from the cavernous sinus and the internal carotid artery.

Nerve supply

The nerve supply is from the ophthalmic division of the trigeminal nerve through the posterior ethmoidal nerve.

ROOT OF THE NECK

Knowledge of anatomy of the root of the neck is essential to perform procedures such as subclavian vein catheterisation, brachial plexus block and to understand the effects of a Pancoast tumour (Pancoast syndrome).

The root of the neck is the junctional area between the thorax and the neck and contains all the structures going from the thorax to the neck and vice versa (Fig. 13.19).

Suprapleural membrane (Sibson's fascia)

The apex of the lung and the apical pleura project into the neck from the thorax. This is covered by a fascia known as the suprapleural membrane or Sibson's fascia. Sibson's fascia is attached to the inner border of the first rib and to the transverse process of the sixth cervical vertebra. It functions to prevent the lung and pleura rising further into the neck during respiration. The subclavian artery and vein and the brachial plexus lie on the suprapleural membrane.

Subclavian artery

The right subclavian artery is a branch of the brachiocephalic trunk, and the left arises directly from the arch of the aorta beyond the origin of the left internal carotid artery. On both sides this artery arches laterally over the cervical pleura (and Sibson's fascia) and the apex of the lung to reach the surface of the first rib. It lies posterior to the insertion of the scalenus anterior on the first rib. The subclavian vein runs parallel to the artery but in front of the scalenus anterior at a slightly lower level. The roots and the trunks of the brachial plexus lie behind the subclavian artery on the first rib between the scalenus anterior and the scalenus medius muscles. The artery beyond the first rib continues into the axilla as the axilla artery.

The pulse of the subclavian artery can be felt at the medial third of the clavicle near the lateral border of the SCM on deep palpatation against the first rib.

The branches of the subclavian artery are as follows:

- the vertebral artery
- the internal mammary (thoracic) artery
- the thyrocervical trunk
- the costocervical trunk.

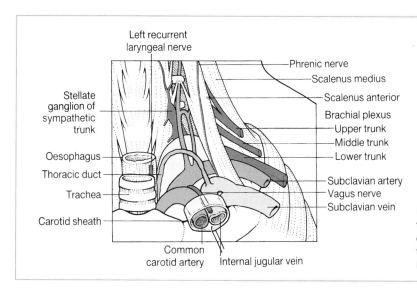

Fig. 13.19 **The structures of the thoracic inlet.** The carotid sheath and contents are cut and reflected to show the deep structures in the neck. From Rogers op. cit.

The vertebral artery is the first branch of the subclavian artery. It enters the foramen transversarium at the sixth cervical vertebra and ascends through the foramina transversaria of the sixth to the first cervical vertebrae and enters the cranial cavity and branches to supply the brain and spinal cord. At the root of the neck the vertebral artery lies deep to the carotid sheath. The stellate ganglion lies behind it near its commencement.

The internal thoracic (mammary) artery passes vertically downwards a fingers breadth lateral to the sternum. In the sixth intercostal space it divides into the musculophrenic artery and the superior epigastric artery.

The thyrocervical trunk is a branch of the subclavian artery medial to the scalenus anterior. It divides into the inferior thyroid artery, the transverse cervical and the suprascapular arteries. The inferior thyroid artery lies behind the carotid sheath and ascends in front of the scalenus anterior. At the level of the transverse process of the sixth cervical vertebra the artery arches medially and enters the posteromedial aspect of the capsule of the thyroid gland at its lower third. The recurrent laryngeal nerve is closely related to the the artery and its branches near the lower pole of the thyroid gland.

Subclavian vein

The subclavian vein follows the course of the subclavian artery in the neck, but lies in front of the scalenus anterior on the first rib. Veins accompanying the branches of the subclavian artery drain into the external jugular, the subclavian vein or its continuation, the brachiocephalic vein (formed by the union of the subclavian and the internal jugular veins).

Subclavian venepuncture can be carried out using an infraclavicular or supraclavicular approach. In the former the needle is inserted below the clavicle at the junction of its middle and medial thirds and advanced upwards and medially behind the clavicle towards the sternoclavicular joint. In the supraclavicular approach the needle is inserted about 2 cm above the clavicle at the junction between its middle and medial thirds at the lateral border of the sternocleidomastoid. The needle is advanced downwards and medially towards the sternoclavicular joint and aspirated for the free flow of blood from the vein. There is the risk of pneumothorax and an inadvertent puncture of the subclavian artery in both of these approaches.

Brachial plexus

The anterior primary ramus of C5 and C6 join to form the upper trunk of the brachial plexus, C7 forms the middle trunk and the C8 and T1 join to form the lower trunk. The nerves lie sandwiched between the scalenus anterior and the medius (Fig. 13.19) above and lateral to the subclavian artery.

A number of approaches are described to block the brachial plexus in the supraclavicular region. In the supraclavicular perivascular method the needle is inserted at the middle of the clavicle just lateral to the subclavian artery pulsation and directed backwards, downwards and inwards. Pneumothorax and/or haematoma are complications. In the interscalene approach the needle is inserted at a higher level, at the level of the cricoid cartilage and advanced towards the transverse process of the sixth cervical vertebra and the local anaesthetic is injected deep to the prevertebral fascia (the plane containing the nerves). The risk of pneumothorax is less in the interscalene approach. Phrenic nerve paralysis and/or inadvertent injection into the vertebral artery are complications.

Thoracic duct

This duct carries lymph from the whole body except that from right side of thorax, right upper limb, and right side of head and neck. It arises in the abdomen, passes through the thorax and enters the neck lying on the left side of the oesophagus. At the root of the neck it arches laterally lying between the carotid sheath and the vertebral artery (Fig. 13.19) and enters the junction between the internal jugular and the subclavian veins. Inadvertent puncture or laceration of the thoracic duct will cause escape of lymph into the surrounding tissue and occasionally chylothorax.

Stellate ganglion

The sympathetic trunk is continued into the neck from the thorax. There are three cervical ganglia: superior, middle and inferior. The sympathetic trunk lies embedded on the posterior wall of the carotid sheath. The superior ganglion lies at the level of C2 and C3, the middle at the level of C6, and the inferior ganglion at the neck of the first rib behind the vertebral artery. Often the inferior ganglion is fused with the first thoracic ganglion to form the stellate ganglion. Grey rami from this reach the upper limb through the roots of the brachial plexus mostly through C7 and C8. The preganglionic input to the cervical ganglia (including the stellate) are from the upper thoracic white rami. In sympathectomy to denervate the upper limb the T2–T4 ganglia and the white rami are severed, preserving the T1 connection and the stellate ganglion to avoid Horner's syndrome. The thoracic part of the sympathetic chain can be seen lying on the heads of the upper ribs through a thoracoscope after deflating the lung. Resection of T2–T4 segment is carried out to produce a dry hand in patients suffering from hyperhidrosis.

Cervical rib

This is a condition in which an extra rib or part of a rib may develop as a prolongation of the transverse process of the seventh cervical vertebra. It can be bony, fibrous, or partly fibrous and partly bony; and, if complete, it will extend up to the tubercle of the first rib. The components of the brachial plexus which normally lie on the first rib get displaced upwards by the extra rib, leading to compression of the lower trunk (C8–T1). In addition the subclavian vessels may also be stretched, giving rise to Raynaud's phenomenon in the hand.

Diagnosis of the cervical rib is not difficult, as it is seen on x-ray if it is bony. But when it is a fibrous band, diagnosis depends on the absence of any cervical spine abnormality and the presence of vascular and neuritic symptoms.

LYMPH NODES OF THE HEAD AND NECK

The lymph nodes of the head and neck can be classified into a superficial and a deep group. The deep nodes outnumber the superficial nodes (Fig. 13.20).

Superficial nodes

The few nodes which lie superficial to the deep fascia are in two subgroups:

- the anterior cervical nodes along the anterior jugular vein
- the superficial cervical nodes along the external jugular vein.

Afferents to these nodes are from the superficial tissues of the regions drained by the veins along which they lie.

Efferents from the superficial nodes join the deep cervical nodes.

Deep lymph nodes of the head and neck

Most of the deep lymph nodes are arranged roughly in a vertical chain along the internal jugular vein and a circular chain.

Vertical chain

The most important of this group are the deep cervical nodes, which constitute the terminal group for all lymphatics in the head and neck. All tissues in the head and

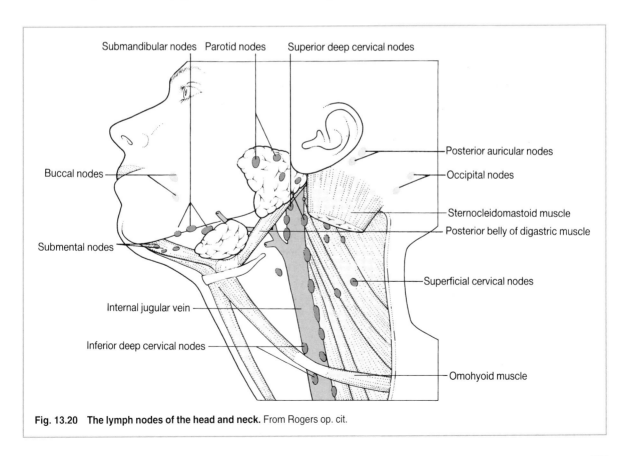

Fig. 13.20 The lymph nodes of the head and neck. From Rogers op. cit.

Submandibular nodes Parotid nodes Superior deep cervical nodes

Buccal nodes

Submental nodes

Internal jugular vein

Inferior deep cervical nodes

Posterior auricular nodes

Occipital nodes

Sternocleidomastoid muscle

Posterior belly of digastric muscle

Superficial cervical nodes

Omohyoid muscle

neck drain into intermediary groups and then into the deep cervical nodes. The deep cervical nodes lie covered by the fascia of the carotid sheath, closely related to the internal jugular vein. They are subdivided into:

- the superior deep cervical nodes
- the inferior deep cervical nodes.

The superior group lies in the region where the posterior belly of the digastric crosses the internal jugular vein, and hence nodes here are also known as the jugulodigastric nodes. This group is closely related to the spinal accessory nerve. They drain the tonsil and the tongue, and the efferents go to the lower deep cervical nodes and/or to the jugular trunk.

The lower group lies where the omohyoid crosses the internal jugular vein and hence are called the juguloomohyoid group. These drain the tongue, oral cavity, trachea, oesophagus and the thyroid gland.

A few nodes in the deep cervical group extend into the posterior triangle and lie along the course of the accessory nerve. There are also a few nodes in the root of the neck — the supraclavicular nodes which enlarge in late stages of malignancies of thorax and abdomen. A classical example is Virchow's node associated with gastric carcinoma (Troisier's sign).

Circular chain

The circular chain of lymph nodes consists of:

- the submental nodes
- the submandibular nodes
- the buccal or facial nodes
- the parotid nodes
- the posterior auricular nodes
- the occipital nodes.

Submental nodes The afferents to this group come from the tip of the tongue, the floor of the mouth and the central part of the lower lip. Efferents go to the submandibular and the jugulo-omohyoid groups.

Submandibular nodes These nodes lie inside the capsule of the submandibular salivary gland. Afferents are received from the side of the nose, upper lip, lateral part of the lower lip, cheek, gums, and the anterior two-thirds of the margin of the tongue. The efferents go to the upper and lower deep cervical nodes.

Buccal or facial nodes These lie on the buccinator along the facial vein and drain the eyelid, conjunctiva, nose and cheek. Efferents drain to the submandibular group.

Parotid nodes There are few nodes in this group, some lying superficial and others deep to the parotid cap-

sule. The superficial nodes drain the eyelids, front of the scalp, external ear and the middle ear. The pre-auricular node is superficial and drains the pinna of the ear and the side of the scalp. The deep nodes drain the parotid gland.

Posterior auricular nodes or the mastoid nodes A few nodes lying on the mastoid process drain the back of the scalp, back of the auricle and the external auditory meatus.

Occipital nodes Situated on the upper attachment of the trapezius, they drain the back of the scalp.

Besides those mentioned above, there are lymph nodes closely related to the pharynx, trachea and the larynx. These are:

- retropharyngeal nodes
- pretracheal and prelaryngeal nodes.

The retropharyngeal nodes lie between the pharynx and the prevertebral fascia and drain the back of the nasal cavity, nasopharynx and the Eustachian tube. Efferents go to the deep cervical nodes. The pretracheal and prelaryngeal nodes drain the adjoining viscera and also receive afferents from the anterior cervical nodes. Their efferents also go to the deep cervical nodes.

Block dissection of the neck

In this all the lymph nodes in the anterior and posterior triangles of the neck, along with the associated structures, are removed *en bloc*. It extends from the mandible above to the clavicle below and the midline anteriorly to the anterior border of the trapezius posteriorly. All the structures from the platysma to the pretracheal fascia are removed, leaving only the carotid arteries, the vagus nerve, the sympathetic trunk, and the lingual and the hypoglossal nerves. The sternocleidomastoid, the posterior belly of the digastric and the omohyoid are all removed along with the internal jugular and the external jugular veins, the submandibular gland and the lower part of the parotid gland. The accessory nerve to which lymph nodes are related in the posterior triangle is also sacrificed.

EYE

Eyeball

The eyeball is a sphere about 24 mm in diameter and consists of a prominent anterior segment, the cornea, which forms one-sixth of the sphere, and a larger posterior segment, the sclera, forming the remaining five-sixths. A line joining the anterior pole and the posterior pole is the optic axis. The optic nerve leaves the eyeball about 3 mm to the nasal side of the posterior pole (Fig. 13.21).

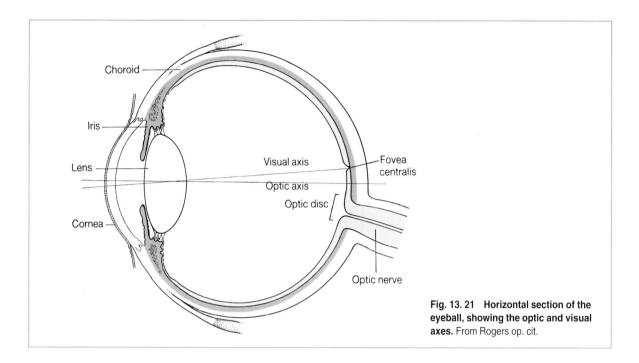

Fig. 13. 21   Horizontal section of the eyeball, showing the optic and visual axes. From Rogers op. cit.

The wall of the eyeball has three distinct coats:

- an outer fibrous coat consisting of sclera and cornea
- a middle vascular coat consisting of the choroid, the ciliary body and the iris
- an inner neural coat formed by the retina.

Sclera
Sclera is normally white and is made of collagen. The tendons of the extraocular muscles fuse with the sclera. The lamina cribosa is an area posteriorly pierced by the optic nerve. The dura of the optic nerve becomes continuous with the sclera. The ciliary vessels and nerves and the venae verticosae that drain blood from the eyeball also perforate the sclera.

Cornea
The curved surface of the cornea is the main refracting site of the eye contributing to about 40 dioptres out of the 58 dioptres the eye can produce. Structurally the cornea consists of collagen, the regular orientation of which makes it transparent. The conjunctiva ends at the sclerocorneal junction, its epithelium becoming continuous with that of the cornea. The cornea is avascular and receives its nutrition from the aqueous humour. It is very sensitive to touch and pain and is innervated by ciliary nerves which are branches of the nasociliary branch of the ophthalmic division of the trigeminal nerve.

Choroid
This thin vascular membrane lines the inner surface of the sclera and is continuous anteriorly with the other vascular components of the eye, namely the ciliary body and the iris. The junction between the choroid and the ciliary body is the ora serrata, which has a serrated appearance when viewed from inside. The choroid has two layers. The outer layer in contact with the sclera is heavily pigmented with brownish-black melanin. The inner layer contains blood vessels and branches of the ciliary nerves.

Ciliary body
The ciliary body consists of the ciliary ring, ciliary processes and ciliary muscles. The ciliary ring is a fibrous ring flattened against the sclera externally (anteriorly) and the vitreous humour or vitreous body internally (posteriorly). It extends forwards from the choroid to the sclerocorneal junction. It is triangular in section with a thicker anterior circumference. Posteriorly it thins out to merge with the choroid at the ora serrata.

The anterior part of the surface of the ciliary ring facing the vitreous (internal or posterior surface) has 60–80 radially arranged ridges. These are the ciliary processes (Fig. 13.22). These are vascular structures and they produce the aqueous humour. A number of delicate fibrils extend from the ciliary processes to be attached to the lens. These form the suspensory ligament (Fig. 13.23).

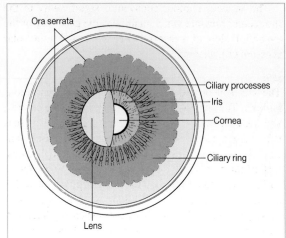

Fig. 13.22   The ora serrata and lens — posterior view.
From Rogers op. cit.

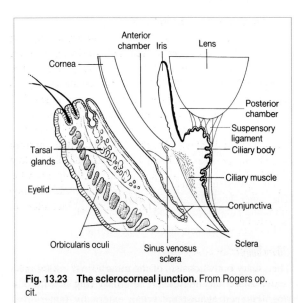

Fig. 13.23   The sclerocorneal junction. From Rogers op. cit.

The ciliary muscles lie between the ciliary ring and the sclera. They take origin from the scleral spur, which is an inner projection from the sclerocorneal junction. Muscles consist of radial and circular fibres. Their contraction relaxes the suspensory ligament, making the lens more convex during accommodation. Both parts of the muscles are supplied by the Edinger–Westphal nucleus through the oculomotor nerve (third nerve). The preganglionic fibres synapse in the ciliary ganglion, and the postganglionic fibres enter the eye via the short ciliary nerves.

Iris

This is the disc surrounding the pupil. The iris divides the anterior segment of the eyeball into anterior and posterior chambers; the former between the iris and the cornea, and the latter between it and the lens (Fig. 13.23). Its periphery is attached to the ciliary body. The main bulk of the iris is formed by blood vessels. The connective tissue stroma has pigment cells which give the iris its colour. There are two sets of muscles in the iris. The circular muscle, the sphincter muscle, supplied by the parasympathetic fibres from the Edinger–Westphal nucleus through the oculomotor nerve (similar to the ciliary muscles) constricts the pupil. Radial muscle fibres, the dilator pupillae, are supplied by postganglionic sympathetic nerves.

Retina

The retina, which developed originally from the optic cup of the embryo, has an outer and inner layer. The outer layer is one cell thick, is heavily pigmented, and it lines the choroid, the ciliary body and the posterior surface of the iris.

The inner layer of the retina varies with position. Anterior to the ora serrata, the inner layer becomes a simple layer of pigmented cells lining the posterior surfaces of the ciliary body (pars ciliaris retinae) and iris (pars iridis retinae). Posterior to the ora serrrata the inner layer is multilayered, forming the pars optica retinae. This part has three layers of neurons:

- an outer layer of rods and cones applied to the pigment layer
- an intermediate layer of bipolar neurons
- an inner layer of ganglionic cells whose axons become the optic nerve.

The details of the retinal structure are shown in Figure 13.24.

When the pars optica retinae is examined with an ophthalmoscope, it looks homogenous, except for two areas posteriorly:

- the optic disc
- the macula lutea.

The optic disc is approximately circular. It is paler in colour than the rest of the retina, which looks brick-red in the living eye. It lies medial to the (nasal) posterior pole. At the disc the axons of the ganglionic cells leave to enter the optic nerve. The central artery of the retina emerges from the disc and divides into upper and lower branches, each of which in turn divides into a nasal and temporal branch. There is effectively no anastomosis between the

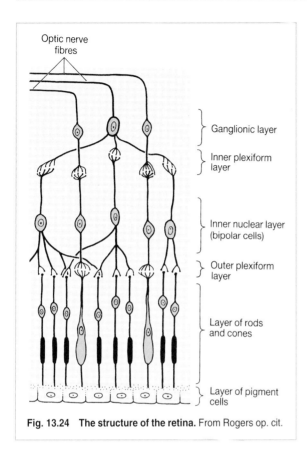

Optic nerve
fibres

} Ganglionic layer

} Inner plexiform
layer

} Inner nuclear layer
(bipolar cells)

} Outer plexiform
layer

} Layer of rods
and cones

} Layer of pigment
cells

Fig. 13.24   The structure of the retina. From Rogers op. cit.

adjacent arteries. The branches of the arteries are accompanied by veins. When seen with an ophthalmoscope the veins appear darker than arteries.

The macula lutea lies lateral to the optic disc almost at the posterior pole. This pale yellowish area is the site of central vision. No large retinal vessels cross the macula. A depression in its centre is the fovea centralis.

Refracting media of the eye

The refracting media of the eye are the cornea, the aqueous humour, the lens and the vitreous humour. As mentioned already the surface of the cornea makes the greatest contribution to the refraction of light.

Aqueous humour

This watery fluid is formed in the posterior chamber (space between the lens and the iris) by filtration and secretion at the ciliary processes. Passing through the pupil the aqueous humour enters the anterior chamber (between the iris and the cornea). At the iridocorneal angle the fluid is absorbed into the canal of Schlemm (sinus venous sclerae) and via the canal into the scleral veins.

The aqueous humour contributes significantly to the intraocular pressure which maintains the geometry of the eyeball. Failure of reabsorption causes raised intraocular pressure or glaucoma.

Lens

The lens is biconvex and is placed in front of the vitreous humour. The posterior surface of the lens is more convex, and the anterior surface is relatively flattened. The lens lies within a capsule which resembles a thick basal lamina. The refractive index of the lens is much higher than that of the vitreous or aqueous humours. It contributes some 15 dioptres to the total refractive power of which the eye is capable (about 58 dioptres). The lens is suspended from the ciliary body by the suspensory ligament. Tension in the suspensory ligament flattens the lens. Contraction of the ciliary muscles reduces the circumference of the ciliary ring and slackens the suspensory ligament, allowing the lens to be more spherical, altering its refractive power.

Vitreous humour or vitreous body

The vitreous humour occupies the posterior segment of the eyeball. It is a transparent gel consisting of water (about 99%) with electrolytes and glycoproteins. The peripheral zone of the vitreous is condensed into a tougher vitreous membrane which is firmly attached to the optic disc posteriorly and to the ciliary processes anteriorly. It is also in contact with the lens and the retina but is not firmly attached to them. The concavity in front which accepts the lens is the hyaloid fossa. The hyaloid canal is a narrow, fluid-filled canal extending from the optic disc to the hyaloid fossa. In embryonic life this houses the hyaloid artery, a branch of the retinal artery to supplying the lens.

Muscles of the orbit

The levator palpebrae superioris, and the extraocular muscles are the muscles of the orbit (Fig. 13.25). The extraocular muscles consist of:

- the medial, lateral, superior and inferior recti
- the superior and inferior obliques.

The four recti arise from the tendinous ring around the optic foramen and the medial part of the superior orbital fissure. They are inserted to the sclera anterior to the equator. The superior oblique arises superior and medial to the tendinous ring. It runs forward and its tendon winds round a fibrous pulley (the trochlea) to run posteriorly and laterally to be inserted to the posterolateral quadrant (behind the equator) on the superior surface of the sclera. The inferior oblique originates from the floor of

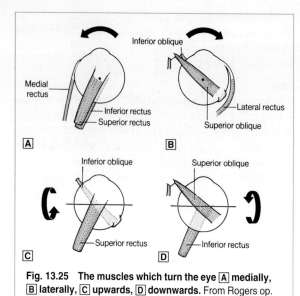

Fig. 13.25 **The muscles which turn the eye** [A] **medially,** [B] **laterally,** [C] **upwards,** [D] **downwards.** From Rogers op. cit.

Nerve supply of the muscles of the orbit

All the muscles are supplied by the oculomotor nerve except the lateral rectus (abducent nerve) and the superior oblique (trochlear nerve).

Eyelids

Each eyelid from without inwards consists of the following layers:

- the skin
- loose connective tissue
- fibres of the orbicularis oculi muscle
- the tarsal plate
- the conjunctiva.

Within the tarsal plate there are a number of tarsal glands (Meibomian glands), which when blocked produce Meibomian cysts. Medially and laterally the upper and lower tarsal plates fuse to become the medial and lateral palpebral ligaments. The medial palpebral ligament is thicker and it anchors the tarsal plates to the anterior lacrimal crest.

The upper eyelid is larger and more mobile than the lower lid. It also receives the attachment of the levator palpebrae superioris. When the eye is closed, a complete conjunctival sac lies between the posterior surfaces of the eyelids and the front of the eyeball. The upper and lower limits of the sac are called the superior and inferior conjunctival fornices. The two eyelids meet at the medial canthus and lateral canthus. In the medial canthus lies a small elevation, the lacrimal caruncle. The plica semilunaris is a triangular fold extending laterally from the caruncle.

The conjunctiva lines the inner surface of the eyelids (palpebral part) and is reflected over the sclera (orbital

the orbit on the orbital surface of the maxilla lateral to the crest of the lacrimal bone. It passes posteriorly and laterally under the eyeball to be inserted behind the equator to the postero-inferior lateral quadrant on the sclera.

The actions of the extraocular muscles are summarised in Table 13.1.

Levator palpebrae superioris

This takes origin from the roof of the orbit posteriorly (lesser wing of the sphenoid, just superior to the tendinous ring). It passes forwards between the superior rectus and the roof of the orbit, to be inserted into the upper eyelid.

Table 13.1 Movements[a] produced by individual extraocular muscles		
Muscle	Movement of pupil	Rotation around optical axis[b]
Medial rectus	Medially	None
Lateral rectus	Laterally	None
Superior rectus	Superiorly and medially	Medially and down
Inferior rectus	Inferiorly and medially	Laterally and down
Superior oblique	Inferiorly and laterally	Medially and down
Inferior oblique	Superiorly and laterally	Laterally and down

[a]These are the movements produced by each muscle acting alone, with the eye in the anatomical position.
[b]Rotation is described as the movement of the 12 o'clock point of the iris.
From Rogers op. cit.

part) along the two conjunctival fornices. The palpebral part is thick and highly vascular, whereas the orbital part is thinner and its extension over the cornea only a single layer of epithelium. The superior conjunctival fornix laterally receive the ducts of the lacrimal gland.

The size of the palpebral fissure (the area between the edges of the two lids when the eye is opened) depends on the tone of the orbicularis oculi and the levator palpebral superioris. Contraction of the former, which is supplied by the facial nerve, shuts the eye. Most of the levator palpebrae superioris is supplied by the oculomotor nerve. However, it has some smooth muscle fibres in its deeper aspect innervated by postganglionic sympathetic fibres. Paralysis of the oculomotor nerve produces marked ptosis, whereas mild ptosis is a feature of Horner's syndrome.

Lacrimal apparatus

The lacrimal gland is situated in the lateral part of the orbit. It has a large orbital part, related to the roof of the orbit, and a smaller palpebral part which extends onto the upper lid. 8–12 ducts open into the lateral aspect of the superior conjunctival fornix. Tears are spread over the surface of the eye by the blinking action of the lids produced by the contraction of the palpebral fibres of the orbicularis oculi. It is drained by the superior and inferior lacrimal canaliculi into the lacrimal sac. The canaliculi and the lacrimal sac are at the medial angle of the eye. Openings of the canaliculi on the eyelids are known as the lacrimal puncta. The lacrimal sac is lodged in the lacrimal fossa between the anterior and posterior lacrimal crests on the medial wall of the orbit. It continues into the inferior meatus of the nasal cavity as the nasolacrimal duct. The sac lies behind the medial palpebral ligament. Blinking alters the tension in the ligament, producing intermittent compression of the lacrimal sac, which aids its emptying.

Sensory innervation of the eyelids and conjunctiva

The skin over the upper eyelid and the palpebral conjunctiva receives sensory supply from various branches of the ophthalmic division of the trigeminal nerve (infratrochlear, supratrochlear, supraorbital and lacrimal nerves). The lower eyelid, including its palpebral conjunctiva, is supplied by the palpebral branches of the infraorbital nerve (from the maxillary division of the trigeminal nerve).

EAR

The ear can be divided anatomically and clinically into three distinct parts (Fig. 13.26):

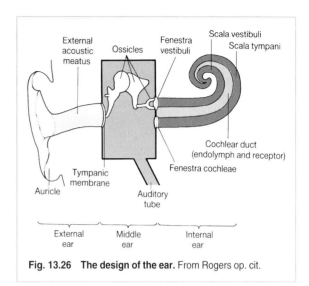

Fig. 13.26   The design of the ear. From Rogers op. cit.

- the external ear, which collects sound waves at the tympanic membrane (ear drum)
- the middle ear, an air-filled space, across which the vibrations of the tympanic membrane are transmitted by a chain of three ossicles to the internal ear
- the internal ear, the membraneous fluid-filled sac containing receptor cells, enclosed in the petrous temporal bone and separated from it by a fluid-filled space.

The external and middle ears are primarily concerned with transmission of sound. The internal ear functions both as the organ of hearing and for balancing the body.

External ear

The external ear comprises two parts:

- the auricle or pinna, which collects the sound waves
- the external auditory meatus, leading from the exterior to the tympanic membrane.

Auricle

This has a framework of elastic cartilage covered on each surface by skin (Fig. 13.27). The skin on the lateral surface is closely adherent to the perichondrium. The lobule has no cartilage and contains fat and fibrous tissue. The auricle is attached to the skull by anterior and posterior ligaments and functionless auricular muscles.

External auditory (acoustic) meatus

In the adult the external auditory meatus is about 2.5 cm long. It is not straight. The S-shaped meatus curves anteriorly and downwards as well as medially as it

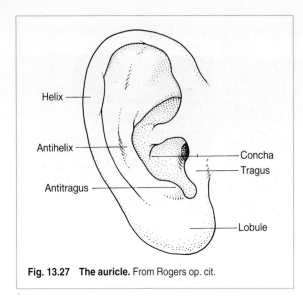

Fig. 13.27 The auricle. From Rogers op. cit.

approaches the tympanic membrane. The lateral third of the meatus is cartilaginous, and the medial two-thirds is bony — the tympanic part of the temporal bone. There are two constrictions in the canal: one at the junction of the cartilaginous and bony part, and the second one in the bony part. The meatus may be partially straightened by pulling the auricle upwards laterally and backwards.

The external auditory meatus is lined by skin except for the outer surface of the tympanic membrane where the stratified squamous epithelium is not keratinised. The skin is closely adherent to underlying tissues; hence, furuncles and other infections are extremely painful, especially in the cartilaginous portion, as tension is increased in the tissues during infection.

The outer part of the meatus is guarded by ceruminous glands in the wall of the meatus producing secretions with antibacterial properties. The tympanic membrane faces laterally, downwards and forwards.

The external auditory meatus lies very close to the temporomandibular joint. Severe blows to the chin can fracture the bony walls of the meatus. Extensions of the parotid gland lie antero-inferior to the meatus.

Nerve supply

The medial or posterior surface of the auricle and the lateral surface below the tragus is supplied by the great auricular nerve (C2 & C3). The auriculotemporal nerve (branch of the mandibular division of the trigeminal nerve) supplies the rest of the lateral surface of the auricle and most of the external auditory meatus and the tympanic membrane. The auricular branch of the vagus also contributes to the supply of the latter two.

Blood supply

This comes from the superficial temporal and the posterior auricular arteries. The meatus receives a further supply from the deep auricular branch of the maxillary artery. The veins accompany the arteries.

Lymphatic drainage

The auricle and the external auditory meatus drain to preauricular nodes (parotid) anteriorly and posteriorly to the glands in the posterior triangle (along the external jugular vein) and also to the mastoid glands. Involvement of the mastoid or retroauricular glands in infections of the scalp and ear may mistakenly be diagnosed as mastoiditis.

Middle ear (tympanic cavity)

The middle ear lies between the tympanic membrane laterally and the cochlea medially. It is described as having a roof, floor, anterior wall and a posterior wall besides the medial and lateral walls. The latter two bulge into the middle ear cavity which is therefore narrower in the middle than peripherally. The tympanic cavity extends anteriorly as the Eustachian tube, which connects it to the nasopharynx. Posteriorly the aditus leads to the mastoid antrum and mastoid air cells. The part of the cavity extending above the tympanic membrane is known as the epitympanic recess.

Lateral wall — the tympanic membrane

The tympanic membrane (Fig. 13.28) separates the external auditory meatus from the middle ear (Fig 13.26). It is attached to the tympanic annulus, which is a sulcus on the tympanic plate of the temporal bone. The membrane has an outer layer of stratified squamous epithelium continuous with that of the meatus, a middle layer of fibrous tissue, and an inner layer of mucous membrane continuous with the lining of the middle ear. The membrane is circular and 1 cm in diameter. It is concave towards the meatus and faces downwards forwards and laterally, forming an angle of 55° with the meatus. The handle of the malleus produces a small depression on the external surface — the umbo (Fig. 13.29). When the drum is illuminated for inspection a cone of light is seen radiating from the umbo in this antero-inferior quadrant. Two malleolar folds diverge from the lateral process of the malleus. The segment of the membrane between the malleolar folds is the pars flaccida or Shrapnell's membrane. This part of the tympanic membrane is crossed by the chorda tympani nerve, which is seen through the tympanic membrane when it is illuminated. The rest of the membrane is tense — the pars tensa.

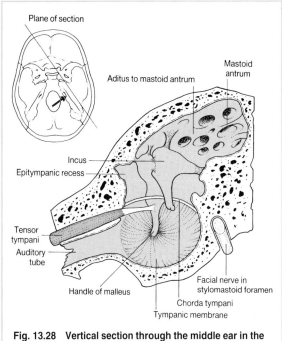

Fig. 13.28 Vertical section through the middle ear in the axis of the petrous temporal bone: medial view. From Rogers op. cit.

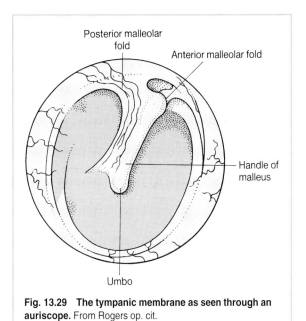

Fig. 13.29 The tympanic membrane as seen through an auriscope. From Rogers op. cit.

Nerve supply The lateral (meatal) surface is supplied by the auriculotemporal nerve supplemented posteriorly by the facial and vagus nerves. The medial surface (middle ear) is supplied by the glossopharyngeal nerve.

Blood supply The deep auricular branch of the maxillary artery supplemented by branches from the posterior auricular artery and the tympanic branch of the maxillary.

Medial wall

The medial wall (Fig. 13.30) separates the tympanic cavity from the inner ear. The central part of this wall is the promontory which overlies the first turn of the cochlea. Above and posterior to the promontory is the fenestra vestibuli or oval window occupied by the footpiece of the stapes. Below and posterior to the promontory is the round window or fenestra cochlea. This is closed by the secondary tympanic membrane. Above the promontory is a linear projection which contains the facial nerve.

Roof

The roof of the tympanic cavity is the tegmen tympani, a thin plate of bone forming the anterior surface of the petrous temporal bone. This separates the middle ear from the middle cranial fossa. The tegmen tympani is easily fractured. If the dura and the tympanic membrane

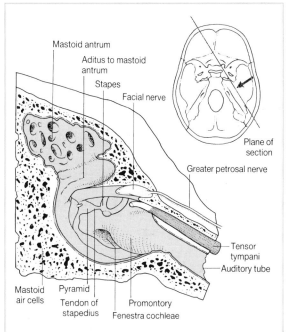

Fig. 13.30 Vertical section similar to Figure 13.28. Here, the medial wall of the middle ear is seen form the lateral side. From Rogers op. cit.

are also ruptured, it is associated with CSF otorrhoea (CSF draining from the ear).

Posterior wall

The upper part of the posterior wall has the aditus which connects the middle ear to the mastoid antrum. Below this it has a shallow depression which houses the short process of the incus (the fossa incudis). The pyramid is an elevation on the posterior wall, from inside which the stapedius muscle takes origin. The canal for the chorda tympani opens below the pyramid.

Anterior wall

The bony part of the Eustachian (auditory) tube opens into the anterior wall. Above this is the canal for the tensor tympani muscle.

Ossicles of the middle ear

The three ossicles (Fig. 13.31) are the malleus, incus and stapes. These transmit the vibrations produced by sound from the tympanic membrane to the cochlea. The joints between them are synovial joints.

The malleus has a handle which is attached to the tympanic membrane (producing the umbo). Its head and narrow neck lies in the epitympanic recess. The malleus is connected to the walls of the tympanic cavity by the malleolar ligaments extending from its anterior and lateral processes. The head of the malleus articulates with the incus. The incus has a body which articulates with the malleus and two projections: the short process posteriorly into the fossa incudis on the posterior wall and the long process projecting down parallel to the handle of the malleus to articulate with the head of the stapes.

The stapes, which is derived from the 2nd branchial arch (malleus and incus from the 1st), has a head which articulates with the incus. Its footplate articulates with the fenestra vestibuli.

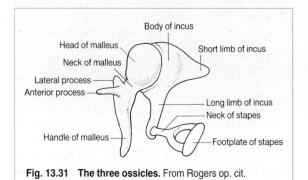

Fig. 13.31 The three ossicles. From Rogers op. cit.

Labels: Body of incus; Head of malleus; Short limb of incus; Neck of malleus; Lateral process; Anterior process; Long limb of incus; Neck of stapes; Handle of malleus; Footplate of stapes

Movements of the ossicles

The malleus and the incus rotate about an anteroposterior axis. When the tympanic membrane moves medially, carrying with it the handle of the malleus, the head of the malleus and the body of the incus move laterally. As the body of the incus moves laterally, its long process and the stapes are carried medially. Thus the handle of the malleus and the long process of the incus and stapes move in parallel.

Muscles of the middle ear

The tensor tympani and the stapedius are the two muscles of the middle ear. The tensor tympani arises from the wall of the canal for the tensor tympani in the anterior wall of the middle ear. The tendon emerges from the canal and turns medially, to insert to the upper part of the handle of the malleus. Contraction of the muscle moves the tympanic membrane medially, tensing it to dampen vibrations produced by loud sounds. This muscle is supplied by a branch from the mandibular division of the trigeminal nerve.

The stapedius also dampens the movements of the ossicles in response to loud sounds. It arises from the inner wall of the pyramid on the posterior wall, and the tendon inserts into the neck of the stapes. It is supplied by a branch of the facial nerve.

Nerve supply of the middle ear

The sensory supply is by the tympanic branch of the glossopharyngeal nerve which contributes to the tympanic plexus on the promontory of the medial wall. Sympathetic fibres from the internal carotid plexus also contribute to the tympanic plexus.

Blood supply

Branches from the maxillary, middle meningeal, ascending pharyngeal and the internal carotid arteries supply the middle ear. Veins drain into the pterygoid plexus and the superior petrossal sinus. Lymph drainage is into the parotid lymph nodes.

Eustachian tube (auditory tube)

This connects the middle ear and the nasopharynx. The posterior and lateral third is bony and is part of the petrous temporal bone. The anterior and medial two-thirds are cartilaginous and lie in the base of the skull in the groove between the petrous temporal bone and the greater wing of the sphenoid.

The cartilaginous part is normally closed except during swallowing, when the communication between the nasopharynx and the middle ear allows the pressures on either side of the tympanic membrane to equalise. Tensor veli

palatini and the levator palatini muscles are attached to
the tube, and their contraction during swallowing opens
the tube. The salpingopharyngeus muscle is attached to
the end of the tube in the nasopharynx. Here cartilage is
prominent posterosuperior to the opening forming the
tubal elevation in the nasopharynx. The tubal end is surrounded by the lymphoid tissues, the tubal tonsil until
adolescence. In the infant the auditory tube is almost
horizontal, shorter and wider.

Mastoid antrum and the mastoid air cells

The mastoid air cells lie within the mastoid process,
opening into the mastoid antrum. They are variable in
extent. In infancy they do not exist, and the infantile type
of mastoid may persist into adult life in about 20% of
people. On the other hand large cells may occupy much
of the mastoid process and extend into the adjoining
bones. The layer of bone separating the air cells from the
posterior cranial fossa and the sigmoid sinus is thin or
even deficient in places, allowing the spread of infection
to the cranial cavity, and thrombosis of the sinus. Acute
mastoiditis arises from an acute otitis media by extension
of infection from the mastoid antrum to the air cells.
Severe infection may spread anteriorly into the external
auditory meatus, simulating a discharging furnucle.

The mastoid air cells communicate with the middle ear
through the mastoid antrum and the aditus. It lies medial
to the suprameatal triangle. Mastoid air cells open into
the floor of the antrum. The roof of the antrum is the
tegmen tympani separating the antrum from the middle
cranial fossa.

Internal ear

The internal (Fig. 13.32) ear consists of a bony labyrinth
inside which is enclosed the membraneous labyrinth.
The membraneous labyrinth contains endolymph and the
sensory end organs for hearing and vestibular functions.
The bony labyrinth contains perilymph which surrounds
the membraneous labyrinth.

The inner ear has three parts: the cochlea (bony),
containing the cochlear duct anteriorly, the three semicircular canals (bony) with the three semicircular ducts
(membraneous) at the posterior aspect, and the vestibule
(bony labyrinth) with the utricle and saccule (membraneous labyrinth) in between the cochlea and the semicircular canals.

Cochlea

The cochlea (Fig. 13.33) is concerned with hearing. It
comprises two and three-quarter turns of a bony canal
around a bony pillar known as the modiolus. The cochlea

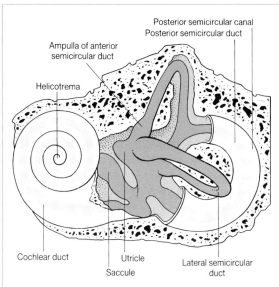

Fig. 13.32 The membraneous labyrinth superimposed on the osseous labyrinth. From Rogers op. cit.

lies at right angles to the long axis of the petrous temporal
bone.

Projecting from the modiolus is a spiral-shaped shelf,
the osseous spiral lamina. It has a canal which is continuous with the canal of the modiolus. From the free edge of
the osseous spiral lamina the basilar membrane extends
to the wall of the cochlea. The basilar membrane forms
the lower wall of the cochlear duct, the membraneous
labyrinth of the cochlea. Its upper wall is formed by the
vestibular membrane (Reissner's membrane). The cochlear
duct thus divides the cochlea into two compartments.
Above the duct is the scala vestibuli, and below the scala
tympani. Both these contain perilymph. Both the scala
vestibuli and scala tympani are continuous with each
other at the apex of the cochlea known as the helicotrema.

The vestibular end of the scala vestibuli is directed
against the fenestra vestibuli of the middle ear. However,
the scala tympani does not open into the vestibule but is
separated from it by the commencement of the osseous
spiral lamina and the basilar membrane. Perilymph of the
scala tympani is separated from the middle ear by the
membrane closing the fenestra cochlea or the round window. From the scala tympani, a minute duct, the cochlear
aqueduct passes through the petrous temporal bone to
open into the posterior cranial fossa allowing communication between perilymph and the CSF. The composition
of perilymph is similar to that of CSF; however, the
details of its formation are not known.

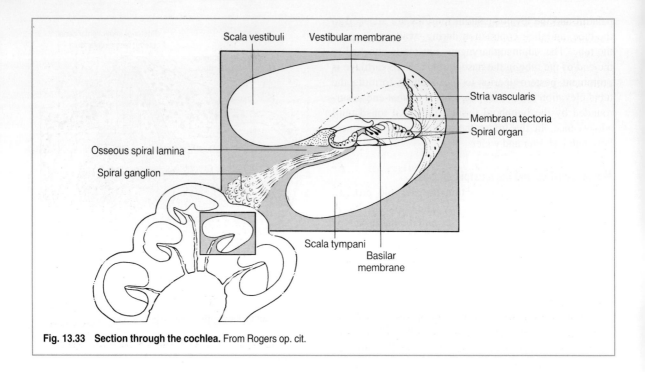

Scala vestibuli   Vestibular membrane

Stria vascularis

Membrana tectoria
Spiral organ

Osseous spiral lamina

Spiral ganglion

Scala tympani

Basilar
membrane

Fig. 13.33   Section through the cochlea. From Rogers op. cit.

Cochlear duct

This is also known as the scala media and has the same shape as the bony cochlea. It separates the scala vestibuli from the scala tympani, and is surrounded by perilymph of the bony cochlea. The organ of Corti, a spiral organ, the sense organ of hearing, is situated inside the cochlear duct on the basilar membrane (Fig. 13.33). The organ of Corti has hair cells and supporting cells. The hair cells are covered by gelatinous membrana tectoria and are innervated by the cochlear nerve.

The mechanism by which sound waves are converted to nerve impulses is not well understood. It is possible that the movements of the footplate of the stapes produce vibratory oscillations in the perilymph of the scala vestibuli which are transmitted at the helicotrema to the scala tympani and ultimately to the membrane at the fenestra cochlea. These vibrations of the perilymph produce corresponding movements of the basilar membrane. Movements of the basilar membrane are detected by hair cells of the organ of Corti and are relayed to the brain by the cochlear nerve (auditory nerve).

Vestibule, utricle and saccule

Vestibule   The vestibule accommodates the utricle and saccule and lies between the cochlea and the semicircular canals. The lateral wall of the bony vestibule has the fenestra vestibuli closed by the footpiece of the

stapes. The medial wall of the vestibule lies at the depth of the internal acoustic meatus and is perforated by a number of holes through which branches of the vestibulocochlear nerve (eighth nerve) enter the internal ear. From the anterior wall of the vestibule the first turn of the cochlea arises. The three semicircular canals open into the vestibule by five orifices on the posterior and lateral walls.

Utricle and saccule   The utricle and saccule are parts of the membranous labyrinth inside the vestibule. They contain endolymph and are surrounded by perilymph of the vestibule. They carry receptors registering positional sense. These end organs are known as maculae. They carry hair cells which project into a gelatinous cap which contains calcium salt, the otoliths or ear stones.

The utricle, which is posterior to the saccule, receives the five openings of the semicircular ducts. From the utricle a small duct joins the endolymphatic duct from the saccule. The endolymphatic duct extends to lie between the layers of the dura mater and ends on the posterior surface of the petrous temporal bone as the endolymphatic sac. The saccule is linked to the cochlear duct by the ductus reuniens.

Semicircular canals

There are three semicircular canals.

● The anterior, also known as the superior semicircular canal, is vertical and is at right angles to the long axis of the petrous temporal bone. It raises the arcuate eminence on the anterior surface of the petrous temporal bone.

- The posterior canal is also vertical but is orientated in the long axis of the petrous temporal bone.
- The lateral semicircular canal is horizontal. It raises a small swelling on the medial wall of the middle ear.

The anterior and posterior semicircular canals share a common crus and a common opening to the vestibule. All four open separately. Just before the opening, each canal has a dilated end called the ampulla.

The long axis of petrous temporal bone is at 45° to the midsagittal plane. Therefore the anterior canal of one side is in a plane parallel to the posterior canal of the other side. The two lateral canals lie in the horizontal plane.

Semicircular ducts

These form the membraneous labyrinth portion of the semicircular canals. They have the same shape as the bony semicircular canals and are separated from the bony wall by perilymph. The semicircular ducts contain endolymph. The semicircular ducts open into the utricle by five openings. The anterior (superior) and posterior semicircular ducts share a common opening. Each semicircular duct also has a swelling near its opening, the ampulla, corresponding to the ampulla of the bony semicircular canals. The ampulla has neuroepithelium called the crista ampullaris. The hair cells of the crista have long filaments which project into a mass of gelatinous material called the cupula. Movement of the endolymph in the ducts bends the cupula and hair cells, and the sensation is transmitted by the terminal fibres of the vestibular nerve.

Vestibulocochlear nerve

The eighth cranial nerve (Fig. 13.34) attaches to the brainstem lateral to the seventh nerve (facial nerve) at the cerebellopontine angle and enters the internal acoustic meatus. At the base of the internal acoustic meatus the vestibulocochlear nerve breaks up into many rootlets, which pierce the thin medial wall of the vestibule. The vestibular fibres have the vestibular ganglion from which fibres pass to innervate the maculae of the utricle and saccule and the cristae of the semicircular ducts. The cochlear fibres pass into the core of the modiolus and enter the osseous spiral lamina where the nerve has its spiral ganglion. From this ganglion, fibres pass through the osseous spiral lamina to innervate the hair cells of the organ of Corti.

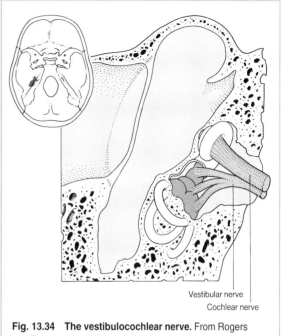

Vestibular nerve
Cochlear nerve

Fig. 13.34   The vestibulocochlear nerve. From Rogers op. cit.

PHYSIOLOGY

SALIVARY GLANDS

All the salivary glands consist of secretory end pieces, the acini, and an elaborate duct system to transport the secretion to the oral cavity. The acini of the parotid are predominantly serous: the sublingual mucous and the submandibular mixed.

About 1.5 L of saliva is secreted daily. The pH of saliva varies from 7 to 8. Saliva contains α-amylase, which initiates digestion of starch, as well as lipase (mostly from the lingual glands) which acts on triglycerides. Saliva also contains mucins (glycoproteins) to lubricate the food and protect the oral mucosa. A dry mouth makes swallowing difficult. Saliva also contains bacteriostatic agents such as IgA, lysozyme and lactoferrin, as well as proline-rich proteins which protect tooth enamel.

The saliva secreted by the acini is isotonic, with concentrations of Na^+, K^+, Cl^- and HCO_3^- close to those in plasma. As the primary secretion passes through the duct system the duct cells remove Na^+ and Cl^- in exchange for K^+ and HCO_3. It also becomes hypotonic. Thus the saliva that reaches the oral cavity is hypotonic, alkaline and rich in K^+ but depleted of Na^+ and Cl^-. As in the renal tubules, aldosterone increases K$^+$ concentration and reduces Na$^+$ concentration.

The salivary secretion is under neural control. Stimulation of parasympathetic nerves increases secretion of watery saliva low in enzymic contents. The transmitter for this is acetylcholine. Nerve stimulation also produces vasodilatation through VIP, another transmitter released by the postganglionic parasympathetic neurons. Atropine and other cholinergic antagonists reduce salivary secretion. Food in the mouth and stimulation of vagal afferents increase secretion.

Saliva performs a number of important functions. It keeps the mouth moist, facilitates swallowing, stimulates taste buds and aids speech. It has a bacteriocidal function. Any condition reducing salivary secretion increases the incidence of dental caries. Saliva also has a buffering action and helps to neutralise the effect of acid regurgitation on the oesophageal mucosa.

MECHANISM OF SWALLOWING

See Chapter 17.

PHONATION AND THE MECHANISM OF SPEECH

Production of sound by the larynx, phonation, and the articulation of that sound into understandable vowels and consonants are all acheived by the controlled and coordinated activity of muscles, nerves, neuronal circuits and large areas in the cerebral cortex. The following is only a simplified and concise account of the mechanism of speech, avoiding complex and often conflicting details.

Phonation

We breathe while we speak. The natural rhythm of respiration has to be altered so that the voice production and its articulation are not disrupted by inhalation at inappropriate times. The rate of respiration is about 12–14 times per minute, and the time taken for quiet inhalation and exhalation are about equal. During speech, however, the inspiration is shorter and the time taken for expiration is more prolonged. Muscles involved in inhalation and exhalation of air are the same as in quiet respiration. In phonation the muscular tone of the diaphragm and intercostals is gradually reduced to achieve a controlled expiration. Patients with spinal injuries who rely entirely on the diaphragm for breathing often break sentences up in order to inspire, and hence have a charcteristic speech impediment. Training the diaphragm by speech therapy can overcome some of the problems.

At the laryngeal level the major event in phonation is adduction of the vocal cords. This involves the transverse arytenoid muscle and the recurrent laryngeal nerve. Adduction of the vocal cords raises the subglottic pressure. When the air is exhaled, it pushes the cords apart. The consequent drop in infraglottic pressure adducts the cords again, and the cycle is repeated. The movements of the tensed cords will produce sound.

There are three important variables in sound:

- loudness
- pitch
- quality of sound.

Loudness

This varies with the level of infraglottic pressure needed to separate the cords and the degree of adduction of the cords. Loudness is increased by tightly adducting the cords and building a higher infraglottic pressure. The latter can be increased further by the contraction of expiratory muscles (as in shouting).

Pitch

This is determined by the frequency of vibration. Higher pitch is achieved by increasing the tension of the cord. The cricothyroid muscle stretches the cord by reducing the cricothyroid interval. Simultaneous isometric contraction of the thyroarytenoid muscle increases the muscle tone contributing to an increase in the tension of the cord. The vocalis muscles are important in the fine adjustment of the vertical depth over which the two cords meet, as well as the gradation of their thickness. These too are important factors in regulating the pitch. Voice training involves a certain degree of hypertrophy of the vocalis and thyroarytenoid muscles. Tension of the cords depends on a number of myotatic reflexes. There are a large number of muscle spindles in the laryngeal muscles; their density is second only to that in the extraocular muscles.

The pitch of the voice also alters with the length of the cords. At birth the cords are only 7 mm long, but they increase to 14 mm by puberty. The adult female cord is 15–16 mm long whereas the adult male cord is about 18–21 mm.

Quality of sound

The size and relationship of the resonating chambers such as the larynx, the pharynx and the paranasal sinuses contribute and maintain the quality of sound. People with a good quality voice are born with it. They cannot be trained to produce it.

Articulation of sounds

Articulation of sound produced by the larynx into understandable vowels and consonants is done by varying the size and shape of the oral cavity as well as interrupting the flow of exhaled air by lips, tongue and palate. Speech sounds are classified according to the structures used in modification of the expired jet of air. The vowels are produced by altering the shape of the oral cavity by adjusting the jaws, cheek, tongue and palate. Consonants are produced by exhalation through the mouth, isolating the nasal cavity by raising the soft palate. By blocking the exhaled air by lips, labial consonants such as P and B are articulated, whereas T and D, which are lingual consonants, need approximation of the tongue against the palate. In nasal sounds such as M and N the soft palate is relaxed and air passes through both the nasal cavity and the oral cavity.

Abnormalities in any structures involved in articulation can produce a speech defect. In cleft palate, air always enters the nasal cavity, giving nasal quality for the voice and affecting sounds which require contact between tongue and palate.

Speech defects are a sequence of a number of neurological problems. In unilateral paralysis of the recurrent laryngeal nerve the vocal cord on the paralysed side is in the cadaveric position and cannot be adducted. Aphonia results at the onset of paralysis. Within a few days the opposite cord will cross the midline on phonation and approximate itself to the paralysed cord and the voice will return. However, complete apposition of the two cords is impossible, especially posteriorly. The voice will be harsh and low and it will never return to its normal quality.

Bilateral recurrent laryngeal nerve paralysis results in aphonia due to inability to adduct the vocal cords.

External laryngeal nerve paralysis, which rarely happens in thyroid surgery, paralyses the cricothyroid muscle, resulting in inability to produce certain high-pitched sounds.

Disturbances in coordination of motor pathways, as in cortical damage and extrapyramidal lesions, produce dysarthria. In Parkinson's disease the tremor and muscular rigidity affect the muscles involved in speech, causing rapid and monotonous speech with slurring of consonants and repetition of syllables. Slurred speech is also characteristic of cerebellar lesions.

Dysphasia results from lesions in the sensory cortex and some of the associated areas connected with speech. The speech in these patients sounds normal but makes little sense. They are unable to comprehend what was heard or seen and hence produce inappropriate responses and often are unable to find appropriate words or formulate sentences. Such patients are capable of initiating speech but are unable to converse. Problems affecting the lower region of the primary sensory cortex (Wernicke's area) and auditory association area will produce dysphasia.

VISUAL PATHWAYS

Impulses produced in the rods and cones in the retina by light reach the visual cortex through the visual pathway. The visual pathway consists of:

- the optic nerve
- the optic chiasma
- the optic tract
- lateral geniculate body
- optic radiation
- visual cortex.

Optic nerve

The optic nerve commences at the lamina cribosa, where the axons of the ganglion cells of the retina (p. 397) pierce the sclera. The nerve fibres, about 1–1.2 million of them, acquire a myelin sheath at this point. The optic nerve, covered by the dura, arachnoid and pia, runs posteromedially in the orbit to enter the optic canal.

The nerve, which is longer than the distance it has to transverse, lies loosely in the orbital fat surrounded by the four recti muscles. The ophthalmic artery accompanies the nerve. The artery, which is superolateral to the nerve posteriorly crosses above the nerve to its medial side. It gives off the central artery of the retina, which sinks into its inferomedial aspect.

In the optic canal the ophthalmic artery lies superolateral to the optic nerve. More proximally the nerve has a short course in the middle cranial fossa before uniting with the nerve of the opposite side at the chiasma.

Optic chiasma

At the chiasma, nerve fibres from the temporal half of the retina lie laterally and those from the medial half lie in the middle. The middle fibres decussate. All the fibres that arise from the ganglion cells medial to a line passing through the fovea centralis cross from the optic nerve of that side to the optic tract of the opposite side (Fig. 13.35). The left optic tract thus contains fibres from the temporal half of the left retina and nasal half of the right retina. As the temporal half of the retina perceives light from the nasal half of the visual field, and the nasal half of the retina from the temporal visual field, the left optic tract transmits data from the right half of the visual field (and the right tract from the left half of the visual field).

Inferior to the optic chiasma lies the sella turcica containing the pituitary gland. The diaphragma sellae

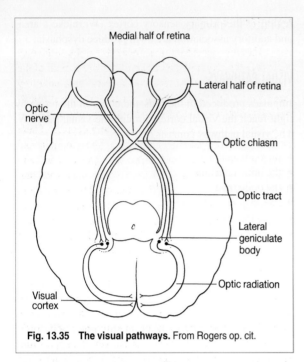

Medial half of retina

Lateral half of retina

Optic nerve

Optic chiasm

Optic tract

Lateral geniculate body

Optic radiation

Visual cortex

Fig. 13.35 The visual pathways. From Rogers op. cit.

cortex. The upper half of the retina is represented on the upper lip of the calcarine fissure and the lower half on the lower lip. The macular region has greater cortical representation than the peripheral retina, facilitating acuity of vision for the macular region.

Lesions of the retina or optic nerve result in unilateral blindness of the affected segment. Lesions of the optic tract and optic radiations produce contralateral homonymous hemianopia. Lesions of the middle fibres of the optic chiasma, as caused by a pituitary tumour, will cause bitemporal hemianopia.

PHYSIOLOGY OF HEARING

Alternate phases of condensation and rarefaction of molecules produce sound waves. The loudness of the sound is proportional to the amplitude of the wave and its pitch is correlated with the frequency. The ear converts sound waves in the air to action potentials in the auditory (cochlear) nerves. The waves are transmitted by the tympanic membrane (ear drum) through the movements of the auditory ossicles into the internal ear. These produce movements in the fluid in the internal ear, which in turn produce waves of movement of hair cells of the organ of Corti, which generate action potentials in the nerve fibres.

Liquid is more difficult to move than air. The sound pressure in the air as it passes through the middle ear must therefore be amplified. Because the tympanic membrane is so much larger than the oval window, the pressure (force per unit area) is increased 15 to 20 times when transmitted from the larger membrane to the smaller. The lever action of the ossicles also accentuates the pressure.

The auricle collects the sound waves and they pass along the external auditory meatus to produce vibrations of the tympanic membrane. The tympanic membrane is most efficient when the pressure on either side of it is equal. This is acheived by opening of the auditory tube, which equalises the middle ear air pressure to that of the external auditory meatus. The vibrations of the tympanic membrane are transmitted to the malleus, incus and stapes. The malleus rocks on an axis through its long and short processes. When the handle of the malleus moves medially with the tympanic membrane the head of the malleus and the body of the incus move laterally. As the body of the incus moves laterally its long process moves medially and transmits the movement to stapes. The stapes does not move in and out of the oval window like a piston, as the fluid in the internal ear cannot be compressed. Movement of the head of the stapes swings its

separates the pituitary gland from the optic chiasma. A tumour of the hypophysis cerberi may bulge the diaphragma sellae or break through it and press on the optic chiasma. The internal carotid artery lies lateral to the chiasma. Aneurysm of the artery at this level will compress the lateral fibres in the chiasma.

Optic tract

The optic tract passes posterolaterally from the chiasma. The tract forms the anterolateral boundary of the interpeduncular fossa, crossing the cerebral peduncle to terminate in the lateral geniculate body.

Not all fibres of the optic tract end in the lateral geniculate body. Some enter the midbrain, ending in the superior colliculus or the pretectal nucleus. These fibres form the afferent limb of the light reflex.

Lateral geniculate body and the optic radiation

The great majority of the fibres in the optic tract end in the lateral geniculate body. The six-layered lateral geniculate body has point-to-point representation at the retina. From the lateral geniculate body, fibres of the optic radiation sweep laterally and backwards to the visual cortex in the occipital lobe.

The visual cortex lies above and below the calcarine sulcus as well as on the walls of the sulcus. There is point-to-point representation of the retina in the visual

footpiece to and fro like a door hinge at the posterior edge of the oval window. Movements of the ossicles amplify the sound system 1.3 times.

The vibrations transmitted by the stapes produce displacement of the basilar membrane and movements of the hair cells and tectorial membrane of the organ of Corti, which initiate nerve impulses in the auditory nerve. The greater the degree of displacement of the basilar membrane the more hair cells and hence the more nerve fibres are stimulated. The basal portion of the cochlear duct responds to high frequency sounds while the apical part responds to low frequency stimuli. The nerve fibres supplying each part of the cochlea, thus, are stimulated by different frequencies. Impulses from the auditory nerve reach the auditory nuclei in the brainstem and are transmitted to the inferior colliculus and medial geniculate body of both sides, through the trapezoid body and the lateral leminisci, from where they reach the auditory cortex through auditory radiations.

Tympanic reflex

When the middle ear muscles — the tensor tympani and stapedius — contract, they pull the malleus inwards and the stapes outwards, thus decreasing sound transmission. Loud sounds initiate a reflex contraction of these muscles, known as the tympanic reflex. It prevents strong sound waves from causing excessive stimulation of the hair cells and thus protects them from being damaged.

Bone and air conduction

Normal conduction of sound waves through the tympanic membrane and ossicles is known as air conduction. Bone conduction is the transmission of vibrations of the bones of the skull to the fluid of the inner ear. This plays a role in transmission of very loud sounds. Air conduction is much more efficient than bone conduction.

Conductive deafness results from failure of the conductive mechanism to transmit sound waves from the external ear to the inner ear. This can be due to various diseases of the external ear and middle ear. Sensory neuronal deafness is due to diseases of the organ of Corti, cochlea or the auditory nerve or its central pathway.

Rinne's test is one of the tuning fork tests where air conduction is compared with bone conduction. If the sound-conducting pathway is normal, the tuning fork is heard much louder by air conduction than by bone conduction and Rinne's test is said to be positive. If the sound-conducting pathway is disrupted, bone conduction is better heard than air conduction, and the Rinne's test is negative. In conductive deafness, Rinne's test is negative.

PHYSIOLOGY OF SMELL

The olfactory receptors are located in the olfactory mucosa in the roof and upper part of the lateral wall of the nasal cavity and nasal septum in a small area covering about 5 cm^2. The olfactory mucosa contains the supporting cells (sustenacular cells) and receptor cells as well as cells which are progenitor cells for the receptors. There are about 10–20 million receptor cells. They are neuronal cells. Each receptor has a dendrite with an expanded end called the olfactory rod. Cilia project from these rods into the mucus on the surface of the mucosa. There are about 10–20 cilia per neuron. The axons of the neurons (olfactory receptors) pass through the cribriform plate of the ethmoid to enter the olfactory bulb. The lifespan of the receptors is short, and they are constantly replaced by the progenitor cells.

Olfactory receptors respond to substances which are dissolved in the mucus. Humans can recognise about ten thousand different odours. Thresholds for various odours vary widely. The concentration required to smell artificial musk is much less than that for oil of peppermint. However, the ability to recognise the various intensities for the same odour is poor. To appreciate the difference in intensity the concentration of odour-producing substance must be changed by more than 30%. In comparison, visual differentiation is possible with a change in intensity as low as 1%.

The olfactory mucus, produced by the Bowman's glands in the olfactory mucosa, may contain odour-binding proteins which will facilitate the passage of lipophylic odour-producing substances through hydrophilic mucus. These proteins thus act as carrier proteins.

In the olfactory bulbs, axons of the receptors synapse around dendrites of the mitral cells to form glomeruli. Each receptor neuron activates only one or two glomeruli. The axons of mitral cells pass posteriorly to the olfactory cortex as the various olfactory striae.

How olfactory neurons can discriminate between a wide variety of odours is not clearly understood. It is possible that there are many different types of odour receptors, or it may be that each receptor is capable of producing a different type of neuronal activity in the brain depending on the substance which stimulates it.

Taste and smell are closely related functionally. Flavours of various foods are a combination of taste and smell. One cannot taste substances adequately without having the aroma. Food tastes different when one has a cold!

Most of the air passing through the nasal cavity will not come into contact with the olfactory mucosa. It passes mainly through the respiratory portion of the mucosa. The turbinate warms the air, and some of it rises by convection to come in contact with the olfactory region in and around the roof. Sniffing, done by compression of the ala against the nose helps to deflect the air upwards. It is a reflex response which occurs when a new or pleasant smell attracts attention.

Adaptation and desensitisation occur when one is constantly exposed to the same odour. Adaptation is specific for the odour smelled and does not affect other odours. Olfactory thresholds increase with advancing age, and many old folks have an impaired ability to identify smells. Several dozen anosmias (absence of the sense of smell) may be present normally. They are probably due to the absence or disrupted function of one of the many different types of odour receptors in the olfactory mucosa.

PATHOLOGY

DISEASES OF THE ORAL CAVITY

Inflammatory disorders

Herpes simplex infections

Infections with the herpes simplex virus result in vesicles surrounded by a red margin appearing on the gingiva, cheek, lips, or tongue. The vesicles break down to form shallow ulcers. They may become encrusted and are frequently secondarily infected. These lesions are often very painful but heal spontaneously. The lesions are commonly associated with infections of the upper respiratory tract and pneumonia. The virus may be in a dormant state in the squamous cells of many individuals and is activated by febrile illness. They also occur in the immunocompromised patient.

Oral candidiasis (thrush)

Seen in neonates and in immunocompromised patients such as those suffering from AIDS or those who are on immunosuppressant drugs and/or long term antibiotics, this is caused by the fungus *Candida albicans*. Lesions, seen as white plaques in the mucous membrane, are confined to the epithelium and comprise fungal hyphae, polymorphs and fibrin.

Aphthous stomatitis

This relatively common condition manifests as recurrent small ulcers of the oral mucosa. Ulcers are shallow with a necrotic base and a haemorrhagic periphery. They heal spontaneously. The exact aetiology is unknown but some cases are associated with inflammatory bowel disease and coeliac disease, suggesting an immunological aetiology.

Epulis

Epulis is a small pedunculated fibrovascular swelling in the oral cavity, caused by repeated minor trauma. It starts as a scar tissue in the submucous layer, which later develops a stalk probably by suction forces generated during deglutition.

Leukoplakia

Leukoplakia is seen as white patches on the oral mucosa, its importance being that it may be a premalignant condition. Histologically there is hyperkeratosis and hyperplasia of the epithelium. The presence of dysplasia in addition to these may suggest the onset of malignancy. Traditionally the condition is thought to be associated with the six 'S's: smoking, sepsis, spirits (or excessive alcohol), spices (or the habit of chewing betel nut and lime wrapped in betel leaf as practised in the Indian subcontinent), sharp teeth causing repetitive trauma, and syphilis. Though syphilis is now rare, candidiasis has become an additional factor.

Tumours

Squamous cell carcinoma is the most common malignant tumour of the oral cavity, the most frequent sites being the lower lip and tongue. Carcinoma of the cheek is very prevalent in the Indian subcontinent. Oral cancers occur more in elderly men. Social and environmental factors such as pipe and tobacco smoking, betel nut and tobacco chewing as practised in Asian countries, as well as prolonged exposure to strong sunlight (lower lip cancers) are contributing factors.

Tumours commonly develop in areas of leukoplakia. They are initially painless and hence may be missed until late, especially those occurring in the posterior third of the tongue. Malignant ulcers in the oral cavity characteristically have an indurated base and a raised and everted margin. Microscopically, squamous cell carcinoma appears as epithelial clusters showing active keratinisation. Lymphatic spread to the cervical nodes is common. In late stages it may also spread to bone, liver and lungs through blood.

Carcinoma of the lower lip is more common than that of the upper lip. This may be because the lower lip gets more exposure to sunlight than the upper. Tumour of the lip has better prognosis because of early detection. 75% of lingual cancers arise on the anterior two-thirds of the tongue. Metastasis occurs unilaterally to the submental, submandibular and then to the lower deep cervical lymph nodes. Rarer posterior one-third tumours spread bilaterally to the upper deep cervical nodes. Poor prognosis of this variety is due to late detection.

SALIVARY GLANDS

Inflammatory diseases

Mumps

Mumps is more common in children (4–12 years) than in adults. The incubation period is about 21 days, and the active state of the disease, when viruses are present in the saliva, lasts about 10 days. There is diffuse interstitial parotid inflammation in mumps which is usually bilateral but occasionally unilateral. In 20% of cases the submandibular and other salivary glands are involved. Epidydimitis, orchitis, and occasional meningo-encephalitis may occur.

Acute bacterial sialoadenitis

Acute bacterial sialoadenitis is often caused by infection spreading into the parotid or submandibular gland from the oral cavity. The condition is associated with poor dental hygiene, periodontal disease, hyposecretion of saliva due to any cause, and stones in the duct causing obstruction. Neonates, elderly and postsurgical patients have a higher risk of developing this condition. Acute bacterial sialoadenitis manifests with fever, trismus, dysphagia and painful enlargement of parotid or submandibular gland. The common organisms involved are *Staphylococcus aureus*, *Streptococcus viridans* and *Escherichia coli*. The condition usually responds to treatment with broad spectrum antibiotics and restoration of good oral hygiene. Duct stones should be removed surgically. If an abscess is formed, it may need drainage.

Sialolithiasis

Primary calculi are more commonly seen in the submandibular gland ducts than in the parotid. They contain phosphate and carbonate. They may be caused by stasis of salivary secretion associated with changes in its physicochemical characteristics. Secondary salivary gland stone formation may occur in hyperparathyroidism, hyperuricaemia and hypercalcaemia.

Sialolithiasis will manifest as recurrent and progressive glandular swelling which in the early stages is associated with meals. Palpation may reveal a stone along the course of the Wharton's or Stensen's duct. Calculi are usually radio-opaque. Stones in the distal part of the duct can be excised, and the opening may be stented or marsupialised. Stones in the proximal region are best treated by excision of the gland and the duct. Acute sialoadenitis with suppuration may occur as a complication.

Sjögren's syndrome

This condition comprises a clinical syndrome affecting the salivary glands and lacrimal glands associated with dry eyes (keratoconjunctivitis sicca) and a dry mouth (xerostomia). It is often associated with rheumatoid arthritis, systemic lupus erythematosus and other systemic autoimmune diseases. The affected glands are painless and have progressively enlarged. Microscopical features include glandular atrophy, lymphocyte infiltration and duct proliferation. The disease usually follows a slow, benign progression, but there is a significant risk of development of lymphoma.

Tumours

Tumours of the salivary glands account for less than 4% of all tumours of the head and neck. 80% occur in the parotid, and 60% of these are benign.

Pleomorphic adenoma or mixed parotid tumour

About 70% of the benign salivary gland tumours are of this type. The lateral or superficial lobe of the parotid gland (lying superficial to the facial nerve) is most commonly affected. The tumour manifests as a slow-growing painless mass. The facial nerve is not involved.

Histologically the mixed parotid tumour consists of epithelial and stromal cells. The stroma, rich in proteoglycan, is thought to be derived from myoepithelial cells surrounding the acini and early duct system. Connective tissue and gland tissue are compressed around tumour tissue to form a false capsule. Surgical excision is performed, preserving the facial nerve and its branches. However, recurrence may occur if the pseudocapsule is ruptured during dissection. Recurrent tumour may encapsulate the facial nerve, and its removal will necessitate sacrificing the nerve, and its branches.

Warthin's tumour

About 10% of the benign tumours of the parotid gland are of this type. Warthin's tumour is rare in the submandibular gland and in the minor salivary glands. It is an adenolymphoma characterised by cystic spaces surrounded by eosinophilic columnar cells. The stroma in between these cysts contain lymphoid tissue, including lymphoid follicles. Malignant transformation is rare, and the treatment of choice is surgical removal.

Muco-epidermoid tumour

This is the most common malignant tumour of the parotid gland. Histologically the tumour consists of sheets of squamous cells and mucus-secreting cells surrounding cystic spaces. Additionally there are small intermediate cells which are precursors of the mucous and squamous cells. Pathological grading of malignancy depends on the proportion of the various cell types in the tumour. A highly malignant variety has more squamous and intermediate cells than mucous cells. The tumour may metastasise into regional lymph nodes, brain and lungs.

Adenocystic carcinoma

Derived from myoepithelial cells and cells of the intercalated ducts, it affects the submandibular gland and the minor salivary glands more frequently than the parotid gland. Histologically the tumour shows a characteristic cribiform appearance having blobs of basophilic material interlaced by myoepithelial cells. The second variety of cells, the duct cells, form strands, cords and islands. These undergo microcystic changes revealed by eosinophilic material. Early perineural invasion occurs causing facial palsy. Metastasis may occur to brain and lungs but is a late event. Total eradicaton by surgical excision is difficult because of extensive infiltration into local tissues and perineural infiltration.

14

Endocrine system

George Proud

The purpose of this chapter is to give a précis of endocrinology as it is most likely to affect the surgeon. Emphasis is given to those aspects of endocrinology which are likely to impinge upon the trainee surgeon at an early stage of training and those hormones which have a broad physiological effect. Other hormones are best considered in the various systems: thus, for example, gut hormones are dealt with in Chapter 17.

WHAT IS A HORMONE?

A hormone is produced by an endocrine gland and it is a chemical messenger. This messenger may be produced by one cell and act locally on adjacent cells (paracrine action). Other hormones act on cells to which they are carried by the blood stream (endocrine action). Some hormones are produced by the brain and reach the pituitary via the hypothalamic–pituitary portal system (neuroendocrine), and yet others, such as adrenaline and acetylcholine, are released at nerve endings and facilitate neurotransmission. Endorphins also modify neurotransmission: there are several opioid peptides produced quite widely in the brain.

Hormones act by binding to receptor proteins on the target cell. There are cell membrane receptors and there are intracellular receptors. Examples of hormones binding to the cell membrane are insulin and adrenaline. Hormones which diffuse into the cell, and which bind with intracellular receptors, include thyroxin and the steroids. The biochemical and transcriptional changes which occur as a result of hormone binding can be reviewed in any textbook of physiology, but are beyond the scope of this chapter.

CONTROL OF HORMONE PRODUCTION: FEEDBACK CONTROL

Regulation of hormone production is clearly essential if endocrine homeostasis is going to be achieved. Frequently, more than one hormone may be involved in the production of the effector hormone. For example, glucocorticoid production from the adrenal gland is modified by adrenocorticotrophic hormone (ACTH) from the pituitary, and the secretion of ACTH is in turn modified by corticotrophin-releasing hormone (CRH) produced by the hypothalamus. In this system, a rise in ACTH production will result in a raised glucocorticoid output. A higher glucocorticoid secretion from the adrenal cortex results in higher levels of circulating steroid hormones and, in turn, this is inhibitory to ACTH secretion — and to CRH secretion also. This is a negative feedback system and allows an elegant method for the body to maintain homeostasis around a predetermined normal level of activity. In disease the knowledge of the feedback system allows one to determine the level at which the pathology exists.

Output of hormone may also be modified by a metabolite. For example, insulin production and release depends on blood glucose concentration. As blood glucose levels rise, so does insulin production: as blood glucose is cleared to normal levels the output of insulin falls. This is a positive feedback system.

THYROID

STRUCTURE

The thyroid is a bilobed structure lying in the base of the neck, with the lobes being joined by an isthmus of varying size. The isthmus lies across the trachea usually just below the cricoid cartilage. A pyramidal lobe is sometimes seen: this is a remnant of the thyroglossal duct and may be seen as a midline extension from the isthmus of the thyroid gland extending cephalad for a variable distance over the thyroid cartilage. The lobes are very variable in size but can each be up to 5–6 cm in length, 2–3 cm in width and about 2 cm thick. The total weight of the normal adult gland will be about 20–40 g. The thyroid is effectively wrapped around the front and sides of the larynx and is bound to it by investing layers of deep cervical fascia. It will be remembered that during swallowing there is elevation of the larynx. Therefore any structure bound to the trachea at this level will also move up during swallowing, i.e. the thyroid gland. This is an important factor in clinical examination.

EMBRYOLOGY

The gland develops in the floor of the pharynx, migrating in front of the developing trachea to its permanent site in the base of the neck. First differentiation of the thyroid begins at about 4 weeks and its development and migration is completed by about 6 months. The track associated with thyroid migration is called the thyroglossal duct. It lies in the midline passing from the foramen caecum in the tongue via the hyoid bone to its usual position in the neck. Remnants of the duct persist as the foramen caecum of the tongue, the pyramidal lobe of the thyroid and a fibrous cord — sometimes known as the 'levator glandulae thyroidiae' — within which epithelial remnants may proliferate and become cystic, i.e. thyroglossal cysts (Fig. 14.1). The thyroid may fail to migrate and remain embedded within the tongue -- the lingual thyroid. This is a rare event, and the patient is usually hypothyroid.

BLOOD SUPPLY AND IMPORTANT RELATIONS

The thyroid gland has a very rich blood supply. There are two main arteries. The superior thyroid artery enters the upper pole of the gland and is associated with a leash of veins draining from this area — the superior thyroid pedicle. The superior thyroid artery is usually a branch of the external carotid artery. The inferior thyroid artery enters the posterior aspect of the midregion of each thyroid lobe. This is a branch of the thyrocervical trunk of the subclavian artery. The inferior thyroid artery also normally supplies the parathyroid glands: bilateral ligature of the inferior thyroid arteries in subtotal thyroidectomy can result in ischaemia of the parathyroids and is not recommended. Unilateral ligature of the inferior thyroid artery is less likely to result in this problem. Total thyroidectomy, with the need for ligatures to each inferior thyroid artery, may result in parathyroid ischaemia even when the artery is ligated at a thyroid capsular level. Transient hypocalcaemia needing calcium supplementation to the diet will occur in around 30–40% of patients undergoing total thyroidectomy (with preservation of parathyroids), although by 3 months only about 2% will still need this. A small artery may enter the thyroid isth-

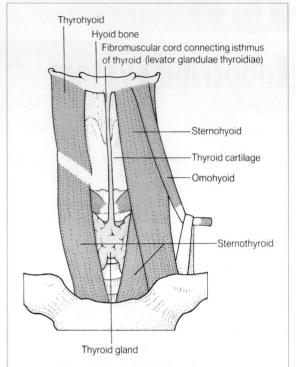

Fig. 14.1 The infrahyoid muscles related to the thyroid gland. The sternohyoid muscle has been removed on the right hand side. From Rogers A W 1992 Textbook of anatomy; Churchill Livingstone, Edinburgh.

Labels: Thyrohyoid; Hyoid bone; Fibromuscular cord connecting isthmus of thyroid (levator glandulae thyroidiae); Sternohyoid; Thyroid cartilage; Omohyoid; Sternothyroid; Thyroid gland

mus from below — the thyroidea ima artery coming from the brachiocephalic artery (Fig. 14.2).

The venous drainage is of some surgical importance. It is extensive and variable, but generally three main groups are identified. The superior thyroid veins tend to coalesce around the region of the superior thyroid artery and are generally ligated by the surgeon in the same ligature used for the artery. The inferior thyroid veins can be many, and they generally drain towards the subclavian or brachiocephalic veins. Veins draining the middle portion of the gland can drain either to the superior and inferior thyroid vein clusters, or may form a short venous trunk draining directly to the internal jugular vein. This middle thyroid vein is not always present, and may sometimes be found only on one side of the neck. Careless handling of the vein during surgery can result in damage to the internal jugular vein and in serious haemorrhage developing. Even traction applied to the thyroid during its dissection can cause this: the surgeon is advised always to identify and manage the middle thyroid vein before the other thyroid blood vessels.

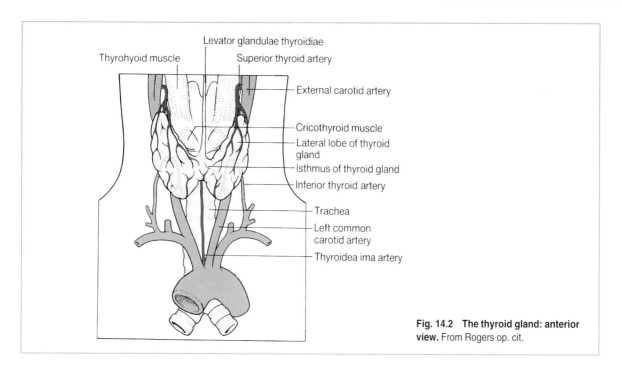

Fig. 14.2 The thyroid gland: anterior view. From Rogers op. cit.

Labels: Thyrohyoid muscle, Levator glandulae thyroidiae, Superior thyroid artery, External carotid artery, Cricothyroid muscle, Lateral lobe of thyroid gland, Isthmus of thyroid gland, Inferior thyroid artery, Trachea, Left common carotid artery, Thyroidea ima artery

Closely related to the superior thyroid vascular pedicle is the external laryngeal branch of the superior laryngeal nerve. Damage to this nerve in surgery can result in voice change, and the nerve should be protected equally with the recurrent laryngeal nerve. The recurrent laryngeal nerve lies deep to the thyroid gland (Fig. 14.3), often in close relationship to the inferior thyroid artery, parathyroid glands and the capsule of the thyroid gland, in the groove between trachea and oesophagus. The nerve must be identified and protected in all lobectomy or total thyroidectomy procedures. In subtotal procedures, where a posterior rim of tissue may be left behind, the nerve should be remote from the surgeon's knife; however, the nerve's position is variable, and it must always be regarded as vulnerable in any thyroid surgery and must be searched for. Damage to one nerve will result in

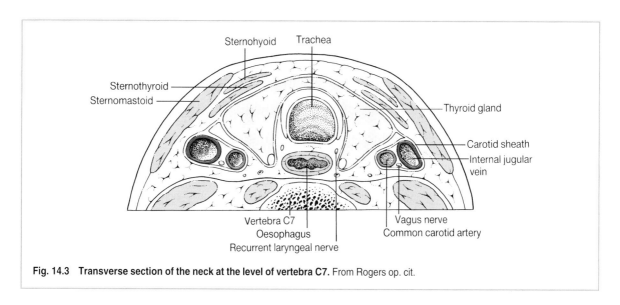

Fig. 14.3 Transverse section of the neck at the level of vertebra C7. From Rogers op. cit.

Labels: Sternohyoid, Trachea, Sternothyroid, Sternomastoid, Thyroid gland, Carotid sheath, Internal jugular vein, Vertebra C7, Oesophagus, Recurrent laryngeal nerve, Vagus nerve, Common carotid artery

paralysis of the vocal cord on that side as well as a sensory deficit in the larynx, and the patient will have a weak, hoarse voice. Bilateral damage will result in the possible need for a permanent tracheostomy. When both cords are paralysed, they are quite motionless, each lying in a midposition. When only one cord is paralysed, the normal one may cross the midline. When operating on the thyroid, there have generally been two schools of thought regarding how best to protect the recurrent laryngeal nerve. One school advocates that the nerve should be sought and protected by maintaining it within direct vision, and the other school has suggested that the nerve is more likely to be damaged if it is deliberately searched for — and therefore its presence should be anticipated rather than deliberately dissecting out the nerve. In fact, there is now a substantial published literature which indicates that the nerve is best searched out and therefore protected by being kept under direct vision. Although the recurrent laryngeal nerve arises differently on each side, it is vulnerable to damage in all thyroid procedures. It can lie very close to the inferior pole of the thyroid, especially on the right side. Its relationship to the inferior thyroid artery is variable — sometimes it courses through the branches of the artery close to the capsule of the thyroid gland, or it may lie in close relationship to the trunk of the artery. Whilst the nerve is vulnerable to injury at these sites in particular, it is especially vulnerable where it enters the larynx below the inferior constrictor muscle: here it lies very close to the thyroid and is often bound up with a dense condensation of fascial tissue binding the thyroid gland to the trachea — the so-called ligament of Berry.

The parathyroid glands should lie close to the inferior thyroid artery and normally derive their blood supply from this artery, although very often the vascular pedicle to the parathyroid appears to arise from the thyroid gland itself. The parathyroid glands frequently lie on the capsule of the thyroid; their presence should be anticipated and they should be preserved. However, if the glands are not seen it may mean that they lie at a site remote from the thyroid — or that they may lie within the thyroid gland itself. It is not a practical proposition always to find the normal parathyroid glands in thyroid surgery.

Managing the inferior thyroid artery in thyroid operations is, therefore, a most important aspect of the procedure. To reduce risk to both the recurrent laryngeal nerve and the parathyroid glands, it is best to carry out a ligation of the radicles of the artery close to the capsule of the thyroid gland rather than at the truncal level of the artery. Even so, approximately 30% of patients undergoing total thyroidectomy will still show hypocalcaemia after

surgery necessitating treatment (although by 3 months this figure has dropped to 2%). Hypocalcaemia is much less common in subtotal procedures.

Recurrent laryngeal nerve injury occurs in 1–3% of all thyroidectomy procedures, although higher figures have been published. All patients should be warned of the risks of nerve injury and of hypocalcaemia as part of the preoperative preparation.

STRUCTURE AND FUNCTION

The gland is composed of follicles which are roughly spherical structures of thyroid epithelial cells surrounding colloid. It is richly supplied with blood vessels. Parafollicular cells may be seen which secrete calcitonin. The actions of calcitonin are considered in the section on calcium metabolism.

In each follicle, the surrounding epithelial cells are cuboidal when 'resting' and 'columnar' when under TSH stimulation (Fig. 14.4). The cells have the following functions (see Fig. 14.5).

- First, they secrete thyroglobulin (TG) and iodine into the colloid.
- Second, they absorb thyroglobulin from the colloid.
- Third, thyroid hormones — triiodothyronine (T3) and thyroxine (T4) — are secreted directly into the blood stream.

The thyroid gland incorporates iodine into the follicle cells in the production of its hormones. Iodine is transported across the basement membrane by a powerful pump mechanism in which I^- follows Na^+. Iodine concentration in the cells is up to 50 times that of the plasma. This active transport mechanism is influenced positively by TSH (thyroid-stimulating hormone) and TSH receptor antibody (found in thyrotoxic Graves' disease). Iodine incorporation into the cell can be blocked or inhibited by various materials, but particularly an excess of iodide, the perchlorate and thiocyanate ions and some drugs — for example, digoxin.

In the cell, iodide is oxidised to iodine by thyroidal peroxidase (TPO). The iodine so produced binds within the cell to tyrosine residues attaching to the glycoprotein thyroglobulin which is also produced within the thyroid cell. Iodine may also bind with thyroglobulin in the colloid. The iodination of thyroglobulin results in the formation of monoiodotyrosyl or diiodotyrosyl (MIT and DIT). MIT and DIT then couple to produce either triiodothyronine (T_3) or thyroxine (T_4) — all occurring within the colloid. The iodination of thyroglobulin through to the production of T_3 and T_4 is under TSH control.

Under continued TSH control, colloid droplets are taken up by the thyroid cell via a process of pinocytosis. Lysosomes fuse with the droplets. Proteolysis occurs, with consequent release of the iodine-bound residues. MIT and DIT are deiodinated, the iodine being neutralised within the cell, whilst T_3 and T_4 are released to the circulation. In the plasma the hormones conjugate to thyroxine-binding globulin (TBG), which is produced by the liver, to thyroxine-binding prealbumin, and to albumin. The function of these hormone-bound complexes is not known. When bound, T_3 and T_4 are inactive and thus are possibly behaving as a 'store' of hormone making T_3 and T_4 available to the tissues.

Whatever their function, the concentration of thyroid-bound hormones in plasma can vary in disease states and in the presences of certain drugs, e.g. aspirin, phenytoin, diazepam, phenylbutazone.

The active hormone is in the 'free' or unbound state. Less than 1% of T_3 is in the free state, and only about 0.05% of T_4 is free. T_3 is considered to be the active hormone. The intracellular T_3 is obtained not from circulating T_3 but from deiodination of T_4, converting it to T_3. This deiodination occurs within the cell. The half life of T_3 is one day and of T_4 is 1 week. This all suggests that T_4 is acting as an immediately available source of T_3 rather than as a hormone in its own right.

CONTROL OF THYROID FUNCTION

The negative feedback control between thyroid hormone production and the stimulating hormones has long been known. Thyroid-stimulating hormone (TSH), from the anterior pituitary, has a stimulating effect on T_3/T_4 production. Thyrotropin-releasing hormone (TRH), which is stored in the hypothalamus, is a stimulator of TSH production. TRH reaches the anterior pituitary via the pituitary venous portal system. Therefore, with increased TRH stimulation, TSH production is raised, with a consequent rise in T_3/T_4 output from the thyroid. Rising levels of T_3/T_4 (primarily a rising T_3 concentration) have an inhibitory effect on the TRH/TSH axis. Thus there is an elegant mechanism in place for the precise control of the production and release of thyroid hormones (Fig. 14.6).

In reality the secretion of thyroid hormones is under a far greater range of control than this simple feedback arrangement. The gland itself can autoregulate according to the supply of iodine (increasing concentrations of iodine are inhibitory), and the thyroid gland itself can produce antibodies which may be either stimulatory or inhibitory to thyroid function. For example, thyroid receptor antibodies may be stimulatory and minimise the effects of

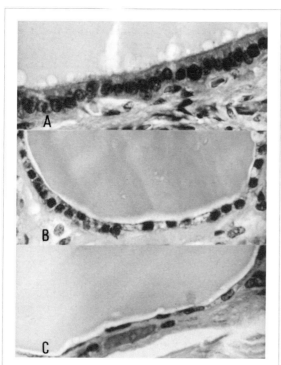

Fig. 14.4 Follicular epithelium of human thyroid.
A increased activity; B normal activity; C inactivity. Haematoxylin–eosin × 560. From Symmers W S C & Lewis P D (ed) Systemic pathology 12: The endocrine system, Churchill Livingstone.

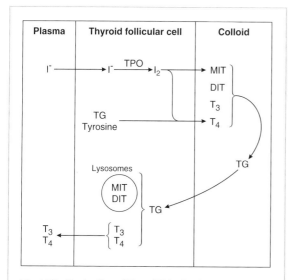

Fig. 14.5 Production of T_3 and T_4 in the thyroid.

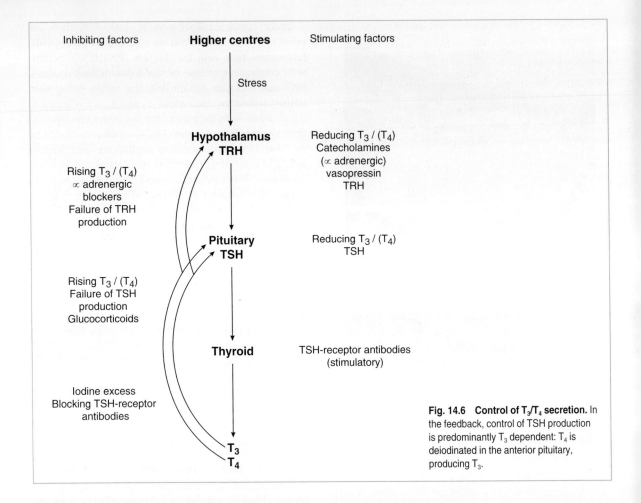

Fig. 14.6 **Control of T₃/T₄ secretion.** In the feedback, control of TSH production is predominantly T_3 dependent: T_4 is deiodinated in the anterior pituitary, producing T_3.

TSH. These stimulatory antibodies are often referred to as long-acting thyroid stimulators (LATS). The receptor antibodies may also have a blocking action — thus reducing the TSH effect. TSH secretion demonstrates a circadian rhythm, with a night time peak.

MECHANISM OF ACTION

T_3 is the active hormone and has many sites of action within the cell. The main effects are seen on the cell membrane, on the mitochondria and on the cell nucleus. At the cell membrane level there is increased uptake of amino acids and glucose via the Na^+/K^+ ATP-ase pump when T_3 stimulation occurs. The effect on mitochondria is to increase energy production. T_3 combines with T_3 receptors within the nucleus. These cause a change of activity, either increased or decreased, on mRNA, with consequent effects on protein synthesis.

Effects of thyroid hormone

These are widespread. They range over energy and heat production, an overall catabolic effect — particularly on glucose and fat metabolism, cardiovascular and adrenergic effects, effects on other hormone production, effects on bone and effects on fetal development and growth. These are now briefly discussed.

Heat production

Heat production is brought about by the T_3 effect on mitochondria: there is increased O_2 uptake by the mitochondria with production of ATP in most tissues, although not in the brain. This function of thyroid hormone is responsible for the basal metabolic rate rise which is seen in hyperthyroidism. It will be obvious also that this is responsible for the heat intolerance described by patients with thyrotoxicosis. In hypothyroidism the reverse is true. Heat production is reduced. This is why the combination of untreated hypothyroidism and a cold environment such as a winter day can be so dangerous.

Catabolic effects

In carbohydrate metabolism thyroid hormones stimulate glycogenolysis in the liver, increase insulin breakdown, stimulate glucose absorption in the gut and also increase the glycogenolysis of catecholamines. In practice, thyrotoxicosis will 'unmask' diabetes mellitus or may make the control of diabetes more difficult.

Thyroid hormones also have a lipolytic effect: in thyrotoxicosis cholesterol is lowered; it is raised in myxoedema. In the breakdown of fats, free fatty acids are produced; their oxidation contributes to the increase in heat associated with thyrotoxicosis. Some of the effects on fat metabolism may be due to the potentiating effect of thyroid hormones on other hormones, including glucocorticoids, growth hormone, adrenaline and glucagon.

Cardiovascular and adrenergic effects

Thyroid hormones have a positive inotropic effect, and there is increase in the number of β adrenergic receptors in cardiac muscle. Cardiac output and rate both rise in thyrotoxicosis. The β adrenergic receptor increase is also seen in many other tissues, including skeletal muscle. The management of the tachycardias and dysrhythmias associated with thyrotoxicosis is most logically carried out with a β adrenergic receptor blocker. Propranolol is often used.

Effects on bone

T_3 and T_4 increase the metabolic activity in bone. This is predominantly a catabolic effect with the result of a net breakdown of bone tissue. Hypercalcaemia and hypercalciuria can be seen in thyrotoxicosis; there may even be radiological change in the bones. However, the hypercalcaemia should not be confused with hyperparathyroidism: the PTH level will be suppressed in the former.

Fetal development

Virtually no T_3 or T_4 will reach the fetal circulation from the mother. The fetus depends on its own thyroid gland for thyroid hormones. The thyroid gland is fully differentiated by approximately 11 weeks gestation, although it is probably not until about 18 weeks that thyroid hormone production commences. Thyroid hormone is essential for normal differentiation and maturation of fetal tissues. A failure of thyroid gland development, or of hormone synthesis, will result in cretinism: there is gross mental retardation due to failure of brain development, and there is a failure of skeletal development leading to dwarfism. Some antithyroid drugs can cross the placenta, i.e. carbimazole and propylthiouracil, and if given in high dose

may also block fetal thyroid function. Radiolabelled iodine given to the mother will also damage the fetal thyroid. Women who are pregnant must never receive radio-labelled iodine for a thyroid disorder. TSH receptor antibodies may cross the placenta with consequent effects on the fetal thyroid.

Other effects

Patients with thyrotoxicosis frequently complain of diarrhoea, and those with myxoedema suffer constipation indicating an effect on gut motility.

The O_2 carrying capacity of blood increases in thyrotoxic states due to an increase in 2,3-DPG content of red blood cells.

During life there are some normal changes in thyroid function. In pregnancy there is a rise in TBG with a consequent rise in total T_3 and T_4 levels: however, the free unbound T_3 and T_4 levels are little changed. The thyroid gland may also increase in size in pregnancy.

In children, thyroxine turnover is high until puberty and then stabilises at somewhat lower adult levels. It is only in old age that a further change occurs in normal thyroid function, when the thyroxine turnover rate declines a little. This is of some practical importance in patients taking thyroxine as replacement therapy: whilst the average adult may have a stable thyroxine need, variations may occur. The patient needs to have regular checks of blood thyroid hormone levels.

TESTING THYROID FUNCTION

In evaluating thyroid function the major interest will be in establishing the level of thyroid hormones in blood, and in evaluating the pituitary–thyroid axis, or even the hypothalamic–pituitary–thyroid axis. Free T_4, total T_4 and total T_3 can be determined and the significance of their levels evaluated against the TSH level of blood. Essentially one is looking for an aberration of the normal relationship between circulating thyroid hormones and the trophic hormones. A high level of thyroid hormones and a low level of TSH will ordinarily reflect a problem within the thyroid gland, i.e. thyrotoxicosis. A high TSH combined with a low level of circulating thyroid hormone will reflect an unresponsive gland.

An assessment of thyroid autoantibody status should also normally be made. TSH receptor antibodies which stimulate may be indicative of Graves' disease, and the presence of thyroglobulin or thyroidal peroxidase (TPO) antibodies might be useful in myxoedema.

Iodine is stored in the thyroid gland in combination with thyroid hormones and their precursors, and iodine is sometimes used in the diagnosis of thyroid disease. For example the uptake of radiolabelled iodine, i.e. ^{123}I, by the gland can be measured and may give an indication of the metabolic activity of the gland. This is done now much less frequently than previously.

Scanning of the thyroid gland with ^{123}I is sometimes indicated. Where doubt exists about a thyroid nodule's nature an isotope study may show whether it is functioning, perhaps with suppression of normal thyroid by suppression of TSH and thus suggesting an autonomous functioning nodule, or the scan may show an area of no uptake corresponding to the nodule — the so-called 'cold nodule'. This may represent a cyst, or tumour, of the thyroid.

Thyroglobulin can also be estimated in peripheral blood. This test is really only useful in one situation: that is, when using thyroglobulin as a tumour marker. After complete eradication of the thyroid in the management of a patient with well-differentiated thyroid cancer (i.e. papillary or follicular cancer) thyroglobulin may be detectable and rise in the presence of recurrent or secondary disease.

These are all tests of thyroid function. Thyroid structure can be assessed with fine needle aspiration cytology, ultrasound, MRI, or CT.

ABNORMALITIES OF THE THYROID

The reader is reminded that this text is not designed to give a comprehensive knowledge of thyroid disease. Some of the more important physiological — and pathophysiological — aspects of thyroid disease and embryological problems are, however, discussed briefly here.

Relating to thyroid development

There may be a failure of thyroid development, possibly due to transplacental crossing of maternal blocking antibodies to TSH receptors, or of thyroid descent, the thyroid lying within the tongue. In this situation, the thyroid usually has seriously inadequate function resulting in hypothyroidism of the newborn ('cretinism'). Neonatal hypothyroidism is rare from whatever cause — other causes include antithyroid drugs and radioactive iodine administration to the mother. A low serum T_4 and a higher serum TSH give the diagnosis.

More commonly, there is aberrant thyroid tissue. Nodules can lie in the neck close to, but separate from, the thyroid gland.

The most common embryological remnant is the thyroglossal cyst — this lies in the midline in the upper part of the neck and is a mucus-filled cyst lined by epithelium

which is usually squamous. Normally the cyst lies above the thyroid cartilage — it may even lie at the level of or above the hyoid bone. The thyroglossal cyst usually elevates on protrusion of the tongue because of its association with the levator glandulae thyroidiae and thus the hyoid bone.

Relating to function

With a knowledge of the function of thyroid hormones the effects of over- or underfunction can be anticipated. Equally, knowing the homeostatic control of the hormones' release, the site of endocrine malfunction can be identified. For example, when a patient presents with hypothyroidism and low blood T_4 levels, and who is also found to have a low TSH release, the assumption can be made that the problem is going to lie at the pituitary or hypothalamic level. If the problem was at the thyroid gland level, then the low T_4 would be associated with a high TSH. Conversely, when a patient presents with thyrotoxicosis and a high blood thyroxin level, but with suppressed TSH levels, the problem lies at the thyroid gland part of the feedback axis. Once the underlying problem has been pinpointed, appropriate investigation and treatment can ensue. It would be quite inappropriate to treat the myxoedematous patient with thyroxine alone if the cause of the myxoedema is in the pituitary gland — for example, where there might be an infiltrating or expanding tumour causing failure of TSH production.

Myxoedema

In myxoedema there is a very widespread effect of the deficiency of thyroid hormones. Coldness, weight gain, anaemia and constipation are frequently present. Markedly slowed reflexes and a husky voice can usually be demonstrated. In the tissues there is increased hyaluronic acid: in the skin this causes 'puffiness', and hyaluronic acid is also present in both striated and cardiac muscle. The increase is due to a slower breakdown than normally occurs and not to any active process of deposition. When the patient is investigated in myxoedema of thyroid origin there will be a high concentration of TSH and a low concentration of thyroid hormones in the blood. The presence of TSH receptor-blocking antibodies confirms the presence of Hashimoto thyroiditis when the gland is enlarged. Patients often present to surgeons with a goitre, a positive thyroid autoantibody test and a humoral profile suggesting early myxoedema. By and large these patients are not candidates for surgery. They are best managed medically. Occasionally, on account of compressive symptoms, an isthmusectomy may be indicated. However, thyroiditic glands are *not* immune from malignant change. Nodules developing in a thyroiditic gland must be viewed with suspicion and aggressively investigated.

The surgeon reading about myxoedema will be aware of the many manifestations of the disease. There will be recognition of the need to do thyroid function tests in some patients presenting with constipation, for example. However, the surgeon is also reminded of the complications — particularly 'myxoedema coma'. Generally occurring in the elderly with coexisting cardiopulmonary problems, it has a very high mortality. The patient has profound hypothermia, may be very weak, and might demonstrate hypoglycaemia, water retention, confusion and hypoventilation. It can come about as the end stage effect of autoimmune thyrotoxicosis or as a result of Hashimoto thyroiditis as well as many other less common clinical problems. It can also come about as a result of failure to take thyroxine medication. There is a greater tendency to 'aggressive intervention' in thyrotoxicosis either by gland ablation with ^{131}I or by thyroidectomy. For reasons beyond the scope of discussion in this book, more total thyroidectomies are being performed than previously. Therefore in the future there will be an increasing number of the population entering the 'old-age' phase of life already taking thyroxine — and therefore a greater number potentially at risk of this very serious complication of myxoedema.

Thyrotoxicosis

In thyrotoxicosis there are also very widespread effects of the excess of circulating thyroid hormones, and the discussion, above, of the effects of thyroid hormones gives an indication of these (see Box 14.1). Thyrotoxicosis is caused by a number of conditions, but the commonest is Graves' disease, an autoimmune condition in which TSH receptor site antibody can be identified which

is stimulatory to the thyroid cell. The clinical features include a diffuse thyroid enlargement, systemic manifestations of raised thyroid hormone levels in blood, and an ophthalmopathy. Some patients demonstrate a pretibial myxoedema and not all have a demonstrable ophthalmopathy. Mild cases of ophthalmopathy may be demonstrated by lid retraction and lid lag which might be arising as a result of catecholamine stimulation. Severe cases include proptosis, muscle paresis, ocular keratitis and blindness from optic nerve involvement. The aetiology of the eye disease has been investigated for many years. Whilst the histological findings in the tissues of the orbit are well described (inflammatory changes in muscles, fibroblast changes and oedema), the exact trigger for the changes is still under investigation. However, the intrathyroid T cells may be important in this by processing antigen resulting in cytokine-dependent B lymphocyte stimulation and thus antibody production and by inducing cytokine stimulation of the fibroblasts. As the aetiology of the changes cannot be described with certainty, it must come as no surprise that the management of thyrotoxic Graves' disease is debated still.

The options for management include:

- medical control with antithyroid drugs
- radio-iodine treatment
- surgery.

Medical control It will be recalled that there are a number of opportunities to block the production of thyroid hormones. The thioamides — carbimazole and propylthiouracil — are most commonly used. They block thyroid peroxidase activity. They can be used either to block, and then control, thyroid hormone production, or they can be used in a blocking dose and, once the gland is blocked as far as hormone production is concerned, thyroxine is introduced and the patient then remains on this block-and-replace therapy for a variable period of time — but possibly up to a year or more. If the size of the thyroid gland is reduced and TSH receptor antibody is no longer detectable, the long term prognosis is good, with 50% or more of patients enjoying long term remissions.

When thyrotoxicosis has been treated in this way and has then relapsed, or where the gland is large, or where the thyrotoxicosis may be arising from another pathology, e.g. multinodular goitre, or a toxic adenoma, then alternatives of treatment need to be considered. These are either radiolabelled iodine treatment or surgery.

Iodine is a very useful agent in the management of thyroid disease. Whilst iodine is secreted by a number of organs, including salivary glands, it is only within the thyroid that iodine concentration occurs. This property

---

Box 14.1 Some presenting complaints and findings suggesting thyrotoxicosis

Presenting complaint	Findings
Nervousness	Elevated thyroid hormones
Irritability	Tachycardia
Sweating	Cardiac dysrhythmia — usually, atrial fibrillation
Heat intolerance	Hypertension
Insomnia	Goitre
Exophthalmos	
Ophthalmoplegia	
Weight loss	
Irregular menstruation	

enables the delivery of iodine which has been modified to be radioactive, ^{131}I, and therefore has the capacity to cause interstitial irradiation from within the thyroid cells. Its use is more liberal in the USA than in Britain. There are some restrictions on its use — for example it must not be used in pregnancy — and patients, male and female, are advised against achieving a pregnancy within the next year or two. Depending on the dose given, there will be restrictions on social contact between the patient and others — especially children. When an adequate dose is given to control the thyrotoxicosis, around 80% of patients will eventually become hypothyroid.

Surgery, therefore, is an alternative treatment and probably indicated when there is a large goitre, when treatment is needed during pregnancy, in the presence of eye disease when surgery is otherwise indicated, i.e. a large gland, or when there is a possible cancer. Surgery or iodine treatment can be considered in some patients, i.e. after failed medical treatment, or if the patient prefers it. A knowledge of the physiology of the thyroid is crucial in planning a safe operation for the patient. Operating on the uncontrolled thyrotoxic patient is unacceptable.

First it is necessary to control the effects of the thyrotoxicosis. Block (with thioamides) or block-and-replace (with thioamides and thyroxine) therapy will produce the euthyroid state, but this can take some months to achieve. The catecholamine effects of thyrotoxicosis can be controlled by β-blockade, i.e. using propranolol, and this approach has the advantage of considerably foreshortening the pretreatment period. Traditionally iodine was added to the pretreatment protocol — and the reader ought now to be aware of the theoretical reasoning behind this. In practice, however, there is no evidence that iodine is beneficial to the patient or surgical outcome in any way. Iodine is just not necessary. Most patients will face surgery on block-and-replace treatment when thyroid function is optimally controlled.

Next the choice of operation should be considered. For Graves' disease subtotal thyroidectomy or total thyroidectomy will be the choice — as it is for toxic multinodular goitre. Total lobectomy is possible for the autonomous functioning nodule. Many patients with Graves' disease will do well with subtotal thyroidectomy. However, it will be recalled that this is an autoimmune condition and therefore there is the potential for recurrence of the disease — or of hypothyroidism occurring in the long term because of the emergence of blocking TSH receptor antibodies. In subtotal procedures the amount of thyroid tissue left in situ is important to the risk of hypothyroidism occurring — either immediately or in the long term. There is little evidence to suggest that the

subtotal procedure — in which a 3 or 4 g posterior rim of thyroid tissue is retained on each side — is protectant to the recurrent laryngeal nerves compared with a total procedure, provided the nerves are identified perioperatively (the risk of permanent nerve injury is around 1–3%), but there is a very significantly enhanced risk of postoperative hypocalcaemia after the total procedure: around 30% but which reduces to around 1–2% by 3 months. For many patients, subtotal operations, retaining around 6–8 g of thyroid tissue in total, will be appropriate, but long term follow-up is essential.

When the gland is very large in Graves' disease and there is a high antibody level, when the patient is a child, or where there is associated ophthalmopathy, total thyroidectomy is indicated. The author's preference for total thyroidectomy in many cases of thyrotoxic Graves' disease is rising, and this is especially so for patients with eye problems. It eliminates the risk of recurrent thyrotoxicosis, which can cause deterioration in any residual ophthalmopathy, and there may be a more immediate improvement in the eye disease after total procedures than with subtotal ones, for reasons already discussed.

MALIGNANT THYROID DISEASE

Approximately 1% of all malignant disease arises in the thyroid. There are several types of malignant thyroid tumours — these are listed in Box 14.2.

Papillary cancer is the commonest tumour. Normally it is non-functioning and appears as a 'cold-spot' on isotope scanning. It is often multifocal within the thyroid, and early spread to pre- and paratracheal nodes can occur. However, it is a very indolent disease, particularly in younger adult patients. It is more aggressive in children and the elderly. Peak incidence is around the third decade. The patient usually presents with a lump in the thyroid gland — or with an enlarged lymph node in the neck.

Follicular cancer presents more commonly in the fourth and fifth decades. Histologically it causes great problems of diagnosis in some instances, for the cells may be indis-

Box 14.2 Incidence of thyroid cancer	
• well-differentiated thyroid cancer:	
— papillary cancer	75%
— follicular cancer	15%
• medullary cancer	6%
• 'undifferentiated' cancer	3%
• others — including lymphoma and secondary cancer	1%

tinguishable from benign tumour cells: the only clue to malignancy may be a small area of capsular, or vascular, invasion. The patient generally presents with a lump in the thyroid. Occasionally the follicular cancer may present as a functioning nodule (see Box 14.1). The prognosis of the well-differentiated cancers is good — particularly for the papillary tumours. Adverse factors include increasing age at presentation (excluding children, in whom prognosis may be less good), male sex, presence of secondary disease.

Undifferentiated cancer covers many types of tumour — small cell, spindle cell, giant cell tumours — and usually affects the elderly. Prognosis is very poor and surgery has little part to play in their management.

Medullary cancers are considered later.

Physiological principles can be applied to the management of well-differentiated thyroid cancer. First, TSH is a potent growth factor to thyroid cells. Second, well-differentiated thyroid cancer cells frequently take up iodine — particularly under a strong TSH drive. Surgical ablation of the thyroid cancer (total thyroidectomy with removal of all affected nodal tissue) is the essential first procedure. The patient is allowed to convalesce whilst on thyroxine replacement therapy, and then this is temporarily discontinued. The patient is subsequently scanned — once the TSH levels have risen — with a short-acting isotope of iodine to identify residual thyroid tissue, usually in the neck. An ablation dose of ^{131}I is then given whilst the TSH drive is high, and the patient is then put on a dose of thyroxine sufficient to suppress TSH. The patient will need to be rescanned in about 6 months, but many can be monitored by looking for the emergence of thyroglobulin in the peripheral blood. It will be recalled from earlier in this chapter that thyroglobulin can be a very useful tumour marker in this situation. Adequate initial surgery, iodine ablation of any residual thyroid tissue, and TSH suppression by thyroxine represents the gold standard treatment of well-differentiated thyroid cancer.

(Disorders of the C-cell are considered in the section on calcium homeostasis, and medullary cancer is discussed briefly under MEN syndromes.)

The one condition not yet considered is the multinodular goitre. This is a very common problem — probably arising as a result of dyshormonogenesis and, as a result, an increased TSH drive with hyperplasia of the thyroid cells — which can be focal within the thyroid gland. Iodine deficiency used to be a potent cause of this, but in the USA and most of Europe this no longer applies. Some cases are familial. It is said that thyroxine administration, and resultant TSH suppression, will slow the progression of the increase in size of the thyroid gland.

Surgery is indicated if the gland is large and with compressive symptoms, and when there is a toxic multinodular goitre. Total thyroidectomy will usually be the preferred surgical procedure.

PARATHYROID GLANDS

NORMAL STRUCTURE AND FUNCTION

There are usually four glands, two on each side of the neck. The glands generally lie deep to the thyroid gland. Their total mass is approximately 120–150 mg. They develop from the third and fourth branchial pouches, migrating down into the neck during development. The glands from the fourth pouch become the superior or upper parathyroids, and those from the third pouch become the inferior glands. The surgeon generally recognises the superior and inferior glands in their relationship to the inferior thyroid artery — those lying cephalad being the superior parathyroids, and those caudally placed being the inferior glands. The blood supply of the glands is usually derived from the inferior thyroid artery.

The position of the glands is very variable. Whilst the upper one is normally just above the inferior thyroid artery and the inferior normally towards the deep aspect of the lower pole of the thyroid gland, the glands can in fact lie in many positions in the neck as well as in the mediastinum. Not infrequently the inferior glands may be found in the thymus. The glands have been seen by the author lying as high as the hyoid bone, in the carotid sheath, paravertebrally, behind the oesophagus or between oesophagus and trachea, above and below the arch of the aorta, and even on the wall of the right atrium.

Not only is the position of the glands very variable, their number also varies. In a few people, only three glands are present, whilst around 6% of the population will have five glands and about 0.5% will have six.

STRUCTURE AND FUNCTION

The histological features of the parathyroid glands are rather uninspiring. The gland consists of epithelial cells and fat. The epithelial cells are of two types: the chief cell, which has a clear cytoplasm, and the oxyphil cell, which has an eosinophilic granular cytoplasm. Both produce parathyroid hormone.

Parathyroid hormone (PTH) has a sequence of 84 amino acids and a molecular weight of 9300. It is formed by cleavage from a 'pro-PTH' with 90 amino acids, and this in turn is cleaved from a pre pro-PTH of 115 amino acids. The cleavage process occurs quite rapidly, with cleavage from pro-PTH to PTH taking about 15 min. When secreted from the cell, intact PTH has a half-life of only 2 or 3 min. There is a very limited amount of stored PTH in the cells — perhaps only an hour or so of PTH. In other words, metabolic changes can occur very swiftly if PTH secretion is modified, i.e. the removal of para-thyroid glands for disease, or inadvertently as might accompany thyroidectomy. The intact PTH is cleaved into two fragments: the amino terminal fragment and the carboxyl terminal fragment. The amino fragment is biologically active; the carboxyl fragment may also be active. PTH is broken down in the circulation, liver and kidney.

The PTH assay depends on identifying intact PTH in plasma. It is essential, therefore, when taking blood samples for PTH analysis to ensure that they are immediately stored in ice and transferred quickly to the laboratory.

Control of PTH secretion

There is a negative feedback control mechanism. Higher levels of free ionised Ca in plasma inhibit PTH secretion and vice versa. The relationship is very sensitive. A small change in Ca^{2+} levels results in large changes in PTH concentration.

Physiological effects of PTH

PTH regulates the serum calcium levels by an effect on bone, kidney and the gut. In bone the effect is to produce resorption via osteoclastic activity. The osteoclast binds to the bone surface and dissolves bone by two mechanisms. Acid is secreted which dissolves out the bone mineral, and proteases are released which break down the bone matrix. In the gut the effect is indirect, being mediated by 1,25 dihydroxyvitamin D which is produced in the kidney proximal tubule under the predominant control of PTH. This is the most active form of vitamin D and is derived from precursors produced in the skin (cholecal-ciferol) and the liver (cholecalciferol → 25,hydroxy-vitamin D). The vitamin D effect on the gut is to enhance calcium absorption.

In the kidney proximal tubule, PTH increases the urinary excretion of phosphate. This in turn causes an increase in the degree of ionisation of calcium. There is also a direct effect on calcium resorption in the kidney, with PTH increasing Ca^{2+} reabsorption in the distal tubule. PTH may also reduce, or inhibit, bicarbonate resorption in the renal tubules, resulting in an acidosis which will increase the degree of calcium ionisation and consequent resorption of calcium from bone. This will be reflected in a hyperchloraemic acidosis.

Therefore the biochemical changes in blood which can accrue from an abnormal, i.e. raised, PTH level include:

- hypercalcaemia
- hypophosphataemia
- hyperchloraemia.

PATHOPHYSIOLOGY OF DISORDERS OF PARATHYROID HORMONE FUNCTION

Some of the commoner conditions recognised include:

- primary hyperparathyroidism
- familial benign hypocalciuric hypercalcaemia
- secondary hyperparathyroidism
- tertiary hyperparathyroidism
- ectopic hyperparathyroidism
- hypoparathyroidism.

Primary hyperparathyroidism is almost invariably caused by a benign adenoma. Parathyroid carcinoma is extremely rare. Symptoms are related to the hyper-calcaemia: renal calculi, polyuria, polydipsia, pancreatitis, bone pains, proximal myopathy. In the elderly particu-larly, confusion and personality change may be present. Pathological fractures can occur but are now extremely rare. Indeed most of the potential symptoms and signs are usually absent, although renal calculous disease remains as a major presenting ailment of hyperparathyroidism. Most cases are detected by the chance finding of hypercalcaemia on biochemical blood analyses. The bio-chemical changes in blood, favouring a diagnosis of hyperparathyroidism, include:

- hypercalcaemia in the presence of a non-suppressed or elevated PTH level (hypercalcaemia is best diagnosed using the ionised form of Ca^{2+} in blood) — this is essential in establishing the diagnosis
- hypophosphataemia
- hyperchloraemia
- (mild) acidosis
- (possible) raised alkaline phosphatase

All or some of these may be present.

Radiological changes include a generalised demineral-isation of bone (which can now be measured and moni-tored), a 'ground-glass' appearance to the skull, a loss of lamina dura around the teeth (a sign almost pathogno-monic of hyperparathyroidism), a loss of the bone 'tufts' of the terminal phalanges of the fingers, and the presence of 'bone cysts' — which are more likely to be tumours comprising osteoclastic cells.

Familial benign hypocalciuric hypercalcaemia is a descriptive name given to an inherited disorder presenting with a mild hypercalcaemia and, quite often, a slight elevation of PTH level. It is an autosomal dominant inheritance and is usually completely asymptomatic. The condition may be biochemically indistinguishable from hyperparathyroidism, but a known family history can assist in distinguishing the two complaints. Surgery has no part in the management of these patients.

Hyperparathyroidism is also seen in the MEN syndromes — especially MEN I (parathyroid adenoma, pancreatic tumours, pituitary tumours, carcinoid and adrenal tumours) and MEN IIa (parathyroid hyperplasia, medullary carcinoma of thyroid and phaeochromocytoma).

Secondary hyperparathyroidism is usually seen in patients with renal failure. A combination of a failure to synthesise 1-alpha dihydroxyvitamin D, and a retention of phosphate by the reduced number of renal tubules, results in a lowered blood Ca^{2+} level and a stimulated elevation in PTH level. The physiological responses to hypocalcaemia are shown in Figure 14.7. The glands show a hyperplastic response, and normally all four will be affected. The condition is now seen less often by the

surgeon, because of improved patient management — in particular, reducing the phosphate content of the diet and prescribing 1-alpha dihydroxyvitamin D to patients who are developing renal failure. Investigating the patient will usually show normal Ca^{2+} levels, high phosphate levels and, not infrequently, very high levels of PTH, when the blood levels are analysed. Ectopic hyperparathyroidism is usually seen in patients with tumours producing a PTH-like substance.

Hypoparathyroidism is, for most practical purposes, an acute-onset iatrogenic condition arising either from a deliberate decision to remove all the parathyroid glands, as might happen in the management of secondary hyperparathyroidism, or as a result of the accidental removal or ischaemic injury of the parathyroid glands during thyroidectomy. Other causes include autoimmune conditions where circulating antibodies to PTH can be detected, congenital conditions of failed branchial arch development (DiGeorge syndrome) and in some conditions of metal deposition, e.g. copper in Wilson's disease. These are rare. Biochemical changes in blood include reduced

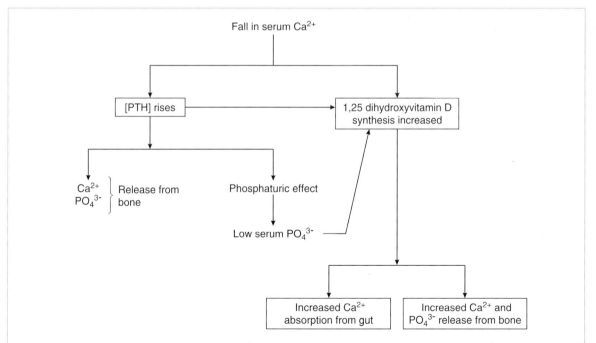

Fig. 14.7 Physiological response to a low serum Ca^{2+}. By utilising this simple chart, the effects of disease on Ca^{2+} homeostasis can be postulated. For example, in renal failure there is (a) PO_4^{3-} retention and (b) reduced 1,25 dihydroxyvitamin D synthesis. As a result Ca^{2+} depletion will occur, and there is a consequent rise in PTH due to chronic hypocalcaemia. There can be no 1,25 dihydroxyvitamin D response in vivo because of the renal disease. Therefore the administration of 1,25 dihydroxyvitamin D is logical. To combat the hyperphosphataemia a low PO_4^{3-} diet might be constructed. In this way the effects of a possible secondary hyperparathyroidism may be prevented or ameliorated.

or absent PTH, hypocalcaemia and hyperphosphataemia. When hypoparathyroidism occurs acutely the patient will complain of paraesthesia, i.e. tingling in the fingers or in the lips, and soon after may demonstrate carpopedal spasm which may lead on to convulsions and tetany. Acute treatment includes the administration of a calcium infusion and, in the long term, management is with 1-alpha dihydroxyvitamin D, with dietary and calcium supplementation if necessary.

Management of hyperparathyroidism is normally surgical. Removal of an adenoma is the treatment for primary disease. It will be recalled that the position of the glands is variable, and the adenoma may be in a wide range of sites in the neck or mediastinum. Attempts to localise the lesion preoperatively have been made and include ultrasound, thallium/iodine subtraction scanning, T_c-subtraction scanning, sestamibi scanning, CT and MRI. Whether an attempt at preoperative localisation is indicated or not is a topic hotly debated by endocrine surgeons. None of the investigations is sufficiently sensitive or specific to be relied upon totally, and the experienced surgeon will probably detect the lesion in about 95% of cases at primary neck exploration. Although it is an ideal circumstance to be able to locate a lesion preoperatively the cost and effort is probably not justified. Where a patient is to undergo reoperation after a failed exploration, further investigations to try and localise a lesion are indicated. These include MRI, radio-isotope scanning and selective venous sampling. In secondary disease, total parathyroidectomy and the maintenance of the patient on 1-alpha dihydroxyvitamin D, usually without calcium supplementation, or subtotal parathyroidectomy preserving about 100–150 mg of parathyroid tissue for adequate function, are both practised. In the latter, surgery may still result in hypoparathyroidism or may permit the eventual re-emergence of hyperparathyroidism. Total parathyroidectomy is increasingly preferred (but not universally practised). Transplantation of parathyroid tissue to the forearm after total parathyroidectomy in the neck was popular, but is now rarely carried out.

Maintenance of calcium ion homeostasis

In the body the main calcium store is in bone. Lesser amounts are present in the soft tissues and extracellular fluid. Only a tiny fraction of the total body calcium is found in the intracellular compartment. There is a very tight regulation of both intra- and extracellular calcium concentrations. Calcium is important in a variety of physiological processes, including:

- bone formation and growth

- nerve synapse function
- muscle contractility, both striated and cardiac
- cell division
- blood clotting cascade.

In the extracellular fluid it is found in a bound form, with albumin predominantly, but also with phosphate and citrate, and in the free form as ionised calcium, Ca^{2+}. The bound form is biologically inactive. The ionised form is the one which is closely regulated in plasma.

In general terms, the concentration of Ca^{2+} is maintained by the bone, extracellular fluid exchange and by the gut and the kidneys.

Regulation of calcium is mainly by three hormones: parathormone, calcitonin and 1,25 dihydroxyvitamin D. Disturbance of calcium can occur as a result of

- a disordered hormone balance, i.e. hyperparathyroidism
- disseminated malignancy
- sarcoidosis (due to production of $1,25(OH)_2$ vitamin D from its inactive form by a hydroxylase enzyme in the macrophages of sarcoid tissue)
- patients on vitamin D preparations, and those on absorbable antacids for dyspepsia (milk-alkali syndrome)
- thyrotoxicosis, where there is a catabolic effect of thyroxin on bone and where there is also a hyperdynamic state of bone.

The functions of parathyroid hormone have already been discussed, and the effect of 1,25 dihydroxyvitamin D on the gut has also been described. The effect of vitamin D on bone itself is complex: at normal concentrations osteoblastic activity is favoured. In excess, however, hypercalcaemia can arise from osteoclastically derived bone resorption. A deficiency of vitamin D results in osteomalacia.

This leaves calcitonin which is produced in the parafollicular cells of the thyroid. It is a polypeptide hormone which is produced in response to hypercalcaemia. It appears to inhibit bone resorption by an inhibiting effect on osteoclasts. It also favours the increased excretion of Ca^{2+} in the renal tubules, with conservation of Mg^{2+}. It is probably of much greater physiological importance in seawater fish than in humans. Patients who have had total thyroidectomy do not appear to have any calcitonin deficiency syndrome identifiable. Patients with medullary carcinoma may have levels several hundred times the normal upper limit and yet do not have any problems with Ca^{2+} homoeostasis. Calcitonin is used therapeutically to reduce hypercalcaemia, particularly in metastatic disease of bone and the management of Paget's disease — the effects being mediated via its inhibitory effect on osteoclasts.

Therefore, in humans, Ca^{2+} homoeostasis is predominantly a function of parathormone and 1,25 dihydroxy-vitamin D. Of these two, it is parathormone which is the more important for the immediate control of extracellular Ca^{2+} concentration.

MULTIPLE ENDOCRINE NEOPLASIA (MEN)

Although comparatively rare, clusters of endocrine tumours have become recognised and classified (Box 14.3). In both MEN I and MEN IIa hyperparathyroidism is part of the syndrome. In MEN I, a parathyroid adenoma is the commonest tumour, whereas in IIa it is medullary thyroid carcinoma. In IIa the hyperparathyroidism is usually hyperplasia rather than an adenoma. Despite the association of the various endocrine tumours in MEN syndromes, hyperparathyroidism is generally seen in the absence of the syndrome. However, one should always be aware of the MEN syndromes when dealing with any endocrine tumour that could be associated with one or other of them. One's index of suspicion should be raised, for example, when parathyroid hyperplasia is encountered in an apparently otherwise well individual. Patients should be screened for medullary thyroid cancer (MTC) (blood calcitonin) and phaeochromocytoma. All cases of MTC should be screened preoperatively for phaeochromocytoma. Families can also be screened for MEN syndromes — in particular, type II patients and their families for the RET proto-oncogene on chromosome 10.

Box 14.3 Syndromes of multiple endocrine neoplasia

- MEN I
  - parathyroid adenomata
  - pituitary tumours (various)
  - pancreatic tumours (insulinoma, gastrinoma)

- MEN IIa
  - medullary thyroid cancer
  - hyperparathyroidism (hyperplasia > adenoma)
  - phaeochromocytoma

- MEN IIb
  - medullary thyroid cancer
  - phaeochromocytoma
  - mucosal (mouth) neuromata
  - marfanoid appearance

MTC is a tumour of the thyroid parafollicular cells (C cells). Less than 10% of thyroid tumours are due to MTC. It is diagnosed by finding cytological evidence for it on aspiration biopsy of a thyroid nodule, and on an elevated blood calcitonin. It spreads early to nodes in the neck. Generally, if there are any systemic symptoms, the commonest symptom is diarrhoea. The adequacy of surgical treatment can be monitored by calcitonin estimations in blood.

ADRENAL GLANDS
DEVELOPMENT AND ANATOMY

There are two glands: one on each side of the abdomen, lying just above or medial to the upper pole of each kidney. On the right side the adrenal gland posteriorly lies against the diaphragm, anteriorly lies against the bare area of the liver and by peritoneum of the hepatorenal pouch of Rutherford Morrison, and medially lies against the inferior vena cava. On the left the adrenal lies against the crus of the diaphragm, and it lies behind the parietal peritoneum of the lesser sac. Below this it lies in direct contact with the pancreas and with the splenic artery and vein (see Fig. 14.8). Their combined mass is only 10 g approximately. Each gland comprises two main parts: a cortex and a medulla.

The adrenal glands differentiate early in the fetus and by 2 months gestation are recognisable as separate structures each comprising two parts. One part differentiates to be the adrenal cortex, the so called definitive zone. This is of mesodermal origin. The other part of the adrenal gland is infiltrated at about 6 weeks by cells derived from neural crest tissue. These cells differentiate into phaeochromocytes and form the adrenal medulla. The cortex and medulla are quite distinct entities physiologically, but share a blood supply. Not infrequently islands of cortical tissue may be seen within the medulla.

The glands are well endowed with blood. There are three main sources: the superior adrenal arteries (from the inferior phrenic artery on each side), the 'middle' adrenal arteries from the aorta, and inferior arteries from the renal artery. The venous drainage is by a central vein. On the left side, the vein drains into the left renal vein, whereas, on the right, drainage is to the inferior vena cava, usually entering the cava just superior to the renal vein. The right adrenal vein is very short and can be difficult to handle when operating on the right adrenal gland. The left adrenal vein is longer. The arteries mainly form a plexus under the cortical capsule but with some branches

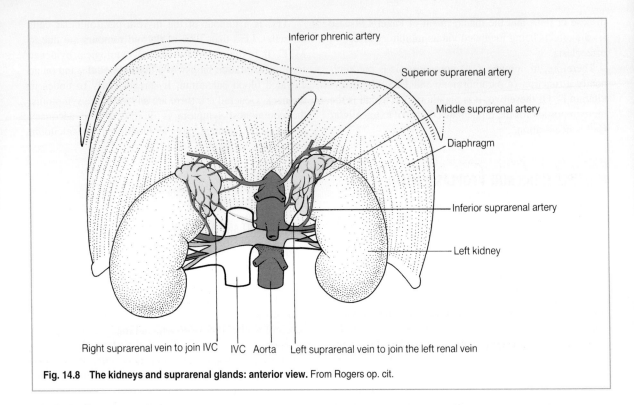

Inferior phrenic artery

Superior suprarenal artery

Middle suprarenal artery

Diaphragm

Inferior suprarenal artery

Left kidney

Right suprarenal vein to join IVC   IVC   Aorta   Left suprarenal vein to join the left renal vein

Fig. 14.8   The kidneys and suprarenal glands: anterior view. From Rogers op. cit.

penetrating directly to the medulla. Within the adrenal glands there appears to be a portal system, for the cortical vessels form into capillaries which then drain to the central vein, giving blood supply to the medulla as they do so.

The medulla additionally has a nerve supply — this is composed of preganglionic sympathetic nerves which terminate in relation to the phaeochromocytes. From a surgeon's point of view, the adrenal gland is rarely going to be handled. Even the specialist endocrine surgeon will see a limited number of cases only. The adrenal glands are, however, supremely important to the surgeon, particularly if they are diseased, producing either an excess or a deficiency of hormone — or if the function of the glands is modified by the administration of exogenous adrenal products. For example, the glucocorticoids, when produced in excess (Cushing's disease) or when deficient (Addison's disease), or when suppressed (by exogenous corticosteroid administration), will, in each instance, modify the patient profoundly from any surgical aspect.

This section will, therefore, consider those aspects of adrenal physiology which impinge on the surgeon and will attempt to illustrate how surgery might be more appropriately conducted adopting sound physiological principles. The adrenal cortex and adrenal medulla effects will be considered separately.

ADRENAL CORTEX

Three layers are recognised: the zona glomerulosa, zona fasciculata and zona reticularis. The zona glomerulosa lies just beneath the capsule of the adrenal gland and produces aldosterone. The zona reticularis surrounds the adrenal medulla and produces androgens and cortisol. Both of these layers are thin and are separated from one another by a thicker layer, the zona fasciculata, which also produces cortisol and androgens. Both fasciculata and reticularis layers are ACTH-responsive. Hormones are produced 'on demand' — they are not stored. It is possible that the zona fasciculata maintains normal homeostasis of cortisol, but that the zona reticularis is the one which responds to the acute situation where hormones are 'required' in excess.

Synthesis of adrenal hormones

The major hormones are: cortisol (glucocorticoids), aldosterone and androgens (and therefore, also, oestrogen). A simplified chart outlining their synthesis is shown in Figure 14.9. All steroid hormone synthesis begins with cholesterol. ACTH has its main influence on the adrenal at the cholesterol–pregnenolone conversion level. Under normal circumstances adrenal androgen and oestrogen

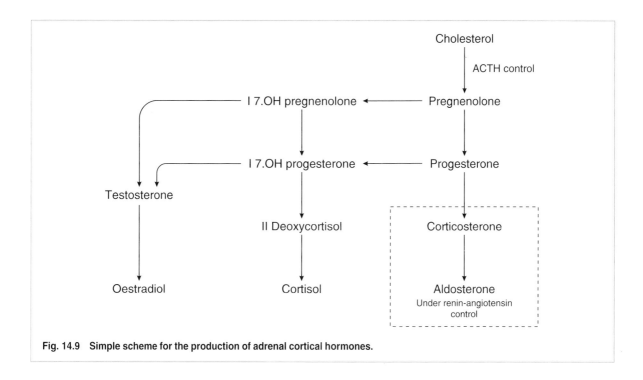

Fig. 14.9 Simple scheme for the production of adrenal cortical hormones.

have no bearing on reproductive function. However, in excess, a profound effect can be observed.

GLUCOCORTICOIDS (CORTISOL)

Functions
The effects of glucocorticoids are widespread. In the plasma over 90% of cortisol is carried bound either to a globulin or to albumin. It is the free cortisol which is biologically active. The bound cortisol may act as a 'circulating' reservoir of cortisol. The half life of plasma cortisol is about 90 min, although much less for the unbound form.

Free cortisol enters the cells, binds with DNA and affects mRNA, and thus protein synthesis. In the liver, this causes an increase in protein synthesis: in most other tissue cortisol is inhibitory to mRNA and has a catabolic effect.

Effects on intermediary metabolism
In the liver, gluconeogenesis is increased. There is a direct mechanism via enzymes such as glucose-6-phosphatase and an indirect effect whereby cortisol has a facilitatory effect on the gluconeogenic actions of glucagon and catecholamines. In skeletal muscle, and in fat tissues, there is a catabolic effect of cortisol. Glucose uptake is reduced

in muscle and fat and there is increased lipolysis resulting in the production of glycerol and free fatty acids. The fatty acids are then incorporated into the gluconeogenic process within the liver. Liver glycogen synthesis is increased. In glucocorticoid excess there is hyperinsulinaemia; this is almost certainly due to the effect of cortisol on glucose metabolism and not a direct cortisol effect on insulin synthesis.

In the normal state, the glucocorticoids are catabolic to fat. In conditions of glucocorticoid excess there is always an associated obesity — generally of a centripetal distribution, the limbs being spared. Overall, though, there is an increase in body fat. This is due probably to the increased insulin response and to hyperphagia, both of which are associated with cortisol excess.

Effects on central nervous system
Normal cortisol synthesis and release is based on a diurnal mechanism and is discussed later in this chapter. In disease states this diurnal variation is readily lost. In excess, glucocorticoids have a number of effects. Appetite is increased and there can be sleep disturbance. In the early stages of cortisol excess, there is usually a feeling of wellbeing. A more serious problem — although seen relatively infrequently — is of steroid-associated psychosis. Regardless of whether the excess cortisol is

endogenous or exogenous, a severe psychosis can be very difficult to manage. The patient may be suicidal and, if this is arising in a patient needing steroid treatment for, say, an organ transplant rejection, the situation may be critical, for the steroid administration may need to be discontinued.

Effects on musculoskeletal and connective tissues

As has already been observed, glucocorticoids inhibit many cells. In the presence of excess glucocorticoids there is inhibition of fibroblastic activity, with a net loss of collagen. Many of the 'classic signs' of Cushing's syndrome are due to this phenomenon, with an apparent thinning of the skin, striae formation, and increased tendency to bruising ('steroid purpura'). Of particular importance to the surgeon is the fact that wounds will heal badly.

Bones are affected in a variety of ways when there is an excess of glucocorticoids. Bone matrix reduces and bone resorption increases. There is also a permissive effect of cortisol on parathormone action — which is potentiated. There is a further effect on parathormone as calcium absorption from the gut is reduced by cortisol excess. The effects on bone are most often seen in patients who have been on long term exogenous steroids — transplant recipients are probably the prime example. It is often forgotten that glucocorticoids are readily absorbed from creams prescribed for eczema and one sees sometimes patients who have developed severe bone disease from nothing more than eczema management. Bony changes include vertebral body collapse, fractures and avascular necrosis — especially of the femoral head. Children show growth retardation — often severe — in cortisol excess.

Haematological and immunological effects

It has long been recognised that the glucocorticoids have immunosuppressive and anti-inflammatory actions. The clinical use of exogenous glucocorticoids was originally based on their apparent clinical efficacy and not as a result of a knowledge of their pharmacological or physiological activity. The glucocorticoids had an observed useful effect and were therefore used. They are easy to synthesise. They are easy to administer in tablet, liquid, injectable, ointment, cream and other forms. This pragmatic approach resulted in their widespread use in a huge range of conditions — for example, inflammatory bowel disease, rheumatoid arthritis and other degenerative joint disorders, allergic disorders including eczema and asthma, as well as in organ transplantation. This has led to a significant overuse of the steroids — with sometimes serious consequences — and now, fortunately, their therapeutic usage is much more selectively applied.

Box 14.4 Some immunological effects of glucocorticoids

- effects on cells
  - lymphocyte, monocyte, eosinophil reduction in blood
  - increase in circulatory polymorphs
  - inhibition of accumulation of inflammatory cells at sites of inflammation
  - inhibition of lymphocyte production

- effects on cell function
  - inhibition of prostaglandin synthesis
  - inhibition of interleukins
  - inhibition of T cell proliferation

The immunological effects are summarised in Box 14.4.

Other effects of glucocorticoids

These include effects on the cardiovascular system, and may be related to the permissive effects of glucocorticoids or catecholamines and catecholamine receptors. In the kidney, a glucocorticoid deficiency is associated with a lower glomerular filtration rate. In the gut, glucocorticoids have been associated with an increase in peptic ulcer disease. This association is not universally accepted, and it is more likely that corticosteroid excess is associated with an enhanced complication rate of pre-existing ulcers (i.e. perforation).

CONTROL OF GLUCOCORTICOID PRODUCTION AND RELEASE

Control is exerted via a negative feedback system, with rising levels of glucocorticoid inhibiting adrenocorticotrophic hormone (ACTH) output from the anterior pituitary directly and inhibiting corticotrophin releasing hormone (CRH) from the hypothalamus, resulting in ACTH inhibition within minutes. In addition, long term administration of glucocorticoids results in a suppression of ACTH and CRH and consequent atrophy of the zona fasciculata and zona reticularis in the adrenal cortex. The feedback control on cortisol production is only part of the story, for there is a strong neurological influence. First, there is a circadian rhythm, with greatest ACTH and glucocorticoid output being observed towards the end of sleep. Higher cortisol levels are found in the morning prior to wakening. The rhythm in any individual can vary. In Cushing's syndrome the diurnal variation is lost. In sleep disturbance the rhythm is modified. Major disease and trauma, and psychological stress will all cause a modification — or loss — of the diurnal variation. The stress effect is mediated through the hypothalamus, with

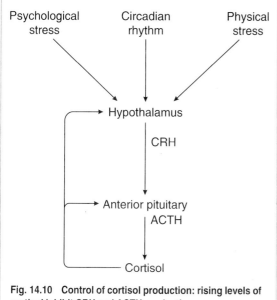

Fig. 14.10 Control of cortisol production: rising levels of cortisol inhibit CRH and ACTH production.

increased CRH production. The control of cortisol production is shown in simplified form in Figure 14.10.

Although adrenal androgens are of little clinical note in the normal individual, their production parallels that of cortisol. Thus there is a circadian rhythm to the production of adrenal androgens. Females with an ACTH-producing tumour may demonstrate some of the clinical effects of an excess of androgens, with hirsutism and acne, although no effect will be seen in men. Prepubertal boys may demonstrate early onset of secondary sexual characteristics.

DIAGNOSIS OF GLUCOCORTICOID DYSFUNCTION

The diagnosis depends on identifying that there is an adrenal cortical dysfunction and determining the site within the hypothalamic/pituitary–adrenal axis at which the dysfunction is occurring.

Plasma cortisol levels may be determined. A single estimation is of less value than estimations performed on first wakening (or as soon as possible thereafter) and again later in the day (usually taken in the evening). Levels two to three times normal can be found in pregnancy and in acutely ill or traumatised patients.

Urinary corticosteroids can also be ascertained using a 24 h urine collection. It is the urinary free cortisol which is measured.

Tests of adrenal axis function will determine the nature of the corticoid dysfunction. The administration of glucocorticoids should, in the normal person, reduce ACTH production and, therefore, endogenous cortisol in plasma should be suppressed. Dexamethasone is generally used — the dexamethasone suppression test — and the test is normally conducted overnight. If cortisol suppression fails to occur and plasma cortisol level remains high, the pituitary–adrenal axis is abnormal, suggesting Cushing's syndrome. A low dose of dexamethasone is usually used.

To test adrenal cortical reserve, synthetic ACTH can be administered and the cortisol response measured. Similarly the ability of the anterior pituitary to secrete ACTH can be assessed by giving CRH. Clearly these tests are done when assessing pituitary–adrenal insufficiency.

Another test of adrenal insufficiency is the response to the administration of metyrapone. Metyrapone inhibits cortisol synthesis, leading to a rise in cortisol precursors in plasma and a rise in ACTH. If this occurs after metyrapone administration, the pituitary adrenal axis is working normally.

The response to stress will test the hypothalamic component of the axis and therefore, potentially, the complete hypothalamic/pituitary–adrenal axis. Hypoglycaemia is the stress test used, and a rise in plasma cortisol and ACTH in response to the insulin-hypoglycaemic stress will demonstrate a normal axis.

ALDOSTERONE

Aldosterone is a mineralocorticoid and the other main product of the adrenal cortex. It is produced in the zona glomerulosa and is predominantly under the control of the renin–angiotensin mechanism. However, ACTH does also stimulate a rise in aldosterone production, as does hyponatraemia, hyperkalaemia and hypovolaemia, i.e. haemorrhage.

Renin is produced in the juxtaglomerula apparatus of the kidney and is released by three main stimuli:

- reduction in renal perfusion pressures via baroreceptors in the afferent arterioles
- arterial receptors which stimulate the sympathetic nervous system and increase catecholamine concentration
- hyponatraemia effect on the juxtaglomerular apparatus.

Renin acts on angiotensinogen, which is secreted by the liver, cleaving angiotensin I from it. Angiotensin I is then converted to angiotensin II by angiotensin-converting enzyme (ACE). ACE is present in many tissues, but particularly in the lungs. Angiotensin II is a powerful vasoconstrictor acting on arteries; it has an inotropic effect on the heart and has a strongly vasoconstrictive effect on arteries within the kidney. In addition, Na$^+$ reabsorption increases in the renal tubule, and the glomerular filtration rate is reduced by constriction of the renal arterioles and the mesangial cells around the macula densa. It also acts on chromaffin cells, causing a release of adrenaline, and stimulates vasopressin release from the pituitary.

Within the adrenal gland aldosterone synthesis is stimulated. Both aldosterone and angiotensin II conserve Na$^+$ and H$_2$O in the gut, and aldosterone itself has a Na$^+$ and H$_2$O conserving effect in the distal renal tubule.

At this point it is pertinent to consider briefly two drugs used in the management of hypertension. The first, spironolactone, is an aldosterone antagonist — it competes for the aldosterone receptor sites — and is therefore used as a K$^+$ sparing diuretic. The second to mention is a group of drugs which act to inhibit the angiotensin-converting enzyme — the so-called ACE inhibitors. This group of agents can be expected to be effective vasodilators and thus lower blood pressure and, of course, this is what they do. However, one of their most potent effects is vasodilatation within the kidney — especially in the efferent arterioles from the glomerulus. Therefore they are effective in patients with renal-related hypertension and are now being seen as especially useful in diabetic patients with hypertension, promoting a more favourable outlook to the management of diabetic nephropathy. However, it can also be seen that a reduction in efferent arteriolar constriction with a fall in intraglomerular pressure may be associated with a serious outcome, i.e. acute renal failure in patients with renal artery stenosis.

DISORDERS OF FUNCTION OF ADRENAL CORTEX

Insufficiency

The condition may arise as a primary problem of the adrenal cortex or as a secondary problem of the cortex, the cause lying elsewhere — for example, a failure of ACTH. Primary insufficiency was described by Thomas Addison ('Addison's disease') in the mid-19th century when the commonest cause of the condition was tuberculosis. This is now a much rarer cause — indeed Addison's disease itself is rare. The causes now include metastatic disease of the adrenal gland, haemorrhage into the adrenals, and autoimmune disorders. Secondary insufficiency is due to a failure of the pituitary adrenal axis — for example, a destructive lesion of the pituitary, or surgery to the pituitary, can result in adrenal failure. The most common cause of secondary insufficiency is exogenous glucocorticoid therapy which results in

suppression of ACTH production, although a similar situation is present in the patient with a cortisol-producing tumour, for the adrenal cortical tissue not involved in the tumour process will also be suppressed. Removal of the tumour will produce an immediate Addisonian state because of this suppression.

Adrenal insufficiency can therefore arise acutely or chronically. In the acute situation there will be hypotension and shock. There is likely to be hypoglycaemia. It must not be forgotten that acute adrenal insufficiency is not a glucocorticoid phenomenon: mineralocorticoid synthesis may also be affected — patients are likely to have, therefore, sodium depletion and dehydration.

In the chronic situation the patient with primary deficiency will demonstrate anorexia and weight loss; there may be muscle weakness and there may be hypotension. The striking feature of primary adrenal insufficiency will be skin pigmentation (and pigmentation of mucosa). This arises because of the high ACTH level present, which includes the shared peptide sequence of melanocyte-stimulating hormone, MSH. The diagnosis of the hypofunctioning adrenal cortex has already been discussed and is not dealt with further.

In practical terms, most patients with Addison's disease will be known to have the disease and already be on replacement therapy — usually a glucocorticoid, such as prednisone, and a mineralocorticoid. These patients, and those on long term glucocorticoid therapy for other reasons, and who will almost certainly have suppressed ACTH levels — and therefore suppressed adrenal corticoids — will be at risk of an acute adrenal crisis when subjected to stress — such as an emergency or elective surgical procedure. These patients will need additional glucocorticoid therapy over the period of their operations — and will also need careful evaluation, both preoperatively and postoperatively, of their state of hydration, electrolytes and blood pressure. An excess of adrenal cortical function results in Cushing's syndrome (glucocorticoid excess), Conn's syndrome (mineralocorticoid excess) and hirsutism and virilism (sex hormones).

Cushing's syndrome

The clinical effects of an excess of glucocorticoids can be predicted from the earlier description of the hormone. Usually the patients are obese and may demonstrate weaknesses of muscle, myopathies may be present, psychiatric disturbance and skin changes with bruising, striae and hirsutism. Investigations will show a loss of bone density and disturbances of glucose metabolism — the patients may be frankly diabetic. They are likely to demonstrate blood lipid elevation.

The causes of Cushing's syndrome may lie within the adrenal cortex — for example, adrenal tumours or adrenal hyperplasia — or outside the cortex, the condition being driven by ACTH arising from a pituitary tumour (Cushing's disease) or from an ectopic source of ACTH production. The laboratory diagnosis has already been discussed: the level of the lesion within the pituitary–adrenal axis can be established. Once this has been established, further investigations may be needed to determine, for example, the nature of the lesion. CT or MRI scanning will evaluate the adrenal glands and should be able to identify tumour or hyperplastic disease.

The management of an adrenal adenoma is to remove it surgically. Where there is primary adrenal hyperplasia this, too, may be removed by bilateral adrenalectomy. Malignant disease of the adrenal cortex can be very aggressive; the tumours are large and often have metastasised before the diagnosis can be made. It can be difficult, therefore, even after adrenalectomy to control the Cushingoid state. The author has used Mitotane, a synthetic agent which is lytic to adrenal cortical cells, in this situation but with no discernable success.

When a functioning adenoma is removed, it will be realised that the 'normal' adrenal cortical tissue will be suppressed and that the patient will need glucocorticoid treatment for at least some months afterwards. Usually it is possible to discontinue this ultimately, although the timing of this will depend upon ACTH recovery and on the ability of the remaining adrenal tissue to respond to ACTH.

After bilateral adrenalectomy, maintenance with glucocorticoids and mineralocorticoids will be needed in perpetuity. Nelson's syndrome may develop; this is almost certainly due to an ACTH-producing tumour of the pituitary, the presence of which is suppressed during the period of increased glucocorticoid synthesis. Surgery to the pituitary to remove the tumour is required, possibly combined with irradiation to the pituitary. Pituitary surgery is also the recommended approach for lesions of the pituitary gland producing ACTH — especially the microadenomata, when it can be expected to be successful with most patients eventually developing a normal pituitary–adrenal axis. The large macroadenoma is less often curable by resection of the adenoma. Patients will need to be maintained on glucocorticoid treatment until it is certain that the normal axis has been re-established.

Conn's syndrome

Primary aldosteronism is a rare condition. Known as Conn's syndrome, it is usually due to a benign adenoma of the adrenal gland producing aldosterone. The syndrome is associated, as might be predicted, with hypertension, Na^+ retention and water retention. In line with these there is K^+ loss and hypokalaemia and, with the intracellular shift of H^+, and a loss of H^+ in the kidney, an alkalosis develops. The loss of K^+ may be marked, and the patient may even describe polyuria and polydipsia. When an adenoma is present, and is identified to one adrenal or the other, adrenalectomy is the treatment of choice. However, the surgeon will recognise the need for preoperative preparation, and the logic of using spironolactone will not escape his or her attention. This should be used with two aims in mind: (a) to treat the hypertension — although other agents may also be needed — and (b) to restore K^+ homeostasis to normal. To do otherwise would be unsafe. Where no adenoma is identified, management is based on spironolactone treatment — although subtotal adrenalectomy, which might be regarded as the operation in the adrenal analogous to the subtotal procedures in the thyroid, is sometimes recommended as a way of controlling the clinical problem.

ADRENAL MEDULLA

The medulla comprises cells originating in neural crest tissue. Preganglionic sympathetic nerve fibres are present and are in close relationship to the chromaffin cells. The medulla produces the catecholamines, adrenaline and noradrenaline. In contradistinction to other sympathetic ganglia the medulla produces adrenaline ('epinephrine') predominantly and, to a much lesser extent, noradrenaline ('nor-epinephrine'). The hormones are synthesised from tyrosine via dopa and dopamine to noradrenaline and thence adrenaline. Once produced, the hormones are stored as granules — causing the appearance of the chromaffin cells. The catecholamines are stored in sympathetic nerve cells and therefore are found widely in the body, and not just in the adrenal medulla.

Secretion of catecholamines from adrenal medulla

This is a function of the cholinergic preganglionic sympathetic nerve fibres. Hypoglycaemia, anoxia, pain, haemorrhage and many other factors stimulate their release. Adrenaline rather than noradrenaline is the major hormone released. Once released, some of the catecholamine output is taken up by sympathetic nerve endings and thus inactivated. Catecholamines are also inactivated by monoamine oxidase and by catechol 0-methyltransferase (with production of hydroxy methyl mandelic acid which is excreted in urine), and some is also directly excreted by the kidneys.

Mode of action

The hormones mediate their effects through two groups of receptors: the α and β receptors. Each is divided into two subgroups, although β_3 receptors are now recognised in adipose tissue. The receptors are found widely but the adrenergic response is dependent on the type of receptor present within the organ tissue. α_1 Receptors are post-synaptic and are concerned particularly with smooth muscle contraction, i.e. uterus and blood vessels. α_2 Receptors are found widely in smooth muscle, fat, on platelets and within the nervous system both presynaptically — where activation will inhibit adrenaline release — and post-synapetically. Beta receptors are found widely. β_1 Receptors are found in cardiac tissue and, when stimulated, cause a rise in the force and rate of myocardial contraction. β_2 Receptors, when stimulated, generally cause smooth muscle relaxation: they are found in blood vessels, the uterus and the bronchioles. β_3 Receptors are found in fat and are associated with increased lipolysis.

Dopamine is a precursor of noradrenaline — but there are also dopamine receptors found in many tissues, including the brain, kidney, heart, pituitary and the mesentery. They are also found presynaptically.

Although this description implies that adrenergic receptors are found selectively they are, in fact, demonstrable in most tissues of the body. Adrenergic responses are very widespread. In addition to the effects describes above, responses in many other tissues can be demonstrated. For example, α receptor stimulation causes decreased insulin and glucagon release in the pancreas, with the opposite effect being seen on β receptor stimulation (Table 14.1). In general, noradrenalin has greater α_2 activity than adrenalin and, vice versa, adrenalin has greater β_2 activity than noradrenaline. α_1 and β_1 activities are roughly similar between the two hormones.

Diagnosis of malfunction

Plasma or urinary catecholamines can be measured. However, it is essential that these be measured in an individual who is calm and rested.

Biological functions of catecholamines

For many years adrenaline has been regarded as the hormone involved in the 'flight or fight' response. The secretion of adrenaline causes shunting of blood to the muscles away from the skin, dilates bronchioles and increases cardiac rate and contractility. A deficiency of catecholamines is a most unlikely clinical scenario. Even after bilateral adrenalectomy the patient is unlikely to notice any ill-effects unless there is an autonomic neuropathy present. This is especially important in diabetes mellitus. There may be quite severe problems with postural hypotension, and the symptoms of hypoglycaemia may be masked.

Phaeochromocytoma

This is the commonest problem of the adrenergic system – even so, it is a rare tumour. Commonly it arises in the adrenal medulla but it can rise in any chromaffin tissue of the sympathetic nervous system. It is also seen in patients with other endocrine neoplasm — for example, with hyperparathyroidism and medullary carcinoma of the thyroid. These syndromes of multiple endocrine neoplasia (MEN) are associated with a genetic abnormality in which there is a genetic mutation on chromosome 10 — the RET proto-oncogene. The symptoms of phaeochromocytoma, and its presentation, will depend largely on whether adrenaline or noradrenaline secretion predominates, although the tumours can produce many other active peptides. The disease should be considered in any patient with severe hypertension or hypertension presenting at an early age, or in an unusual fashion. The symptoms and signs can be paroxysmal and include sweating, anxiety and panic, tremor, headache, nausea and tachycardia. The patients may exhibit hyperglycaemia.

Phaeochromocytomata may be solitary tumours or multiple. They can be small or large, benign or malignant. CT or MRI scanning ought to localise the tumour(s) once the biochemical diagnosis has been made. Radio-labelled MIBG (metaiodobenzylguanidine) can also be used for identifying tumours, although it may take up to 72 h for useful images to be obtained.

Surgery is the treatment of choice. Removal of the tumour(s) will return the patient to normal. However, in

Table 14.1 Distribution of adrenergic receptors in selected tissues		
Structure	Receptors	Response
Blood vessels	α β_2	Constrict Dilate
Heart	β_1	Force and rate of contraction rise
Pancreas	α_2 β_2	Insulin decrease Glucagon increase
Skin	α	Sweating increase
Lungs	β_2	Bronchiolar dilatation
Gut	α_2 α_1	Decreased motility Increased sphincter tone

the ill-prepared patient the operative and perioperative morbidity and mortality may be high. Handling the tumour during surgery can cause very profound cardiovascular responses, as can anaesthesia itself — therefore the physiological responses of the tumour must be fully controlled before surgery is contemplated. It should be assumed that both α and β catecholamine activity is increased — and that both need to be controlled. It is the author's preference to have the patient fully α and β blocked prior to surgery, using phenoxybenzamine, an alpha-adrenergic antagonist, and propranolol. Hyperglycaemia, if not controlled by this preparation, requires insulin therapy. Postural hypotension produced by this regime may be a problem but is sometimes partially ameliorated by the use of compression hose to the legs. During the operation the tumour is handled as little as possible and the tumour's draining vein is ligated as early in the procedure as feasible.

Once the tumour(s) is/are extirpated, the effects of the preparation must not be forgotten. If the patient has been on insulin, hypoglycaemia may develop within a short space of time. The effects of full adrenergic blockade mean that the patient's intravascular compartment may expand very rapidly, and large transfusions of fluid including colloid will be needed in the course of an hour or two to compensate for this.

Malignant tumours may already have metastasised. Radiotherapy and chemotherapy can be used — but in the author's experience ^{131}I-labelled MIBG is also useful. Although anecdotal, one young patient with secondary disease at the time of removal of a large primary involving the left adrenal gland, spleen and greater curve of stomach is well and tumour free 14 years later after treatment of the secondaries with ^{131}I MIBG.

ENDOCRINE PANCREAS

The pancreas is a large organ lying retroperitoneally in the upper abdomen. The head of the pancreas lies in the concavity created by the C-shape of the duodenum, the body and tail extending laterally and rostrally towards the hilum of the spleen. Most of its blood supply comes from branches of the coeliac axis, although the inferior pancreaticoduodenal artery, derived from the superior mesenteric artery, supplies part of the head of the pancreas (the posterior lobe). Venous drainage is to the portal vein. The greatest part of the mass of pancreas is associated with its exocrine digestive function. However, the pancreas also has an endocrine function, with the production of insulin, glucagon and somatostatin. A pan-

creatic polypeptide is also recognised, but its function is unknown. The cells producing these agents are clustered together into islands scattered throughout the pancreas — the Islets of Langerhans. The bulk of the insulin- and glucagon-producing cells are contained within the body and tail of pancreas. Insulin is produced by the beta cells and glucagon by the alpha cells. Somatostatin is synthesised in the delta cells.

INSULIN

Insulin is cleaved from pro-insulin (which is itself cleaved from a larger molecule known as pre pro-insulin) via the rough endoplasmic reticulum of pancreatic β cells. The cleavage of pro-insulin produces two compounds: insulin and C-peptide. C-peptide has no identifiable function. Within the β cells insulin is stored in the secretory granules. Approximately 5 mg of insulin is stored in the normal adult in this way. Once into the circulation it has a short half-life of approximately 5 min. Insulin is unbound in the plasma. Insulin is released into the portal circulation, and about half of this will be removed by the liver. Insulin in the systemic circulation is predominantly broken down in the kidney. Patients with developing endstage diabetic nephropathy usually require less insulin than before the nephropathy developed.

Secretion

Glucose is the strongest and most important stimulus to insulin release. A rising blood sugar level is associated with a rise in circulating insulin. The circulating insulin is derived from two sources: the secretory granules release stored insulin and there is a release of newly produced insulin. Pro-insulin and C-peptide are also released. Diminishing blood sugar levels are associated with lower levels of insulin secretion, and below about 4 mmol/L there will be no glucose-stimulated insulin release. Carbohydrate is not the only stimulus to insulin release: there are many substances known to cause insulin secretion. Amino acids stimulate insulin release, as do some fatty acids. Vagal stimulation and β-adrenergic stimulation also increase insulin secretion. Various hormones will also release insulin, including gut hormones and secretin.

Actions and effects of insulin

Insulin receptors are found on cells in many tissues. They can be found on the cell membranes of fat, liver and muscle cells. Once insulin binds to the cell, glucose is taken up into the cell. The receptor–insulin complex on the cell membrane undergoes autophosphorylation which then stimulates glucose transporter systems permitting diffusion of glucose into the cell. It is known that the insulin–receptor complex becomes incorporated into the cell. Once inside the cell the complex is broken down; whether the insulin then remains active or is simply metabolised and broken down is not known.

It is also known that, in the presence of high insulin concentration, the number of receptors is reduced. Conversely, when insulin levels are low there is an upgrading of the number of cell-membrane receptors for insulin. This probably comes about as a result of the receptor–insulin complex internalisation which occurs — but the importance of this change in receptor concentration in modifying the effects of insulin, and thus modifying the metabolism of glucose in high or in low concentrations, can readily be understood.

Insulin is released in response to rising blood sugar levels, and its predominant action is to promote the cellular uptake of glucose. In liver and muscle, glucose is converted to glycogen. Liver stores of glycogen amount to about 100 g, and the muscle store of glycogen is approximately 400 g in the average adult male. Muscle glycogen is an immediate source of energy in exercise but it does not contribute to the maintenance of blood sugar levels. Liver glycogen is a major store of carbohydrate but is also readily depleted when glucose intake is inadequate, i.e. in states of fasting or vomiting.

Glycogen represents an immediately available store of energy, but within the body the major source of stored energy is fat, i.e. triglycerides. Insulin acts on fat cells in several ways: it increases glucose transport into the cells and thus increases triglyceride synthesis; it induces lipoprotein lipase activity which then acts to break down circulating chylomicrons to free fatty acids and glycerol — which in turn are taken up by fat cells and reconverted back again to triglycerides, and insulin also inhibits the breakdown of triglyceride within the adipocytes by inhibiting the action of lipolytic lipase.

Within muscle there is an additional effect of insulin independent of glucose metabolism, and this favours the uptake of amino acids into skeletal muscle and proteins.

Therefore insulin is strongly anabolic. It is also anti-catabolic by inhibiting glycogenolysis within the liver, and gluconeogenesis.

Another effect of insulin is on potassium. Insulin reduces extracellular K^+ levels; the intracellular shift of K^+ is substantial and significant. This property of insulin is used in situations where hyperkalaemia is a problem — for example, acute renal failure, shock and septicaemia — an infusion of insulin and glucose lowering the extracellular K^+ concentration. A low K^+ concentration inhibits insulin secretion — thus any condition, or drug

therapy, which results in a depleted K^+ may cause a deterioration in blood sugar control.

Insulin has another effect within the Islet of Langerhans. It has a direct inhibitory effect, i.e. it has a paracrine action on the glucagon-producing cell (the A cell), thus reducing glucagon secretion.

GLUCAGON

Glucagon is produced by the pancreatic A cell. It is a polypeptide molecule (of 29 amino acids) and is stored in the A cell prior to release into the circulation. Glucagon is found in several unbound forms in plasma. It has a circulation half-life of only a few minutes.

The most potent stimulus to glucagon release is hypoglycaemia. Glucagon is inhibited by high glucose levels in blood. However, glucagon, as well as insulin, is stimulated by amino acids. Thus the ratio of glucagon and insulin release after eating will depend on the food content of the meal.

As mentioned earlier, insulin has a direct effect on the glucagon-producing A cell of the Islet and glucagon is also inhibited by somatostatin produced by the Islet D cells. Many gut hormones stimulate glucagon: vagal stimulation and β-adrenergic sympathetic stimulation are also associated with increased glucagon release.

Effects of glucagon

In broad terms glucagon has the opposite effects of insulin. Its effects are probably confined to the liver. Glycolysis occurs with the production of glucose, and this action is probably responsible for the homeostatic maintenance of blood sugar in the normal individual between meals and with normal glycogen levels. It stimulates gluconeogenesis and the production of ketone bodies within the liver.

SOMATOSTATIN

Somatostatin is produced in the D cells of the pancreatic islets. It is also produced in the gut and found widely in brain tissue. The stimulus for its secretion follows very closely the same substances as for insulin. It inhibits growth hormone, delays gastric emptying and reduces gastrin secretion. It also reduces pancreatic exocrine secretions and has been used therapeutically to reduce the output of pancreatic fistulae.

GROWTH HORMONE

Before considering the homeostatic control of blood sugar, and the effects of insulin perturbations, it is useful to consider, briefly, the physiology of growth hormone. Growth hormone — also known as somatotropin — is produced in the anterior pituitary, and its secretion comes largely under the control of growth-hormone-releasing hormone produced by the hypothalamus and released into the hypothalamic–pituitary portal system. Growth hormone release is greatest when asleep — an effect seen most in children.

Growth hormone release is modified by a large range of agents in addition to GRH. It is inhibited by somatostatin, fatty acids, amino acids and glucose. Hypoglycaemia stimulates growth hormone release.

Growth hormone stimulates the production of insulin-like growth factor (IGF-1) in the liver and in other tissues, including cartilage, fat and muscle. This indirect effect of growth hormone is associated with bone growth, protein synthesis and the production of free fatty acids.

Growth hormone also has a direct effect: on fat it is lipolytic, producing free fatty acids, and in muscle it has an anti-insulin effect evidenced by gluconeogenesis. In this way growth hormone may be diabetogenic: patients with excess growth hormone production will have an abnormal response to glucose, and 10% or more will be diabetic.

A failure of growth hormone can be familial, due to pituitary causes or due to hypothalamic causes. In children the result is dwarfism.

An excess of growth hormone causes gigantism in children, with particular emphasis on limb growth due to the effects on the cartilaginous epiphyses. In adults an excess of growth hormone is associated with local bone growth, particularly in the skull and mandible, and soft tissue proliferation with a characteristic increase in hand and finger size (sometimes described as a shovel-like hand) and increase in foot size. The skin is thickened and coarse. Carpal tunnel compression of the median nerve may occur and, secondary to the bone changes, hypercalcaemia and hypercalciuria may be present — the patient presenting with renal calculi. There can be many metabolic changes. The commonest is impairment of glucose metabolism and hyperinsulinism, which have already been referred to.

In the normal individual, growth hormone is suppressed by rising glucose levels. Single one-off measurements of growth hormone may, in the presence of a 'typical picture' of acromegaly, be enough to suggest the diagnosis of acromegaly; however, growth hormone may be physiologically high in a variety of other conditions, including stress, and, in these situations, suppressible by glucose. In addition there is, even in acromegaly, a variation in hormone output. However, in acromegaly, the output of growth hormone will always remain elevated in the presence of a high sugar level. As a result the glucose suppression test has emerged as a specific test for acromegaly.

Most cases of acromegaly are due to a pituitary tumour, and the presentation and diagnosis of such lesions is discussed elsewhere in this chapter. Excess growth hormone is sometimes seen from ectopic sites, such as tumour of the lung, pancreas (islet cells) and the gut, i.e. carcinoid.

Now it is appropriate to consider glucose homeostasis and situations which might result in disturbances of glucose metabolism.

CONDITIONS RESULTING IN LOW BLOOD SUGAR LEVELS

Commonly these are associated with excessive insulin concentration. They include an inappropriate level of insulin administered by the diabetic patient (including deliberate overdosage) and excessive insulin production, i.e. an insulinoma (tumour of β cells of pancreatic islets). Hypoglycaemia, with hyperinsulinism, may also be seen with oral hypoglycaemic agents.

Much less commonly, hypoglycaemia may be seen in patients with severe liver disease, high alcohol intake in someone not eating, and also those indulging in strenuous exercise. The current popularity of 'fun runs' of marathon or half-marathon length can result in depletion of glycogen reserves and hypoglycaemia. Runners become uncoordinated, confused and even unconscious. Exercise-induced hypoglycaemia in the diabetic on insulin treatment can be of very rapid onset, and may be very profound. It is dangerous. In the normal individual, insulin secretion falls with lowered blood sugar levels but in the insulin dependent diabetic there will be continued absorption of the injected insulin as the blood sugar level declines with resulting more severe hypoglycaemia.

A reactive hypoglycaemia after gastric drainage procedures is well recognised and is of importance in surgical practice. The stomach drains rapidly after a meal, presenting the small bowel with a high carbohydrate load: rapid absorption of carbohydrate occurs and high levels of insulin are produced, with resulting hypoglycaemia. This problem is known as 'dumping'.

A low blood sugar level presents with similar symptoms regardless of the cause, and these are the consequences of the low sugar levels on neurological tissue.

As blood sugar levels decline, symptoms develop. The first are related to activation of autonomic neurotransmitters: vagal stimulation can be associated with hunger or nausea; adrenergic stimulation with anxiety, sweating and palpitations. The diabetic patient with an intact autonomic nervous system relies on these early symptoms to warn of developing hypoglycaemia. A number of diabetic patients develop hypertension as part of the disease; the wisdom — or otherwise — of presenting adrenergic blocking agents to manage the high blood pressure must be very carefully considered. There should be special caution with the β-adrenergic blockers. If the blood sugar levels fall further, the individual becomes confused, lethargic and uncoordinated, eventually losing consciousness.

In the normal individual, insulin secretion switches off as blood sugar levels fall, and the catecholamine secretion increases. The overall effect is to increase glucose by reduction of glycogen and increase free fatty acid availability — all increasing available energy — and reducing muscle uptake of glucose.

The adrenergic effect is mainly β-adrenergic and it is the same mechanism which stimulates glucagon secretion. Glucagon is also secreted as a result of the direct effect of a low blood sugar level on the pancreatic A cells. Relatives of diabetic patients prone to hypoglycaemia should have glucagon available and know when and how to administer it.

The adrenergic response also results in raised ACTH production; thus cortisol production increases, with gluconeogenesis occurring. Growth hormone secretion rises as a direct result of hypoglycaemia, and this, too, favours an increase in blood sugar levels.

The management of hypoglycaemia is urgent. Patients presenting to hospital unconscious should have a blood sugar estimation performed. This is especially important when there is no history of trauma. Patients with intermittent attacks of impaired consciousness — for example, patients alleged to have 'temporal lobe epilepsy' — should have glucose estimations done during an attack. They may have an insulinoma. If the patient is conscious, then oral glucose may be given; if unconscious, intravenous glucose should be given, i.e. 50 mL of 50% dextrose should be given over 2 to 3 min. The unconscious diabetic at home should be given glucagon by a family member if it is feasible to do so. Failure to treat severe hypoglycaemia urgently may result in death or permanent brain damage.

CONDITIONS ASSOCIATED WITH HIGH BLOOD SUGAR LEVELS

The commonest of these by far is diabetes mellitus, but there are others, including Cushing's syndrome, which may be resulting from endogenous or exogenous (i.e. corticosteroid treatment) causes, acromegaly, phaeochromocytoma and glucagon-producing tumours. Post-pancreatectomy patients may develop diabetes, and some drugs may also be associated with impaired glucose homeostasis, for example thiazide diuretics.

A full discussion of the pathophysiology of diabetes mellitus is not appropriate here; a full account can be gained in any medical textbook. However, it is useful to consider the physiological consequences of high blood sugar levels and the effect of impaired glucose metabolism on metabolism as a whole.

When there is no insulin it must now be obvious to the reader that the patient will be catabolic. There will be no cellular uptake of sugar, there will be no storage of glycogen, and the patient will be hyperglycaemic. Any stored glycogen will be broken down and amino acids will be utilised as an energy source by gluconeogenesis and there will be lipolysis with the production of an acidosis and ketone bodies. There will be an osmotic diuresis secondary to the hyperglycaemia, and there will be a net loss of K^+ to the body. There is profound weight loss.

Type I diabetes — insulin-dependent diabetes mellitus — is more often seen in children and younger adults. It can present with a ketoacidotic coma — although there will almost always be a longer period of a few weeks, or a month or two, when the patient has polyuria, polydipsia, weight loss, tiredness and during which there may be recurring opportunistic infections of the skin (staphylococci and yeast especially) arising as a direct result of high tissue sugar levels. This form of diabetes may be autoimmune: it may be genetically linked, with a number of HLA antigens being associated with it. It appears probable that, in susceptible individuals, a viral infection may result in diabetes developing. Some viruses, i.e. Coxsackie and mumps, which are known to be β cell toxic, may initiate the disease.

Type II diabetes — non-insulin-dependent diabetes mellitus — is much commoner than Type I. It is usually associated with older people, although its presentation in teenagers and young adults is also recognised. The vast majority of patients are obese, have an insensitivity to insulin and overfeed. When the overeating is corrected the levels of insulin may fall; the number of insulin receptors will thus return towards normal and the insulin sensitivity will improve. Non-obese Type II diabetics will usually respond to dietary control also, although all Type II diabetics will respond to oral hypoglycaemic agents.

Treatment of the diabetes will depend upon the type: treatment will be with insulin, oral hypoglycaemic agents, or diet alone. However, regardless of the type of diabetes from which the patient is suffering, there will be an impact on the management of the patient for surgery.

The diabetic patient can present a challenge to the surgeon in several ways. The disease itself — or its control / lack of control — can be a problem; the management of diabetes over the perioperative period may be the challenge; the surgery may be for one of the complications of the disease.

In the preoperative assessment of the diabetic patient the nature of the surgery will influence what can or must be done. It is clear that diabetic patients must be optimally controlled over the period of surgery. Unfortunately, some diabetic patients may not have been optimally controlled prior to presentation with a surgical problem and may be at enhanced risk. Even the well-controlled diabetic will not be as well controlled as the non-diabetic. Insulin, when given, is not given to the portal circulation but to the systemic circulation (even those patients who have had pancreatic transplants for diabetes mellitus will never achieve ideal blood sugar control, for this insulin will also be released to the systemic circulation). It is inevitable, therefore, that diabetic patients will all be susceptible to disorders of metabolism, particularly intermediary metabolism and may, therefore, suffer some of the consequences such as atherosclerotic vascular disease, microangiopathies and neuropathy, renal disease and ischaemic heart disease.

Clearly a patient presenting for a minor procedure under local anaesthetic will need less investigation than the patient presenting for major elective surgery. In the latter case a thorough clinical examination and specific investigations to check cardiac function, i.e. ECG and echocardiography, and renal function, i.e. check for proteinuria and estimations of blood urea, creatinine and electrolytes with a creatinine clearance or inulin clearance if renal function is thought to be impaired. A measurement of overall diabetic control can be achieved by assessing the amount of sugar incorporation into the red cells — the glycosylated haemoglobin. A random one-off blood sugar estimation is useless in determining overall control, for even the well-controlled diabetic will show figures varying from as low as 3–4 mmol/L to 15 mmol/L of blood glucose.

For surgical procedures, when there is major trauma to the patient, there is an inevitable glucocorticoid and catecholamine response, and these responses will produce substantial changes in blood sugar levels even in non-diabetic patients. It is critically important to anticipate problems in the diabetic, and at the time of surgery frequent estimations of blood sugar is imperative. The aim should be to keep the blood glucose level in the range 4–10 mmol/L. Hypoglycaemia must be avoided. Hyperglycaemia must be avoided also — the risks to the

patient of ketoacidosis, hypokalaemia and dehydration are great.

During major surgery, most patients, irrespective of their diabetes type, will require management with insulin. Intravenous administration of insulin, glucose and potassium will be needed, the amount of insulin given being determined by the blood glucose levels measured at frequent intervals in the peri- and postoperative periods. In general the frequency of blood glucose measurements should be hourly (or more often) during theatre, two hourly in the early postoperative period, and then reduced as feeding commences until the patient is on normal diet and the usual insulin dose or other diabetic treatment is being administered.

A patient undergoing minor surgery under local anaesthetic needs no modification of his or her regular treatment but the surgery should be deferred if it is clear that the patient is not adequately controlled.

The final major way in which the diabetic patient presents to the surgeon is for treatment of the complications of the disease — particularly the chronic complications. Complications can occur irrespective of the type of diabetes, and by the time a patient presents with one or other problem it is more than likely that others will coexist. A list of the commoner complications is found in Box 14.5.

The influence of glycaemic control on the development of complications is less controversial now than it used to be. It is almost certain that better blood sugar control is, overall, going to lead to fewer complications than when the control is poor. However, diabetes is such a long term chronic disease that the full influence of good blood sugar control may not be fully evident for some time yet. It is only in recent years that more intensive monitoring of blood sugar on a domiciliary basis by the patient has been widely available, and it is also only relatively recently that reliable glycosylated Hb estimations have been feasible. It is only when these factors have been fully and widely available for 20 to 30 years that the true impact of good glycaemic control will become apparent. Nevertheless, the signs are encouraging. One group of patients has been intensively studied — this is the group with diabetic nephropathy receiving a transplant of the kidney and the pancreas. When successful, pancreatic transplantation achieves very good blood sugar control — although it is never completely normal, as the islets contained within the transplant drain to the peripheral circulation. These patients are in a 'tough group' to assess, for by the time they develop end-stage renal failure they are likely to have developed many other related clinical problems. Nevertheless, there is evidence

Box 14.5 Some of the commoner long term complications of diabetes mellitus

- cardiovascular disease
  — macrovascular
  — microvascular
  — cardiac
- nephropathy
- neurological disease
  — autonomic neuropathy
    — stomach and gut
    — vascular/postural hypotension
    — impotence
    — bladder
  — peripheral neuropathy
    – distal sensory
    – motor neuropathy
    – mono neuropathies
- skin/subcutaneous tissues
  — necrobiosis lipoidica diabeticorum
  — infections, i.e. candida,
  — otitis externa
  — ischaemia
- bones and joints
  — neuropathic joints
  — diabetic cheiroarthropathy
- eye
  — retinopathy
  — cataracts

now emerging that the successful pancreatic transplant is beneficial to the patient in terms of slowing down, arresting, or even improving the developing complications. This at least strengthens the view that good glycaemic control is likely to result in fewer long term complications.

The complications listed in Box 14.5 embrace many surgical specialties, and most surgeons will inevitably be called upon to treat them. In some areas great strides have already been made — the intensive monitoring by photography of the retina in diabetes, and early intervention by the ophthalmologist to treat the proliferative retinopathy has had a great impact on preventing blindness. In other areas, progress is much slower. Some of the complications may have common aetiologies. For example, microvascular disease may lead to skin ischaemia but it may also lead to neuropathy with the small nutrient vessels to the nerves becoming diseased, resulting in infarction of the nerve. However, whatever the complication the surgeon may be faced with, he must remember that diabetes

is a systemic disorder and that the patient may well have other, often occult, complications.

A note on the drug treatment of diabetes mellitus

Insulin is used for all Type I diabetics and also in those Type II diabetics who are poorly controlled on oral hypoglycaemic agents. All diabetic patients require an adequate carbohydrate intake: strict carbohydrate restriction is neither appropriate nor required and in any case can readily lead to disorders of lipid metabolism. Nevertheless the diabetic patient will need to take a reasonably stable carbohydrate diet in order to make some sense of his/her insulin management. A typical adult sedentary worker may have a carbohydrate baseline intake of:

- breakfast   30 g
- morning snack   10 g
- lunch   30 g
- afternoon snack 10 g
- evening meal   40 g
- bedtime snack   20 g.

Available insulin is derived either from pork/beef sources, or is synthetic human insulin produced by recombinant DNA technology. It is available in short-, medium- or long-acting forms and is injected subcutaneously. Most short-acting insulins have a duration of peak activity lasting about 2 h, usually with an onset about 2 h after injection. Long-acting insulin will have peak activity commencing 6–8 h after injection and lasting up to 12–16 h.

The patient will need to be able to deal with the postprandial surges in sugar and also have a background of insulin availability. Therefore patients will normally be on a combination of short-acting and long-acting insulins. For some a single daily injection of a combination of insulins may be used — especially in the elderly patient who may not be able to cope with more frequent injections. This is not ideal, and most diabetics will be taking multiple injections of insulin per day. This could be in the form of twice daily injections of a combination of short and medium duration insulins — but in these patients there is a need for some discipline over meal times and the content of the meal.

For an active diabetic in employment a better regime may be to take a long-acting insulin at bedtime, and short-acting insulin before each meal. The average normal adult produces about 50 units of insulin per day, and the average normal adult diabetic patient will be taking 50 to 60 units per day. Thus the diabetic may take 10 units of short-acting insulin before each main meal and 30 units of long-acting insulin at night. This gives the patient greater flexibility and he/she soon learns how to adjust the short-acting insulin dose to suit the needs of the meal. The reusable pen has assisted the patient enormously to achieve this greater flexibility. A cartridge of short-acting insulin is loaded to the pen and the patient then has several days' supply in his pocket.

Oral hypoglycaemic agents (OHA)

There are two main groups: the sulphonylureas and the biguanides. As with Type I diabetes, those needing OHAs must also have a discipline to their diet.

The sulphonylureas act by stimulating insulin secretion from the β cells of the pancreas. The biguanides, on the other hand, do not affect insulin secretion but appear to block gluconeogenesis, increase glycogen storage in muscle and reduce carbohydrate absorption from the gut. Other oral agents include drugs which inhibit α-glucosidase (thus reducing the breakdown of carbohydrate to monosaccharides, with consequent reduced absorption in the gut) and so-called insulin action enhancers. It is important to remember that patients taking oral hypoglycaemics can suffer from hypoglycaemic episodes.

PITUITARY AND HYPOTHALAMUS

The pituitary gland lies within the cranial cavity in a bony fossa known as the hypophyseal fossa. There are two main parts: the anterior pituitary ('adenohypophysis'), which is developed from the oral cavity, and the posterior pituitary ('neurohypophysis'), which is developed from neural tissue, i.e. a downward extension of the hypothalamus. (There is a tiny intermediate 'lobe' producing melanocyte-stimulating hormone.)

During development, the anterior pituitary develops an extensive blood communication with the hypothalamus and the posterior pituitary: the hypothalamo–hypophyseal portal system. Various trophic hormones, for example TRH and CRH, are released in response to neural stimuli and drain into the portal system from the hypothalamus to the anterior pituitary with resulting stimulation of TSH and ACTH secretion. The posterior pituitary secretions — oxytocin and vasopressin — are synthesised in hypothalamic nuclei, pass down the axons of the neurohypophyseal tract, and are released at the nerve endings in the posterior pituitary (Fig. 14.11).

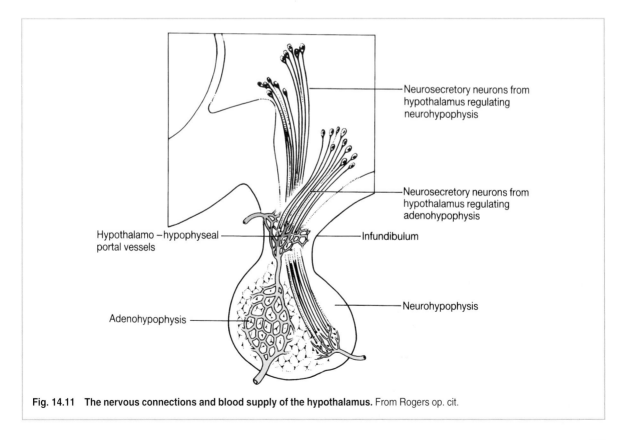

Fig. 14.11   The nervous connections and blood supply of the hypothalamus. From Rogers op. cit.

The hypothalamus not only has this close and inter-related connection with the pituitary gland, it has extensive connections with other parts of the brain, including the brainstem, higher centres, cerebral cortex and spinal cord. Through these connections the hypothalamus can receive and transmit 'information' which allows for the coordination of many autonomic and visceral functions. The neuroendocrine control of many hormones is a function of the hypothalamus (e.g. growth hormone, TSH, ACTH, vasopressin, oxytocin). Temperature regulation is mediated by the hypothalamus. The hypothalamus contains osmoreceptors, satiety and hunger centres, and cells sensitive to glucose levels — all giving the hypothalamus an important role in thirst and feeding responses. Other functions attributed to the hypothalamus include responses to fear, the regulation of rage, and an influence on sexual behaviour.

PITUITARY GLAND HORMONES

The anterior pituitary has six main hormones: these are ACTH, TSH, GH (growth hormone), prolactin (PRL), luteinising hormone (LH) and follicle-stimulating hormone (FSH). The posterior pituitary secretes oxytocin and vasopressin (ADH). Of the anterior pituitary hormones, a number are discussed elsewhere in this chapter. Prolactin is a hormone associated with lactation: excess of the hormone can be associated with galactorrhoea — a persistent and troublesome discharge from the breast. This excess can be due to a tumour — prolactinoma — hence, in a patient with galactorrhoea a prolactin level should be obtained.

LH and FSH have functions in both the male and female. In the female, LH stimulates ovarian oestrogen and progesterone, and it is responsible for ovulation. FSH is responsible for the development of the follicle. In the male, LH stimulates testosterone production. Testicular growth is a function of FSH. Both LH and FSH are associated with the maturation of spermatozoa.

If there is an excess, or deficiency, of a pituitary hormone the evidence for disease will depend upon the hormone affected. In the posterior pituitary–hypothalamic axis, vasopressin and oxytocin are the hormones involved. When there is damage to the posterior pituitary, there is reduced vasopressin (ADH-antidiuretic hormone) release with resulting inability of the renal tubules to conserve water. Diabetes insipidus results — with polyuria, polydipsia and a raised haematocrit due to haemoconcentration.

Disturbed function of the anterior pituitary–hypothalamic axis will produce changes according to the system involved. For example an ACTH-producing lesion will result in excess cortisol production but inhibited CRH levels (from hypothalamus). A failure of ACTH will result in Addison's disease. There is a low blood cortisol and a high blood CRH level. A knowledge of the regulating system for each hormone cascade enables logical investigation of the site of the disease to be established. The pituitary lies within the hypophyseal fossa, the walls and floor of which are bony: the roof is soft — the diaphragma sellae (after sella turcica, the old name for the hypophyseal fossa) — through which the infundibulum (hypophyseal stalk) emerges linking the pituitary gland to the hypothalamus (Fig. 14.12). The infundibulum lies immediately behind the optic chiasm. Any tumour of the pituitary will, of necessity, cause pressure through the diaphragma sellae in the optic chiasm. Before this happens, pressure may have built up within the hypophyseal fossa as a result of the tumour. Thus patients with a tumour of the pituitary may present in many ways. If it is producing a hormone, then there may be symptoms of excess. The tumour may grow and, as a result of either increasing pressure, or infiltration, other hormone production may fail. Finally, upward pressure, or infiltration, may cause visual disturbances as the optic chiasma becomes affected. The final picture produced by a pituitary tumour can be very complex.

Treatment of the tumours may be surgical, via the transsphenoidal route, but subsequently hypopituitarism may result and the patient need multiple endocrine replacement.

GYNAECOMASTIA

It is worth considering this common condition briefly, for most trainee surgeons will be confronted with it. It is common, and usually self limiting, in neonatal children and pubertal boys. However, it can occur also at any time in adult life. It is generally held to be due either to an excess of oestrogen, an inadequate androgen concentration (or androgen insensitivity), or an imbalance of the two. A huge range of drugs is associated with it, including antiulcer drugs, e.g. cimetidine; cardiovascular drugs, e.g. digoxin; ACE-inhibitors; Ca^{2+}-channel blockers and spironolactone; sedatives and tricyclic drugs; antiepileptics and many more. It can also be associated with testicular tumours (human chorionic gonadotrophic (hCG)-producing tumour), hyperprolactinaemia, cirrhosis (with failure of oestrogen breakdown) and thyrotoxicosis. However, many cases never reveal an underlying cause. When there is no obvious cause for the gynaecomastia, an endocrine screen should be performed; this might include HCG, LH, prolactin, testosterone, oestradiol and thyroxine/TSH.

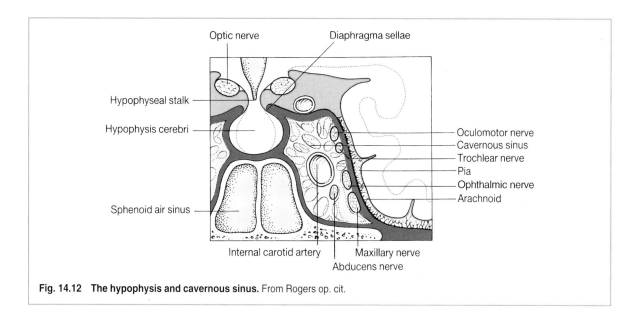

Fig. 14.12 The hypophysis and cavernous sinus. From Rogers op. cit.

Pubertal gynaecomastia may resolve, although many cases persist. Some boys respond to tamoxifen. If there is no resolution, surgery may be considered for these patients, and any other with established gynaecomastia, assuming there is no other aetiology for the condition.

15

Breast

Clive R G Quick

ANATOMY

'The breasts from their prominence, the colour of their skin, and the red colour of the nipples, by which they are surmounted, add great beauty to the female form' (Sir Astley Paston Cooper, On the anatomy of the breast, 1840).

DEVELOPMENT AND STRUCTURE

Breasts are skin appendages arising from ectodermally derived mammary ridges in the embryo. Accessory nipples, sometimes with underlying breast tissue, can be found along a line beneath the breast, and these occasionally function during lactation. The breast is a bilateral structure which is vestigial in the male and fully formed in the adult female; this account largely refers to the female breast. It is a domed structure, variable in size, shape and pendulousness, overlying approximately the third to the seventh ribs on the anterolateral part of the chest wall. It lies predominantly on the pectoralis major muscle, extending over part of the serratus anterior laterally, the external oblique inferolaterally, the rectus sheath inferomedially and the costal cartilages medially and superiorly. The nipple projects forwards and outwards to a variable degree but may be congenitally inverted. In the female, the function of the breast is to supply milk by secretion to nourish the infant soon after it begins to breathe.

The breast is essentially a conglomerate gland consisting of 6–12 branching glands which radiate towards the nipple. The secretions also drain centripetally towards the nipple. The ducts of the various gland units are interwoven and intermixed with each other. The glandular structure is supported by a collagenous and inelastic membrane which penetrates the surface of the gland and sends fibres into all its interstices, uniting the glandules and ducts to each other. This was formerly known as the 'fascia mammae' and, along with the ligaments of Astley Cooper, forms the suspensory mechanism for the breast by its attachment to the periosteum of the ribs and the skin anteriorly. The anterior part of the fascia mammae forms a fibrous covering but not a true capsule for the breast. It sends two sets of fibrous processes from its two surfaces. On its deep surface, the fascia spreads over the anterior of the gland, supporting numerous folds of glandular tissue, penetrates the substance of the organ, and everywhere connects the portions of the gland to each other. It extends to the nipple, where it forms a firm support for the ducts. On its superficial surface, the 'ligamenta suspensoria' are large, strong and numerous and are inserted into the posterior surface of the skin. The projections spread out to form a white, firm irregular surface of folds between the skin and the gland (Fig. 15.1).

Adipose tissue forms the remainder of the breast tissue, and here the arteries, veins, lymphatics and nerves run and are distributed throughout the structure. The areola is a pigmented area of thin skin containing numerous sebaceous glands as well as sweat glands. A number of small swellings or *Montgomery's tubercles* are visible around the areola, and these are overly enlarged sebaceous glands. The areola is surmounted by the nipple, which contains the terminations of milk ducts, blood vessels and nerves united by fibrous and cellular tissue. There are many strands of smooth muscle beneath the areola and nipple, which contract when stimulated by touch or cold, making the nipple more protuberant for ease of suckling. The relative predominance of each of the main structural elements of the breast changes with age, pregnancy and hormonal status and, along with that, the size and shape of an individual's breasts.

Glandular structure

The breast consists of 6–12 branching glands radiating from the nipple and extending outwards to unequal lengths (Fig. 15.2); this is important to remember when attempting to achieve a complete mastectomy. The

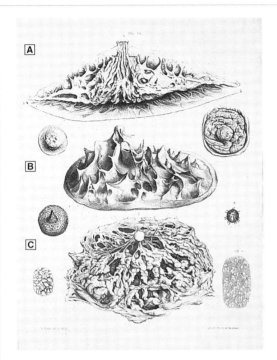

Fig. 15.1   The suspensory mechanism of the breast.
[A] A vertical section through the breast demonstrating the fanning out of the ligaments into the skin ('ligaments of Astley Cooper'). On the deep surface of the breast, fibrous processes from the ligamenta pass into the aponeurosis over pectoralis major. Thus the breast is slung between pectoral fascia and skin by a complex architecture of fibrous tissue. [B] The fibrous ligamenta suspensoria with glandular tissue removed. [C] The glandular structure of the breast which is supported by the ligamenta suspensoria. Individual ducts can be seen converging on the nipple. (Reproduced by kind permission of the President and Council of the Royal College of Surgeons of England.)

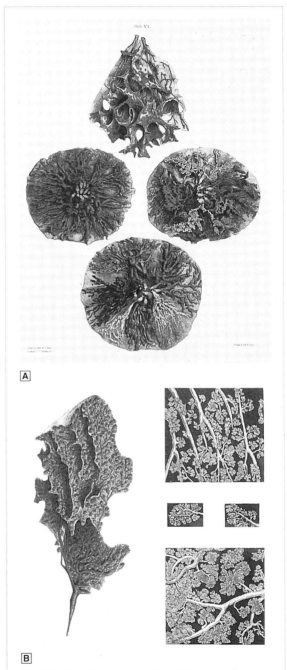

Fig. 15.2   The glandular structure of the breast. The breast consists of 6–12 branching glands radiating from the periphery towards the nipple. [A] In this case 9 glands are shown. In most of the breast, there is only a single gland, but in certain parts, ducts lie two deep. [B] On a larger scale, the arborescent structure of the glandules is evident.
(Reproduced by kind permission of the President and Council of the Royal College of Surgeons of England.)

ducts of individual glands do not communicate with each other. The thickness of glandular tissue varies greatly in different parts, with the lateral and inferior margins very dense and compact compared with the superior and medial parts. In the superolateral quadrant, the number of ducts and glandules is greater than elsewhere and several glands lie one on top of one other. In other parts, the glands are usually of single thickness. Medially, the disc is very irregular in outline, and superolaterally the edge of the breast disc is turned up like a hem. The oft described 'axillary tail' is not a separate part of the gland but merely an extension of the distal part of the superolateral gland units towards the axilla.

This structure and the age and hormonal status of the patient affects its palpation characteristics. At puberty, the breast texture is dense, compact, smooth and homogeneous. During lactation, the glands separate into separate small bodies with indentations around them, i.e. become lobulated. This also occurs in childless women towards the menopause. This lobulation must be distinguished from 'lumps', particularly malignancy, and this may require the assistance of imaging and biopsy. Beyond the menopause, the lobulation becomes less as a result of atrophy of the glandular structure. During pregnancy, the glandular elements become hypertrophied, the blood supply increases and the breasts become full, heavy, tense and often painful.

Blood supply

The blood supply of the breast arises from the axillary artery, via its lateral thoracic and acromiothoracic branches, and the internal mammary via its perforating branches, which pierce the first to fourth intercostal spaces then traverse the pectoralis major muscle to reach the breast along its medial edge. Internal mammary branches ramify from the pectoral surface of the breast to meet the axillary branches from the superficial surface.

The venous drainage corresponds to the arterial supply. There is a venous circle beneath the areola which drains towards the axillary vein in the hypodermis overlying the breast. Other veins drain via the second and third intercostal spaces towards the internal mammary vein.

Lymphatic drainage

The lymphatics of the nipple (Fig. 15.3) are large and numerous and drain along the surface of the breast towards the cribriform axillary fascia, and penetrate the fascia to reach the lymph nodes. From the medial part of the breast, lymphatics drain towards internal mammary nodes via the second and third intercostal spaces. From most of the breast, lymph drains into lymphatics passing superficially through the fat on the surface of the gland towards the axilla. The majority of lymph from the breast first enters a node near the first rib, descending from there towards axillary nodes at the third/fourth rib level, then ascending towards nodes near the second rib. From there, efferent lymphatics join a plexus around the axillary vein then enter nodes overlying the first rib. From here, efferents form a lymphatic trunk lying close to the inner part of the axillary vein. On the right, this passes between the first rib and the clavicle to join the junction of the internal jugular and subclavian vein along with lymphatics draining the right arm and right side of the neck. On the left, a similar trunk joins the jugular/subclavian vein confluence along with the thoracic (lymphatic)

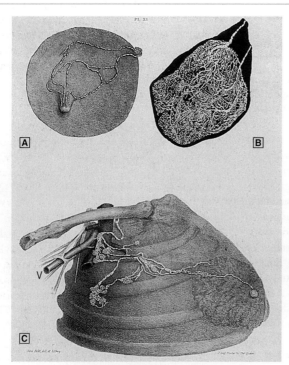

Fig. 15.3 The lymphatic drainage of the breast.
[A] The lymphatics of the nipple are large and numerous and drain along the surface of the breast beneath the skin. [B] The deeper lymphatics of the breast interconnect and drain chiefly into main channels directed towards the axilla. [C] Some lymph is routed inferiorly before progressing towards the axilla. The main lymph nodes lie around the axillary vein (V). (Reproduced by kind permission of the President and Council of the Royal College of Surgeons of England.)

duct. Other lymphatic channels take a different route from the lower axillary nodes, passing behind the axillary artery, vein and nerve to join the brachial lymphatic channel. This may explain the occasional case of breast cancer where higher axillary nodes are involved but lower ones are not — so called 'skip' node involvement. This has implications for determining axillary node status if sampling rather than clearance is performed.

In treating breast cancer, the axillary node status is one of the most important prognostic indicators, as well as helping determine the most appropriate therapy. Sampling of the lowest axillary nodes can be useful but is unreliable in determining nodal involvement. Most surgeons therefore prefer to remove more axillary nodes. 'Axillary clearance' implies total clearance of axillary nodes and is difficult and hazardous to achieve. Current practice involves standard operations known as Level I, II and III dissections. Level I dissection involves removing nodes in the axillary tail (if present) and clearing the axillary vein of nodes superficial to pectoralis minor muscle. Level II includes nodes deep to pectoralis minor and Level III clears nodes up to the apex of the axilla. About 4–8 nodes are usually retrieved at Level I, 10–15 at Level II and up to 30 at Level III. With Level I dissection, there is about a 25% chance of higher 'skip node' involvement; with Level II this falls to about 3%.

Nerves

The sensory and sympathetic nerves are derived from the anterior and lateral cutaneous branches of the fourth, fifth and sixth thoracic nerves. Branches proceed alongside the arteries to the nipple. The nipple is supplied by a dense nerve plexus with various types of nerve endings, including free nerve endings which play a part in signalling suckling to the hypothalamus.

PHYSIOLOGY

At all stages of female life, the breast is under hormonal control. Oestrogen leads to ductal elongation and branching as well as fat deposition; progesterone governs alveolar formation and prepares the breast for lactation. During pregnancy, prolactin (along with oestrogen and progesterone) develops the alveoli for secretion and, after parturition, (along with cortisone) triggers milk production and release.

FETAL AND NEONATAL

Breast development is identical in both sexes during fetal life and is not influenced by sex hormones until the seventh intrauterine month. Epithelially derived precursor tissue resembling sweat glands passes through a branching stage to form 15–25 epithelial strips which later canalise to form ducts. This primitive duct system starts peripherally and grows towards the nipple. After the seventh month, the duct system becomes arranged into lobules with end-vesicle formation under the prime influence of maternal progesterone. After birth, the abrupt withdrawal of female sex steroids allows endogenous prolactin to act directly on the alveolar epithelium, resulting in colostrum production. This colostrum or 'witches milk' can be expressed from the breasts of both sexes in about 90% of newborn infants. After birth, the breast tissue regresses because of a lack of sex steroids. This is manifest as a loss of end vesicles and the breasts then remain dormant until puberty.

PUBERTY

In the female at puberty, the breast tissue is again exposed to increasing levels of sex steroids. Early menstrual cycles are anovulatory, so that oestrogens are produced without progesterone. The effects of oestrogen (predominantly oestradiol) are to promote breast development, with branching and elongation of existing breast structures. There are also obvious increases in the supporting mesenchymal elements and in fat deposition. In ovulatory cycles, progesterone is secreted by the corpus luteum, promoting development of the lobular-alveolar structures, and the breast gradually develops its mature size and shape.

MENSTRUAL CYCLE

Between menarche and the menopause, there are monthly cyclical changes in ovarian hormone production, ostensibly in preparation for pregnancy. During the proliferative phase of the cycle, oestrogens are secreted by the maturing Graafian follicle, promoting breast development with duct proliferation and budding and causing a cyclical increase in breast size of 15–30 mL. This results from increased blood flow, lobular oedema, thickening of the basement membrane, and especially enlargement of the alveolar diameter and the appearance of secretions. Failure of ovular implantation, i.e. an unsuccessful cycle, is marked by rapidly falling levels of sex steroid production by the corpus luteum. This liberates the hormonal inhibition of prolactin, sometimes promoting a little milk production in the premenstrual phase. After each menstruation, regressive changes occur, with shrinkage of the lobular-alveolar units.

PREGNANCY

During pregnancy, there is intense stimulation of development and differentiation of breast tissue under the influence of sex steroids (luteal and placental), as well as prolactin, human placental lactogen (HPL, a growth-hormone-like substance) and human chorionic gonadotrophin. The relative importance of each phase is different in the three trimesters of pregnancy.

First trimester There is marked ductular sprouting and elongation which far exceeds that seen in the menstrual cycle. Noticeable breast enlargement is seen from around the sixth week of pregnancy, with venous engorgement in the overlying skin and a sensation of breast heaviness. The nipple and areola becomes more pigmented and the areola enlarges.

Second trimester Progesterone levels rise, inhibiting ductular sprouting and promoting development of the lobular units. The lobular alveolar epithelium becomes single layered in preparation for secretion, and colostrum, which contains little fat, accumulates. Progesterone also promotes growth in the mesenchymal supporting tissues and a massive increase in blood supply. From mid-pregnancy, the proliferative phase decreases and the differentiation of existing structures progresses in anticipation of secretory function.

Third trimester Breast size increases dramatically as a result of dilatation of existing alveoli with colostrum. The average increase in weight of each breast is 350 g.

LACTATION

Milk production is a complex process under the hormonal control of the hypothalamus, anterior pituitary, ovary, placenta and adrenals. Periodic release of milk is under the control of the posterior pituitary.

Prolactin or lactogen is the most powerful hormone responsible for milk production, but the secondary actions of cortisol, insulin and growth hormone are also required. Prolactin is produced in the anterior pituitary and is similar in structure to growth hormone. During pregnancy, the high oestrogen levels inhibit the development of prolactin receptors on the mammary alveoli. After birth, this inhibitory effect is removed. Prolactin levels return to near normal, but suckling produces periodic surges of prolactin release from the anterior pituitary. Suckling can maintain lactation indefinitely.

For the first few days after birth, colostrum is secreted, later replaced by mature human milk with its high content of lactose and fat. Colostrum is a thick yellow substance which differs from mature milk in containing a high protein content in the form of lactoglobulin. IgG is secreted into the colostrum and is absorbed intact by the newborn intestinal tract, although its role in transmitting immunity is not clear.

Milk letdown

Milk cannot be produced by suction alone. A complex neurohumoral mechanism exists whereby suckling or tactile stimulation of the nipple is transmitted to the hypothalamus via spinal reflexes and results in the release of oxytocin from the posterior pituitary. Oxytocin causes contraction of myoepithelial cells surrounding the breast alveoli, moving milk into the major ducts. This is known as *milk letdown*. Emotional factors such as pain and anxiety can inhibit this reflex and result in failure to eject milk. When suckling stops, milk letdown ceases. Accumulation of milk probably then causes reduced secretory activity. Prolactin levels are not stimulated by suckling, and the duct system involutes to its prepartum state. The increased fat and connective tissue within the breast often remain, so that the breasts remain larger. Sometimes, however, there is atrophy of all elements of the breast, resulting in shrinkage to a size smaller than before.

PATHOLOGY

The normal lobular unit consists of a series of acini surrounding an intralobular terminal ductule that leaves the lobular unit to become an extralobular terminal duct. The terminal-duct–lobular units are the site of origin of most proliferative breast lesions, including most cancers. The extralobular terminal ducts join together in a branching fashion to form eventually into a single duct emerging on the summit of the nipple. The lobules are embedded in a loose specialised connective tissue stroma which is itself altered in certain disease states.

INFECTIONS AND INFLAMMATIONS OF THE BREAST

Inflammation and infection of the breast occurs almost exclusively in adult females. Most occur during lactation. The others occur in the perimenopausal phase, largely in women with mammary duct ectasia, and is often sterile, at least initially. Infections during or soon after lactation are usually pyogenic, most commonly due to staphylococci. Infection is said to be introduced via cracked or traumatised nipples during suckling. Infection probably starts within milk ducts, initiating local inflammation, then a spreading cellulitis which is localised to one radial section of the breast. At this stage, before pus formation, the infection can often be successfully treated with anti-staphylococcal antibiotics. Once pus has formed and an abscess or abscesses develop, standard principles of surgical drainage apply. If not drained, the combination of inflammation and scarring can destroy a large part of the functioning breast tissue. Incisions need to be placed some distance from the areola, otherwise there is a danger of opening a duct and, if lactation continues, risking the development of a milk fistula to the skin surface.

BENIGN CONDITIONS OF THE BREAST AND THE RELATIVE RISK OF MALIGNANCY

Classification of benign breast disorders

There have been several attempts to classify or group benign breast disorders, but these have mostly developed in a haphazard and piecemeal manner. Terms such as fibrocystic disease usually describe only a small element of the histological picture and do not match any recognisable clinical picture. In order to be useful, any system of description needs to incorporate both the clinical patterns and the histopathological picture. Many of the breast complaints of pain, nodularity and nipple discharge may result from normal physiological changes taking place at the different stages of reproductive life and with changes in the hormonal environment during the monthly cycles. From both the clinician's and the pathologist's point of view, the aims are to decide whether a patient's symptoms are due to normal physiological changes, or abnormal changes. Abnormalities might be graded into 'disorders' and 'diseases' according to severity and histopathological findings. Clinicians and patients also want to know the likely natural history, and the risk of malignancy over

the years. The ANDI concept (Aberrations of Normal Development and Involution) was introduced by Hughes, Mansel & Webster in 1987 to provide a framework on which to place many of the benign breast conditions (Table 15.1). This was offered as a framework, accepting that, as understanding increased, conditions might move from one category to another.

The common presentations of breast pain and nodularity fall either into normality or benign disorder depending on severity, assuming malignancy can be excluded. Mild hyperplastic conditions such as fibroadenoma, which do not carry an increased risk of cancer and which tend to regress spontaneously with involution of the breast, can be classified as disorders, behaving as they do in an archetypal manner for normal endocrine responsive tissues. Small fibroadenomas are so common they can be regarded as variants of normal. Similarly, microcystic changes are so common in the involuting, premenopausal breast as not to cause comment. Duct ectasia is difficult to place within this classification, but mild ectasia is so common in the perimenopausal breast that it can be regarded as an involutional condition.

Mastalgia and nodularity

These extremely common symptoms have an uncertain aetiology, but the evidence points to disturbed responses of the breast to the hormonal environment, as evidenced by the following.

- The changes do not occur before the menarche and are rare for some years afterwards.
- Symptoms are greatest in the premenstrual phase, when levels of oestrogen and progesterone are highest.
- Symptoms remit after the menopause unless hormone replacement therapy is given.

Table 15.1 Aberrations of normal development and involution			
	Normal	Benign disorder	Benign disease
Development	Ductolobular growth	Fibroadenoma	Giant fibroadenoma
Cyclical change	Hormonal cycles Premenstrual swelling Epithelial hyperplasia	Mastalgia Nodularity Intraduct papilloma	Hyperplasia with atypia
Pregnancy/lactation	Lactation	Inappropriate lactation	
Involution	Lobular involution Ductal involution	Cysts Sclerosing adenosis Duct ectasia	Periductal mastitis with suppuration and/or fistula formation

After Hughes L E, Mansel R E, Webster D J 1987 Aberrations of normal development and involution (ANDI): a new perspective on pathogenesis and nomenclature of benign breast disorders. Lancet ii(8571): 1316–1319.

Most of these sufferers undoubtedly have physiological changes but with exaggerated symptomatology, and, provided malignancy can be excluded, patients can often be managed conservatively. Certain proliferative changes in these patients and in others with lesions discovered mammographically increase the long term risk of developing malignancy, and it is clearly important to quantify this risk in those undergoing breast biopsies. Long term studies have compared the risks of malignancy of various non-malignant histological patterns with age-matched normals, and results have been used to predict the malignant potential relative to control women of the same age (Box 15.1). However, it is important to remember that these risk assessments describe probabilities and not the risk in an individual. Overall, the risk of developing breast cancer for any woman in the Western world is about one in ten.

Mastalgia and nodularity or 'lumpiness' are common symptoms. If histological specimens are examined, they show a range of fibrocystic changes in varying degree. The main purpose of making a diagnosis is to exclude premalignant or malignant change. Non-neoplastic hyperplasia of the breast occurs chiefly in the upper outer quadrant of the breast. Clinically, the nodularity is often indistinguishable from breast tissue elsewhere, but it may be more obviously nodular. At operation, the tissue is usually seen to be dense and white, often with obvious cyst formation. Histology shows a combination of:

- *fibrosis* (an increase in collagen rather than an overgrowth of fibrous tissue)
- *cyst formation* (usually multiple cysts, varying in size from microscopic to several centimetres across). Cysts

are extremely common. The stimulus is unknown, but cyst formation is thought to occur as lobular units unfold and coalesce with loss of specialised connective tissue. The lining epithelial cells are often large with abundant cytoplasm, and this is known as *apocrine metaplasia.* The presence of these cells in needle aspirates confirms the diagnosis of cystic change. Large cysts may refill after incomplete aspiration drainage. If no proliferative components are found and there is no family history of breast cancer, there is no increased risk of cancer. However, clinicians must be aware that cancer can occur in other parts of the breast independently

- *adenosis* — an increase in the number and size of lobules without thickening of the ductular epithelium
- *sclerosing adenosis* — a localised proliferation of both stroma and acini, often with marked mitotic activity but no dysplasia. Sclerosing adenosis refers to lobular units which have deformed sclerotic glandular elements. They often contain microcalcifications and are frequently detected on mammography. The main concern is that sclerosing adenosis can clinically and pathologically mimic invasive cancer
- *epithelial proliferative breast disease* — this is the main factor in determining the malignant potential of an apparently benign breast lesion and is described in the next section.

Epithelial proliferative breast disease

The normal terminal ductule (acinus) has a double cell lining; any increase in the number of cells above the basement membrane is termed hyperplasia. Epithelial hyperplasia represents a spectrum of changes ranging from mild and clinically insignificant to severe, resembling carcinoma in situ (CIS). Specific histological criteria allow classification and stratification of the hyperplasias. Thus hyperplasia is graded mild, moderate, florid, or atypical, with consequent risk implications. A specific pattern of lobular hyperplasia known as *atypical lobular hyperplasia* is easily recognised and may be found in association with lobular CIS.

The surgical pathologist has responsibility for recognising a borderline group of lesions (which are not malignant but with an increased risk of later cancer development), subclassifying non-invasive cancer, that currently represents up to 20% of newly diagnosed lesions, and predicting the behaviour of malignant lesions.

So-called ductal hyperplasia (there is little evidence to support its ductal origin) is represented by common patterns of hyperplasia designated *ordinary hyperplasia* or *hyperplasia of the usual type* and is found in 96% of

---

Box 15.1 Relative risk of later malignancy of benign histological patterns

- no increased risk
  - adenosis
  - apocrine metaplasia
  - mild hyperplasia
  - cysts, microscopic and macroscopic
  - mastitis
  - duct ectasia
- slightly increased risk (1.5–2 times)
  - hyperplasia, moderate or florid
  - intraduct papilloma
  - fibroadenoma
  - sclerosing adenosis
- moderately increased risk (4–5 times)
  - atypical ductal hyperplasia
  - atypical lobular hyperplasia

cases with hyperplasia. The severity ranges from *mild,* with spaces lined by only 3–4 cells thick, to *florid* with proliferating cell masses distending and distorting the involved spaces. These ordinary patterns feature irregularity of cells with nuclei that vary in size, shape and position. There is no increased risk of malignancy from mild hyperplasias, but moderate or florid hyperplasia doubles the risk, i.e. to similar levels brought about by early menarche, late menopause, or a positive family history.

About 4% of biopsies from the premammographic era show hyperplasia falling into a borderline category, with some features of CIS but other clearly benign features. This is known as *atypical ductal hyperplasia.* Criteria for this are precisely described by histopathologists. In brief, there is normal polarity of cells around the periphery of the space but sharply defined secondary spaces and rigid cellular bars which in themselves would suggest CIS (Fig. 15.4).

Criteria for the diagnosis of epithelial hyperplasias in general have been clearly defined on the basis of cytological features, the patterns and the extent of lesions. Using these criteria, reproducibility between histopathologists is strong. In atypical ductal hyperplasias (ADH), the risk of carcinoma in either breast lies between that predicted for usual pattern hyperplasia and ductal CIS, but if the patient also has a first degree relative with invasive carcinoma, the risk increases to 8–9 times that

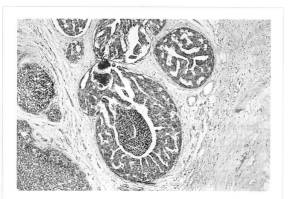

Fig. 15.4 Ductal carcinoma in situ of comedo type. The thickness of the ductular epithelium is much greater than normal, and the cells exhibit malignant characteristics: namely, variations in size and shape of cells and nuclei and a broad range of nuclear staining. Mitoses are also evident, but there is no invasion of the basement membrane in this section. One duct is seen to be filled with cellular debris.
Photomicrograph kindly supplied by Dr M Harris, Consultant Histopathologist, Hinchingbrooke Hospital, Huntingdon, Cambridgeshire.

of the normal population, i.e. similar to the risk found in lobular CIS.

GYNAECOMASTIA

Gynaecomastia is a benign enlargement of male breast tissue, unilaterally or bilaterally, which is often reversible. The enlargement is predominantly due to an increase in stromal tissue rather than to ductal proliferation. Physiological gynaecomastia is seen in the newborn (under the influence of maternal hormones) and at puberty, resulting from sex hormone stimulation. Pathological gynaecomastia occurs in cirrhosis, renal failure, chronic obstructive airways disease and HIV infection. Certain drugs can also cause gynaecomastia. These include spironolactone, tamoxifen, cimetidine, digoxin, marijuana and anabolic steroids.

The histological appearance is similar whatever the aetiology. Initially, in the active proliferative phase, there is an excess of stromal tissue with some ductal proliferation. The breast is often tender during this phase. Later the breast tissue becomes fibrotic, with the pain disappearing but the lump persisting. Clinically, it is important to distinguish these benign causes from carcinoma.

CARCINOMA OF THE BREAST
CARCINOMA IN SITU

Carcinoma in situ (CIS) is defined as a condition where malignant cells are confined within existing ductal or lobular units. However, it is a complex disease with heterogenous biological behaviours. The histological diagnosis of ductal or lobular CIS is based purely on the histological pattern rather than on the tissue of origin, which is uncertain. Lobular CIS (LCIS) tends to present in a readily recognised 'pure' form, whereas ductal CIS (DCIS) is more heterogenous and is usually diagnosed by excluding LCIS. DCIS is now thought to be a spectrum of disease, ranging from the tiny mammographically detected lesion that can be properly treated by simple excision to widespread DCIS which cannot be excised conservatively.

Comedo DCIS is a variant so called because of the gross appearance of caseous material dotting the cut surface of the lesion. This corresponds to necrotic debris within ductule lumens. Comedo DCIS frequently calcifies, producing characteristic coarse linear branching patterns on mammography. The combination of necrosis with pleomorphic, hyperchromatic nuclei make the diagnosis. Non-comedo types of DCIS compose several architectural

DERMOID CYSTS

Dermoid cysts develop at an area where fusion of sections of the embryo has occurred, and are most common in the midline of the neck, at the external angle of the eye, and behind the pinna. They should be removed to prevent secondary infection.

CLEFT LIP AND PALATE

This is one of the more common congenital anomalies, occurring in 1 in 600 live births.

The face forms during the fifth to the eighth week, from the maxillary and mandibular prominences of the first branchial arch. They grow and fuse together, and if this fusion is incomplete, unilateral or bilateral cleft lip may arise (Fig. 16.2).

The palate develops after the eighth week, and fusion occurs between the primary palate (the anterior section of the premaxilla and attached four front teeth) and the secondary palate (the hard and soft palate). The palate may be cleft posteriorly only, a cleft soft palate, or it may extend anteriorly to include the hard palate, cleft palate only, and more commonly it extends further anteriorly to join up with either a unilateral or bilateral cleft lip (Fig. 16.3).

Surgical correction of cleft lip and palate needs to take the embryological origins and in particular the blood supply into consideration, in order to allow an optimum repair and subsequent growth.

CYSTIC HYGROMA (LYMPHANGIOMA)

The primitive lymph sacs develop in the mesenchyme in the sixth week, and the largest is in the neck, and should resolve, but persistence and sequestration produces a

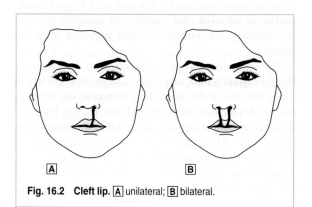

Fig. 16.2   Cleft lip. [A] unilateral; [B] bilateral.

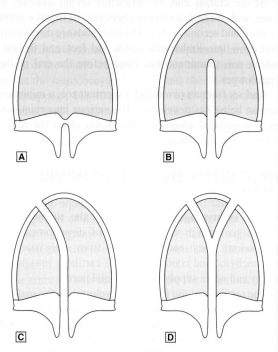

Fig. 16.3   Types of cleft palate. [A] cleft of soft palate; [B] partial cleft palate; [C] unilateral complete cleft palate; [D] bilateral complete cleft palate.

multicystic swelling within the neck which is a lymphangioma, a benign hamartoma (overgrowth of normal tissue), which is also called a cystic hygroma when it occurs in the neck. Occasionally this is very large and causes respiratory distress in the neonatal age group, but more ususaly is just a soft swelling in the neck which may extend into the axilla, or even the chest. A degree of spontaneous resolution can be hoped for, but often it comes to surgical debulking — a difficult prospect because of the multicystic nature, which makes it difficult to be sure that every bit of the abnormal tissue is removed. If there is a haemangiomatous element as well as the lymphangiomatous part, spontaneous resolution is unlikely. An MRI scan is recommended to delineate the full extent and nature of the lesion, and the normal structures which are involved, to help plan surgical excision.

CONGENITAL DIAPHRAGMATIC HERNIA

The diaphragm develops between the thoracic and abdominal cavity, and this is a complex process which is finished before the end of the eighth week (Fig. 16.4). As the embryo folds and carries the primitive heart and

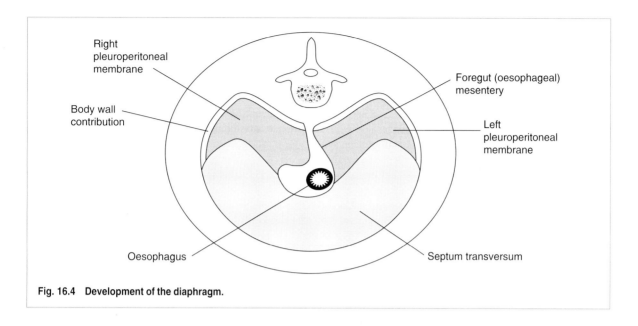

Fig. 16.4 Development of the diaphragm.

Right pleuroperitoneal membrane

Body wall contribution

Foregut (oesophageal) mesentery

Left pleuroperitoneal membrane

Oesophagus

Septum transversum

septum transversum caudally and ventrally, it carries part of the yolk sac dorsally to develop as the foregut. The lateral mesenchyme develops into the pericardioperitoneal canals, from which the pericardial cavity and the lungs develop, and is separated from the peritoneal cavity by the closure of the diaphragm. The motor nerve supply travels with the diaphragm as it descends, and so comes from a more cranial region than may be expected: C3–5. This explains the clinical observation that diaphragmatic inflammation/irritation, e.g. due to intraperitoneal blood, can demonstrate referred pain and can cause shoulder tip pain (which area is also supplied by C4).

The diaphragm develops from the fusion of four parts:

- the septum transversum (the fibrous central tendon)
- the mesentery of the foregut (the area adjacent to the vertebral column becomes the crura and median part)
- ingrowth from the body wall (the peripheral muscular portion)
- the pleuriperitoneal membrane (a small dorsal part).

There are different types of congenital diaphragmatic hernia, depending on which section has failed to close.

The most common defect is the posterolateral Bochdalek hernia (through the pleuroperitoneal canal) which is more common on the left, as that side closes last. Absence of the diaphragm can also occur, or absence of the central tendon. These three hernias tend to present early with respiratory distress soon after birth. The presence of the intestines within the pleural cavity antenatally prevents the normal development of the lung on the ipsilateral

side, and mediastinal shift also prevents normal development of the contralateral lung. If the lung hypoplasia is severe, it is not compatible with life. Urgent supportive ventilation is required, and nasogastric aspiration of the gut, to decrease direct pressure on the lungs.

These diapragmatic hernias must be dealt with surgically, after resuscitation of the patient (this is sometimes not possible in a neonate because of the severity of the lung hypoplasia) — up to 50% of babies born with congenital diaphragmatic hernias will die even today with all the modern management possibilities of oscillatory and jet ventilation, or extracorporeal membrane oxygenation (bypass).

Morgagni hernias are small defects in the anterior diaphragm close to the sternum, and are rarely associated with lung hypoplasia. They may be a coincidental finding on a chest x-ray taken for another reason. These hernias also require surgical repair.

GASTROINTESTINAL TRACT

The foregut develops from the yolk sac which folds in to the embryo at its cephalad end during the fourth week. From this foregut is derived the:

- pharynx (and from the floor of that the thyroid)
- airways and lungs
- oesophagus
- stomach

- duodenum (proximal to the opening of the bile duct)
- liver, biliary system and pancreas.

OESOPHAGEAL ATRESIA

The foregut starts to divide into the oesophagus and the laryngotracheal tube during the fourth week. If it fails to do so correctly, there can be pure oesophageal atresia (in 8% of cases), or atresia associated with tracheo-oesophageal fistula — the commonest (in 80% of cases), being a fistula between the lower trachea and the distal oesophagus (Fig. 16.5).

The baby presents soon after birth, unable to swallow saliva, and an attempt to pass a tube into the stomach fails. An x-ray taken then will show the tube in the proximal oesophagus, and either no gas below the diaphragm (in pure oesophageal atresia) or gas below the diaphragm (in patients with oesophageal atresia and tracheo-oesophageal fistula). There is a high incidence (50% of babies) of associated anomalies described by the acronym VACTERL:

- Vertebral anomalies (e.g. hemivertebrae)
- Anorectal anomalies (eg. imperforate anus)
- Cardiac anomalies
- Tracheal anomalies (e.g. fistula, tracheomalacia)
- Esophageal anomalies (the American version!)
- Renal anomalies
- Limb anomalies (e.g. radial aplasia).

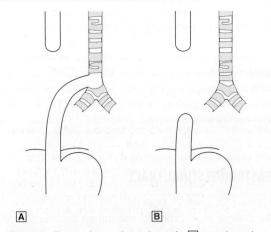

Fig. 16.5 Types of oesophageal atresia. A oesophageal atresia with distal tracheo-oesophageal fistula — the usual type, with an incidence of 80%; B isolated oesophageal atresia — the second commonest form, with an incidence of 8%.

Management involves protection of the lungs from aspiration of saliva prior to surgical repair. This is usually by a right thoracotomy to ligate the fistula, freeing the distal oesophagus which is then anastomosed primarily to the upper oesophageal pouch. If primary repair is not possible, a feeding gastrostomy is performed to feed the baby until it has grown enough to perform a delayed primary anastomosis or oesophageal substitution, e.g. with stomach, colon, or small bowel.

CONGENITAL HYPERTROPHIC PYLORIC STENOSIS

The stomach develops from a simple tubular part of the foregut by localised dilatation. The stomach rotates clockwise so that the vagus which followed the left side of the oesophagus supplies the anterior stomach. The mesentery which suspends the stomach from the posterior abdominal wall enlarges and becomes the greater omentum. The exit of the stomach into the duodenum is the pyloric canal.

All of the gastrointestinal tract has two layers of muscle: circular and longitudinal. The circular muscle only of the pylorus can become hypertrophied in some babies. This is often called 'congenital' hypertrophic pyloric stenosis, but does not actually exist at birth. The baby usually presents after 10–50 days (most commonly 3–5 weeks), as the pyloric canal is narrowed by the hypertrophied muscle, and milk is prevented from leaving the stomach. The stomach becomes full and peristalses vigorously to try to empty. This peristalsis may be visible on the baby's abdomen. The baby will then vomit forcefully, which is described as projectile.

As the baby vomits fluid and gastric hydrochloric acid, he/she becomes dehydrated, hypochloraemic and alkalotic. This is reflected in the baby's electrolytes and blood gases at presentation. The diagnosis is made by feeding the baby, to relax him/her. The visible peristalsis may be seen, and the abdomen is palpated to feel for the pylorus, which can be felt as a lump in the right upper quadrant, about the size and shape of an olive. After rehydration and correction of the acid–base balance, the baby is taken to theatre for a laparotomy, and the hypertrophied muscle is split, without opening the mucosa — a pyloromyotomy. This is a curative operation, and the baby will be fully fed within 24–36 h postoperatively and discharged home.

DUODENAL OBSTRUCTION

The duodenum develops from both the fore and the midgut. The caudal part of the foregut, which is supplied by the coeliac artery, develops into the first and second parts of the duodenum, up to the ampulla of Vater — where the bile and pancreatic ducts enter. The cephalad part of the midgut, supplied by the superior mesenteric artery, develops into the second part of the duodenum after the entry of the bile and pancreatic ducts, and the third and fourth parts.

The embryology of duodenal obstruction is different to that of atresias lower in the intestine, and has a greater number of associated other anomalies. During the fifth and sixth week, the duodenum becomes occluded by proliferation of its endodermal lining. It then recanalises by the end of the eighth week, but if this recanalisation is incomplete, either atresia (complete occlusion) or stenosis (narrowing) of the duodenum occurs. 30% of babies with duodenal atresia have Down's syndrome.

The pancreas develops (Fig. 16.6) from two outgrowths of the foregut, one ventral and one dorsal. Due to rotation, the ventral bud and the adjacent gallbladder and common bile duct rotates so that the ventral and dorsal buds lie adjacent to each other and fuse. The two ducts also usually fuse, and the main pancreatic duct enters the duodenum adjacent to the entry of the common bile duct at the ampulla of Vater. The proximal part of the dorsal bud duct may persist as the accessory duct, which opens proximally into the duodenum. Occasionally the pancreas appears to encircle the duodenum — annular pancreas — and appears to be causing duodenal obstruction. This annular pancreas is invariably associated with an abnormality of the development of the duodenum, which makes it appear to be causing the obstruction, but is in fact an apparent effect rather than the true cause. This is supported by the fact that annular pancreas has also been recorded without associated obstruction.

Babies with duodenal atresia present in the first few days of life, vomiting every feed. Babies with duodenal stenosis present later — how much later depends on the degree of the stenosis. The most common part of the duodenum to be obstructed is just distal to the ampulla of Vater, and so the vomit is most likely to be bilestained. Plain abdominal x-ray in duodenal atresia reveals a 'double bubble' — the first bubble being air in the distended stomach, and the second bubble being air in the distended duodenum. The diagnosis may have been made antenatally, as the mother may have had ultrasound scans. This reveals a double cystic structure — similar to the double bubble, but the appearance is not due to swallowed air but to swallowed amniotic fluid which is prevented from passing through the gastrointestinal tract by the obstructed duodenum. This can lead to polyhydramnios.

Due to the common association of duodenal atresia and stenosis with other congenital anomalies, the baby must

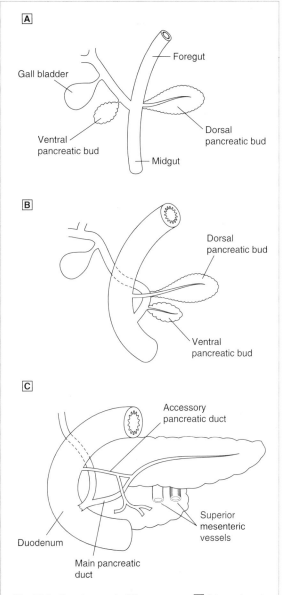

Fig. 16.6 Development of the pancreas. [A] A large dorsal bud develops from the duodenum and a smaller ventral bud from the side of the common bile duct. [B] The ventral bud rotates posteriorly to fuse with the lower aspect of the dorsal bud. [C] The ducts of the two buds communicate, the duct of the smaller ventral bud forming the main duct, while the original duct of the larger dorsal bud forms the accessory duct.

be checked thoroughly, e.g. for Down's syndrome, for cardiac and renal anomalies, etc.

After rehydration, the baby undergoes laparotomy, and a duodenoduodenostomy — which is the most physiological operative correction. Duodenojejunostomy might bypass the obstruction, but leaves a blind part of the duodenum, which often fails to work and causes later problems.

MALROTATION

The midgut is supplied by the superior mesenteric artery, and develops into the duodenum distal to the entry of the bile/pancreatic duct, all of the small bowel, and the colon from the caecum to two-thirds of the way along the transverse colon.

Between the sixth and eleventh week, the midgut develops and rotates. As the midgut lengthens, it forms a loop which projects and herniates into the base of the umbilical cord. While the midgut is within the cord, it rotates through 90°, counterclockwise around the superior mesenteric artery. This brings the third and fourth part of the duodenum across to the left of the midline, behind the superior mesenteric artery, and this duodenum is fixed retroperitoneally. The midgut returns to the abdomen during the tenth week, and during this time it continues to rotate counterclockwise through a further 180°, which brings the ascending colon to the right side of the abdomen, with the caecum and appendix to the right iliac fossa. The ascending colon also becomes retroperitoneal. The mesentery of the small bowel stretches from the duodenojejunal flexure in the left upper quadrant to the right iliac fossa (Fig. 16.7).

Malrotation occurs when the normal rotation sequence described above does not occur, or is incomplete. This results in the duodenojejunal flexure not becoming fixed retroperitoneally in the left upper quadrant, but hanging freely from the foregut, and tending to lie on the right of the abdomen.

The caecum is also free, and may obstruct the second part of the duodenum because of fibrous bands which stretch across the duodenum from the caecum. The base of the mesentery of the midgut is then very narrow, as it is not fixed at either end, and the whole of this midgut can undergo twisting around its own blood supply, with resultant ischaemia. This is malrotation volvulus, a true surgical emergency.

These patients classically present in the first week or two of life with bilious vomiting. In neonates and infants, bilious vomiting has a surgical diagnosis in origin until proved otherwise. Plain abdominal x-ray may show the small bowel on the right of the abdomen, and the large bowel on the left, suggesting malrotation. This requires urgent resuscitation, and then laparotomy and correction, before a volvulus occurs. Even more worrying is an x-ray with no gas distal to the stomach — suggestive of a vol-

vulus of the midgut. This is potentially fatal if the whole of the midgut is ischaemic, and again requires emergency laparotomy after urgent resuscitation. If the plain x-ray cannot confirm the diagnosis, a contrast meal will demonstrate the position of the duodenojejunal flexure and subsequent lie of the jejunum. The diagnosis and management of malrotation of the midgut is one of the very few causes for true emergency neonatal laparotomy for a congenital anomaly.

SMALL AND LARGE BOWEL ATRESIA

Duodenal atresia is thought to be due to a defect in recanalisation during the eighth week of embryonic development. Atresia of the small and large bowel is thought to occur later during fetal life, in the second trimester (fourth to sixth months of pregnancy), and to be due to an ischaemic vascular accident of the mesentery. This is confirmed by the presence of bile (first produced in the eleventh week) and squames which have been swallowed (swallowing first occurs after the third month) being found in the bowel distal to an atresia.

Jejunal atresia is twice as common as ileal atresia, and both present in the first few postnatal days with increasing bilious vomiting and abdominal distension. The atresias may be multiple, and apart from surgical correction, the main problem is any associated dysmotility of the bowel proximal to the atresia, short bowel syndrome, and complications of the total parenteral nutrition required to maintain the baby whilst the intestines function normally, if ever. Colonic atresia is very rare, and presentation and treatment is similar to that of small bowel atresia.

MECONIUM ILEUS

Meconium ileus is the term given to ileal obstruction due to inspissated meconium in the terminal ileum in neonates. In 95% of cases, this is found to be due to cystic fibrosis. The intestinal secretions in babies with cystic fibrosis are abnormal, producing very thick and viscid meconium. In combination with abnormal pancreatic enzymes, this produces meconium which produces an intraluminal obstruction in the terminal ileum. The obstruction may be simple, and presents at birth with failure to pass meconium, abdominal distension, and bilious vomiting. In some cases the obstruction is complex, with intrauterine perforation, volvulus, or atresias. Management includes treatment of the obstruction, and then investigation and treatment of the baby for cystic fibrosis.

Cystic fibrosis is the most commonly inherited gene of

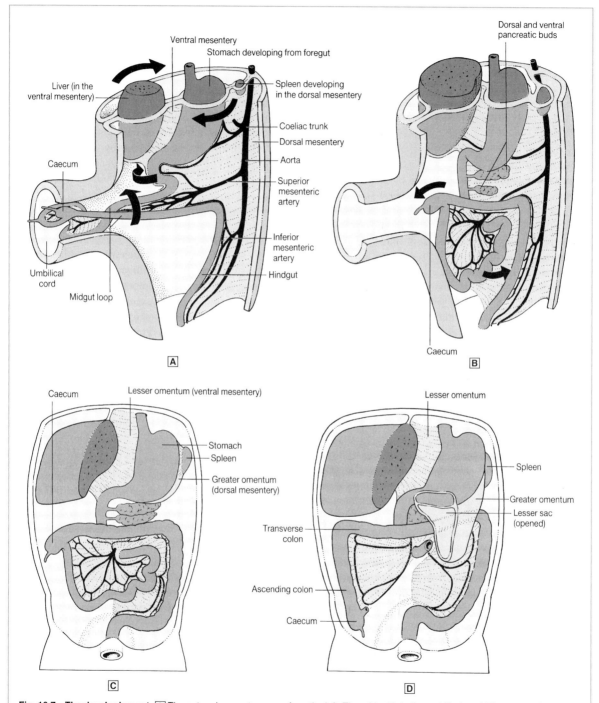

Fig. 16.7 The developing gut. [A] The gut and mesentery seen from the left. The midgut is in the umbilical cord. The arrows show the direction of rotation of the foregut and midgut. [B] Anterolateral view, after the return of the midgut back into the abdominal cavity. From this position the caecum and transverse colon will rotate to the right, bringing the transverse colon in front of the superior mesenteric artery; the small intestine will move to the left behind the artery (see arrows). [C] Anterior view, after the return of the midgut and a stage further on from [B] . Note that the caecum is now on the right side under the liver. [D] Final position. The caecum has now descended to the right iliac fossa. From Rogers op. cit.

a potentially lethal congenital disorder. It has an auto-somal recessive inheritance, meaning that one in four pregnancies will be affected in a family. The genetics are now more fully identified, and the diagnosis is made by DNA testing, looking for the delta F508 mutation on gene 7.

ANTERIOR ABDOMINAL WALL DEFECTS

These comprise exomphalos and gastroschisis. The embryology of these two defects is not understood, and various theories have been postulated, but with no defini-tive outcome, except that they are separate clinical enti-ties. The closure of the anterior abdominal wall muscles occurs between the fourth and seventh week, and failure of this could explain exomphalos, but not gastroschisis where the anterior abdominal wall muscles are in com-plete existence but with a defect.

Exomphalos is the herniation of a variable amount of the intra-abdominal contents through the open umbilical ring into the base of the umbilical cord. It differs from an umbilical hernia, which is skin covered, as it is covered by a thin double membrane of peritoneum on the inside, and an outer layer of amniotic membrane. The size of the exomphalos varies from a single loop of bowel within it (minor exomphalos) to a giant exomphalos containing stomach, all of the small and large intestine, liver, spleen, pancreas and urinary bladder, leaving the peritoneal cavity almost empty.

Gastroschisis babies have a full thickness defect in the abdominal wall, usually adjacent to the right side of the umbilical cord. The intestines may be outside the defect to a varying degree, and the stomach, but never the liver. There is no sac or membrane covering the defect, and the intestines have been exposed to the amniotic fluid during pregnancy, and this often produces a very thickened and dysmotile bowel wall, from which the baby may not recover. The defect is much narrower in gastroschisis, and there may be vascular ischaemic insults to the exteri-orised bowel, causing atresias, or even complete absence.

Babies with exomphalos may have other associated congenital malformations, some of which may be incom-patible with life, for instance major lethal cardiac or chromosomal anomalies. Gastroschisis is rarely asso-ciated with other anomalies, although there may be gastrointestinal atresias or bowel malfunction.

The principle of management of both anterior abdo-minal wall abnormalities is to replace the exteriorised bowel/organs into the abdominal cavity, and then to feed the baby intravenously until his/her own guts tolerate enteral nutrition. If there is no other gross congenital abnormality in an exomphalos baby, the problem is clo-sure of the abdominal wall defect. Once this is complete, the guts usually function well. In a gastroschisis baby, the problem is that even though it is usually easier to get the guts back into the peritoneal cavity, the bowel may be slow to, or may never, function.

Antenatal diagnosis of both these anomalies is very common these days, and, if there is an exomphalos, chro-mosomal analysis will be recommended, with scanning for other major anomalies. A baby with gastroschisis rarely has other anomalies, but regular scanning is carried out during pregnancy to watch for intestinal catastrophes.

UMBILICAL REMNANTS

Meckel's diverticulum

The vitello-intestinal duct is the remnant of the yolk sac which is attached to the primitive midgut in the first few weeks of embryonic development. It should completely obliterate during the sixth week, but may persist com-pletely or in part (Fig. 16.8). If it persists completely, there is a diverticulum, the Meckel's diverticulum, which arises from the terminal ileum. The classical description in adults is that it is present in 2% of the population, is 2 inches (5 cm) long, and 2 feet (60 cm) from the ileocae-cal valve. A persistent vitello-intestinal duct can present at birth, as a swelling at the base of the umbilical cord, or as a fistulous connection to the umbilicus, or as an umbilical polyp, which does not respond like simple granulation tissue to cautery, because it has a mucosal surface. Surgical excision is required. It may be lined by ileal mucosa, or contain ectopic gastric mucosa, which may undergo peptic ulceration with subsequent bleeding. It may present with diverticulitis (like appendicitis), or with adhesion/band obstruction and volvulus because of its persistent attachment to the umbilical cord.

Management is by excision after the diagnosis has been made — which is often only at laparotomy, although it may be suspected beforehand. There is no definitive scan or investigation to confirm the existence of a Meckel's diverticulum. A radiolabelled technetium scan looking for ectopic gastric mucosa (that is, outside the stomach) is only positive in about 70% of patients with a Meckel's diverticulum who present with rectal bleeding.

Urachus

The urachus is the embryonic remnant of the connection between the urinary bladder and the allantois at the umbilicus (Fig. 16.9). It can also persist, either in part — as a cyst or fine cord, or completely — as a mucosa-covered structure at the umbilicus, from which urine

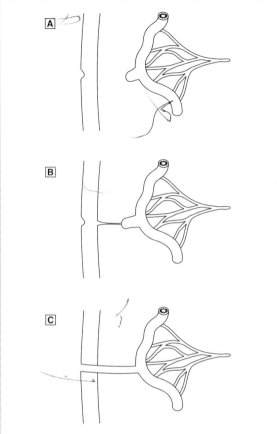

Fig. 16.8 Congenital abnormalities associated with the vitello-intestinal duct. [A] Meckel's diverticulum; [B] congenital band adhesion between Meckel's diverticulum and umbilicus giving rise to risk of volvulus; [C] a persistent patent vitello-intestinal duct.

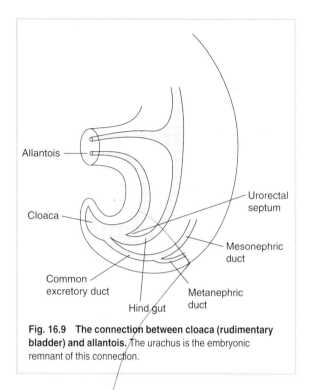

Fig. 16.9 The connection between cloaca (rudimentary bladder) and allantois. The urachus is the embryonic remnant of this connection.

comes. Treatment is by surgical excision after accurate diagnosis.

ANORECTAL ANOMALIES

The structures of the rectum, anus and genitourinary tracts are created by the end of the ninth week of gestation, by separation of these structures within the cloaca. The exact mechanism of these events has never been clear, and there is still no consensus.

The cloaca contains the hindgut and the urogenital passage (Fig. 16.9). The cloacal membrane should extend from the genital tubercle anteriorly to the tail dorsally and initially separates the future gut and urinary passages from the amniotic cavity. The urorectal septum is a mass of mesenchymal tissue between these two passages. As the cloacal membrane thins dorsally and the tail regresses, the hindgut and urogenital passages open into the amniotic cavity. The distance between these passages increases as the urorectal septum broadens, with the urogenital passage maintaining close proximity to the genital tubercle anteriorly, and the gut passage moving relatively dorsally (Fig. 16.10). The mesenchyme of the urorectal septum develops into the muscles of the pelvic floor and sphincter mechanisms. If the cloacal membrane does not reach the tail groove, abnormalities of the anorectum occur — with the many types of anorectal anomalies which exist.

The varieties of anorectal anomalies can be broadly divided into low, intermediate and high, in males and females (Figs. 16.11 and 16.12). The high lesions commonly have a fistula, which goes anteriorly — to the urinary system in a boy, or to the vagina in a girl.

The division into high or low is dependent on the amount of mesenchymal tissue which existed in the urorectal septum, from which the sphincter mechanisms developed. If most or all the sphincter muscles develop it is a low lesion; or, if very little, a high lesion. A high lesion is associated with poor continence, even after surgical reconstruction, but even the low lesions often have

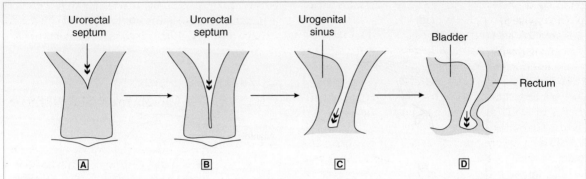

Fig. 16.10 The development of the perineum, and urogenital and rectal cavities. The urorectal septum is indicated by the double arrows.

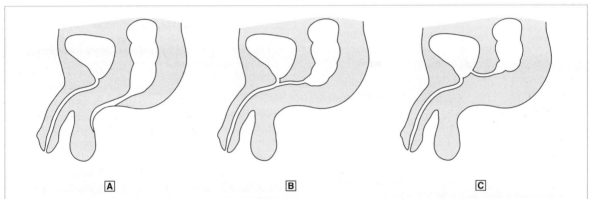

Fig. 16.11 Types of anorectal anomalies in the male. Ⓐ low — with covered anus and anoperineal fistula; Ⓑ intermediate — anal agenesis with rectourethral fistula; Ⓒ high — anorectal agenesis with rectovesical fistula.

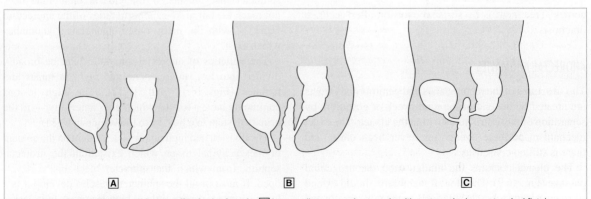

Fig. 16.12 Types of anorectal anomalies in the female. Ⓐ intermediate — anal agenesis with rectovaginal or rectovulval fistula; Ⓑ high — anorectal agenesis with rectovaginal fistula; Ⓒ persistant cloaca (rare) — bladder, vagina and rectum open into the cloaca.

problems of continence; and both types have associated problems with the urinary system.

After birth, all babies must be examined for the presence of a normally sited anus. If the anus is imperforate, assessment and investigations may help identify the lesion to be high or low. In the former case, a fistula is looked for, and the parents are warned about the long term difficulties in achieving normal continence. The baby may have a colostomy formed, and a definitive pullthrough operation at the age of a few months; or it is becoming more common for that definitive procedure to be done at the first operation if the baby is healthy, and the surgeon experienced. A low imperforate anus is dealt with by a local procedure, and long term followup still needs to be maintained until the child has developed continence.

HIRSCHSPRUNG'S DISEASE

Although Hirschsprung described two patients with this disease in 1887, it was not until 1948 that the histopathological abnormality of aganglionosis was identifed. The aganglionosis is in the colonic wall, always involving the distal rectosigmoid, and extending proximally for a variable length (total colonic aganglionosis occurs, as does total gastrointestinal aganglionosis). The aganglionosis does not allow normal gut peristalsis, and is nonpropulsive, thereby producing a functional intestinal obstruction. Proximal to the abnormal section is a transitional zone which is hypoganglionic, and then the normally ganglionic bowel is chronically distended — a megacolon — because of the functional obstruction. As well as aganglionosis, the other histological abnormality is hypertrophied nerve trunks in the bowel wall, which stain densely for acetylcholinesterase. The combination of these two histological techniques — cholinesterase staining and routine histology for ganglion cells — enables the diagnosis of Hirschsprung's disease to be made on a suction rectal biopsy on a newborn baby who classically presents at the age of 36 h with abdominal distension, bilious vomiting, and failure to pass meconium (they should pass meconium within 24 h of delivery).

Treatment is aimed at decompression of the bowel, either with a stoma in ganglionic bowel just proximal to the transitional zone, or by regular washouts, until a definitive operation is performed. On this occasion, the aganglionic bowel is excised and normal ganglionic bowel brought down to the anus, to prevent the functional obstruction. The operative procedures available are many and variable, indicating as ever that the perfect procedure is still elusive.

Most cases are sporadic, but occasional cases are familial. In these cases, the affected segment tends to be longer, and increases in length as the number of affected children increases. There is still no gene probe available to test antenatally.

RENAL, URETERIC AND URETHRAL ANOMALIES
EMBRYOLOGY

The development of the kidneys, ureters and reproductive system is an overlapping process which consists of the development and degeneration of various organs and ducts (Fig. 16.13). It starts in very early fetal life (the third week) with the first 'kidney' — the pronephros, which does not function. The second 'kidney' appears in the fourth week, as the pronephros is degenerating, and is the mesonephros with its mesonephric duct. This mesonephros also degenerates, but the mesonephric duct persists (the Wolffian duct), which in males persists and develops into the epididymis, vas deferens, ejaculatory ducts and seminal vesicles. In females, this Wolffian duct degenerates, but the paramesonephric ducts (Mullerian ducts) grow and develop into the female genital tract. The Mullerian ducts do not persist in the male (due to the secretion of Mullerian inhibiting substance), apart from the most cranial end which persists as the appendix testis

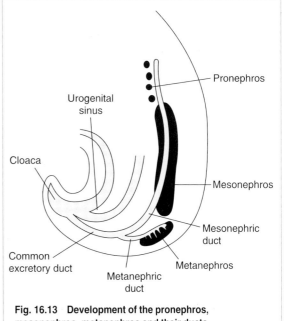

Fig. 16.13 Development of the pronephros, mesonephros, metanephros and their ducts.

(hydatid of Morgagni) on the upper pole of the testis — which may undergo torsion and the patient present with acute scrotal pain.

The third and final kidney starts development in the fifth week, as metanephric mesoderm in both sides of the pelvis is invaginated by the metanephric duct on that side — which is the ureteric bud, or diverticulum growing from the caudal end of the mesonephric duct. The ureter continues to grow into the renal tissue, and undergoes repeated branching until it has developed into the full collecting system of ureter, renal pelvis, calyces and collecting tubules. These collecting tubules fuse with the nephrons, the renal tubules of the metanephric tissue, to form the definitive kidney and collecting system.

Abnormalities of the collecting tubules can lead to polycystic disease of the autosomal recessive variety, which can be lethal (usually within a year or so of birth), or the autosomal dominant variety, which is more likely to present in the third decade of life (Fig. 16.14).

These definitive kidneys are initially close together in the pelvis, but then, as the abdomen grows, the two kidneys separate and move cranially until they lie in their final position in the lumbar region. As the kidney moves cranially, its blood supply also moves cranially. The artery comes from more and more cranially, initially from the iliac artery and then from the aorta. The venous drainage also goes into the inferior vena cava in a more cranial position. Although each kidney may have only

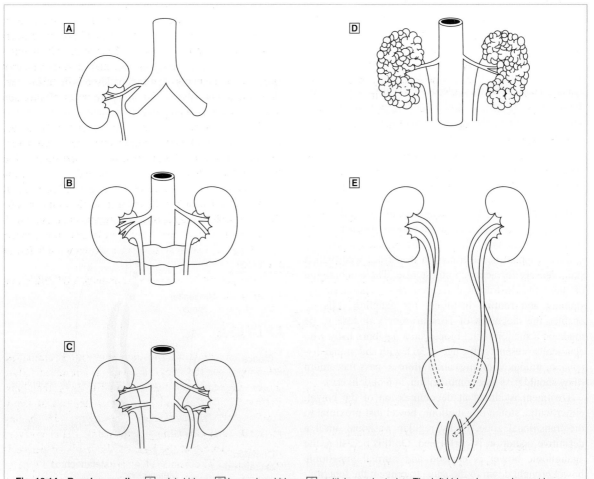

Fig. 16.14   Renal anomalies. [A] pelvic kidney; [B] horseshoe kidney; [C] multiple renal arteries. The left kidney has an aberrant lower polar artery 'tenting' the ureter and causing hydronephrosis. [D] polycystic kidneys; [E] ureteric anomalies. The right kidney has a bifid ureter. The left kidney has a double ureter with one ureter having an ectopic orifice into the vagina. Note that it is the ureter draining the upper part of the kidney that drains more caudally.

one artery and vein, their blood supply is very variable, especially to the lower pole if the previous vessels have not degenerated (Fig. 16.14).

ANOMALIES

This complex developmental process explains the various congenital anomalies of the renal tract which are seen. If the kidney fails to ascend to its normal position, it can be ectopic, anywhere along the normal line, although pelvic is most common (Fig. 16.14). If the kidneys fuse whilst they are close together in the pelvis, they can remain fused by a bridge of tissue connecting each lower pole — a horseshoe kidney (Fig. 16.14). Abnormalities of reflux and urinary drainage are more common in these abnormal kidneys. Division of the ureteric bud at an early stage leads to a divided, or duplex kidney. This duplex kidney itself is not necessarily associated with abnormalities of reflux or obstruction. If the ureters draining the two parts of the kidney are completely separate, the cranial part of the kidney invariably drains more caudally, either lower into the bladder, or even into the urethra in a boy or the urethra or vagina in a girl, causing problems of continence due to this ectopic ureter if it drains outside the urethral sphincter (Fig. 16.14).

The existence of urinary tract anomalies is commonly detected during routine antenatal scanning. It has not been found helpful to intervene antenatally, as the renal damage from anatomical changes has occurred before the date of the early antenatal scans in the 14th–20th week.

It is essential however to accurately investigate the baby postnatally, especially if bladder outflow obstruction is possible, which may lead to bilaterally damaged kidneys. The usual initial investigations include a urine for culture, an ultrasound of the urinary tract, and close monitoring. The urea, electrolytes and creatinine may be measured if poor renal function is suspected, remembering that the figures in the first 24 h of life only reflect the mother's renal function, due to placental clearance of the baby's waste products.

The commonest abnormalities of the urinary tract of paediatric surgical relevance are vesico-ureteric reflux, or obstruction.

Vesico-ureteric reflux (VUR) is the retrograde flow of urine from the bladder into the ureters. If the child gets a urinary tract infection (UTI), there is a chance of infected urine refluxing into the kidneys, risking renal cortical damage and scarring. Reflux is treated energetically with prophylactic antibiotics to prevent UTIs and thus to prevent renal damage. Surgery is rarely performed for simple reflux these days. If it is required, the surgical principle is to reimplant the ureter with a long submucosal tunnel, to prevent the reflux.

Unilateral obstruction is most commonly seen at the junction between the renal pelvis and the upper ureter — pelvi-ureteric junction (PUJ) obstruction — or less commonly at the junction between the lower ureter and the bladder, vesico-ureteric junction (VUJ) obstruction, the causes of which are unknown. Bilateral PUJ or VUJ obstruction does occur, but less commonly. PUJ obstruction may be due to a ureteric kink, a high ureteric insertion, a narrow area of ureter, extrinsic bands, or an aberrant blood vessel. Surgical treatment, if required, consists of a pyeloplasty, where the narrow upper end of the ureter is excised, along with the distended renal pelvis. The remaining collecting system is anastomosed to the ureter, with a wide drainage channel.

Unilateral obstruction to urine drainage can cause deteriorating renal function on that side, and operative intervention is undertaken if that is happening. Commonly, however, the obstruction is incomplete and the renal function is maintained. Many children will 'grow out' of the obstruction over the first few years of life, and surgery can be avoided.

Bladder outflow obstruction can occur in boys, but rarely, due to posterior urethral valves, which are membraneous mucosal folds in the posterior urethra distal to the veru montanum. This serious anomaly can be lethal if the valves cause severe obstruction leading to renal failure. If there is only mild obstruction, they may only be detected in childhood during investigations of a boy with a urinary tract infection, or with difficulty in becoming dry. Surgical treatment involves endoscopic ablation of the valves.

Some patients can have a combination of reflux and obstruction.

HYPOSPADIAS

This is one of the commonest congenital anomalies, affecting 3 per 1000 boys. It occurs as a result of failure of complete fusion of the urogenital folds on the penis. Eighty-five percent will have minor degrees of hypospadias only (i.e. glandular). This leaves 15% having moderate (urethral opening on the penile shaft) or severe (urethral opening at the base of the penis or perineal) hypospadias. The degree of severity dictates the type of surgical correction performed, but it is expected that, eventually, most boys will pass urine from a near terminal meatus. In severe cases, especially if the testes are impalpable, intersex must be considered and excluded, and also congenital adrenal hyperplasia syndrome.

Surgical correction involves construction of a neo-urethra, and is a complicated process, especially in the more proximal hypospadias. The urethral meatus should end on the glans, and should enable the boy to stand and pass urine normally in a good stream.

EPISPADIAS

This is very rare, the urethral opening being on the dorsal surface of the penis. It is usually associated with more complex penile anomalies, which may require very complex surgical correction.

HERNIA, HYDROCELE AND IMPERFECT DESCENT OF THE TESTIS

The gonads in both sexes develop from the urogenital ridges. Up to the seventh week of the embryo, it is not possible to differentiate between the sexes, but then the Y chromosome in the male leads to testosterone production and to the differentiation of the gonad into a testis. The mesonephric duct (Wolffian duct) becomes the epididymis, vas deferens and ejaculatory duct. Males also release Mullerian-inhibiting substance, which inhibits the development of the paramesonephric ducts (Mullerian ducts) — which become the reproductive organs in female embryos.

At the time the second kidneys — the mesonephric kidneys — are degenerating, the gonads descend from the abdomen into the pelvis. A peritoneal diverticulum protrudes through the internal ring of the anterior abdominal wall, as the processus vaginalis. This occurs by the 15th week. After the 28th week, the gubernaculum with its adjacent patent processus vaginalis (PPV) migrates into the scrotum, with the testis posterior to the PPV. Once complete testicular descent has occurred, the PPV should obliterate. If it remains patent, a congenital hydrocele is found clinically (Fig. 16.15). Fluid migrates up and down the PPV to and from the peritoneal cavity, allowing the size of the hydrocele to alter. The PPV can obliterate in part, leaving an encysted hydrocele of the cord (Fig. 16.15). If the PPV is large enough, it allows abdominal contents to prolapse into the scrotum — an inguinal hernia.

Surgical correction of congenital inguinal hernia and PPV ligation are two of the commonest paediatric surgical procedures. The principle is to explore the inguinal region, to locate the hernial sac or PPV either within or as it leaves the inguinal canal, to separate that sac from the spermatic cord in a boy, and to ligate the sac.

Failure of the testis to descend fully is known as an

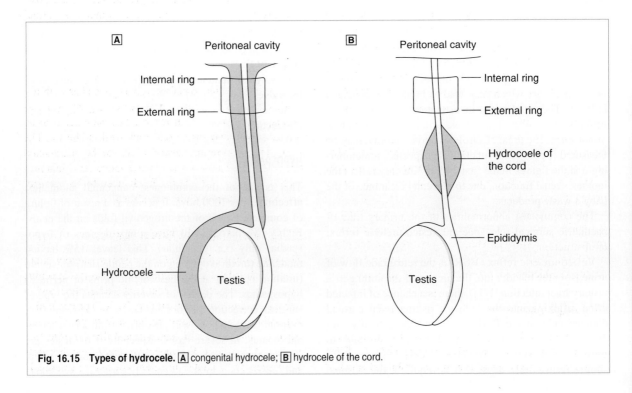

Fig. 16.15 Types of hydrocele. A congenital hydrocele; B hydrocele of the cord.

undescended testis. This can lead to the testis being located anywhere along the line of normal descent, down the posterior abdominal wall, in the inguinal canal or in the upper scrotum. If the testis descends, but to an abnormal position, it is called ectopic. Ectopic testes are very uncommon, but can be found in the perineum, in the upper part of the femoral triangle in the thigh, at the base of the penis, or in the anterior abdominal wall. An undescended testis usually has a patent processus vaginalis associated with it.

The surgical procedure for an undescended testis, an orchidopexy, is similar in principle to a hernia operation. The operation is done via a groin approach, the testis is located, and separated from the PPV. The testis is then mobilised further on the spermatic cord to allow enough length for the testis to be placed in a scrotal pouch.

PHYSIOLOGICAL RESPONSE OF THE NEONATE TO ANAESTHESIA AND SURGERY

It is the greater understanding and application of the knowledge of the physiology of the neonate, of their response to life, illness and surgery, which has played the greatest part over the last 10–20 years to decrease the morbidity and mortality associated with surgery in the neonate.

From the moment of birth, the neonate has to adapt to extrauterine life, and this affects all physiological parameters and control mechanisms. These mechanisms are not as well developed as in adults, especially in a premature neonate, and these factors influence the response of the neonate to anaesthesia and to the stress of surgery.

APNOEA

Neonates have only just learnt to breathe independently, and their mechanisms to keep breathing under all conditions are not 100% reliable; this is even more so in premature neonates.

Apnoea is more likely if the baby has been hypoxic, is hypothermic, is septic, is under postsurgical stress or following anaesthesia. They must be kept under close monitoring and observation – especially if they have any analgesia which might depress their respiratory centre.

CARDIOVASCULAR SYSTEM

In utero, blood flows from the umbilical arteries to the placenta, where it is detoxified, oxygenated and filled with nutrition, and then returns via the umbilical vein and the ligamentum venosum, past the liver, to the inferior vena cava and the right atrium. From there most of it goes via the foramen ovale into the left atrium and ventricle, and via the ascending aorta and so on up to the head and upper limbs. Venous drainage from here returns to the heart via the superior vena cava and into the right ventricle and the pulmonary artery. From there most of it goes via the ductus arteriosus into the descending aorta to the body and lower limbs and on back to the placenta via the umbilical arteries (which arise from the iliac arteries). There is very little flow of blood through the pulmonary circulation.

Following delivery, umbilical blood flow stops after the cord is clamped, so there is no flow through the umbilical vein and right atrial pressure falls. At the same time, due to the baby's first breath, the pulmonary vascular bed opens and there is a decrease in pulmonary vascular resistance which leads to an increase in pulmonary flow (in utero this was unnecessary, as the blood was oxygenated via the placenta), and left atrial pressure consequently rises. This allows the functional closure of the foramen ovale. The ductus arteriosus also closes and normal neonatal circulation is established. Both the foramen ovale and the ductus arteriosus are initially only closed physiologically, and can reopen, especially under hypoxia, acid–base disturbance and stress — and these must be avoided during anaesthesia and surgery and postoperatively in order for the neonate to maintain normal circulation.

HEAT CONTROL

A large surface area to bodyweight ratio, and an inability to shiver (even when not paralysed during anaesthesia) predisposes neonates to heat loss. The baby needs to be nursed in an incubator, or under an overhead heater. The room temperature in theatre needs to be maintained above 26°C for a term neonate and above 30°C in a premature neonate. All infused fluids need to be warmed, and inspired gases must be humidified.

METABOLIC RESPONSE TO SURGICAL TRAUMA

The endocrine and metabolic response to surgery is not as well defined yet in babies and children as it is in adults. There is an increase in circulating adrenaline and a decrease in insulin, which initially leads to postoperative hyperglycaemia. The stress response to surgery is abolished by small doses of fentanyl, and this can lead to a more stable patient. Postoperative energy requirements are increased in adults, but they are only increased in children for the first 12 h. After those 12 h the resting energy requirements (REE) are the same as preoperatively, for the baby diverts growth energy to wound repair and healing. Consequently, unlike adults, children do not require an increase in their usual nutritional requirements postoperatively, but growth stops while healing occurs.

SEPSIS

All neonates are prone to sepsis, and their susceptibility is increased postoperatively. Sepsis alters their fluid balance requirements, their ability to resist apnoea, and their ability to control their acid–base equilibrium. The baby must be tested for sepsis at any time it is suspected, and appropriate broad spectrum antibiotics commenced intravenously before the culture results are available.

LIVER

The neonatal liver is immature, and cannot prevent hypoglycaemia as successfully as in older infants, and so their blood sugar level needs to be monitored regularly and maintained with dextrose infusions.

The liver is slower at breaking down drugs used in anaesthesia, analgesics and others, including antibiotics, and appropriate doses or dose intervals should be used. These are to be found in a neonatal formulary.

Clotting mechanisms are not fully developed, and haemorrhagic disease of the newborn can arise; all neonates must have intramuscular vitamin K preoperatively. If blood transfusions are given, calcium must be administered and the clotting checked and fresh frozen plasma prescribed if necessary.

PAIN CONTROL

It used to be thought that neonates did not feel pain, but this has now been disproved, and neonates are now also given adequate pain control.

This may be in the form of local or regional anaesthetic blocks, oral or rectal paracetamol (which is a very effective analgesic in babies), or opiates. It is essential to remember the effect of the latter on the respiratory centre and apnoea, and to keep the baby under close monitoring in a specialised unit with pulse oximetry and an apnoea alarm.

FLUID AND ELECTROLYTE BALANCE

The management of fluids and electrolytes and nutrition is crucial to the successful outcome of surgery at all ages. However, the smaller and the younger the patient, the less is the margin for error, and the understanding of fluids and electrolytes in neonatal and paediatric surgery is therefore of paramount importance.

From the moment of birth, the neonate has to adapt to extrauterine life, and requirements of fluid, calories and nutrients vary daily. Gestational age at birth also affects the ability of the neonate to adapt to the stresses of life, to sepsis and to surgery. In the normal full term neonate, 75% of the body is water, of which 35% is extracellular. In a 26 week gestation premature neonate, 86% of the body is water, of which 50% is extracellular. The fluid requirements for these two extremes vary when they are healthy, and vary more so if they are sick. The smaller the baby, the greater surface area it has relative to body weight, the more heat it loses and the more insensible water losses occur.

Maintenance fluid requirements are both age and weight dependent (Box 16.1), but maintenance electrolyte requirements are fairly constant (Table 16.1).

The circulating blood volume in a baby is 80–90 mL/kg, in an infant and child 80 mL/kg, and in an older child 70–80 mL/kg.

In a small baby, all fluid lost or gained must be recorded in order to keep an accurate balance. Frequent blood sampling for tests requiring 0.5–1.0 mL blood each time will soon lead to hypovolaemia as well as anaemia in an 800 g premature neonate, who has only about 75 mL of circulating blood. Infusions or bolus injections of antibiotics or other drugs (e.g. dopamine, morphine) will also soon add up and need to be subtracted from maintenance fluid, and is of course not nutritious.

Table 16.1 Maintenance fluid requirements (mL/kg per 24 h)				
(a) In normal neonates				
Day of life	Body weight			
	< 1000 g	1000–1500 g	1500–2000 g	> 2500 g
Day 1	100–120	80–100	60–80	50–70
Day 2	120–150	110–130	90–110	80–100
Day 3	150–170	140–160	120–140	100–120
Day 4	180–200	160–180	140–160	120–140
Day 5 +	180–200	180–200	150–180	140–160

(b) In children of 6 months and over
- 100 for up to 10 kg
- 50 for next 10 kg
- 25 for each subsequent kg

Table 16.2   Maintenance intravenous electrolyte requirements (all ages and weights)

Electrolyte	(mmol/kg per 24 h)
Sodium	2–5
Potassium	2–4
Chloride	2–4
Calcium	0.5–1.0
Magnesium	0.25–0.5
Phosphate	0.25–1.0

The reason babies needs less fluid when first born is that their renal function is not normal and they cannot excrete a water load. The reason a tiny baby needs more fluid than a heavier one is that the former's surface area is larger relative to its weight, and its insensible losses are greater. This applies also to full sized babies in comparison to larger children and young adults. Insensible losses are also increased, and must be compensated for, in babies who are under overhead heaters or under photo-therapy lights for jaundice. Sick or ventilated babies (who lie still!) have less insensible losses, and all these factors must be taken into account when calculating the baby's fluid requirements.

MAINTENANCE FLUID AND BASIC ELECTROLYTES

See Table 16.1 and Box 16.2. Maintenance fluid in a 1 week old, full term 3 kg neonate consists of 0.18% sodium chloride in dextrose solution, at 150 mL/kg per 24 h. This will provide maintenance water requirements, as well as normal sodium requirements at 4 mmol/kg per 24 h. Potassium is added (as potassium chloride) at 10 mmol per 500 mL of the dextrose/saline solution, and this will supply normal potassium requirements of 3 mmol/kg per 24 h.

The strength of dextrose used in a neonate is always 10% dextrose solution, as they need all the calories they can get; in older children, who have greater nutritional reserves, a 4% dextrose solution is used. The veins of babies and young children are much more tolerant of hypertonic solutions, and can therefore tolerate 10% dextrose solutions in their peripheral veins without problem. The fluid used for a neonate is therefore 0.18% sodium chloride in 10% dextrose solution with 10 mmol potassium chloride added to every 500 mL bag, infused at 150 mL/kg over 24 h.

Additional electrolytes

All neonates, but premature infants in particular, have low calcium and magnesium reserves, and will soon become hypocalcaemic and hypomagnesaemic unless this is also included in the maintenance fluids.

NUTRITION

A neonate's nutritional reserves are non-existent, and this is why any neonate that will not receive enteral nutrition (i.e. milk) for more than a day if premature, or 2 days if full term, must have parenteral nutrition. This will supply all the electrolytes, vitamins, trace elements as well as calories and protein that they need to allow survival, to improve postoperative healing as well as brain growth and development.

Babies that are sick or ventilated will require less water, as mentioned above. If they have cardiac or renal problems as well, they may also not handle water volume, and need less — but they still require their nutrition. Although the total fluid input may be decreased until they become able to handle water, their nutrition (electrolytes, calories, protein, trace elements and vitamins) must still be supplied in the reduced fluid volume available — remembering the water used to give the drugs needed. It is always a case of bartering between the fluid available and their nutritional needs.

Fortunately, as babies become infants and get bigger and older, they have more reserves, but they still need parenteral nutrition as soon as it becomes apparent that they will not be getting any oral nutrition for a few days.

Any patient who has had a surgical condition requiring

operation will have additional water and electrolyte losses which need to be considered on top of the maintenance requirements. If there are fluid losses from nasogastric tubes or into stoma bags, these can be measured, and must be replaced mL for mL — nasogastric losses with 0.9% sodium chloride solution, and stoma losses with 0.45% sodium chloride solution with 10 mmol potassium choride in each 500 ml. The effect of a postoperative ileus on any abdomen is to encourage sodium into the static loops of bowel, and the patient becomes effectively hyponatraemic. This is compensated for by using 0.45% sodium chloride rather than 0.18% as the maintenance fluid for a baby or child with postoperative ileus.

This leads to a very simple postoperative fluid regime for those patients who have an ileus: 0.45% sodium chloride in 5% or 10% dextrose solution (the concentration depends on age, 10% dextrose being used up to the age of 6 months) with 10 mmol potassium chloride in every 500 mL. The basic volume is weight dependent (see Table 16.1). All additional losses need to be replaced as described above.

Regular monitoring of the serum electrolyte levels and osmolality, as well as urine electrolytes and osmolality, will enable the patient's fluid and electrolyte status to be maintained accurately.

All paediatric patients must be considered for parenteral nutrition early.

17

Alimentary system

Andrew T Raftery

ANATOMY

Although not part of the alimentary system, the anatomy of the abdominal wall and peritoneal cavity is described here, as it is important in the surgical approach to the alimentary system.

ANTERIOR ABDOMINAL WALL

Fasciae of the anterior abdominal wall

There is only superficial fascia on the abdominal wall. This forms two layers in the lower abdomen, a superficial layer of fatty tissue (Camper's fascia) and a deeper fibrous layer (Scarpa's fascia). Scarpa's fascia is attached to the deep fascia of the thigh about 2.5 cm below the inguinal ligament. It extends into the perineum as Colles' fascia, which is attached to the perineal body, perineal membrane and laterally to the rami of the pubis and the ischium. Scarpa's fascia also extends onto the penis and scrotum. These attachments are important when considering the effect of rupture of the bulbous urethra. Urine will track into the scrotum, perineum and penis and into the lower abdominal wall deep to the plane of Scarpa's fascia. However, it does not track into the thigh, because of the attachment of Scarpa's fascia to the deep fascia of the thigh. Likewise, an ectopic testis in the groin does not descend any lower into the thigh because of this attachment.

Muscles of the anterior abdominal wall

A knowledge of the anatomy of the muscles of the abdominal wall (Fig. 17.1) is a prerequisite to understanding the basis of abdominal incisions. The abdominal wall consists principally of three sheets of muscle which are fleshy laterally, and aponeurotic in front and behind. As the aponeuroses pass forward they ensheath the rectus abdominis muscle.

Rectus abdominis

This is a vertical muscle on either side of the midline. It arises from the fifth, sixth and seventh costal cartilages and is inserted into the pubic crest. The anterior aspect of the muscle bears three transverse tendinous intersections: one at the level of the xiphoid, one at the level of the umbilicus, and one half way between these two points. They are adherent to the anterior rectus sheath but not to the posterior sheath.

The lateral muscles of the abdominal wall are the external oblique, the internal oblique, and transversus abdominis.

External oblique

This arises from the outer surface of the lower eight ribs and is inserted into the linea alba (which runs between the xiphoid and the pubis), the pubic crest and pubic tubercle, and into the anterior half of the iliac crest. Between the anterior superior iliac spine and pubic tubercle, its lower recurved aponeurotic border forms the inguinal ligament.

Internal oblique

This arises from the lumbar fascia, the anterior two thirds of the iliac crest, and the lateral two thirds of the inguinal ligament. The majority of its fibres run upwards and medially (at right angles to those of external oblique) and are inserted into the lower six costal cartilages and the linea alba. The lower fibres are attached to the pubic crest by the conjoint tendon common to internal oblique and transversus abdominis.

Transversus abdominis

This arises from the deep surface of the lower six costal cartilages (interdigitating with the diaphragm), the lumbar fascia, the anterior two thirds of the iliac crest, and the lateral third of the inguinal ligament. It is inserted into the linea alba and into the pubic crest by the conjoint tendon.

Nerve supply

The rectus abdominis is supplied by the lower six thoracic nerves, as also is the external oblique. The internal

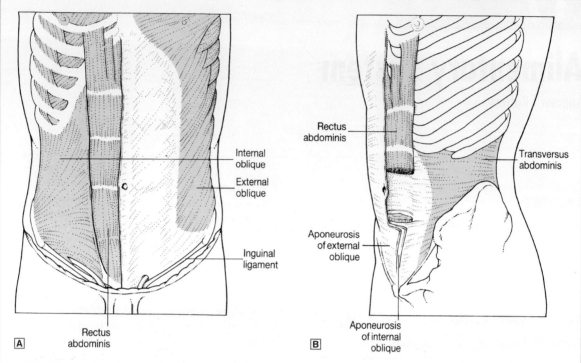

Fig. 17.1 The muscles of the anterior abdominal wall. A anterior view; B oblique view. From Rogers A W 1992 Textbook of anatomy; Churchill Livingstone, Edinburgh.

oblique and transversus are, in addition, supplied by the iliohypogastric and ilioinguinal nerves.

Rectus sheath

The rectus sheath (Fig. 17.2) is composed largely of the aponeuroses of the lateral abdominal muscles. It is deficient in certain areas, as follows.

1. Above the costal margin, the anterior sheath is composed of the external oblique aponeurosis only. The costal cartilages are behind.
2. From the costal margin to a point midway between the umbilicus and pubic symphysis, the anterior rectus sheath is composed of the external oblique aponeurosis and the anterior leaf of the internal oblique aponeurosis. The posterior leaf of the internal oblique aponeurosis and the aponeurosis of transversus abdominis form the posterior rectus sheath.
3. Below a point midway between the umbilicus and pubic symphysis, all aponeuroses pass in front of the rectus to form the anterior rectus sheath. It is deficient behind, where there is only transversalis fascia and peritoneum.

The lower border of the posterior aponeurotic part of the rectus sheath is marked by a crescentic free margin, the arcuate line of Douglas. At this point, the inferior epigastric vessels enter the sheath, passing upwards to anastomose with the superior epigastric vessels. The rectus sheaths fuse in the midline to form the linea alba, which runs from the xiphisternum to the pubic symphysis.

ANATOMY OF ABDOMINAL INCISIONS

The anatomy of the common abdominal incisions only will be described.

Midline incision

This is made through the linea alba skirting the umbilicus. It is an excellent incision for both routine and rapid access to the peritoneal cavity, the linea alba being almost a bloodless line. Structures encountered include skin, subcutaneous fat, linea alba, extraperitoneal fat and peritoneum.

Subcostal incision (Kocher's incision)

The subcostal incision is used most commonly on the

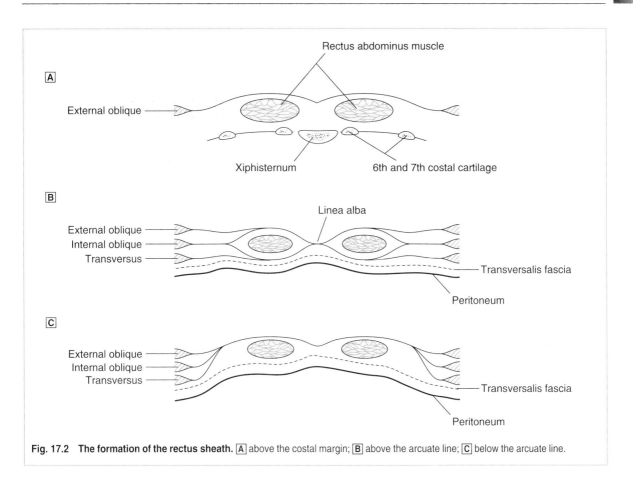

Fig. 17.2   The formation of the rectus sheath. Ⓐ above the costal margin; Ⓑ above the arcuate line; Ⓒ below the arcuate line.

right hand side for open cholecystectomy. On the left side it is used for elective splenectomy. On both sides it may be used to expose the kidneys. The incision is carried out about 2.5 cm below and parallel to the costal margin extending laterally from the midline. Structures encountered include skin, subcutaneous fat, anterior rectus sheath which is opened in the line of the incison, the rectus muscle and the posterior rectus sheath with the adherent extraperitoneal fat and peritoneum. The ninth intercostal nerve is in danger in the lateral part of the wound. Damage to this may cause weakness and atrophy of the rectus, with predisposition to incisional hernia formation.

Grid iron incision (muscle-splitting incision)
The incision is centred on McBurney's point (two thirds of the way along a line drawn from the umbilicus to the anterior superior iliac spine) and at right angles to this line. Structures encountered include skin, subcutaneous fat, Scarpa's fascia (at the lower end of the incision),

external oblique aponeurosis (which is incised in the line of its aponeurotic fibres), the internal oblique and transversus muscles (which are split in the line of their fibres). Finally, extraperitoneal fat and peritoneum are reached.

Paramedian incision
The use of this incision is declining. It is placed about 2.5 cm lateral to, and parallel to, the midline. The anterior rectus sheath is opened, the rectus displaced laterally, and the posterior sheath together with the peritoneum is incised. The anterior rectus sheath adheres to the muscle at the tendinous intersections, and the sheath requires to be dissected off at this point. Bleeding will be encountered in doing this, as the segmental vessels enter at these points. The rectus is not attached to the posterior sheath. The upper posterior rectus sheath is a thick, well-defined structure, but below a point half way between the umbilicus and pubic symphysis it is composed of transversalis fascia only and is relatively thin. The inferior epigastric vessels anastomosing with the superior epigastric ves-

sels, may be seen posterior to the muscle and may require dividing in a lower paramedian incision.

Pararectus incison (Battle incision)

An incision is made at the lateral border of rectus abdominis below the level of the umbilicus, and the rectus is displaced medially. It was once popular for appendicectomy, but the disadvantage is that if the wound is extended vertically it may damage the nerves entering the rectus sheath to supply the rectus muscle. The use of the pararectus incision is increasing for open insertion of a Tenckhoff catheter for continuous ambulatory peritoneal dialysis.

INGUINAL CANAL

The inguinal canal (Fig. 17.3) is an oblique passage in the lower part of the abdominal wall which transmits the spermatic cord and ilio-inguinal nerve in the male, and the round ligament of the uterus and the ilio-inguinal nerve in the female. It is approximately 4 cm long and passes downwards and medially from the deep inguinal ring to the superficial inguinal ring lying above and parallel to the inguinal ligament.

Relations

Anteriorly lie skin, Camper's fascia, Scarpa's fascia and the external oblique aponeurosis along the full length of the canal. The arching fibres of internal oblique form the anterior wall in the lateral third of the canal.

Posteriorly lie the conjoint tendon medially and the transversalis fascia laterally. Above are the arching fibres of internal oblique and transversus abdominis. Below lies the recurved lower edge of the external oblique aponeurosis, i.e. the inguinal ligament.

The deep inguinal ring is a defect in the transversalis fascia lying 1 cm above the midpoint of the inguinal ligament. It lies immediately lateral to the inferior epigastric vessels. The superficial inguinal ring is a V-shaped defect in the external oblique aponeurosis and lies above and medial to the pubic tubercle.

Spermatic cord

As it passes through the canal, the spermatic cord obtains

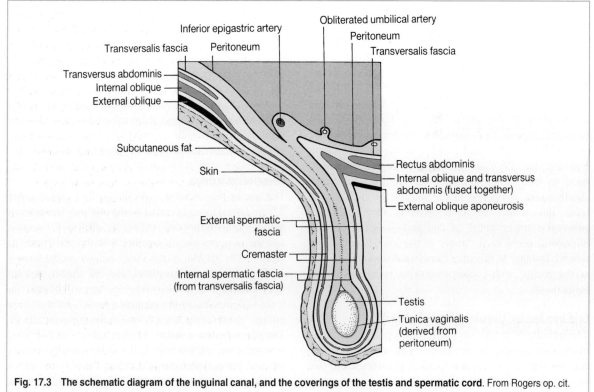

Fig. 17.3 **The schematic diagram of the inguinal canal, and the coverings of the testis and spermatic cord**. From Rogers op. cit.

three coverings: (i) the external spermatic fascia from the external oblique aponeurosis at the superficial inguinal ring; (ii) the cremasteric fascia from the internal oblique containing the cremaster muscle; (iii) the internal spermatic fascia from the transversalis fascia. The cord contains the testicular artery, the pampiniform plexus of veins, and the vas deferens. Other structures include the cremasteric artery, the artery to the vas, the nerve to cremaster, sympathetic nerve fibres and lymphatics. The ilio-inguinal nerve lies on the cord but is not part of it.

FEMORAL CANAL

The femoral artery and femoral vein enter the femoral triangle deep to the inguinal ligament within a prolongation of fascia termed the femoral sheath. This is derived from the transversalis fascia anteriorly, and posteriorly from the fascia covering iliacus. The medial part of the femoral sheath is occupied by the femoral canal. The upper opening of the femoral canal is called the femoral ring and will just admit the tip of the little finger in the male. In the female the pelvis is wider and the canal therefore is larger, and femoral herniae are consequently more common in the female. The boundaries of the femoral ring are:

- anteriorly, the inguinal ligament
- posteriorly, the pectineal ligament (of Astley Cooper); this runs along the pectineal border of the superior pubic ramus
- laterally, the femoral vein
- medially, the lacunar ligament (of Gimbernat). An abnormal obturator artery occasionally runs in close relationship to the lacunar ligament and is a danger during surgery.

The femoral canal contains fat, some lymphatics and a lymph node (Cloquet's node). The canal functions as a dead space for expansion of the femoral vein and secondly as a pathway for lymphatics from the lower limb to the external iliac nodes. The femoral ring is narrow, and the lacunar ligament forms a sharp medial border. Because of this, irreducibility and strangulation occur commonly with femoral hernias. Also, femoral hernias are likely to be of the Richter's type.

SURGICAL ANATOMY OF HERNIAS

An indirect hernia passes through the deep inguinal ring and along the inguinal canal and reaches the scrotum if it is very large. The hernial sac is covered by the layers of the cord. A direct inguinal hernia bulges directly through the posterior wall of the inguinal canal medial to the inferior epigastric artery. It bulges through Hesselbach's triangle, bounded by the inferior epigastric artery laterally, the inguinal ligament inferiorly, and the lateral border of rectus abdominis medially. Distinction between the two types of hernia at operation relates to the relationship to the inferior epigastric vessels. An indirect sac lies laterally, a direct hernia medial to the vessels.

Prior to surgery an attempt may be made to distinguish between the two types of hernia and between a femoral and an inguinal hernia. If an inguinal hernia protrudes through the superficial ring, it can be felt above and medial to the pubic tubercle. A femoral hernia is felt below and lateral to the pubic tubercle. If a hernia descends into the scrotum it is almost always an indirect inguinal hernia. If an inguinal hernia is reducible then application of pressure by the finger over the deep inguinal ring should control the hernia when the patient coughs if it is an indirect inguinal hernia. However, if the hernia appears medial to the point of finger pressure then it is a direct hernia.

PERITONEAL CAVITY

The peritoneum is the serous membrane of the abdominal cavity. It consists of a parietal layer lining the abdominal and pelvic walls, and a visceral layer which more or less covers the contained organs. In the male the peritoneal cavity is a closed sac, but in the female the free extremities of the uterine tubes open into the cavity, constituting a possible pathway of infection from the exterior. The peritoneal cavity is subdivided into a main cavity, the greater sac, and a small cavity, the lesser sac (omental bursa). The greater sac is further divided by the transverse colon into a supracolic and infracolic compartment. The connection between the greater and lesser sac is known as the epiploic foramen or the foramen of Winslow.

The attachments of the peritoneum are complicated. It is convenient to start at the umbilicus and work down. Below the level of the umbilicus, the parietal peritoneum is smooth apart from some folds (Fig. 17.4). These are the median umbilical fold on the median umbilical ligament (which is due to the obliterated urachus passing from the bladder to the umbilicus), the medial umbilical folds on the obliterated umbilical arteries, and the lateral umbilical folds which are further lateral and contain the inferior epigastric arteries. The peritoneum of the pelvis is continuous with that of the abdominal cavity. It completely encloses the sigmoid colon, forming the pelvic mesocolon. It is applied to the front and side of the upper third of the rectum and to the front only of the middle

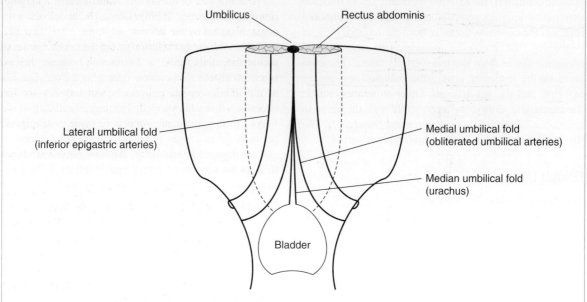

Umbilicus

Rectus abdominis

Lateral umbilical fold
(inferior epigastric arteries)

Medial umbilical fold
(obliterated umbilical arteries)

Median umbilical fold
(urachus)

Bladder

Fig. 17.4   The posterior surface of the lower part of the anterior abdominal wall, showing the median, medial and lateral umbilical folds.

third of the rectum. It is then reflected in the male onto the base and upper part of the bladder, forming the rectovesical pouch. In the female the peritoneum is reflected from the side and front of the rectum, to the upper part of the posterior wall of the vagina and then over the posterior upper and anterior surface of the uterus to the bladder. Between the uterus and the rectum is the recto-uterine pouch (of Douglas). The peritoneum passes off the lateral margins of the uterus to the pelvic wall, forming the broad ligaments, the upper borders of which contain the uterine tubes. The free upper margins of the broad ligament lateral to the uterine tubes form the infundibulopelvic fold.

Returning to the umbilicus, the falciform ligament, the sickle-shaped fold of peritoneum, passes upwards and slightly to the right of the midline to the liver. It contains the ligamentum teres, i.e. the obliterated umbilical vein, in its free edge, and this passes into the groove between the quadrate lobe and left lobe of the liver. Traced superiorly the two layers of the falciform ligament diverge from each other, the right limb joins the upper layer of the coronary ligament while the left layer passes to the left to form the anterior layer of the left triangular ligament. Elsewhere on the anterior abdominal wall, above the umbilicus, the peritoneum sweeps upwards and over the inferior aspect of the diaphragm to be reflected onto the liver and onto the right margin of the abdominal oeso-

phagus. Details of the peritoneal reflections of the liver are described in the section on the liver. After enclosing the liver the peritoneum descends from the porta hepatis as a double layer, i.e. the lesser omentum, and then this separates to enclose the stomach. It reforms again at the greater curve and then loops downwards, again turning upwards and attaching to the length of the transverse colon, forming the greater omentum (Fig. 17.5).

The lower leaf of the greater omentum then continues upwards, enclosing the transverse colon within the peritoneum, and then passes upwards and backwards as the transverse mesocolon, a double layer of peritoneum, to the posterior abdominal wall, where it attaches along the anterior aspect of the pancreas. At the base of the transverse mesocolon, this double layer of peritoneum divides once again, the upper leaf passing upwards over the posterior abdominal wall to reflect onto the liver, while the lower leaf passes over the lower part of the posterior abdominal wall to cover the pelvic viscera and to join with the peritoneum of the anterior abdominal wall. However, the peritoneum of the posterior abdominal wall is interrupted as it is reflected along the small bowel from the duodenal jejunal flexures to the ileocaecal junction, forming the mesentery of the small intestine. The lines of peritoneal reflection on the posterior abdominal wall are shown in Figure 17.6.

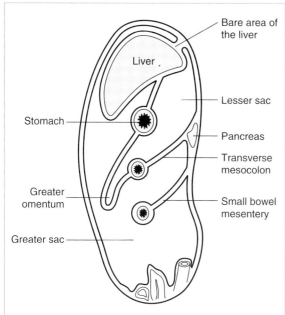

Fig. 17.5 A longitudinal section of the peritoneal cavity, showing the lesser and greater sacs and the peritoneal reflexions.

The lesser sac (Fig. 17.7) is entered via the epiploic foramen or foramen of Winslow. The lesser sac is a potential space lying behind the lesser omentum and stomach and projecting downwards to the transverse mesocolon. Superiorly is the superior recess, whose anterior border is the caudate lobe of the liver. The left wall of the lesser sac is formed by the spleen and the gastrosplenic and lienorenal ligaments. To the right the sac opens into the main peritoneal cavity via the epiploic foramen.

The epiploic foramen has the following boundaries (Fig. 17.8).

- Anteriorly lies the free edge of the lesser omentum, containing the bile duct to the right, the hepatic artery to the left and the portal vein behind. The hepatic artery can be compressed between finger and thumb in the free edge of the lesser omentum. This is known as Pringle's manoeuvre and is useful if the cystic artery is torn during cholecystectomy or there is haemorrhage from the liver following trauma.
- Posteriorly lies the inferior vena cava.
- Inferiorly lies the first part of the duodenum.
- Superiorly lies the caudate process of the liver.

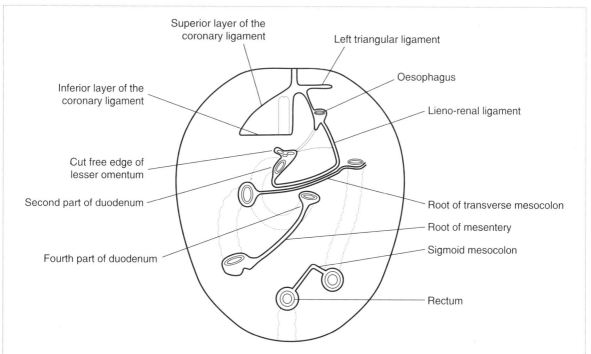

Fig. 17.6 The posterior abdominal wall. The lines of reflexion of the peritoneum are shown. The liver, stomach, spleen and intestines have been removed.

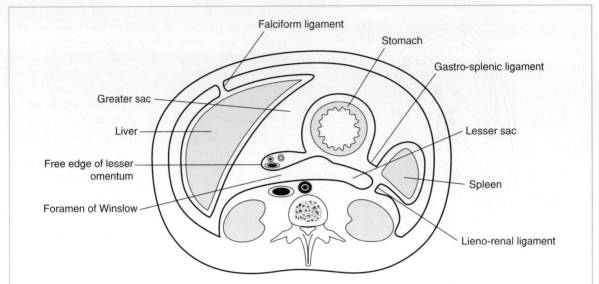

Fig. 17.7 A transverse section through the peritoneal cavity at the level of the foramen of Winslow (epiploic foramen), showing the peritoneal relations.

Subphrenic spaces

There are a number of potential spaces below the diaphragm in relation to the liver which may become the site of abscess formation (a subphrenic abscess). Abscesses may arise from such lesions as perforated peptic ulcers, perforated appendicitis, or perforated diverticulitis. Only two

of the spaces are in fact directly subphrenic, the other two being subhepatic. The right and left subphrenic spaces lie between the diaphragm and the liver and are separated from one another by the falciform ligament. The right subhepatic space (pouch of Rutherford Morrison) is bounded by the posterior abdominal wall behind and by the liver above. The gall bladder, duodenum and right kidney are immediate relations. The left subhepatic space is the lesser sac itself. It may distend with fluid as a result of a perforated posterior gastric ulcer or as a result of acute pancreatitis (pseudocyst of the pancreas). At the present time most subphrenic abscesses are drained percutaneously under ultrasound control. However, the occasional one still requires open surgery and may be accessed if they are posteriorly placed by an incision below or through the bed of the twelfth rib. If they are placed anteriorly they can be drained through an incision below and parallel to the costal margin.

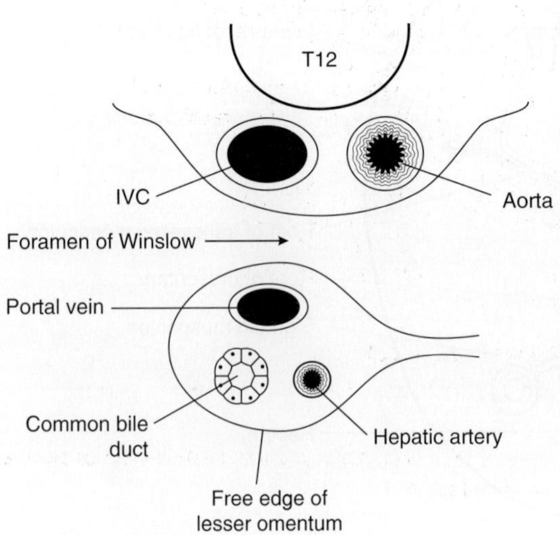

OESOPHAGUS

The oesophagus (Fig. 17.9) extends from the lower border of the cricoid cartilage to the cardiac orifice of the stomach. It is about 25 cm long. It has three parts: cervical, thoracic and abdominal.

Cervical

See Figure 17.10. The oesophagus passes downwards

Fig. 17.8 A transverse section through the foramen of Winslow (epiploic foramen).

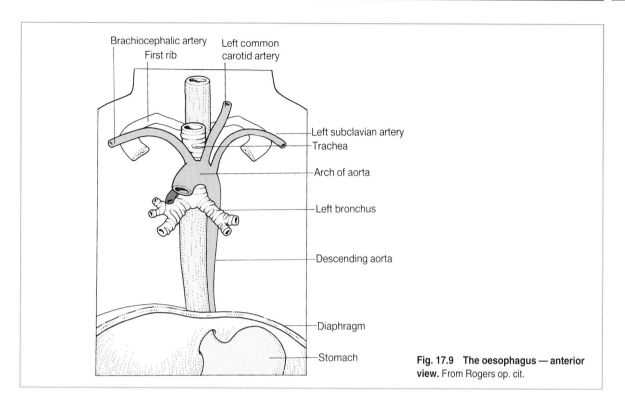

Fig. 17.9 The oesophagus — anterior view. From Rogers op. cit.

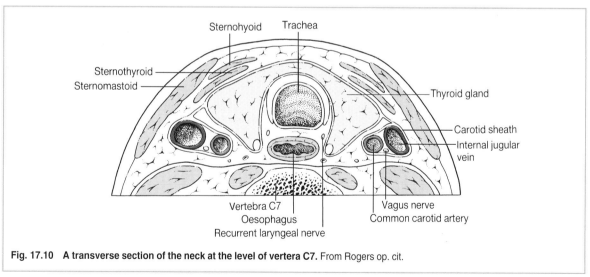

Fig. 17.10 A transverse section of the neck at the level of vertera C7. From Rogers op. cit.

and slightly to the left. Anteriorly lie the trachea and thyroid gland. Posteriorly lie the lower cervical vertebrae and the prevertebral fascia; to the left lie the left common carotid artery, the left inferior thyroid artery, the left subclavian artery and the thoracic duct; to the right the right common carotid artery. The recurrent laryngeal nerves lie on either side in the groove between the trachea and the oesophagus.

Thoracic

See Figure 17.11. The oesophagus passes down through the superior and posterior mediastinum, passing initially

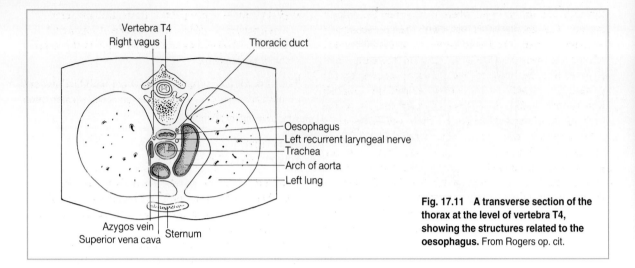

Vertebra T4
Right vagus
Thoracic duct
Oesophagus
Left recurrent laryngeal nerve
Trachea
Arch of aorta
Left lung
Azygos vein
Superior vena cava
Sternum

Fig. 17.11 A transverse section of the thorax at the level of vertebra T4, showing the structures related to the oesophagus. From Rogers op. cit.

to the right to reach the midline opposite T5. It then passes downwards, forwards, and to the left to reach the oesophageal opening in the diaphragm at T10. The two vagus nerves form a plexus on the surface of the oesophagus in the posterior mediastinum, the left nerve being anterior and the right posterior.

Anteriorly lie the left common carotid artery, the trachea, the left main bronchus which constricts it, the pericardium separating it from the left atrium and the diaphragm. Posteriorly lie the thoracic vertebrae, the thoracic duct, the hemiazygos vein, and below, the descending aorta.

On the left side lie the left subclavian artery, the aortic arch, the left vagus nerve and its recurrent laryngeal branch, the thoracic duct and the left pleura. On the right side lie the pleura and azygos vein.

Abdominal

The oesophagus passes through the oesophageal opening in the right crus of the diaphragm at the level of T10. It then lies in a groove on the posterior surface of the left lobe of the liver, with the left crus of the diaphragm behind. It is covered anteriorly and to the left with peritoneum. The anterior vagus nerve is closely applied to its surface behind its peritoneal covering. The posterior vagus nerve is at a little distance from the posterior surface of the oesophagus.

Blood supply

In the neck it is from the inferior thyroid arteries, in the thorax from branches of the aorta, and in the abdomen from the left gastric and inferior phrenic arteries. Venous drainage of the cervical part is to the inferior thyroid veins; of the thoracic part to the azygos veins; and the

abdominal part partly to the azygos vein (systemic) and partly to the left gastric veins (portal).

Nerves

The upper third of the oesophagus is supplied with parasympathetic fibres via the recurrent laryngeal nerve and sympathetic fibres from the middle cervical ganglion via the inferior thyroid artery. Below the root of the lung the vagi and sympathetic nerves contribute to the oesophageal plexus.

Microscopical structure

The oesophagus consists of: (i) a mucous membrane lined by stratified squamous epithelium; occasionally there is gastric mucosa in the lower part of the oesophagus; (ii) a submucosa containing mucous glands; (iii) a muscular layer consisting of inner circular and outer longitudinal muscle; in the upper third it is striated, producing rapid contraction and swallowing; in the lower two thirds it is smooth, exhibiting peristalsis; (iv) an outer layer of loose areolar tissue.

STOMACH

The stomach is approximately J shaped, having two surfaces: the anterior and posterior. It has two curvatures — the greater and lesser curve — and two orifices: the cardia and the pylorus. Initially the stomach projects to the left, the dome-like gastric fundus projecting above the level of the cardia. In the erect living subject the vertical part of the J shape of the stomach represents the upper two thirds of the stomach. The lesser curvature of the stomach is vertical in its upper two thirds but then turns upwards and to the right, where it becomes the pyloric antrum. The junction of the body with the pyloric antrum is marked along the lesser curve by a distinct notch termed the incisura angularis. Between the cardia and pylorus lies the body of the stomach, leading to the pyloric antrum which is a narrow area of the stomach immediately before the pylorus. The left margin of the body of the stomach is the greater curvature. In the erect subject this may reach or lie below the umbilicus. It then passes upwards to the right as the lower margin of the pyloric antrum. To the lesser curvature of the stomach is attached the lesser omentum and to the greater curvature the greater omentum, which to the left is continuous with the gastrosplenic ligament. The thickened pyloric sphincter is easily palpable at surgery and surrounds the pyloric canal. The junction of the pylorus with the duodenum is marked by a constant prepyloric vein of Mayo which crosses it vertically at this level. Unlike the cardiac sphincter of the stomach the pyloric sphincter is well marked anatomically.

Relations of the stomach

Relations are:

- anteriorly — from left to right, the diaphragm, abdominal wall and left lobe of the liver

- posteriorly — it is separated from the diaphragm, aorta, pancreas, spleen, left kidney and suprarenal gland, transverse mesocolon, and colon by the lesser sac of peritoneum.

The stomach lies in the epigastric and umbilical regions of the abdomen but, when distended, encroaches upon the left hypochondrium.

Blood supply

Blood supply (Fig. 17.12) is via:

- the left gastric artery, which is derived from the coeliac axis and runs along the lesser curvature of the stomach, where it anastomoses with the right gastric branch of the hepatic artery
- the right gastric artery from the hepatic artery
- the right gastroepiploic artery; this arises from the gastroduodenal branch of the hepatic artery and anastomoses along the greater curvature with the left gastroepiploic artery
- the left gastroepiploic artery, arising from the splenic artery
- the short gastric arteries arising from the splenic artery.

The veins are named according to the arteries. The venous drainage is into the portal system. The stomach

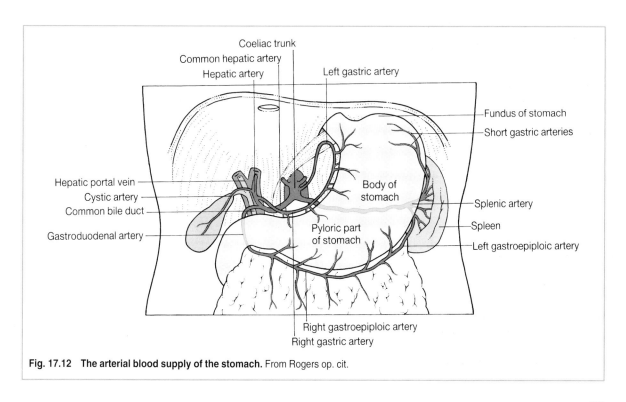

Fig. 17.12 The arterial blood supply of the stomach. From Rogers op. cit.

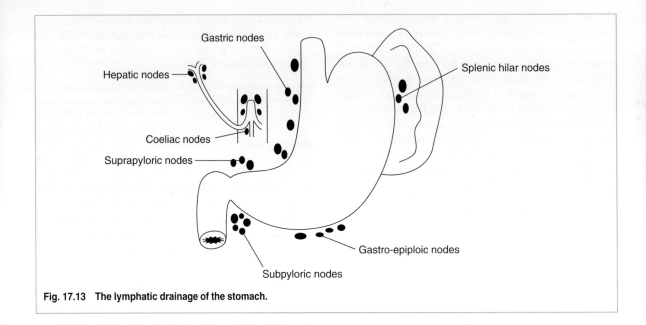

Gastric nodes

Hepatic nodes

Splenic hilar nodes

Coeliac nodes

Suprapyloric nodes

Gastro-epiploic nodes

Subpyloric nodes

Fig. 17.13   The lymphatic drainage of the stomach.

has such a rich blood supply that any three of the four main arteries may be ligated without any compromise of the arterial blood supply to the stomach.

Lymphatic drainage

The arrangements of lymph nodes in relation to the stomach is shown in Figure 17.13. The lymphatic drainage of the stomach accompanies its blood vessels. The area of the stomach supplied by the splenic artery drains via lymphatics accompanying that artery to the lymph nodes of the hilum of the spleen, then to those situated along the upper border of the pancreas and eventually to the coeliac nodes. The cardiac area of the stomach drains along the left gastric artery to reach the coeliac nodes. The remainder of the stomach drains as follows: via branches of the hepatic artery through nodes along the lesser curve to the coeliac nodes and along the right gastroepiploic vessels to the subpyloric nodes and then to the coeliac nodes. Retrograde spread may occur into the hepatic lymph nodes at the porta hepatis. Enlargements of these nodes may cause external compression of the bile ducts to produce obstructive jaundice. The extensive and complex lymphatic drainage of the stomach creates problems in dealing with gastric cancer. Involvement of the nodes around the coeliac axis may render the growth incurable.

Nerve supply

The clinically important nerve supply (Fig. 17.14) of the stomach is the vagus nerves. The anterior and posterior vagus nerves enter the abdomen through the oesophageal hiatus. The anterior vagus nerve lies close to the wall of the oesophagus and upper part of the stomach, but the posterior nerve is at a little distance from it. The anterior vagus runs caudally and supplies the anterior surface and lesser curve of the stomach. Before it reaches the stomach, it gives off a hepatic branch which passes in the lesser omentum to the liver and gall bladder and the pyloric branch to the pyloric sphincter. The posterior vagus nerve gives off a coeliac branch which passes to the coeliac plexus before sending a gastric branch to the posterior surface of the stomach. The gastric divisions of both anterior and posterior vagi reach the stomach at the cardia and descend along the lesser curve between the anterior and posterior peritoneal attachments of the lesser omentum. These nerves are referred to as the anterior and posterior nerves of Latarjet.

The vagus nerves used to be divided in operations for peptic ulceration. However, with the advent of H_2 receptor antagonists and proton pump inhibitors and the discovery of the role of *H. pylori* in the aetiology of peptic ulceration, these operations are performed less and less. However, it is necessary to understand the role of the vagus, as vagotomy is still required in surgery for bleeding peptic ulcer, and also a knowledge of the oesophageal hiatus and the relations of the vagus nerve is required so that these nerves are not inadvertently damaged in repair of hiatus hernia. The vagus nerve constitutes both the

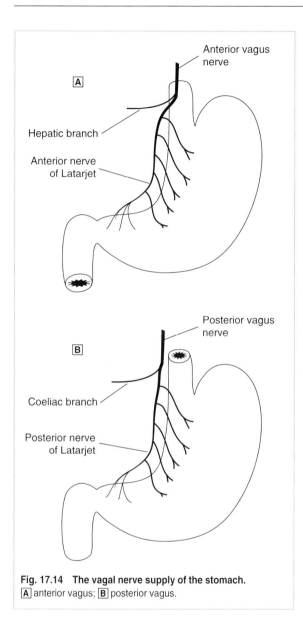

Fig. 17.14 The vagal nerve supply of the stomach.
A anterior vagus; B posterior vagus.

tomy) it is possible to avoid the drainage procedure, as the nerve of Latarjet remains intact and this maintains the innervation of the pyloric antrum and hence its propulsive activity.

Structure of the gastric mucosa

The surface of the gastric mucosa is covered by columnar epithelial cells that secrete mucus and alkaline fluid that protects the epithelium from mechanical injury and from gastric acid. The surface of the mucosa is studded with gastric pits, each pit being the opening of a duct into which the gastric glands empty. The gastric mucosa can be divided into three areas. The cardiac gland area is the small segment located near the gastro-oesophageal junction. Histologically it contains principally mucus-secreting cells, although occasionally a few parietal (oxyntic) cells are present. The remainder of the stomach is divided into the acid-secreting region (oxyntic gland area) and the pyloric gland area. The oxyntic gland area is the portion containing the parietal (oxyntic cells) and the chief (zymogen) cells. The pyloric end area constitutes the distal 30% of the stomach and contains G cells that produce gastrin. In this region there are few oxyntic and peptic cells, mucus-secreting cells predominating. As in the rest of the gastrointestinal tract the muscular wall of the stomach is composed of an inner circular layer and an outer longitudinal layer. However, in addition there is an incomplete inner layer of obliquely situated fibres which is more prominent near the lesser curvature. Figure 17.15 shows the histological features of the mucosa in the oxyntic gland area. Each gastric pit drains between three and seven tubular gastric glands. The neck of the gland contains many mucus cells, oxyntic cells being most numerous in the midportion of the glands and chief cells predominating in the basal portion.

DUODENUM

The duodenum is C-shaped. It curves around the head of the pancreas and is approximately 25 cm long. The first 2–3 cm of the first part of the duodenum is completely covered with peritoneum, but then the duodenum becomes retroperitoneal. The duodenum is divided into four parts.

First part

This is approximately 5 cm long and it ascends from the pylorus, being directed superiorly, posteriorly and to the right. It has a complete investment of visceral peritoneum on its first 2–3 cm. Anteriorly lie the liver and gall bladder. Immediately posterior to it lie the portal vein,

motor and secretory nerve supply for the stomach, i.e. it is responsible for motility and control of gastric secretions. When the nerve is divided in the operation of vagotomy, acid secretion is cut down in the stomach, but so is motility, so that the stomach empties through an intact pylorus only with difficulty. Because of this, total vagotomy (truncal vagotomy) must always be accompanied by some form of drainage procedure: either a pyloroplasty to destroy the pyloric sphincter or a gastrojejunostomy to bypass the pyloric sphincter. In the operation of highly selective vagotomy (proximal selective vago-

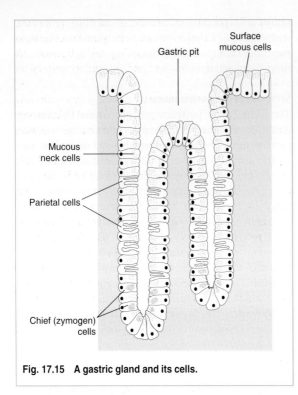

Fig. 17.15 A gastric gland and its cells.

the common bile duct and gastroduodenal artery. Behind these is the inferior vena cava. The relationship of the gastroduodenal artery to the first part of the duodenum is important because erosion of posterior duodenal ulcers into the gastroduodenal artery will cause haematemesis and melaena.

Second part

This descends in a curve around the head of the pancreas. It is approximately 7.5 cm long. The bile ducts and main pancreatic ducts enter the second part of the duodenum together at the duodenal papilla on its posteromedial side. The point of entry marks the junction of the foregut and midgut. The accessory pancreatic duct (of Santorini) opens into the duodenum a little above the papilla. The second part of the duodenum is crossed by the transverse colon and lies anteriorly to the right kidney and ureter.

Third part

The third part of the duodenum is approximately 10 cm long and runs horizontally to the left. It crosses the inferior vena cava, the aorta and the third lumbar vertebra. It is crossed anteriorly by the root of the mesentery and the superior mesenteric vessels.

Fourth part

This is approximately 2.5 cm long and ascends vertically to end by turning abruptly anteriorly and to the left to continue as the jejunum. At the duodenal-jejunal flexure the small intestine leaves the posterior abdominal wall and acquires a mesentery. At surgery the duodeno-jejunal flexure may be identified by the presence of the suspensory ligament of Treitz. This is a peritoneal fold descending from the right crus of the diaphragm to the termination of the duodenum.

Blood supply of the dudoenum

The superior pancreaticoduodenal artery, which arises from the gastroduodenal artery, anastomoses with the inferior pancreatico duodenal artery, which originates from the superior mesenteric artery. These two arteries both lie in the curve between the duodenum and the head of the pancreas, supplying both the duodenum and the head of the pancreas.

SMALL INTESTINE

The length of the small intestine is variable, averaging some 6 m in length. The upper half of the small intestine is termed the jejunum, the remainder being termed the ileum, although the distinction between the two is not sharply defined. The jejunum and ileum lie in the free edge of the mesentery. The mesentery of the small intestine is about 15 cm long and is attached across the posterior abdominal wall. It commences at the duodeno-jejunal juncture to the left of the second lumbar vertebrae and passes obliquely downwards to the right sacroiliac joint. From left to right the root of the mesentery crosses anterior to the following structures:

- the third part of the duodenum
- the aorta
- the inferior vena cava
- the right psoas major muscle
- the right ureter
- the right gonadal vessels
- the right iliacus muscle.

The mesentery contains the superior mesenteric vessels which enter the mesentery anterior to the third part of the duodenum, the lymph nodes draining the small intestine, and autonomic nerve fibres.

At surgery it is necessary to distinguish between the jejunum and the ileum. The following factors serve to distinguish the jejunum from the ileum.

- The jejunum has a thicker wall due to circular folds of mucosa (valvulae conniventes or plicae circulares) which are larger and more numerous in the jejunum than the ileum.

- The jejunum is of greater diameter than the ileum.
- In the mesentery of the jejunum the arteries form one or two arcades some distance from the free edge of the mesentery, and long straight branches from these arcades run to supply the jejunum. In the ileum the arterial supplies form several rows of arcades in the mesentery, and the final straight arteries to the ileum are shorter than in the jejunum.
- In general, the jejunum is most likely to be found at or above the level of the umbilicus, while the ileum tends to lie below the level of the umbilicus in the hypogastrium and pelvis.

LARGE INTESTINE

The large intestine extends from the ileocaecal junction to the anus. It is approximately 1.5 m in length on average. It consists of the caecum, ascending colon, transverse colon, descending colon, sigmoid colon and rectum. The caecum is a dilated blind-ended pouch situated in the right iliac fossa and is usually completely covered with peritoneum. The ileocaecal valve lies on the left side of the junction between the caecum and ascending colon. Tumours may grow to a large size in the caecum without causing any obstruction until they encroach on the ileocaecal junction. The appendix arises from the posteromedial aspect of the caecum about 2.5 cm below the ileocaecal valve. The taenia coli, three flattened bands of longitudinal muscle which pass from caecum to rectosigmoid, converge at the base of the appendix. The taenia are shorter than the length of the bowel hence the sacculated appearance of the large bowel.

The ascending colon extends from the caecum to the undersurface of the liver where, at the hepatic flexure, it turns left to become the transverse colon. It is covered on its anterior and lateral aspect by peritoneum. Posterior relations include iliacus, quadratus lumborum, and the perirenal fascia over the lateral aspect of the kidney.

The transverse colon passes to the left, where it becomes the descending colon at the splenic flexure. It is attached to the anterior border of the pancreas by the transverse mesocolon. Superiorly it is related to the liver, gall bladder, greater curvature of the stomach and the spleen. Inferiorly are coils of small intestine. Anteriorly lie the anterior layers of the greater omentum. Posteriorly lie the right kidney, second part of the duodenum, pancreas, small intestine and the left kidney.

The descending colon passes from the splenic flexure to the sigmoid colon. Peritoneum covers its anterior

and lateral surfaces. Between the splenic flexure and the diaphragm is a fold of peritoneum, the phrenicocolic ligament. Posteriorly to the descending colon lies the left kidney, quadratus lumborum and iliacus. Anteriorly lie coils of small bowel.

The sigmoid colon commences at the pelvic brim and extends to the rectosigmoid junction. It has a mesentery which occasionally is extensive allowing the sigmoid colon to hang down into the pelvis. The root of the sigmoid colon crosses the external iliac vessels and left ureter. The sigmoid loop rests on the bladder in the male and is related to the uterus and the posterior fornix of the vagina in the female. Hence the development of vesicocolic and vaginocolic fistulae in diverticular disease of the sigmoid colon. The taenia coli extend from the base of the appendix to the rectosigmoid junction. There are no taenia on the appendix or rectum. The colon, but neither the caecum, the appendix, nor rectum, possesses fat-filled peritoneal tags scattered along its surface. These are called appendices epiploicae and are most numerous in the sigmoid colon.

APPENDIX

The appendix is attached to the posteromedial aspect of the caecum below the ileocaecal valve. Its length varies considerably from one subject to another but usually is within the range 5–10 cm. It can be as small as 2.5 cm or as long as 25 cm. The position of the appendix is variable. In 75% of cases the appendix lies behind the caecum or colon, i.e. retrocaecal or retrocolic. In 20% of cases it hangs down into the pelvis, and in 5% of cases it is either pre-ileal or retro-ileal (Fig. 17.16). The appendix bears a mesentery containing the appendicular artery, which is a branch of the ileocolic artery. The mesentery of the appendix descends behind the ileum as a triangular fold containing the appendicular artery in its free border. The appendicular artery is functionally an end artery, and therefore in acute appendicitis, if it thromboses, there is a consequent rapid development of gangrene and perforation of the appendix.

RECTUM

The rectum is about 12 cm long, commencing anterior to the third segment of the sacrum and ending about 2.5 cm in front of the coccyx, where it bends sharply backwards to become the anal canal. It is extraperitoneal on its posterior aspect in its upper third and extraperitoneal on its posterior and lateral aspect in its middle third. The lower third is completely extraperitoneal lying below the pelvic

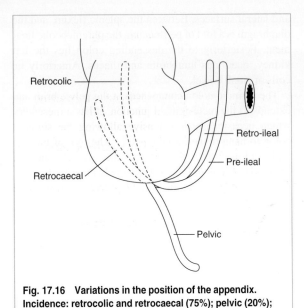

Fig. 17.16 Variations in the position of the appendix. Incidence: retrocolic and retrocaecal (75%); pelvic (20%); pre-ileal and retro-ileal (5%).

Labels in figure: Retrocolic, Retro-ileal, Pre-ileal, Retrocaecal, Pelvic

peritoneum. The rectum is curved to follow the contour of the sacral hollow. There are three lateral inflexions projected to the left, right and left again from above downwards. Each inflexion is capped by a valve of Houston.

The relations of the rectum are important in the understanding of a digital rectal examination and also in the spread of rectal cancer. Anteriorly in the male lies the recto-vesical pouch, the base of the bladder, seminal vesicles and the prostate. A layer of fascia (of Denonvilliers) lies in front of the rectum, separating it from the anterior structure, and this is the plane of dissection which must be sought during abdominoperineal excision of the rectum. In the female lies the recto-uterine pouch (of Douglas) and the posterior wall of the vagina. The upper two thirds of the rectum is covered with peritoneum anteriorly and related to coils of small bowel and the sigmoid colon in the rectovesical or recto-uterine pouch. Posteriorly lie the sacrum, coccyx and middle sacral artery. The lower sacral nerves also lie posteriorly and may be invaded by rectal cancer spreading posteriorly and resulting in sciatic pain. Laterally, below the peritoneal reflection, lie the levator ani and coccygeus.

Blood supply of the large intestine

The arterial blood supply of the large intestine is shown in Figure 17.17. The large intestine is supplied by both branches of the superior and inferior mesenteric artery.

The branches of the superior mesenteric artery are as follows:

- the ileocolic artery, which supplies the caecum and commencement of the ascending colon
- the right colic artery, supplying the ascending colon
- the middle colic artery, supplying the transverse colon.

The branches of the inferior mesenteric artery supplying the colon are:

- the left colic artery, supplying the descending colon
- the sigmoid branches, supplying the sigmoid colon
- the superior rectal artery, supplying the rectum.

Each branch of the superior and inferior mesenteric artery anastomoses with its neighbour above and below, thus establishing a continuous chain of anastomoses along the length of the colon, sometimes known as the marginal artery (of Drummond). A good collateral circulation can thus be established if one or more of the colic arteries is obstructed or divided. The marginal artery is weakest and sometimes deficient where the superior and inferior mesenteric distributions meet just proximal to the splenic flexure. Diminution of the blood supply in this region may lead to the condition known as ischaemic colitis. The marginal artery is also important in allowing the surgeon to transpose large segments of the colon as far as the neck or thorax to replace segments of oesophagus, the bowel depending on the marginal artery for its blood supply.

The superior rectal artery supplies the whole of the rectum and the upper half of the anal canal, while the inferior rectal supplies the lower half of the anal canal. The middle rectal artery is small and supplies only the muscle coats of the rectum. When the superior rectal artery reaches the rectum, it first divides into two branches which run either side and then the right branch divides further into two again. These branches descend to the level of the anal valves, where they anastomose with branches of the inferior rectal artery. They are accompanied by tributaries of the superior rectal vein which drain into the portal system. The position of these vessels, namely one on the left and two on the right, explain why haemorrhoids occur at 3, 7 and 11 o'clock when the anal canal is viewed with the patient in the lithotomy position.

Lymphatic drainage of the large intestine

Lymphatics drain to small lymph nodes lying near, or even on the bowel wall, and these drain to further groups of nodes lying along the blood vessels and then to groups of nodes situated near the origins of the superior and inferior mesenteric arteries. The efferent vessels from these

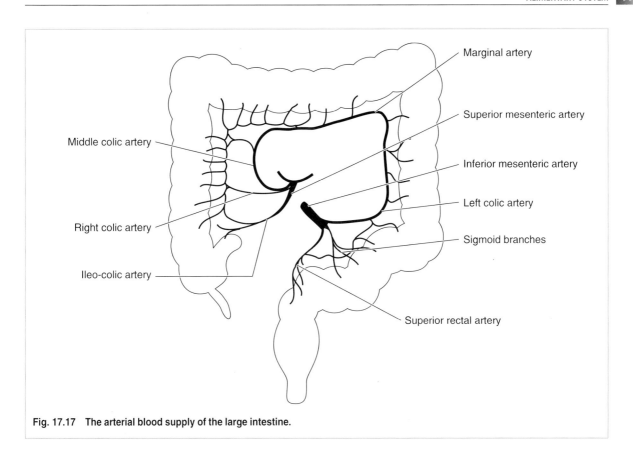

Fig. 17.17   The arterial blood supply of the large intestine.

Labels on figure: Marginal artery, Superior mesenteric artery, Inferior mesenteric artery, Left colic artery, Sigmoid branches, Superior rectal artery, Middle colic artery, Right colic artery, Ileo-colic artery

nodes join to drain into the cisterna chyli. The field of lymphatic drainage of each segment of bowel corresponds more or less to its arterial blood supply. High ligation of the vessels to the involved segment of bowel, with removal of a wide surrounding segment of the mesocolon and bowel wall, will result in the removal of lymph nodes draining that particular area. For example, division of the inferior mesenteric artery and resection of the sigmoid mesocolon would be performed for carcinoma of the sigmoid colon.

ANAL CANAL

The anal canal is about 4 cm long and passes downwards and backwards. It is surrounded by a complex arrangement of sphincters consisting of smooth and striated muscle. The lining of the anal canal is also complex. At the midpoint of the canal there is a series of vertical columns in the mucosa (the columns of Morgani). At their distal end are some valve-like folds (the anal valves of Ball). Behind these small anal valves are the anal sinuses, into which open the anal glands. The epithelium of the upper half of the anal canal is columnar epithelium, but at a point about midway down the canal, just below the anal valves, the epithelium changes to stratified squamous epithelium, and lower down further, near the anal verge, this is transformed into skin. The boundaries between these zones are not clear cut.

The upper half of the anal canal is derived from endoderm, the lower half being derived from ectoderm. Some important anatomical facts with clinical significance result from this derivation of the anal canal, as follows.

- The upper half of the anal canal is lined by columnar epithelium and the lower half with stratified squamous cell epithelium. Consequently a carcinoma of the upper anal canal is an adenocarcinoma, while that arising from the lower part would be a squamous cell carcinoma.
- The upper half of the canal is supplied by the autonomic nervous system; the lower part has somatic innervation from the inferior rectal nerve. The lower part of the canal therefore is sensitive to pinprick sensation, while the upper part is not. This is an important factor when injecting haemorrhoids, where the needle

should be inserted through the upper, insensitive part of the anal canal.

- The upper half of the anal canal drains into the portal venous system, whereas the lower half drains into the systemic venous system. The two systems communicate and therefore this forms one site of anastomosis between the portal and systemic circulation and may result in dilated veins in portal hypertension.
- The lymphatic drainage of the upper half of the canal is along the superior rectal vessels to the abdominal nodes, whereas, below this site, drainage is to the inguinal nodes. This is clinically important, as a carcinoma of the rectum which grows down into the lower anal canal may metastasise to the inguinal nodes.

Anal sphincters

The anal canal is surrounded by a complex arrangement of muscles.

The internal anal sphincter comprises smooth muscle which is continuous above with a circular muscle of the rectum. It surrounds the upper two thirds of the anal canal and it is supplied by sympathetic nerves.

The external anal sphincter is composed of striated (voluntary) muscle which surrounds the internal sphincter but extends further distally, curving medially as the subcutaneous part surrounding the lower part of the anal canal just below the lower edge of the internal sphincter (Fig. 17.18). The muscle is divided into three parts: the subcutaneous; the superficial, which is attached to the coccyx behind and the perineal body in front; and the deep part which is continuous with the puborectalis part of levator ani.

The deep part of the external sphincter, where it blends with the levator ani, together with the internal anal sphincter, are termed the anorectal ring. This is easily palpable with a finger in the anal canal where it forms a ring immediately above which the finger enters the ampulla of the rectum. The subcutaneous portion of the external sphincter is traversed by a fan-shaped expansion of the longitudinal muscle fibres of the anal canal (Fig. 17.18). The nerve supply of the external sphincter is via the inferior rectal branch of the pudendal nerve (S2,3) and the perineal branch of S4.

PELVIC FLOOR AND PERINEUM

The muscles of the pelvic floor and perineum comprise:

- the pelvic diaphragm formed by the levator ani and coccygeus
- the anterior (urogenital) perineum
- the posterior (anal) perineum.

The levator ani is the largest muscle of the pelvic floor. It arises from the back of the body of the pubis, the spine of the ischium, and between these from the fascia on the side wall of the pelvis covering obturator internus. From this origin it passes downwards in a series of loops. One loop forms a sling around the prostate (levator prostatae) or around the vagina (sphincter vaginae) inserting into the perineal body. Another loop forms a sling around the

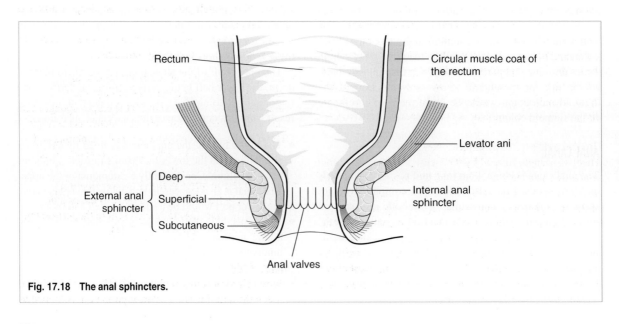

Fig. 17.18 The anal sphincters.

(labels:) Rectum — Circular muscle coat of the rectum — Levator ani — Internal anal sphincter — External anal sphincter { Deep / Superficial / Subcutaneous } — Anal valves

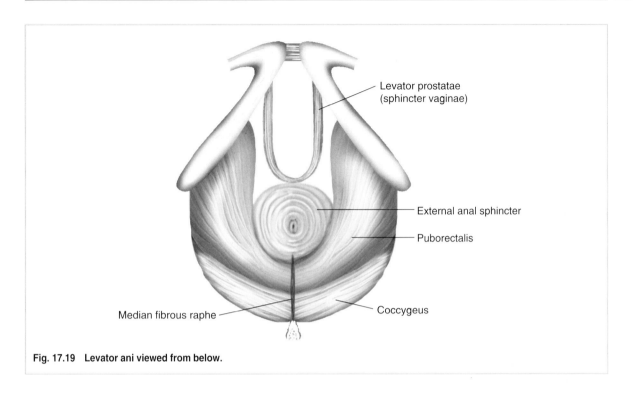

Fig. 17.19 Levator ani viewed from below.

Levator prostatae
(sphincter vaginae)

External anal sphincter

Puborectalis

Coccygeus

Median fibrous raphe

rectum where this passes between the muscle of either side (puborectalis).

The posterior fibres are attached to the side of the coccyx and a median fibrous raphe stretching between the coccyx and anorectal junction (Fig. 17.19). Coccygeus is a small triangular muscle behind and in the same plane as levator ani.

The levator ani muscles form a muscular diaphragm which support the pelvic viscera and oppose the downward pressure of the abdominal muscles. They constrict the rectum and vagina and steady the perineal body. They are supplied by a branch of S4 on the pelvic surface and by a branch of the inferior rectal nerve or perineal division of the pudendal nerve on the perineal surface.

Urogenital triangle (the anterior perineum)

This is a triangle formed by the ischiopubic inferior rami and a line joining the ischial tuberosities which passes just in front of the anus (Fig. 17.20). Attached to the sides of this triangle is a strong fascial sheet, the perineal membrane (inferior fascia of the urogenital diaphragm). The perineal membrane is pierced by the urethra in the male and the urethra and the vagina in the female. Deep to the perineal membrane is the external urethral sphincter which is composed of striated muscle fibres and surrounds the membraneous urethra.

The deep perineal pouch encloses the external urethral sphincter. Below is the perineal membrane, while above is an indefinite layer of fascia, i.e. the superior fascia of the urogenital diaphragm. In the male the pouch also contains the bulbo-urethral glands (of Cowper) whose ducts pierce the perineal membrane to open into the bulbous urethra. The pouch also contains the deep transverse perineal muscles.

Superficial to the perineal membrane is the superficial perineal pouch. In the male this contains:

- the bulb of the penis, which is attached to the undersurface of the perineal membrane; the bulbospongiosus muscle covers the corpus spongiosum
- the crura of the penis, which are attached at the angle between the insertion of the perineal membrane and the ischiopubic rami; each crus is surrounded by an ischiocavernous muscle
- superficial transverse perineal muscle running transversely from the perineal body to the ischial ramus; the same muscles are present in the female but are less well developed (Fig. 17.21).

Perineal body

This is a fibromuscular nodule which lies in the midline between the anterior and posterior perineum. Attached to

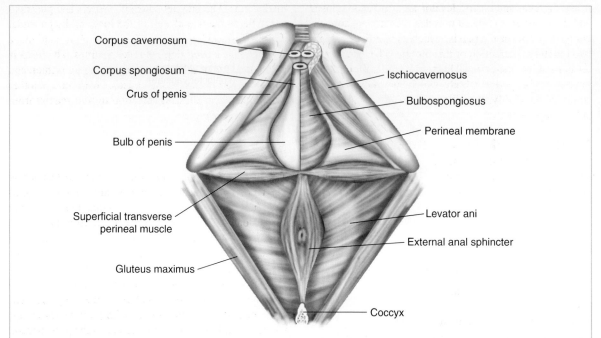

Fig. 17.20   The male perineum viewed from below. On the right side the muscles have been removed to display the crus and bulb of the penis.

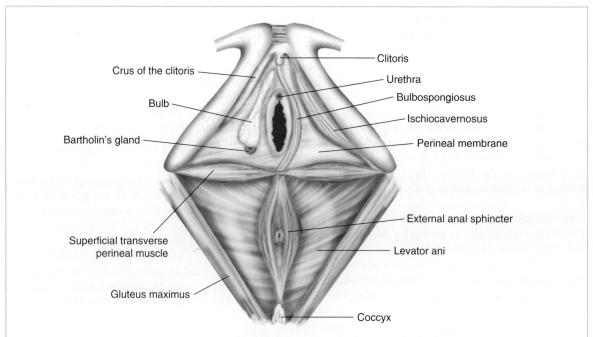

Fig. 17.21   The female perineum. On the right side the muscles have been removed to display the bulb of the vestibule, and Bartholin's glands.

it are the anal sphincters, levator ani, bulbospongiosus and the transverse perineal muscles. Levator ani forms a complete floor for the pelvis, which can be tightened up by voluntary contraction of this muscle. The insertion of levator ani into the perineal body is essential for this, and tearing of the perineal body which may occur during complicated childbirth will considerably weaken the pelvic diaphragm.

Posterior (anal) perineum

This is a triangular area lying between the ischial tuberosities on each side and the coccyx. It contains the anus and its sphincters, the levator ani, and on each side the ischiorectal fossa.

Ischiorectal fossa

This is a space between the anal canal and side wall of the pelvis (Fig. 17.22). Its boundaries are:

- medially, fascia over levator ani and the external anal sphincter
- laterally, fascia over obturator internus
- anteriorly, it extends forwards as a prolongation deep to the urogenital diaphragm
- posteriorly, it is limited by the sacrotuberous ligament and the origin of gluteus maximus from this ligament
- the floor is formed from skin and cutaneous fat.

The ischiorectal fossa contains mainly fat and is crossed by the inferior rectal vessels and nerves from lateral to medial side. The internal pudendal vessels and pudendal nerve lie on the lateral wall of the fossa in the pudendal canal (of Alcock), a tunnel of fascia which is continuous with the fascia overlying obturator internus. The fossa is a common site of infection giving rise to an ischiorectal abscess. The fossae communicate with one another behind the anus, allowing infection to pass readily from one fossa to the other.

LIVER

The liver is the largest organ in the body. It lies across the right hypochondrium, epigastrium and left hypochondrium. It is divided into two unequal lobes by a fold of peritoneum, the falciform ligament (Fig. 17.23). Its superior surface, which is dome shaped, is related to the diaphragm, which separates it from the pleura, lungs, pericardium and heart. Its postero-inferior surface is related to the abdominal oesophagus, stomach, duodenum, hepatic flexure of the colon, right kidney and right suprarenal gland. It is covered with peritoneum except where the gall bladder is attached and at the porta hepatis and the fissure for the ligamentum venosum which gives attachment to the lesser omentum. The posterior surface is connected to the diaphragm over the right lobe of the liver by the coronary ligament, between the two layers of which is a non-peritonealised area, i.e. the bare area. To the left of the bare area is the caudate lobe, which bounds the lesser sac in front. The anatomical right and left lobes

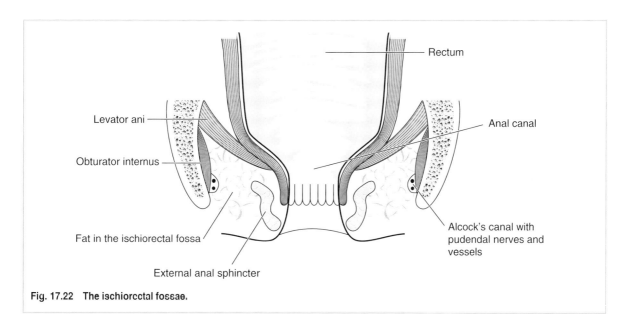

Fig. 17.22 The ischiorectal fossae.

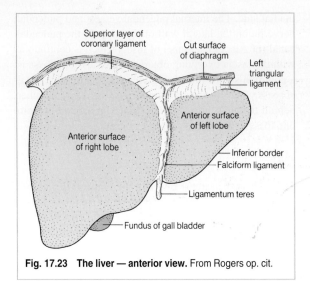

Fig. 17.23   The liver — anterior view. From Rogers op. cit.

of the liver are separated anteriorly and superiorly by the falciform ligament, and postero-inferiorly by the H-shaped arrangement of the fossae (Fig. 17.24).

The porta hepatis is the gateway to and from the liver.

It contains the common hepatic ducts anteriorly, the hepatic artery in the middle and the portal vein posteriorly. It also contains lymph nodes which, when enlarged (usually by malignancy), may compress the bile ducts and cause obstructive jaundice. The ligamentum venosum is a fibrous remnant of the ductus venosus lying in the depth of its fissure and joining the left branch of the portal vein to the inferior vena cava. The ligamentum teres is the obliterated remains of the left umbilical vein, which in the fetus brings blood back from the placenta. The ligamentum teres and ligamentum venosum should be viewed together as a 'bridge' between the umbilicus and the inferior vena cava. In the fetus, oxygenated blood from the placenta can pass via the umbilical vein and ductus venosus to the inferior vena cava, most of the blood bypassing the liver.

Peritoneal relations of the liver

These are shown in Figures 17.23 and 17.25. The liver is almost completely covered by peritoneum except for the bare area in which the inferior vena cava is embedded. The bare area is the area between the upper and lower leaves of the coronary ligament. These leaves fuse to the right to form the right triangular ligament. The falciform

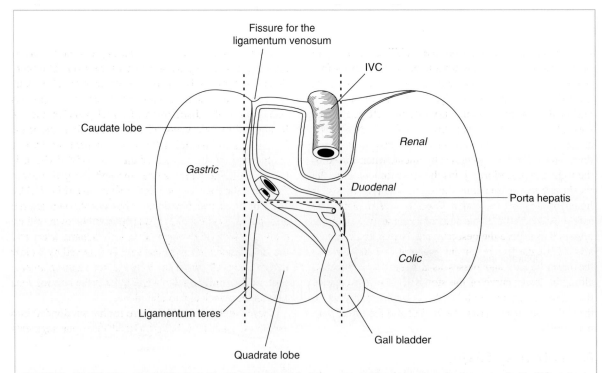

Fig. 17.24   The inferior aspect of the liver. The H-shape (dotted line) demonstrates the various fissures, the groove for the IVC, and fossa for the gall bladder. The sites of the impressions of the various relations are indicated in capital letters.

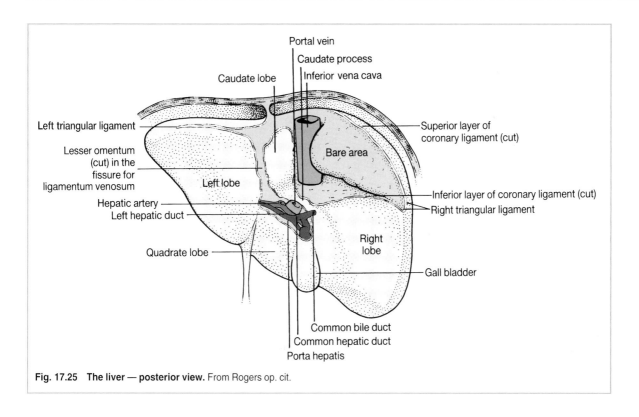

Fig. 17.25 **The liver — posterior view.** From Rogers op. cit.

ligament passes upwards from the umbilicus to the right of the midline, the ligamentum teres running in its free border. The falciform ligament passes over the dome of the liver and separates, its right part joining the upper leaf of the coronary ligament, while the left part forms part of the left triangular ligament, the latter being attached to the peritoneum on the undersurface of the diaphragm. The left triangular ligament, when traced to the right and posteriorly, joins the lesser omentum in the fissure for the ligamentum venosum. The left triangular ligament contains no major blood vessels and may be safely divided so that the left lobe of the liver may be retracted to expose the oesophagus. The lesser omentum arises from the fissure for the ligamentum venosum and the porta hepatis and passes as a sheet to be attached along the lesser curve of the stomach. The free edge of the lesser omentum contains the common bile duct to the right, the hepatic artery to the left and the portal vein posteriorly.

Functional anatomy of the liver

The gross anatomical division of the liver into right and left lobes demarcated by the falciform ligament anteriorly and the fissure for the ligamentum teres and ligmentum venosum postero-inferiorly is not appropriate to understanding of the surgical anatomy of the liver. The functional anatomy is based on the description of hepatic segmentation which divides the liver into segments according to the distribution of portal pedicles and the location of hepatic veins. The functional division of the liver into right and left lobes is not demarcated by any visible line on the surface of the liver. The division is through a plane which passes through the gall bladder fossa and the fossa of the inferior vena cava (Fig. 17.26). Each of these two functional lobes has its own arterial and portal venous blood supply and its own biliary drainage. Surgical division of the right hepatic artery and the right branch of the portal vein is followed by a clear line of demarcation on the liver surface running antero-posteriorly from the gall bladder fossa to the inferior vena cava in the principal vascular plane.

These two functional lobes are further subdivided into segments, each lobe being divided into four segments (Fig. 17.27).

Hepatic veins

There are three main hepatic veins: a right, a central and a left. They pass upwards and backwards from the

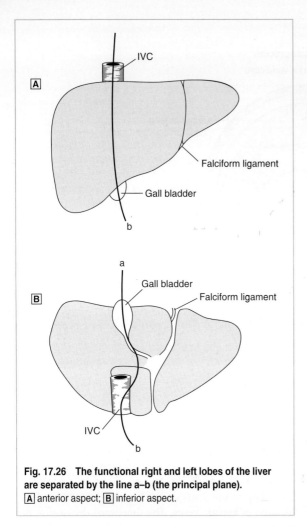

Fig. 17.26 The functional right and left lobes of the liver are separated by the line a–b (the principal plane). Ⓐ anterior aspect; Ⓑ inferior aspect.

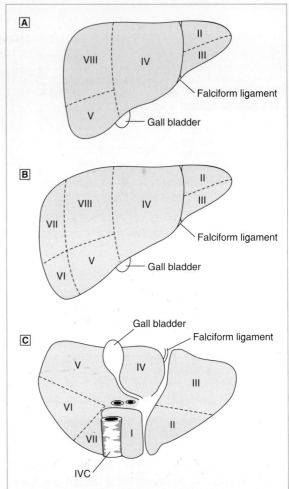

Fig. 17.27 The functional division of the liver into segments. Ⓐ anterior view as seen in the patient; Ⓑ anterior view with the liver 'flattened' in the ex-vivo position (note that segments VI and VII may now be seen — in vivo they appear more laterally and posteriorly); Ⓒ inferior view.

substance of the liver, draining into the inferior vena cava at the superior limit of the liver. Their terminations are variable, the right and left veins usually draining directly into the inferior vena cava while the central vein may join the left vein near its termination. The caudate lobe of the liver has independent hepatic veins which drain directly into the inferior vena cava. The three main hepatic veins divide the liver into four sectors, each of which receives a portal pedicle, with an alternation between hepatic veins and portal pedicles (Fig. 17.28). The middle hepatic vein lies at the line of the principal plane of the liver between its right and left functional lobes. Terminology in liver resection has been confusing, and it is perhaps better to adopt a terminology based on function and segmental anatomy. Hence a right hemihepatectomy would involve segments V, VI, VII and VIII, while a left hemihepatec-

tomy would involve segments II, III and IV. Excision of the anatomical left lobe of the liver would involve only segments II and III, while excision of the functional left lobe of the liver would involve segments II, III, IV and possibly I.

EXTRAHEPATIC BILIARY SYSTEM

The right and left hepatic ducts join at the porta hepatis to form the common hepatic duct. This is joined by the cystic duct to form the common bile duct. The common bile duct is about 9 cm long, commencing on average

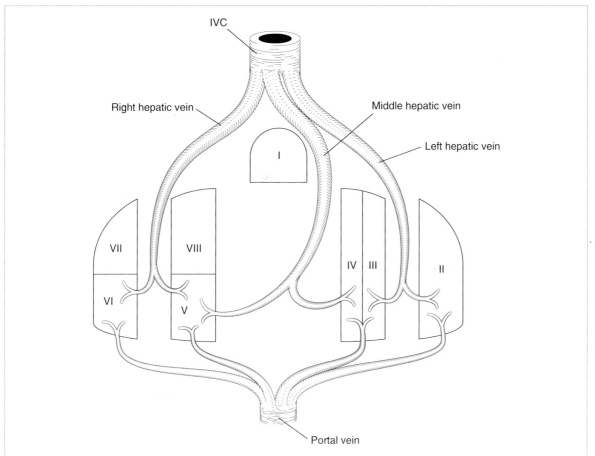

Fig. 17.28 **A schematic representation of the functional anatomy of the liver.** The three main hepatic veins divide the liver into four sectors, each of which receives a portal pedicle.

4 cm above the duodenum and then passing behind it and running in a groove on the posterior aspect of the head of the pancreas before opening into the medial aspect of the second part of the duodenum. Occasionally, the common bile duct is completely buried in the substance of the head of the pancreas. In 90% of individuals the main pancreatic duct joins the common bile duct to form a common dilated channel about 1 cm long, the ampulla of Vater. The opening of the ampulla of Vater into the duodenum is guarded by the sphincter of Oddi (peri-ampullary sphincter). Occasionally the bile ducts and pancreatic ducts open separately into the duodenum. Frequently there is an additional duct which receives ducts from the lower part of the head of the pancreas known as the accessory pancreatic duct. It opens into the medial wall of the second part of the duodenum about

2 cm proximal to the main duodenal papilla. Endoscopists should be aware of these anatomical variations.

The common hepatic duct and supraduodenal part of the common bile duct lie in the free edge of the lesser omentum. The bile duct lies anteriorly to the right; the hepatic artery anteriorly to the left. The portal vein lies posteriorly and is separated more posteriorly from the inferior vena cava by the foramen of Winslow (Fig. 17.8).

Gall bladder

The gall bladder is pear-shaped organ adherent to the undersurface of the liver, lying in a fossa which separates the morphological right and left lobes. It acts as a reservoir for bile, which it also concentrates. It holds about 50 mL of bile when physiologically distended. The gall bladder consists of a fundus, a body and a neck, the latter opening into the cystic duct which conveys bile to and from the common bile duct. The lumen of the cystic duct contains a mucosal valve, the spiral valve of Heister, which offers mild resistance to bile flow. The gall bladder is related inferiorly to the duodenum and transverse colon. An inflamed gall bladder may ulcerate into either of these structures, most commonly the second part of the duodenum. A cholecystoduodenal fistula may result with passage of a gall stone into the small bowel. If the stone is large enough, gall stone 'ileus' will result. A small pouch may be present on the ventral aspect of the gall bladder just proximal to the neck which projects downwards and backwards towards the duodenum. This is called Hartmann's pouch. Originally thought to be a constant feature of the normal gall bladder, it is now recognised as being associated with a dilated and pathological gall bladder. A stone may become lodged in the pouch. The gall bladder is supplied by the cystic artery, which usually arises from the right hepatic artery (Fig. 17.29). It lies in a triangle made up of the liver, the cystic duct and the common hepatic duct, i.e. Calot's triangle. The cystic artery passes behind the common hepatic and cystic ducts to gain the upper surface of the neck of the gall bladder. Occasionally, the cystic artery arises from the main hepatic artery, and crosses in front of or behind the common bile duct or common hepatic duct prior to reaching the gall bladder. Other vessels derived from the right hepatic artery pass directly to the gall bladder from its bed in the liver. Venous drainage is via small veins drain-ing directly through its bed into the liver. Variations in the anatomy of the extrahepatic biliary system are not uncommon (Fig. 17.30).

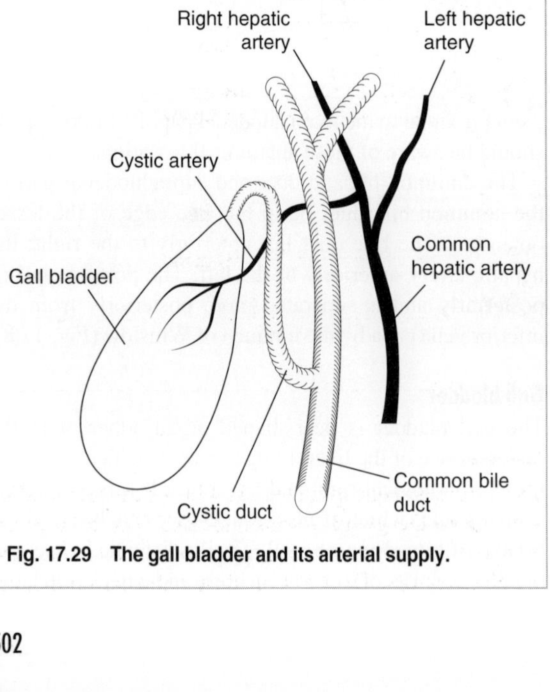

The gall bladder receives parasympathetic innervation, which gives motor nerves to the gall bladder and secretory fibres to the ductal epithelium. Sympathetic afferents mediate the pain of biliary colic.

The gall bladder is lined by columnar epithelium, the luminal surface possessing microvilli to aid its absorptive capacity. When the organ is collapsed the mucosa is thrown into prominent folds. The wall of the gall bladder and cystic duct contains smooth muscle, but this is virtually absent in the bile duct, hence little pain from a gall stone in the bile duct.

PANCREAS

The pancreas (Fig. 17.31) lies retroperitoneally in the upper abdomen in the transpyloric plane. It is divided into a head, uncinate process, neck, body and tail. The head of the pancreas lies in the C-shape of the duodenum and is continuous with the uncinate process below, which passes posterior to the superior mesenteric vessels as they in turn pass from behind the head of the pancreas and into the root of the mesentery.

Relations of the pancreas

The head of the pancreas is adherent to the medial aspect of the C-shaped portion of the duodenum and lies in front of the IVC, renal vessels and superior mesenteric vessels. The uncinate process lies behind the superior mesenteric vessels. The common bile duct passes through a groove on the posterior aspect of the head of the pancreas. The stomach and the first part of the duodenum lie partly in front of the head of the pancreas, separated from it by the lesser sac. The neck merges into the body of the pancreas. Behind the neck lies the junction of the superior mesenteric vein and splenic vein forming the portal vein. The body of the pancreas is in contact posteriorly with the aorta, the left crus of the diaphragm, the left adrenal gland and the left kidney. The tail of the pancreas lies at the splenic hilum. The splenic artery is tortuous and runs along the superior border of the gland. The splenic vein runs behind the gland. The transverse mesocolon is attached along the anterior aspect of the pancreas. Below this attachment, the duodeno-jejunal flexure, the left flexure of the colon, and the small intestine, covered by peritoneum, lie in relation to the gland. The main pancre-atic duct (of Wirsung) passes along the gland from the tail to the head, joining the common bile duct before entering the medial aspect of the second part of the

Fig. 17.29 The gall bladder and its arterial supply.

Right hepatic artery

Left hepatic artery

Cystic artery

Common hepatic artery

Gall bladder

Common bile duct

Cystic duct

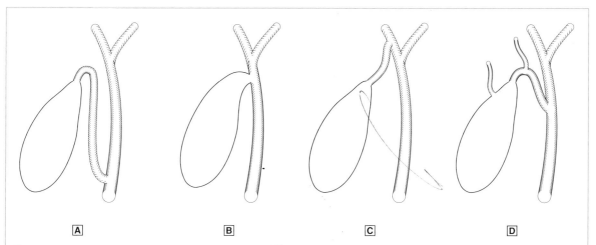

Fig. 17.30 Variations in the extrahepatic biliary anatomy. A A long cystic duct joins the common hepatic duct behind the duodenum. B The cystic duct is short or absent, the gall bladder opening directly into the common hepatic duct. C The cystic duct enters the right hepatic duct. D Accessory hepatic ducts may open into the gall bladder or cystic ducts.

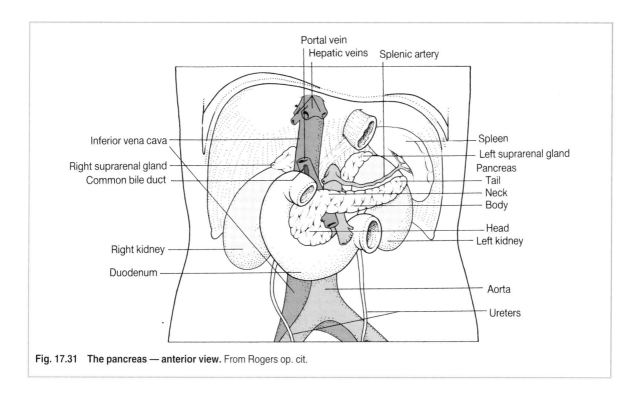

Fig. 17.31 The pancreas — anterior view. From Rogers op. cit.

duodenum at the ampulla of Vater. The accessory duct (of Santorini) passes from the lower part of the head in front of the main duct, usually communicating with it, and, if present, opens into the duodenum approximately 2 cm proximal to the ampulla of Vater (Fig. 17.32).

Structure

The pancreas is encapsulated, the fibrous capsule sending septae into the gland, forming lobules. The lobules are composed of acini of serous cells which secrete the pancreatic enzymes. Ductules lined by cuboidal epithelium

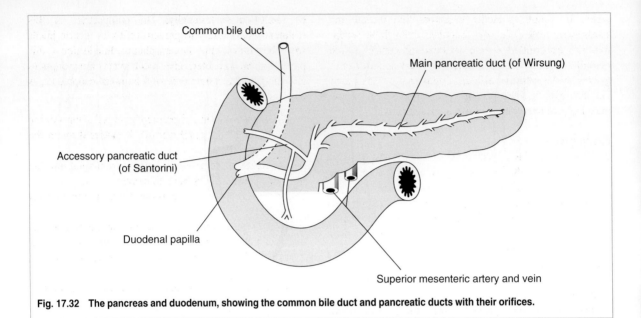

Fig. 17.32 The pancreas and duodenum, showing the common bile duct and pancreatic ducts with their orifices.

drain the secretions into the pancreatic ducts. Scattered throughout the pancreas are the islets of Langerhans, which appear as spheroidal clusters of pale-staining cells with a rich blood supply. These cells secrete insulin and glucagon.

Blood supply

Arterial blood supply is from the splenic artery via the arteria pancreatica magna. Supply to the head and the uncinate process is from the superior pancreaticoduodenal artery, which is a branch of the gastroduodenal artery, and the inferior pancreaticoduodenal artery, which is a branch of the superior mesenteric artery.

Lymphatics

Lymphatics drain into the nodes along the upper border of the pancreas, to those related to the medial aspect of the duodenum and head of the pancreas and to those at the root of the mesentery.

PHYSIOLOGY

OESOPHAGUS

The function of the oesophagus is to transport food from the mouth to the stomach. The upper and lower ends of the oesophagus contain sphincters. Pressures in the mouth and pharynx are atmospheric while pressures in the thoracic oesophagus are subatmospheric, a reflection

of normal intrathoracic pressure. Pressure within the stomach is slightly greater than atmospheric. The upper oesophageal sphincter at the junction between pharynx and oesophagus (pharyngo-oesophageal) prevents the entry of air into the oesophagus. The lower oesophageal sphincter prevents the entry of gastric contents into the oesophagus. The upper oesophageal sphincter is formed by a circular layer of striated muscle, i.e. the cricopharyngeus. The lower oesophageal sphincter is not an anatomical entity, but the lower 4 cm of the oesophagus functions as a sphincter. In normal individuals the pressure at the lower oesophageal sphincter is always greater than that in the stomach. Sphincteric competence is aided by the normal intra-abdominal location of the terminal part of the oesophagus. The lower oesophageal sphincter opens when the wave of peristalsis begins in the upper oesophagus. Opening is vagally mediated. In the absence of oesophageal peristalsis the sphincter remains tightly closed to prevent reflux of gastric contents.

SWALLOWING

Swallowing is divided into three stages: the oral or voluntary stage, the pharyngeal stage and the oesophageal stage. Swallowing can be initially voluntary, but thereafter it is almost entirely under reflex control.

Oral

The tongue propels the bolus of food into the pharynx,

where it stimulates tactile receptors that initiate the swallowing reflex. Sensory impulses from these receptors are transmitted to the swallowing centre in the medulla via the fifth, ninth, and tenth nerves. After integration in the medulla, efferent impulses are transmitted via the twelfth, seventh, fifth and tenth nerves to the muscles involved in the process of swallowing.

Pharyngeal

1. The soft palate is pulled upwards and the palato-pharyngeal folds move inwards towards one another, preventing reflux of food into the nasopharynx.
2. The vocal cords are approximated, the epiglottis covers the opening of the larynx, and the larynx moves upwards against the epiglottis. Food is thus prevented from entering the trachea.
3. The upper oesophageal sphincter relaxes and the superior constrictor of the pharynx contracts to force the bolus onwards.
4. The bolus is then propelled onwards by sequential contraction of the superior, middle and inferior constrictors of the pharynx. This produces a peristaltic wave pushing the bolus towards the upper end of the oesophagus.
5. During the pharyngeal stage, respiration is reflexly inhibited.

Oesophageal

After the bolus has passed the upper oesophageal sphincter, the latter reflexly constricts. The bolus is propelled downwards by the primary peristaltic wave caused by impulses originating in the swallowing centre and conducted via the tenth nerve to the myenteric plexus of the oesophagus. This wave pushes the bolus ahead of it at 2–4 cm/s, i.e. the entire oesophagus is traversed in approximately 10 s. If the primary peristaltic wave is insufficient to clear the oesophagus of food, the distension of the oesophagus initiates another peristaltic wave that begins at the site of distension and moves downwards. This is known as secondary peristalsis. Tertiary contractions may occur. These are stationary, non-propulsive contractions that may occur anywhere in the oesophagus. They are considered abnormal, but are frequently present in the elderly who have no symptoms of oesophageal disease.

LOWER OESOPHAGEAL SPHINCTER

At the lower end of the oesophagus is a high pressure zone where the pressure averages 15–25 mmHg. It extends from approximately 2 cm above the diaphragm to 2 cm below. It is purely a physiological sphincter, as it cannot be identified anatomically. The competence of this sphincter is necessary to prevent reflux of gastric juices from the stomach into the oesophagus. In addition to this physiological sphincter, other mechanisms are thought to contribute to the competence of the lower oesophagus, as follows.

1. The oesophagus is compressed by muscle fibres of the right crus of the diaphragm as it passes through the oesophageal hiatus.
2. The acute angle of entry of the oesophagus into the stomach produces a valve-like effect.
3. Mucosal folds at the gastro-oesophageal junction act as a valve.
4. The intra-abdominal portion of the oesophagus is subjected to intra-abdominal pressure which compresses the walls of the intra-abdominal segment of the oesophagus.
5. The hormone gastrin causes contraction of the muscle at the lower end of the oesophagus.

In some individuals during swallowing the lower oesophageal sphincter fails to relax sufficiently to allow food to enter the stomach — a condition known as achalasia. This is related to the absence of ganglion cells in the lower oesophagus.

Some patients present with diffuse oesophageal spasm, and they have prolonged and painful contraction of the lower part of the oesophagus after swallowing instead of a normal oesophageal peristaltic wave.

Incompetence of the lower gastro-oesophageal sphincter occurs normally during vomiting. The gastro-oesophageal junction rises above the level of the hiatus above the diaphragm at the time of vomiting. This may be due to contraction of the longitudinal muscle of the oesophagus. The gastric contents are expelled up the oesophagus by violent contractions of the muscle of the stomach and the abdominal wall. Following vomiting, the gastro-oesophageal junction descends below the level of the diaphragm. Vomiting is further discussed in the section on the stomach.

STOMACH

Functions of the stomach

1. It acts as a reservoir allowing the ingestion of large meals.
2. It mixes food with gastric secretions, producing chyme which is then delivered to the small intestine for further digestion and absorption to occur.
3. It produces gastric juices which contain hydrochloric acid, pepsin, intrinsic factors, and mucus secretions.

4. The pyloric glands produce the hormone gastrin (G cells).

Gastric secretions

2–3 L of gastric juice are secreted each day. This contains water and ions, hydrochloric acid, mucus, pepsin, gastric lipase, and intrinsic factor. HCl is required for the activation of pepsinogen to pepsin. HCl is formed by active secretion from stimulated parietal cells. Control of gastric secretion is under neural and a hormonal control. The control of gastric secretion is divided into three phases: cephalic, gastric and intestinal.

Function of gastric secretions

Hydrochloric acid   This is necessary for the activation and optimum activity of pepsin. It is secreted by the parietal cells of the body and fundus of the stomach. It activates pepsinogen to pepsin. It allows conversion of ferric iron in the diet to the ferrous form and provides an acid environment in the duodenum to facilitate iron and calcium absorption. The presence of acid in the duodenum stimulates the release of secretin. HCl is also responsible for killing a number of ingested bacteria.

Pepsin   Pepsin is secreted as the inactive precursor pepsinogen by the chief cells of the gastric glands. Pepsinogen is activated to pepsin by the presence of HCl. Pepsin breaks down food proteins into smaller peptides and polypeptides, digesting as much as 20% of protein of an average meal. When the duodenal contents are neutralised, pepsin is irreversibly inactivated.

Mucus   Gastric mucus is produced by the superficial cells of the gastric mucosa, the mucous-neck cells and the mucous cells of the pyloric glands. It is a thick, sticky, glycoprotein material which adheres to the gastric mucosa. It acts as a lubricant and also protects the underlying mucosa from digestion by acid and pepsin.

Intrinsic factor   Intrinsic factor is a glycoprotein secreted by the parietal cells. It is required for the normal intestinal absorption of vitamin B_{12}. Vitamin B_{12} binds to intrinsic factor and passes to the terminal ileum, where receptors in the ileal mucosa bind the complex and B_{12} is absorbed by the ileal mucosal epithelial cells. Intrinsic factor is released by the same stimuli that cause secretion of acid from parietal cells, i.e. vagal, gastrin and histamine. Lack of intrinsic factor may arise from deficient production by parietal cells due to antiparietal cell antibodies, in pernicious anaemia, or following loss of parietal cells, i.e. following gastrectomy. In the absence of intrinsic factor, vitamin B_{12} will not be absorbed in the terminal ileum, and megaloblastic anaemia will result. Removal of more than 1 m of the terminal ileum,

e.g. resection in Crohn's disease, will also result in megaloblastic anaemia.

Regulation of acid secretion

Cephalic phase   This is initiated by the site, smell and taste of food, and occasionally by the thought of food. The effect is vagally mediated and is abolished by vagotomy. Cholinergic vagal fibres are the mediators of the cephalic phase. Acetylcholine released directly stimulates the parietal cells to produce acid. It also stimulates acid secretion indirectly by releasing gastrin from G cells and histamine from enterochromaffin-like cells in the gastric mucosa.

Gastric phase   The presence of food in the stomach releases gastrin by both a mechanical and chemical stimulation. Products of protein digestion are the chemical stimulators. Amino acids in the antrum cause gastrin release directly by stimulation of receptors on G cells. Distension of the body or antrum are the mechanical mediators. The presence of food in the stomach excites vagal reflexes, impulses passing to the brain via vagal afferents and returning via efferents to stimulate the parietal cells. Distension of the pyloric area enhances gastrin release through a local intramural cholinergic reflex. Gastrin then stimulates the parietal cells via its release into the circulation, reinforcing direct parietal cell stimulation. Once the buffering capacity of the gastric contents is saturated, the gastric pH falls rapidly and inhibits further acid release. Gastric secretion is also directly stimulated by calcium ions, caffeine and alcohol.

Intestinal phase   During this phase, gastric secretion is brought about by duodenal distension and the presence of protein digestion products, i.e. peptides and amino acids. The effect is mediated by endocrine mechanisms, largely via G cells in the duodenum and proximal jejunum. Other mechanisms operating during the intestinal phase inhibit gastric secretions. These include the presence of acid, fat digestion products and hypertonicity in the duodenum and proximal jejunum. Acid in the duodenum causes the release of secretin into the circulation. Secretin inhibits gastrin released by G cells and inhibits the response of parietal cells to gastrin. Fatty acids in the duodenum inhibit gastric secretion by releasing two hormones: cholecystokinin and gastric inhibitory peptide (GIP). GIP suppresses gastrin release and also directly inhibits acid secretion by parietal cells. Cholecystokinin inhibits acid secretion by parietal cells.

Pharmacological modifications of gastric acid secretion

Gastrointestinal hormones

The gastrointestinal hormones are peptides produced by

enterochromaffin cells in the gastrointestinal mucosa. They are involved in the control of gastrointestinal secretions and motility. The cells producing these hormones are sometimes referred to as APUD cells (amine precursor uptake and decarboxylation). The major hormones are gastrin, cholecystokinin (CCK), secretin and somatostatin.

Gastrin Gastrin is produced by the G cells contained in the antral mucosa and in the upper small intestine. Factors responsible for gastrin release are: (i) stimulation by the products of digestion, caffeine and alcohol; (ii) extrinsic nerve stimulation during the cephalic phase of gastric secretion; (iii) antral distension, where the release is mediated by local intrinsic nerve reflexes.

Gastrin release is inhibited by increasing gastric acidity, secretin and somatostatin. Gastrin is carried in the blood stream and stimulates gastric secretion of hydrochloric acid, pepsinogen and intrinsic factor. It also enhances gastric motility and may increase the tone of the lower oesophageal sphincter.

Gastrin may be produced by gastrinomas in the gastrointestinal tract, and this can result in increased production of acid, causing peptic ulceration (Zollinger–Ellison syndrome).

Cholecystokinin Cholecystokinin is produced by cells found in the mucosa lining the duodenum and the jejunum. It is released into the blood stream in response to the products of digestion, especially fatty acids, peptides and amino acids. The presence of these in duodenum and jejunum acts either directly on the cells or through local intrinsic nerve reflexes. CCK stimulates an enzyme rich secretion from the acinar cells of the pancreas. It also causes contraction of the gall bladder and relaxation of the sphincter of Oddi. It also delays gastric emptying.

Secretin Secretin is produced by cells lying in the mucosa of the duodenum and jejunum. It is released into the blood stream following increased acidity of the duodenum and jejunum and also by the presence of fatty acids. It causes increased secretion of HCO_3^- by stimulating the duct cells of the pancreas and also of the liver. It also reduces gastric acid secretion by direct action on oxyntic cells and by inhibition of gastrin release.

Somatostatin Somatostatin is produced by the D cells in the intestine and pancreatic islets in response to glucose, fats and bile salts in the intestinal lumen. It has an inhibitory effect on pancreatic enzymes secretion, insulin and glucagon release, gastric acid and pepsin secretion, and gastrin release.

VOMITING

Vomiting is the mechanism by which the upper gastro-

intestinal tract empties its content when it becomes irritated, overdistended and overexcited. Afferent impulses from the gastrointestinal tract reach the vomiting centre in the medulla via general visceral afferents in the vagus and sympathetic nerves. Afferents also reach the vomiting centre from the labyrinth, and the chemoreceptor trigger zone in the fourth ventricle. Efferents from the vomiting centre pass via the fifth, seventh, ninth and twelfth nerves to the gastrointestinal tract and by the spinal nerves to the intercostal muscles, diaphragm and abdominal muscles.

Causes of vomiting

Causes of vomiting are:

- stimulation of the faucial mucosa and posterior oropharynx
- excessive distension of the stomach or duodenum, e.g. excessive food or drink intake, pyloric stenosis, intestinal obstruction
- stimulation of the labyrinth, e.g. motion sickness
- severe pain via extensive stimulation of cerebral centres
- raised intracranial pressure, via direct stimulation of the vomiting centre
- stimulation of the chemoreceptor trigger zone by chemicals, e.g. morphine, toxins from chronic renal failure and liver failure
- bacterial irritation of the upper gastrointestinal tracts.

Process of vomiting

At the commencement of vomiting, a deep inspiratory effort is taken, then the glottis closes to prevent entry of vomitus into the larynx. The soft palate is elevated to close the nasopharynx and prevent vomitus coming down the nose. Relaxation of the lower oesophageal sphincter occurs followed by contraction of the abdominal and thoracic muscles. When descent of the diaphragm coincides with contraction of the abdominal muscles, the elevation of intra-abdominal pressure forces gastric contents out through the mouth.

SMALL INTESTINE

Functions of the small intestine include digestion and absorption. The following substances are either digested or absorbed: carbohydrate, fat, protein, vitamin B_{12}, folate, iron, calcium, water and electrolytes. The small intestine has an enormous surface to allow absorption. Even following extensive resection of small bowel it is possible to survive with approximately 80 cm without the need for total parenteral nutrition. Intestinal circulation of blood and lymph is important in absorption, the blood and lymph flow both being in the region of 1–2 L/min. Active transport mechanisms occur for the absorption of many substances.

Vitamin B$_{12}$

Vitamin B$_{12}$ is present in animal food sources, e.g. liver, meat, cheese, milk, eggs. It does not occur in plant sources. It combines with gastric intrinsic factor produced by the parietal cells of the stomach. The B$_{12}$–intrinsic-factor complex passes to the terminal ileum where the vitamin B$_{12}$ is absorbed. Absorption of vitamin B$_{12}$ is reduced in the following states:

- lack of intrinsic factor, e.g. pernicious anaemia, gastric resection
- resection of the terminal ileum
- diseases of the terminal ileum, e.g. Crohn's
- blind loop syndrome — bacteria compete with the patient for vitamin B$_{12}$.

Folic acid

Folic acid is present in foods, vegetables, fish and liver. It is absorbed in the jejunum. Malabsorption occurs in diseases involved in the jejunal mucosa, e.g. coeliac disease and following jejunal resection. Patients on epanutin, an anti-epileptic drug, may become folate deficient because of the inhibition of a mucosal enzyme system and consequent prevention of folate leaving the mucosal cells.

Iron

Iron is absorbed by active transport in the duodenum and the jejunum. Iron is found in meat, liver, eggs and green vegetables. Most of the dietary intake is in the ferric form, but is converted in the presence of hydrochloric acid in the stomach to the ferrous form for absorption in the duodenum and upper jejunum.

Calcium

Calcium is absorbed by active transport from the upper small intestine, chiefly the duodenum. Absorption is regulated by requirements. Most of the calcium in the diet is in the form of calcium phosphate and is derived from milk and other dairy products. A fall in serum calcium level in the plasma leads to an increased output of parathyroid hormone. This acts on bone, the kidney and indirectly on the gastrointestinal tract through the active form of vitamin D to return the serum calcium to normal. Acidity increases calcium absorption from the gut lumen. Factors influencing calcium absorption include: (i) increased dietary oxalates, phytates and phosphates, which chelate calcium and reduce its absorption; (ii) vagotomy and gastrectomy, which reduce acid secretion and therefore reduce absorption; (iii) steroids (glucocorticoids) which antagonise the effects of vitamin D on the gastrointestinal tract and reduce absorption.

MALABSORPTION

Malabsorption may occur for a variety of reasons, as follows.

1. Defects of mixing of food and digestive juices. This may occur following pyloroplasty, where the gastric contents may be 'dumped' into the small bowel and adequate mixing with pancreatic juices and bile does not occur.
2. Defective production of enzymes. This may occur with abnormalities of the pancreas, e.g. chronic pancreatitis, cystic fibrosis, or carcinoma of the head of the pancreas. Lack of pancreatic enzymes reduce absorption of fats, proteins and carbohydrates.
3. Defective production of bile. This may occur because of blockage of the bile duct by stone, tumour or inflammation. Bile can not enter the duodenum, preventing digestion and absorption of fats with consequent steatorrhoea and malabsorption of fat soluble vitamins. Bile salt reabsorption is impaired by terminal ileal disease, e.g. Crohn's disease, or resection, resulting in defective enterohepatic circulation and consequent reduction in bile salt concentrations in the duodenum.
4. Abnormal luminal conditions. This may result from increased intraluminal pH as a result of reduced gastric secretion, e.g. after vagotomy or gastrectomy. This would result in decreased absorption of iron and calcium. Blind loop syndrome (bacterial overgrowth in areas of stasis) may cause malabsorption. Bacteria may compete with the host for dietary vitamin B$_{12}$, resulting in megaloblastic anaemia.
5. Loss of enterocyte mass (reduction of absorptive area). This usually results from surgical resection, e.g. Crohn's disease, mesenteric infarction, or trauma. The effects depend on the extent of resection as well as the site, proximal or distal.

Consequences of small intestinal resection

After resection of a length of jejunum the ileum can take over some of the functions. However, the reverse is not true, the jejunum being incapable of absorbing bile salts and vitamin B$_{12}$. Following loss of most of the jejunum, absorption of fat, protein and carbohydrates is severely curtailed because of loss of the large absorptive area. Severe diarrhoea occurs with additional loss of water and electrolytes. After a few weeks, ileal adaptation takes place and diarrhoea abates. Loss of body weight and reduced folate and iron absorption occur in the early phase after resection.

With resection of more than 1 m of terminal ileum, absorption of vitamin B_{12} and bile salts is reduced. Malabsorption of vitamin B_{12} results in megaloblastic anaemia. However, with normal stores prior to resection it can take 3–6 years for this to develop. Vitamin B_{12} supplements will then be required parenterally. With loss of the terminal ileum there is a reduced absorption of bile salts and the bile salt pool declines. As the pool normally circulates 6–8 times/day the liver can not make good this loss. Reduction in the bile salts leads to an increased tendency to gall stone formation and poorer emulsification and absorption of fats in the small intestine leading to steatorrhoea and decreased absorption of vitamins A, D, E and K. Decreased absorption of bile salts results in more entering the colon resulting in diarrhoea. With resection of small bowel, calcium deficiency may also occur as a result of decreased absorption of vitamin D.

Consequences of fistula formation

Fistulae involving the small intestine may be external where the fistula opens onto the skin or internal between two pieces of bowel. In both cases there is a loss of absorptive surface, with loss of nutrients, water and electrolytes. A fistula may have a high output or low output depending on its site. High output fistulae occur in the upper small bowel, e.g. duodenal fistula, and low output in the ileum.

High output fistulae

Approximately 3–4 L of fluid is lost per day. This is derived from gastric juice, bile, pancreatic juice and duodenal secretions. This depletes intravascular and interstitial volume and requires replacement with isotonic saline, as the juices lost are mostly isotonic. Loss of alkaline pancreatic juice and bile gives rise to a metabolic acidosis. Any oral intake of food passes out through the fistula; in some cases it is virtually unchanged and, unless replaced by intravenous feeding, would result in starvation. Skin protection is required with external fistulae because activated pancreatic trypsin will digest the keratin of the skin, causing excoriation. Treatment of high output fistulae requires intravenous administration of water and electrolytes commensurate with losses, together with total parenteral nutrition until the fistula closes or is surgically closed.

Low output fistulae

A low small bowel fistula may initially put out up to 1500 mL daily. A low output small bowel fistula is similar to an ileostomy. The proximal ileum can gradually adapt to the loss of any colonic surface distal to it, and more fluid and electrolytes are absorbed. Fluid loss is lower in low fistulae because there is still a large proximal surface area to deal with fluid absorption. Also, loss of nutrients is less because most have already been absorbed in the proximal small bowel. In the initial stages, fluid and electrolyte management is important but nutrition may be maintained by elemental diets.

LARGE INTESTINE

The primary functions of the colon are absorption, secretion, motility and storage.

Absorption

Water and electrolytes are absorbed in the colon. Approximately 1–2 L of ileal contents containing 90% water reach the colon daily. Water is absorbed during transit such that only 100–200 mL of water are lost in the faeces. Some amino acids, fatty acids and vitamins, e.g. vitamin K, may be absorbed in the colon, but only a small amount of these normally reaches the colon, having been absorbed in the small intestine. A proportion of ingested starch reaches the colon, where bacterial action converts it to short chain fatty acids which are absorbed. Sodium is actively absorbed, being potentiated by the action of aldosterone.

Secretion

Potassium is secreted into the intestinal lumen. Aldosterone increases potassium secretion. Potassium is also secreted in mucus, and hypokalaemia may result if large amounts of mucus are lost, e.g. from a large villous adenoma. Bicarbonate is also secreted by colonic cells. It neutralises any acidity of the faeces which may result from bacterial fermentation of carbohydrate. Mucus is secreted by the goblet cells and lubricates the passage of faeces.

Motility

The movement of contents through the large intestine does not occur at constant speed and is dependent on different patterns of motor activity, as follows.

Retrograde peristalsis (antiperistalsis). These are annular contractions moving against flow and occur chiefly in the right colon. This churns the contents, confining them to the caecum and ascending colon.

Segmentation. This occurs chiefly in the transverse and descending colon. Contraction rings occur in the smooth muscle over lengths of approximately 2.5 cm. These occur at different points along the bowel, dividing it into segments of contracted and relaxed areas. Faeces are propelled over short distances in both directions.

Mass movement. This represents a strong peristaltic wave which covers a large distance in the transverse and descending colon, pushing faeces distally. Mass movement occurs only 3–4 times daily, usually after food. Some of the material entering the caecum may pass by faeces remaining from earlier periods. In most people the unabsorbed part of a meal reaches the caecum in approximately 4 h and the descending colon in 24 h. However, because of the complex and variable movements of the colon, approximately 25% of the residue of a meal can remain in the rectum at 72 h. Mass movement occurs following entry of food into the stomach, i.e. the gastrocolic reflex.

Colonic motility is affected by physical activities such as lifting and by emotional states, e.g. irritable bowel syndrome. Colonic transit times are increased by increasing the fibre content of the diet.

Storage

The colon stores faeces until the time for defaecation is appropriate. The primary site of storage is the transverse colon. Gas is also stored in the colon. Colonic gas is largely nitrogen but also contains oxygen, carbon dioxide, methane and some hydrogen sulphide. Only about one-third of the population produce methane. Hydrogen and methane are explosive gases, and caution should be used with diathermy in the bowel. Mannitol has been used in the past to prepare the bowel for surgical procedures. Colonic bacteria ferment mannitol to produce hydrogen. Hence, mannitol should be avoided in bowel preparation. Excessive colonic gas is usually due to hydrogen. Avoidance of lactose, beans and wheat in the diet is appropriate in avoiding excessive colonic gas.

DIARRHOEA

Diarrhoea is an increased frequency of abnormally loose motions for a particular patient. Colonic transit time is reduced, and consequently there is a reduced time for reabsorption of sodium and water, and secretion of potassium. Consequently there is loss of sodium and water in the stools and, if this is severe, dehydration results and may result in hypovolaemic shock. Acid–base disturbances may occur, especially with acute diarrhoea, with loss of bicarbonate and a resulting metabolic acidosis. With chronic diarrhoea resulting in loss of sodium and water, there is an increase in circulating aldosterone levels. This increases loss of K^+ from the kidney and colon, leading to hypokalaemia and a consequent metabolic alkalosis.

Causes

Malabsorption

Abnormalities of digestion and absorption result in undigested products, with associated water being retained in the intestinal lumen which then pass into the colon. Causes include:

- absence of bile
- absence of pancreatic exocrine secretions
- loss of enterocyte mass
- intestinal fistulae
- after gastric surgery
- osmotic laxatives
- intestinal ischaemia.

Infection

Several bacteria produce enterotoxins which stimulate water and electrolyte secretion by the enterocyte of the small intestine. Some bacteria destroy the small bowel mucosa, reducing the surface area for absorption. In both cases, excess volumes of fluid enter the colon, which is unable to absorb it and diarrhoea results.

Reduction in the absorptive capacity of the colonic mucosa

A reduced surface area results in less absorption of sodium and electrolytes. This may occur in surgical removal, e.g. subtotal colectomy, or ulcerative colitis.

Presence of excess bile in the colon

This occurs following resection of the terminal ileum and resultant reduction in salt absorption. Bile salts stimulate secretion of water and eletrolytes into the colonic lumen, resulting in diarrhoea.

Increased peristalsis

This may occur because of the following:

- vagotomy and drainage — lack of vagal reflexes controlling movement of food through the gut, and increased gastric emptying which results in food not being in a suitable format for digestion, contribute to diarrhoea following vagotomy and drainage
- carcinoid via serotonin production
- thyrotoxicosis via thyroid hormones
- irritable bowel syndrome.

Tumours

- carcinoid via 5HT effect on secretion of water and electrolytes
- vipoma via VIP.

Drugs

- antibiotics altering intestinal flora
- laxatives.

Factors ensuring faecal continence

Faecal continence depends upon several factors. The anal canal is surrounded by sphincters (see section on anatomy) which are normally tonically contracted. Sympathetic nerves maintain sphincter tone in the internal sphincter. Parasympathetic innervation is via the pelvic splanchnic nerves (S2, 3, 4). This is inhibitory, causing the sphincter to relax. Rectal distension reflexly causes sphincteric relaxation. The external sphincter is maintained in a contracted state via impulses passing along the pudendal nerve. Contraction of the internal and external sphincters keeps the anal canal closed and maintain a pressure in it of 40–90 mmHg. Continence is also maintained by angulation between the anal canal and rectum, which in the upright position is approximately 90°. This angulation is maintained by the puborectalis muscle. The anal canal is slit-like in an anterior–posterior direction. Intra-abdominal pressure maintains this slit-like state by compressing the rectum laterally at a point just proximal to where the anal canal passes through puborectalis.

Mechanism of defaecation

The lining of the anal canal contains sensory nerve endings which are sensitive to tactile, thermal and painful stimuli. A classical anatomical description suggests that somatic sensation ceases at the dentate line, but often it may extend more proximally. The nerve endings in the anal canal relay information into the CNS, identifying the luminal contents, i.e. whether solid or gas.

When faecal material enters the rectum, causing the pressure to increase above 18 mmHg, a desire to defaecate occurs. This is due to stimulation of receptors within the rectal wall. Afferent impulses pass via the pelvic nerves to sacral segments 2, 3, 4, i.e. the defaecation centre. Efferent impulses then pass back to the rectum to the myenteric plexus where postganglionic parasympathetic nerves are activated. These cause contraction of the rectum, pushing faeces distally. The internal sphincter also relaxes. Afferent impulses from the rectum also activate ascending sensory pathways providing conscious awareness of rectal distension. When faecal material enters the upper anal canal, sensory receptors are stimulated which send impulses to S2, 3, 4 segments of the cord. The effect of these impulses is two-fold: (i) there is reflex activation of the pudendal nerve which sends impulses to the external sphincter to increase its contraction and maintain continence; (ii) there is activation of ascending pathways to the sensory cortex, which differentiates between solid and gas. If it is solid, efferent impulses pass down the cord to reinforce contraction of the external sphincter and maintain continence. If it is gas the sphincter relaxes and flatus is passed.

If the time for defaecation is not appropriate, the desire to defaecate ceases after a few minutes as the rectal muscle relaxes. The reflex does not return until more faeces have entered the rectum and distended it further. If the time for defaecation is appropriate, the initial stages are described above. Whilst in a suitable place for defaecation, the external sphincter relaxes allowing the pressure in the anal canal to fall. Peristalsis in the rectum then pushes the faeces out. This is aided by adopting a squatting position when the rectum and anal canal are now in a straight line. Straining at stool is a voluntary reinforcement of defaecation by performing the Valsalva manoeuvre. Overdistension of the rectum with a pressure of greater than 55 mmHg causes involuntary defaecation. This involuntary mechanism occurs in patients with spinal cord transection above S2, 3, 4. Immediately after transection, spinal shock occurs and there is no reflex activity, with retention of faeces. When reflex activity returns, reflex defaecation occurs although the patient is unaware that the rectum is filling.

Incontinence

Incontinence is the inability to control the passage of faeces and flatus.

Aetiology

The following are aetiological factors.

- ageing
- neurological disorders
- obstetric injury
- trauma
- rectal prolapse
- iatrogenic, e.g. previous anorectal surgery
- overflow secondary to faecal impaction.

Any disease process that interferes with rectal sensation or affects function of the anorectal musculature may produce incontinence. Diagnosis is based on the clinical history, rectal examination, anorectal manometry and electromyography.

In neurogenic incontinence the pelvic muscles are

atonic with laxity of the anal canal. There is lack of sensibility to tactile stimulation, inability to contract the anal musculature voluntarily, and the anal reflexes are absent. In traumatic or postoperative incontinence there is loss of integrity of the anorectal ring.

LIVER

The liver has several functions:

- production of bile
- storage, e.g. glycogen, vitamins A, D, E and K and B_{12}
- metabolism of proteins, fat and carbohydrate
- detoxification and inactivation of hormones, drugs and toxins
- reticulo-endothelial function via Kupffer cells
- haemopoieses (fetus).

Production of bile

Bile is produced at the rate of 500–1500 mL/day by hepatocyte secretion and the addition of secretions from the ducts. Bile is produced continuously, being stored in the gall bladder between meals. Bile contains bile salts and HCO_3^- which aid digestion. In addition, bile acts as an excretory route for bile pigments, cholesterol, steroids and a number of drugs. Bile salts are essential for lipid digestion. HCO_3^- assists in neutralising gastric acid entering into the duodenum. Three factors regulate bile flow: hepatic secretion, gall bladder contraction, and choledochal sphincter resistance. In the fasting state, pressure in the bile duct is 5–10 cm of water, and bile produced by the liver is diverted into the gall bladder. After a meal the gall bladder contracts, the choledochal sphincter (sphincter of Oddi) relaxes, and bile enters the duodenum in squirts as ductal pressure intermittently exceeds sphincteric pressure. During contraction, pressure in the gall bladder reaches 25 cm of water and that in the bile duct 15–20 cm of water. More than 90% of the bile salts secreted into the small intestine are reabsorbed, largely in the terminal ileum, and return to the liver in the portal circulation. The total pool of bile salts is recycled as many as 6–8 times per day. Secretin increases in the production of HCO_3^--rich secretion from the duct epithelium. Also under the effect of secretin, the volume flow of bile increases, but the content of bile acids does not increase.

Bile salts and the enterohepatic circulation

Bile salts are steroid molecules formed from cholesterol by hepatocytes. The major bile salts synthesised in the liver are called primary bile salts. These are cholate and chenodeoxycholate. Intestinal bacteria alter these primary bile salts to produce secondary bile salts by a process of dehydroxylation. Secondary bile salts are deoxycholate and lithocholate. Deoxycholate is reabsorbed and enters bile while lithocholate is insoluble and is excreted in faeces. The function of bile salts is to solubilise lipids and aid their absorption. Bile salts are detergents, i.e. molecules with water soluble and fat soluble groups at opposite poles. In aqueous solution they spontaneously aggregate in groups called micelles. The molecules in the micelles are arranged with a hydrophobic pole in the centre and hydrophilic poles on the surface facing the water. Micelles are capable of solubilising lipids within the hydrophobic centres, whilst still remaining in aqueous solution. Lecithin and cholesterol, other constituents of bile, are transported in bile within micelles. Lecithin increases the amount of cholesterol that can be solubilised in the micelles. If more cholesterol is present in the bile than can be solubilised in micelles, crystals of cholesterol may form in the bile. These crystals may form a nidus for development of cholesterol gall stones. Bile salts, lecithin and cholesterol constitute about 90% of solids in the bile, the remainder consisting of bilirubin, fatty acids and inorganic salts. Bile salts remain in the intestinal lumen throughout the jejunum, where they are responsible for fat absorption. More than 80% of bile salts are actively absorbed in the distal ileum and pass back in the portal blood to the liver, where they are re-secreted. The bile salts that are not absorbed enter the colon, where they are converted to secondary bile salts, some of which are reabsorbed in the colon, the remainder being lost in the faeces. The entire bile salt pool (2.4–4.0 g) circulates twice through the enterohepatic circulation during each meal, recycling occurring 6–8 times per day. About 10–20% of the total bile salt pool is lost in the stool daily, the amount being restored by hepatic synthesis.

Bile pigments

The breakdown of red cells by the reticulo-endothelial system results in the degradation of the haem groups of haemoglobin, with the formation of biliverdin. Biliverdin is reduced to bilirubin which enters the blood stream, attaches to albumin, and is carried to the liver. This is unconjugated bilirubin. In the liver it is conjugated with glucuronic acid, making it into the water soluble bilirubin diglucuronide (conjugated bilirubin). This is excreted in the bile and enters the intestine, where it is reduced by intestinal bacteria, resulting in urobilinogen and stercobilinogen. Urobilinogen is readily absorbed from the gut and passes back to the liver, where it is taken up and released back into the bile. A small amount of absorbed urobilinogen enters the systemic circulation and is excreted in the bile as urobilin. Stercobilinogen is excreted in the faeces as stercobilin.

Storage function

The liver stores glycogen, vitamins A, D, E and K and vitamin B_{12}, iron and copper. The liver contains a large store of vitamin B_{12}. Even if absorption totally ceases, the store will last for 3–6 years.

Metabolism of protein, fat and carbohydrate

Protein

Protein catabolism results in the deamination of amino acids, with the formation of ammonia. Ammonia is dissipated by conversion to urea in the liver. The liver synthesises all non-essential amino acids and all the plasma proteins with the exception of the gammaglobulins, which are produced by plasma cells.

Carbohydrate

Liver and skeletal muscle are the two major sites of glycogen storage. When blood glucose levels are high, glycogen is deposited in the liver (glycogenesis). When blood glucose is low, liver glycogen is broken down to glucose (glycogenolysis), the glucose being released into the blood. The liver therefore helps to maintain a relatively constant blood glucose level. The liver is also a major site of gluconeogenesis, i.e. the conversion of amino acids, lipids, or simple carbohydrates substances, e.g. lactate, into glucose. The liver can thus perform glycogenesis, glycogenolysis, or gluconeogenesis, depending upon the hormonal stimulus to the hepatocytes.

Lipids

Hepatocytes synthesise and secrete very low density lipoproteins. These are then converted to other lipoproteins which are a major source of cholesterol and triglycerides for most tissues in the body. Hepatocytes are the principal source of cholesterol in the body and are the major site of excretion of cholesterol. In certain physiological (starvation) and pathological (diabetic ketoacidosis) states, β-oxidation of fatty acids provides a major source of energy for the body. Ketone bodies are formed and released from hepatocytes and are carried in the circulation to other tissues where they are metabolised. Diabetic ketoacidosis is the result of severe insulin deficiency combined with excessive glucagon production. The altered hormonal state promotes lipolysis, gluconeogenesis and glycogenolysis while inhibiting glycolysis. This results in overproduction of glucose by the liver. Peripheral tissues cease to utilise glucose because of low insulin levels and become dependent on fatty acids and ketone bodies. In diabetic ketoacidosis the production of ketone bodies continues unchecked. This does not occur in starvation, as the level of ketone bodies is controlled by insulin levels which, although low, are sufficient to inhibit further lipolysis.

Detoxification and inactivation functions

The liver is a major site for the degradation and excretion of hormones. Peptide hormones, e.g. insulin, ADH, growth hormone are inactivated in the liver. The liver also inactivates and excretes steroid hormones of the adrenal cortex, ovary and testis. Catecholamines are also inactivated in the liver. Drugs and toxins are also metabolised by the liver. This may occur in two stages. Phase 1 increases the water solubility of the molecule to aid its excretion but does not necessarily detoxify the drug. Occasionally, toxic metabolites may be produced, such as occurs with paracetamol. During phase 2, toxicity and biological activity are reduced and water solubility further increased. The cytochrome P450 system is mainly involved in phase 1. Amongst substrates for this pathway are phenytoin, warfarin, halothane, indomethacin and cyclosporin. Drugs such as barbiturates, phenytoin, and rifampicin can increase activity of the P450 system. This can lead to decreased levels of drugs which are metabolised via the P450 system: e.g. levels of the immunosuppressant drug cyclosporin may be reduced in patients taking barbiturates, rifampicin, or phenytoin. Conversely, drugs which inhibit the cytochrome P450 system can lead to increased levels of other drugs metabolised via the system, e.g. cytochrome P450 inhibitors such as erythromycin and ketoconazole can lead to increased cyclosporin blood levels. Cimetidine can prolong the elimination of drugs by inhibiting the cytochrome P450 system. This can reduce metabolism of such drugs as oral anticoagulants, phenytoin and lignocaine. Close monitoring of patients receiving cimetidine and who are also taking oral anticoagulants or phenytoin is desirable, and a reduction in the dosage of these drugs may be necessary.

Reticulo-endothelial function

The reticulo-endothelial function of the liver is carried out by the Kupffer cells which line the hepatic sinusoids. They remove bacteria and toxins absorbed from the colon and which arrive in the liver via the portal circulation. They also remove effete and abnormal erythrocytes from the blood.

Haemopoiesis

In the embryo, haemopoiesis occurs in the liver, the bone

marrow gradually taking over after the 20th week of gestation. In a number of diseases, e.g. chronic haemolytic anaemia or megaloblastic anaemia, foci of haemopoiesis may appear in the liver (extramedullary haemopoiesis).

GALL BLADDER

The production of bile is dealt with in the section on the liver. Bile enters the gall bladder via the cystic duct and is then stored and concentrated in the gall bladder. In response to ingestion of food, especially fatty food, cholecystokinin (CCK) is released from the duodenal mucosa. This circulates to the gall bladder, causing its contraction and also relaxation of the sphincter of Oddi. Bile flow during a meal is augmented by increased turnover of bile salts in the enterohepatic circulation and stimulation of ductal secretion by secretin, gastrin and CCK.

PANCREAS

Pancreatic juice is secreted at a rate of 1200–1500 mL per day. It contains water, electrolytes and enzymes and has a pH of 8. This highly alkaline secretion, together with bile, neutralises the acid chyme which enters the duodenum from the stomach. Water and electrolytes are secreted mainly by the duct cells, while enzymes come from the acinar cells.

Pancreatic enzymes

The pancreatic enzymes are involved in proteolysis, carbohydrate digestion and fat digestion. The proteolytic enzyme trypsinogen is converted into the active form trypsin by enterokinase, present in the enterocytes of the duodenum. Its release into the duodenal lumen is triggered by CCK. Activated trypsin will itself activate more trypsinogen to trypsin. Trypsin acts on long protein chains, splitting them into smaller polypeptides and peptides. Pancreatic amylase acts on starch and glycogen, aiding absorption. Pancreatic lipase acts on triglycerides to produce monoglycerides and free fatty acids.

Control of pancreatic secretion

This is chiefly hormonal. Secretion of water and electrolytes is under the control of secretin. It is released from the endocrine cells of the mucosa of the upper small intestine in response to the presence of acid in the duodenum and upper small intestine. Secretin also increases bicarbonate secretion by the intrahepatic bile ducts, inhibits gastric secretion, and controls gastric emptying by causing contraction of the pyloric sphincter. Enzyme

secretion is controlled by CCK released from endocrine cells of the mucosa of the duodenum and jejunum. CCK promotes release of pancreatic enzymes stored in the zymogen granules of the acinar cells. It also causes gall bladder contraction and relaxation of the sphincter of Oddi. Vagal stimulation potentiates the effect of CCK on gall bladder contraction and pancreatic enzyme secretion. Inhibition of pancreatic secretion is via release of somatostatin from the D cells of the pancreatic islets. Somatostatin inhibits enzymes, bicarbonate, gall bladder contraction and gastric acid secretion, and decreases splanchnic blood flow. Factors stimulating its release from D cells include elevated blood glucose after meals, and elevated blood levels of glucagon and CCK.

Pancreatic fistula

A pancreatic fistula may develop after operations on the pancreas, trauma to the pancreas, or accidental damage to the pancreas, e.g. damage to the tail of the pancreas during splenectomy. The patient loses up to 1–2 L of pancreatic secretion per day, which is isotonic, and this results in dehydration involving the extracellular fluid compartment. As the pancreatic juice contains bicarbonate, metabolic acidosis results if the losses are not replaced. A pancreatic fistula does not normally cause digestion of the skin, as the enzymes have not come into contact with small bowel contents and therefore remain inactivated. However, if infection occurs, organisms can activate trypsinogen, and skin digestion may occur. Somatostatin, which inhibits pancreatic secretion, is useful in 'drying up' a pancreatic fistula provided there is no obstruction to the proximal duct.

GASTROINTESTINAL HORMONES

These are produced by cells of the gastrointestinal tract and associated organs and control activity of other parts of the tract. They may act distantly via the blood stream, i.e. a true endocrine effect, or locally (paracrine), or by a neurotransmitter effect (neurocrine). Only the more common will be discussed here.

Gastrin

The major site of gastrin production is the antrum of the stomach. It is released from the G cells of the antral mucosa. Secretion is stimulated by antral distension, presence of peptides and amino acids in the antrum, gastrin-releasing peptides and insulin-induced hypoglycaemia. Secretion is inhibited by acid in the stomach, hyperglycaemia, somatostatin, secretin, glucagon and VIP. Gastrin stimulates secretion of acid, pepsin and intrinsic factor. At high concentrations it stimulates gastric motility and increases tone of the lower oesophageal sphincter.

Cholecystokinin (CCK)

CCK is produced by cells of the duodenal and jejunal mucosa. Secretion is stimulated by the presence of fatty acids, peptides and amino acids in the duodenal or jejunal lumen. Secretion is inhibited by somatostatin. CCK stimulates an enzyme rich secretion from the acinar cells of the pancreas; it potentiates the effect of secretin on HCO_3^- secretion by duct cells; and causes contraction of the gall bladder and relaxation of the sphincter of Oddi. It also inhibits gastric emptying.

Secretin

Secretin is produced by cells in the duodenal and jejunal mucosa. The main stimulus to release is an acid intraluminal pH of < 4.5. It is also released by the presence of fatty acids in the duodenum and jejunum. It stimulates the duct cells of the liver and pancreas to produce secretion rich in HCO_3^-. It also inhibits gastric acid secretion.

Gastric inhibitory peptide (GIP)

GIP is produced by cells of the mucosa in the duodenum and upper intestine. It is released by the presence of intraluminal carbohydrate and fat. It releases insulin from the beta cells of the pancreas and inhibits gastric secretion and motility.

Somatostatin

Somatostatin is present in the pancreatic islets and in cells of the intestinal epithelium. Its release is stimulated by the presence of fats, glucose and bile salts in the intestinal lumen. It inhibits gastric acid and pepsin secretion, gastrin release, pancreatic enzyme secretion and insulin and glucagon release.

Enteroglucagon

Enteroglucagon is produced by cells in the distal ileum and colon and released in response to glucose and fat in the ileal and colonic lumen. It inhibits gastric and intestinal motility and has a trophic effect on intestinal crypt cells.

Vasoactive intestinal peptide (VIP)

VIP is widely distributed in the gut, in intestinal neurones and possibly in mucosal endocrine cells. Its physiological role is not clear, although in experimental animals it increases water and bicarbonate secretion by the pancreas, inhibits gastric secretion and causes marked secretion of intestinal fluid. It also causes vasodilatation and hypotension. The main interest in VIP relates to VIP-secreting

tumours (vipomas), usually in the pancreas, which cause watery diarrhoea, achlorhydria and hypokalaemia (the Verner–Morrison syndrome).

Insulin

Insulin is produced by the β cells of the pancreas. Insulin lowers blood glucose by facilitating uptake in muscle and adipose tissue and by inhibiting hepatic glucose output. In the liver it stimulates glycogen and fat synthesis and inhibits glycogen breakdown and ketone body formation. Insulin increases K^+ uptake into cells and consequently can lower plasma K^+. Insulin release is also stimulated by glucagon, secretin, CCK, VIP and gastrin. Tolbutamide and chlorpropamide, oral hypoglycaemic agents, release insulin by acting on the adenyl cyclase system.

Glucagon

Glucagon is produced in the α cells of the pancreas. Its release is stimulated by low blood glucose concentrations, amino acids, catecholamines and CCK. It is inhibited by insulin and hyperglycaemia. It increases blood glucose levels. It acts on the liver to stimulate glycogenolysis and gluconeogenesis.

PATHOLOGY

PERITONEUM

Peritonitis

Peritonitis is an inflammatory or suppurative response of the peritoneal lining to direct irritation. It may be localised or generalised, bacterial or chemical. Localised peritonitis is due to transmural inflammation of a viscus, e.g. acute appendicitis, acute cholecystitis, acute diverticulitis. It may remain localised by being contained by omental wrapping or adhesion of adjacent structures. In many cases, however, it becomes generalised, spreading to involve the whole peritoneum. Sudden perforation of a viscus usually results in generalised peritonitis. In this case, the patient is usually seriously ill. Hypovolaemia results from massive exudation into the peritoneal cavity, and septicaemia may result if the cause is infective, e.g. faecal peritonitis due to perforated diverticulitis. Chemical peritonitis results from gastric or pancreatic juice, bile, urine, or blood in the peritoneal cavity. Bile causes little reaction if it is sterile, but can cause a severe peritonitis if it is infected or mixed with pancreatic juice. Blood and urine, again, cause little reaction if sterile, but a severe reaction usually results if they are infected. The causes of peritonitis are shown in Box 17.1.

Box 17.1 Causes of peritonitis

Acute
- Bacterial
  — Primary (rare)
    • Streptococci, pneumococci
    • Haematogenous spread, occurs in young girls, ascites, nephrotic syndrome and post-splenectomy
  — Secondary (common)
    • Related to perforation, infection, inflammation or ischaemia of the GI or GU tract

- Chemical
  — Gastric juice e.g. perforated gastric ulcer
  — Pancreatic juice e.g. acute pancreatitis
  — Bile e.g. perforated gall bladder
  — Blood e.g. ruptured spleen
  — Urine e.g. intraperitoneal rupture of the bladder

Chronic
- Tuberculosis
- Starch (immunological reaction)

Complications of peritonitis

These may be either systemic or local. Local complications include:

- intraperitoneal abscess, e.g. subphrenic or pelvic
- wound infection
- anastomotic breakdown
- fistula formation
- adhesions.

Systemic complications include:

- hypovolaemic shock
- septic shock
- adult respiratory distress syndrome
- disseminated intravascular coagulation
- immunological failure
- multiorgan failure.

Prognosis

The overall mortality in generalised peritonitis, especially if it is infective, is high. Factors affecting mortality include:

- age — elderly patients with faecal peritonitis have an exceptionally high mortality
- causation — infective causes have a higher mortality than chemical
- duration of symptoms
- degree of bacterial contamination
- concomitant disease processes, e.g. cardiac, renal and hepatic
- organ failure.

OESOPHAGUS

Congenital

These are dealt with in Chapter 16.

Mechanical disorders

Hiatus hernia

This is the commonest mechanical disorder of the oesophagus. It implies that part of the stomach is above the oesophageal opening in the diaphragm. There are two types: sliding and rolling.

Sliding This is the most common type. Obesity and raised intra-abdominal pressure are contributory factors, but loss of diaphragmatic muscular tone may also occur. Pregnancy is also a contributing factor. Occasionally, sliding hiatus hernia may occur in apparently normal people. The stomach 'slides' through the oesophageal opening in the diaphragm. Reflux occurs with consequent chronic oesophagitis.

Rolling The fundus of the stomach passes alongside the oesophagus into the chest. The cardio-oesophageal junction remains intra-abdominal, and reflux does not occur. The presence of the fundus of the stomach alongside the lower oesophagus may lead to dysphagia. The fundus may become incarcerated, and strangulation with perforation may occur.

Achalasia

This occurs most frequently in the fourth decade of life. There is an incomplete relaxation of the lower oesophagus, with increased resting pressure in the lower oesophageal sphincter. Peristalsis is absent over the affected segment. The cause of the condition is unknown, but there is reduction or absence of ganglion cells in the myenteric plexus. Above the involved area, the oesophagus dilates and food collects in the dilated oesophagus. Dysphagia occurs and is worse for liquids than solids. The condition affects 1:100 000 of the population. Overspill from the dilated oesophagus into the bronchial tree may result in pneumonitis and lung abscess. Carcinoma complicates achalasia in 3% of cases. It is usually of the squamous cell variety.

Diverticulae

These are outpouchings of the wall of a hollow viscus. They are uncommon in the oesophagus and may be of the traction (i.e. pulled out by external stimuli) or pulsion (i.e. pushed out by increased intraluminal pressure) variety. They may become distended with food and cause dysphagia.

Inflammatory disorders

Acute oesophagitis

This is fairly rare and is most commonly seen in diabetics and immunocompromised patients. Candidiasis is one of the more common infections, which may give rise to retrosternal pain and dysphagia. Oesophagoscopy reveals white plaques with haemorrhagic margins. In immuno-compromised individuals herpes simplex and CMV may cause oesophagitis. Corrosive substances accidentally ingested by children, or taken with suicidal intent by adults, may cause marked oesophagitis.

Chronic oesophagitis

Non-specific chronic oesophagitis is very common and usually results from reflux of gastric acid. Specific causes are rare, but it may be due to Crohn's disease or tuberculosis.

Reflux oesophagitis

This is usually associated with the presence of a sliding hiatus hernia, although in some patients it may occur with increased intra-abdominal pressure without herniation. Morphologically there is an increased loss of squamous cells with an increased proliferation of cells in the base of the epithelium, and the connective tissue papillae elongate. This is accompanied by a chronic inflammatory cell reaction. Where reflux is severe, ulceration may occur with slow bleeding leading to anaemia. Occasionally, brisk haemorrhage occurs. Rarely, ulceration may occur with a perforation leading to mediastinitis or peritonitis. Healing of oesophagitis occurs by fibrosis, and this may result in a stricture with consequent dysphagia. In some cases squamous epithelial cells are replaced by areas of columnar epithelium, giving rise to a condition known as Barrett's oesophagus.

Stricture

These may be benign or malignant. Malignant strictures are dealt with below. Benign strictures may result from reflux oesophagitis, achalasia, corrosive substances, ionising radiation and trauma. Scleroderma is a rare cause.

Barrett's oesophagus

In this condition, which is usually associated with reflux, the distal part of the oesophagus becomes lined with columnar epithelium. However, there is poor correlation between the degree of reflux and the severity of the epithelial change. Endoscopy reveals reddened columnar epithelium either in islands or extending circumferentially around the lower oesophagus. The condition is recognised as premalignant. Malignancy is considered to be related to the degree of dysplasia, patients with high grade dysplasia having 100-fold risk of developing adeno-carcinoma compared with the normal population. There is some evidence that low grade epithelial dysplasia may regress. Regular endoscopic surveillance is advised, with multiple biopsies to assess the degree of dysplasia. In severe cases of Barrett's oesophagus, ulceration and stricture may develop.

Perforation of the oesophagus

Causes of perforation of the oesophagus include:

- iatrogenic
  — oesophagoscopy (especially rigid oesophagoscopy)
  — dilatation of strictures
  — biopsy
  — insertion of endoprostheses (stent)
- foreign bodies
  — coins
  — bones
  — false teeth
- vomiting
  — Boerhaave's syndrome.

Clinical consequences of perforation include mediastinal emphysema, mediastinitis and empyema.

Chagas' disease

This is due to chronic infection with the parasite *Trypanosoma cruzi*. The organism destroys the ganglion cells of the myenteric plexus, leading to a clinical picture similar to achalasia.

Tumours

Benign tumours of the oesophagus are uncommon. The most frequent is leiomyoma. Dysphagia and bleeding may occur.

Carcinoma

Carcinoma of the oesophagus accounts for about 2% of all malignant disease in the United Kingdom. The incidence is increasing worldwide. The frequency is high in Iran, particularly around the Caspian Sea area, and also in northern China. There is considerable geographical variation in its incidence, being 300 times higher around the Caspian Sea than in the United Kingdom.

Causes

Causes include: high dietary intake of tannic acid, e.g. in strong tea; dietary deficiency of vitamin A, riboflavin and zinc; fungal contamination of food; opium ingestion; and thermal injury. Cigarette smoking and drinking of spirits may be associated with a high incidence. There is some recent evidence to suggest that human papilloma virus (HPV) may be important. There is also a higher incidence with Barrett's oesophagus. Oesophageal stasis may increase the risk of carcinoma, there being a 22-fold increase with lye strictures, 9-fold with oesophageal webs, 7-fold in achalasia, and 6-fold with peptic strictures. Postcricoid carcinoma usually occurs in females and is part of the Plummer–Vinson syndrome.

Types

Most carcinomas of the oesophagus are of the squamous type although, in the lower third, adenocarcinomas are the predominant type. Squamous cell carcinoma usually commences as an ulcer, spreading to become annular and constricting, causing dysphagia. Dysplasia usually precedes malignant change. In countries with a high prevalence of the disease the change may be recognised at regular endoscopy with biopsy or exfoliative cytology. Lymphatic spread within the submucosa occurs beyond the recognisable margins of the tumour viewed endoscopically. Lymphatic metastases occur early. Local extension within the mediastinum occurs and may result in tracheo-oesophageal fistulae. Invasion into the aorta may occur, with fatal haemorrhage. Most patients die of local spread and bronchopneumonia. Haematogenous spread to the liver and lungs may occur. By the time of presentation the tumour has often spread to adjacent organs, and surgical resection is only possible in 30–40%. The remainder require palliation. Prognosis is extremely poor, most patients surviving less than 6 months. The 5 year survival rate is only 5%.

Other malignant tumours of the oesophagus are rare. Malignant melanomas, small cell anaplastic carcinomas, and sarcomas may occur.

Vascular disorders

The veins of the lower oesophagus are a potential site of portosystemic shunting of blood in portal hypertension. The latter may result in development of oesophageal varices, i.e. dilatation and congestion of the veins in the oesophageal submucosa. The dilated veins protrude into the lumen, where they may be traumatised by passing food. Haemorrhage may occur which on occasions is torrential and fatal.

STOMACH

Gastritis

This may be acute or chronic.

Acute gastritis

This is usually an acute response to an irritant chemical agent, e.g. drugs or alcohol. Mucosal inflammation may be caused by steroids, non-steroidal anti-inflammatory agents and aspirin. Their effects are mediated by inhibition of prostaglandin synthesis. Acute gastric erosions arise, an erosion being defined as partial loss of the mucosa, the defect lacking penetration of the muscularis mucosa. Erosions in acute gastritis may be multiple and result in life-threatening haemorrhage.

Chronic gastritis

This occurs in two forms: type A and type B. Type A is an autoimmune disease, while Type B is a response to bacterial infection with *Helicobacter pylori* and is now more commonly known as *H. pylori*-associated chronic gastritis.

Autoimmune chronic gastritis Patients with autoimmune chronic gastritis have serum antibodies against gastric parietal cells and intrinsic-factor-binding sites. They have achlorhydria and a macrocytic anaemia resulting from B_{12} deficiency. Autoimmune gastritis associated with macrocytic anaemia is known as pernicious anaemia.

Histologically there is glandular atrophy and fibrosis of the lamina propria with infiltration of lymphocytes and plasma cells. Intestinal metaplasia may occur. The association between autoimmune gastritis and intestinal metaplasia, and the development of gastric cancer is not clear. There is, however, an increased incidence of gastric cancer in autoimmune chronic gastritis.

H. pylori-*associated chronic gastritis (formerly Type B)* Eighty percent of chronic gastritis is of this type. *H. pylori* is a Gram negative, spirally shaped bacterium which colonises the gastric mucosa, particularly in the antrum and pyloric canal. It is a highly adapted organism which lives only on gastric mucosa. Initially, morphological changes are essentially superficial, with inflammation affecting the upper half of the mucosa. The majority of patients exhibit diffuse involvement of the antrum and body of the stomach, and, with time, progression occurs to glandular atrophy, fibrosis and intestinal metaplasia. These patients are at risk of developing gastric ulcer and gastric carcinoma. In those in which the antrum is mainly involved with little involvement of the body of the stomach, there is an increased acid output and they are at greater risk of developing duodenal ulceration. Patients which chronic gastritis and *H. pylori* usually improve when treated with antimicrobial agents, and relapses are associated with reappearance of the organism.

Peptic ulceration

A peptic ulcer is a breach in the epithelial surface of the

gastrointestinal tract due to attack by acid and pepsin. Peptic ulcers occur in the stomach, duodenum, lower oesophagus, gastrojejunal anastomosis (gastric drainage procedure) and in a Meckel's diverticulum which contains gastric mucosa. Peptic ulcers may be acute or chronic.

Acute peptic ulceration

This may arise as part of an acute gastritis as a response to severe stress and due to severe hyperacidity such as occurs in a Zollinger–Ellison syndrome. Acute ulcers arising following acute gastritis are usually consequent upon ingestion of steroids, non-steroidal anti-inflammatory drugs, aspirin, or excessive alcohol. Stress-induced ulcers may follow severe sepsis, acute pancreatitis, major trauma, head injury (Cushing's ulcer), and burns (Curling's ulcer). Stress-induced ulcers may arise as a consequence of mucosal ischaemia. Hyperacidity associated with Zollinger–Ellison syndrome may lead to multiple acute ulcers in the stomach, duodenum and occasionally the proximal jejunum.

Chronic peptic ulceration

Chronic peptic ulceration occurs when the action of acid and pepsin is not opposed by adequate mucosal protection mechanism. The mucosal defences against acid attack consist of a mucus–bicarbonate barrier and the surface epithelium.

The mucus barrier itself has acid-resistant properties, but these are enhanced by the establishment of a buffering gradient across the mucus layer brought about by bicarbonate ions. The surface epithelium also constitutes a line of defence. Ulceration can result from either destruction or removal of the mucus barrier or a loss of integrity of the surface epithelium. Factors which interfere with mucosal protection are helicobacter-associated gastritis and the ingestion of non-steroidal anti-inflammatory drugs.

Aetiology Several factors show an association with peptic ulceration:

- acid hypersecretion
- helicobacter-associated gastroduodenitis
- non-steroidal anti-inflammatory drugs
- steroids
- smoking
- alcohol
- diet
- stress.

An increased incidence of peptic ulceration, especially duodenal ulceration, has been associated with uraemia, hyperparathyroidism, hypercalcaemia, chronic obstructive airways disease and alcoholic cirrhosis.

Complications of peptic ulceration

Complications include:

- perforation resulting in peritonitis
- bleeding due to an erosion of a vessel in the base of the ulcer
- penetration into underlying structures e.g. pancreas or liver
- scarring — this may result in pyloric stenosis
- malignant change — this may occur rarely in gastric ulcers but never in duodenal ulcers.

Carcinoma of the stomach

Gastric cancer is the second most common fatal malignancy (after lung cancer) in the world. The incidence is declining but it remains a common tumour with a poor prognosis. Widespread geographical variations occur, the incidence being high in Japan, China and certain coastal countries where the intake of dietary nitrate is high. Eating smoked fish and highly spiced foods have been implicated. Causative environmental factors are important, migrant studies showing that when Japanese move to other countries where the incidence is low, the incidence of gastric cancer falls and after only one generation approximates to that of the local population. Other associations with gastric cancer include blood group A, pernicious anaemia, atrophic gastritis, previous gastric surgery, and benign gastric ulcer. More recently a link between *H. pylori* infection and gastric cancer has been established. Epidemiological studies have shown that patients with antibodies to *H. pylori* have a higher incidence of gastric cancer. Several molecular genetic changes have been demonstrated in gastric carcinoma. Changes in the tumour suppressor genes, p53, K-ras, and the APC gene and overexpression of oncogenes, e.g. c-myc, have been demonstrated.

Classification

Gastric cancers are classified as either 'early' or 'advanced' on the basis of direct spread through the stomach wall. 'Early' gastric cancer is confined to either the mucosa or submucosa. 'Advanced' cancer extends into or beyond the muscularis propria. Most cancers are advanced at the time of diagnosis, and potentially curative operations are possible in less then 50%. Patients who have potentially curable resections with radical surgery and extensive lymph node dissection have a better chance of survival, the 5 year survival rate being as high as 60%. Overall, however, the 5 year survival rate is 10%. In countries where there is a high incidence of gastric carcinoma and screening programmes are carried out to detect 'early' gastric cancers, the prognosis is considerably better, the survival rate being as high as 90% at 5 years.

Factors carrying a good prognosis include 'early' gastric cancer, the fewer lymph nodes involved, and the degree of differentiation of the tumour. Factors carrying a bad prognosis include involvement of the resection margins, distant lymph node metastases, and hepatic metastases.

Morphology

High grade dysplasia and intramucosal carcinoma are visible on endoscopy as elevated plaques or shallow depressions. Discovery of either on biopsy is an indication for surgery. As growth progresses, the elevated tumours develop into polypoidal or fungated cancers while the depressed lesions develop into ulcerating carcinomas. Chronic peptic ulcer of the stomach may resemble an ulcerating carcinoma, and therefore biopsy of a chronic ulcer is essential to exclude malignancy. Carcinoma of the stomach may be classified as 'intestinal' or 'diffuse' types. The intestinal type show glandular formation lined by mucus-secreting cells and tend to have a well-demarcated border. The 'diffuse' type infiltrate the wall with a poorly demarcated invasive margin. Mucus secretion is in the form of intracytoplasmic vacules pushing the nucleus to the cell periphery, forming 'signet ring' cells. The intestinal form is more prevalent in higher incidence countries and has an association with *H. pylori*-associated chronic gastritis. Diffuse carcinoma is more prevalent in low incidence countries and has a poorer prognosis.

Spread

Spread may be:

1. direct to adjacent organs, e.g. pancreas
2. lymphatic, initially to local lymph nodes along the right and left gastric artery, then to coeliac nodes; retrograde spread to nodes to the porta hepatis (obstructive jaundice); distant nodes, e.g. to the left supraclavicular fossa (Troisier's sign, Virchow's node)
3. by blood, usually via the portal vein to the liver
4. transcoelemic, e.g. to the ovaries (Krukenberg tumours).

Other malignant tumours of the stomach

These include carcinoid tumours (see small intestine section) and lymphoma.

Lymphoma

The stomach is the commonest site for a primary lymphoma of the gastrointestinal tract. The development of gastric lymphoma is associated with previous *H. pylori* infection. As a result of *H. pylori* infection, lymphoid tissue appears in the gastric mucosa and resembles mucosa-associated lymphoid tissue (Malt), being composed of follicles with germinal centres. This tissue forms the basis for the development of B-lymphomas. Gastric lymphomas have a fair prognosis, the 5 year survival rate being about 50%. Poor prognostic indicators include serosal involvement and involvement of the regional nodes. The stomach may be involved in lymphomas which have arisen elsewhere in the body, in which case the prognosis depends on the overall extent and grading of the disease.

INTESTINES

Infections of the intestine

Bacterial

Bacterial infection of the intestine is a major cause of morbidity and mortality worldwide. Bacterial contamination of water supplies in developing countries is a major cause of diarrhoeal illness, which is a major cause of mortality especially in infancy and old age. Causes include salmonella (food poisoning, usually *Salmonella enteritidis*), bacillary dysentery (*Shigella sonnei, Shigella flexeneri, Shigella dysenteriae*) and cholera (*Vibrio cholera*). All these give profuse, watery diarrhoea with severe colicky abdominal pain. The diarrhoea may be bloody. Severe dehydration and death may occur. The commonest bacterial causes of diarrhoea in the UK include campylobacter, salmonella, shigella, *E. coli, Staph. aureus,* and *Clostridium perfringens.* Campylobacter is now recognised as the commonest cause of infective diarrhoea in the UK. Symptoms vary from a mild illness to a severe illness with dehydration and collapse. *E. coli* is responsible for diarrhoea in neonates and infants, travellers' diarrhoea, and haemorrhagic colitis and haemolytic uraemic syndrome. Staphylococcal enterocolitis is rare but potentially fatal. It usually arises as a result of the use of broad spectrum antibiotics which alter gut flora, allowing organisms that are foreign to the gut or normally present in small numbers to invade and proliferate. In this context *Staph. aureus* is most dangerous; when present in large numbers it produces an endotoxin which produces a severe enterocolitis. It occurs usually as a result of cross infection in hospital from contact with a patient with resistant staphylococcus. This is not to be confused with *Staph. aureus* food poisoning. This is due to ingestion of food contaminated with the endotoxin of *Staph. aureus*. The symptoms are of rapid onset because the disease is due to a preformed toxin in the food. The food may contain toxin but no viable staphylococci.

Many patients taking broad spectrum antibiotics may develop diarrhoea. In most cases it is mild and settles on withdrawal of the antibiotic. Other patients may develop a severe colitis with diarrhoea and dehydration. Sigmoidoscopy reveals the characteristic false membrane of mucus, polymorphs and fibrin, hence the name pseudomembranous colitis. The best method of diagnosis is demonstration of specific toxin in the faeces. *Cl. difficile* may also be isolated from the faeces.

Other bacterial infections of the intestines which are surgically important include tuberculosis and actinomycosis. Tuberculosis is usually seen in the UK as ileocaecal tuberculosis, and presents with thickening and narrowing of the terminal ileum. It may be indistinguishable from Crohn's disease on naked eye examination, although pale tubercles may be seen on the serosa in tuberculosis. Complications include adhesive obstruction, perforation, and malabsorption due to widespread mucosal involvement or lymphatic blockage. Actinomycosis affects the appendix and caecum and is due to *Actinomyces israelii,* a mouth commensal. A chronic granulomatosis infection results, with abscesses and sinus formation. Abdominal actinomycosis may simulate appendicitis. Earlier appendicectomy may be curative but, if the appendix perforates, multiple lesions and sinuses of the abdominal wall may result.

Viral infections

Many causes of gastroenteritis are of viral origin and are self-limiting.

Fungal infection

Fungal infections are rare. Histoplasmosis may occur.

Parasitic diseases

Parasitic diseases include giardiasis, amoebiasis and schistosomiasis. Giardiasis is due to the protozoan parasites *Giardia lamblia.* It is a cause of travellers' diarrhoea, childhood diarrhoea and diarrhoea in those with IgA deficiency. Malabsorption may occur. Diagnosis is based on demonstration of the characteristic trophozoites in faeces, duodenal aspirates, or biopsies.

Inflammatory bowel disease

Crohn's disease

Crohn's disease is a chronic inflammatory disorder of unknown aetiology. It affects the small bowel most commonly, but any part of the gastrointestinal tract from the mouth to the anus may be affected. It is characterised by a transmural inflammation with non-caseating granulomas.

Thickened and fissured bowel leads to intestinal obstruction and fistula formation.

Aetiology Although the aetiology is unknown, several factors have been postulated. It is thought to occur due to genetic predisposition to environmental factors as yet undetermined. It has been postulated that a genetic defect prevents the patient mounting an effective immune response to a causative agent. A genetic influence is suggested by a family history of the disease in 15–20% of patients. This is supported by a Swedish study where 50% of monozygotic twins had Crohn's disease compared with 4% of dizygotic. Genes coding for HLA antigens, e.g. HLA-DR1, HLA-DQw5, are more frequent in patients with Crohn's disease than normal controls. Transmissible agents such as viruses, mycobacteria and Yersinia have been isolated from patients with Crohn's disease, but their role in the pathogenesis of the condition is not yet established.

Morphology Crohn's disease is classically segmental, with areas of involved bowel separated by normal bowel. These segmental areas of disease are termed 'skip' lesions. Small discrete ulcers similar to aphthous ulcers of the mouth, hence often described as aphthoid, develop on the mucosa. Later, more characteristic longitudinal ulcers develop, progressing into deep fissures. Eventually the disease spreads throughout the wall of the affected segment of bowel. Fibrosis occurs subsequently, leading to narrowing of the bowel lumen. This narrowing can be seen on a barium enema where only a narrow column of barium passes through the affected area, giving rise to Cantor's 'string' sign. Where longitudinal fissures cross oedematous transverse folds of mucosa, a cobblestone appearance results. The regional lymph nodes show reactive hyperplasia and occasionally granulomas. Microscopy shows a transmural inflammation, demonstrating collections of lymphocytes, plasma cells and non-caseating granulomas.

Complications Widespread involvement of the small intestine may lead to malabsorption syndromes, and extensive surgery may lead to 'short bowel' syndrome, again causing malabsorption. Fistula formation is common and may lead to enterocutaneous fistulae after surgery. Over 50% of patients have anal lesions: either skin tags, fissures, or fistulae. Acute complications include intestinal obstruction, perforation, haemorrhage, and toxic dilatation. The latter being rarer than with ulcerative colitis. There is also an increased risk of carcinoma in both large and small bowel. Gall stones and renal calculi may occur as a result of malabsorption syndromes. Extra-alimentary manifestations of the disease including finger clubbing, erythema nodosum, pyoderma gangrenosum, and uveitis. Rarely, systemic amyloidosis may occur.

Ulcerative colitis

Ulcerative colitis is a chronic inflammatory disease which involves the whole or part of the colon. The inflammation is initially confined to the mucosa and nearly always involves the rectum, extending to involve the distal or whole colon. In severe cases the inflammation may extend into the muscle coats. Acute complications include toxic dilatation, haemorrhage and perforation.

Aetiology The cause of ulcerative colitis is not known. Current hypotheses includes immunological, dietary and genetic factors. Familial clustering occurs. There is an association with HLA-DR2. Other evidence of a genetic role includes a higher concordance rate in monozygotic twins, and increased prevalence in certain ethnic groups and an association with diseases that are known to have a genetic predisposition, e.g. ankylosing spondylitis and sclerosing cholangitis. Immunological mechanisms may be important. Under normal circumstances the mucosal immune system is tolerant of luminal foreign antigens and this is dependent upon the relationship between colonic epithelium and suppressor T cells. Changes in epithelial cell antigen presentation consequent upon an acquired expression of Class II major histocompatibility molecules activate helper T lymphocytes and induce a sustained mucosal immune reaction. Antigens from gut flora may be responsible for this. This may explain the well-known triggering of ulcerative colitis by enteric infections. Dietary factors may also provide a triggering factor.

Morphology Ulcerative colitis is a diffuse inflammatory disease confined initially to the mucosa. Unlike Crohn's disease it is confined to the large intestine and is continuous in its distribution. In some cases it is confined to the rectum (proctitis), or to the rectosigmoid (distal proctitis). Abscesses form in the crypts of Lieberkuhn, penetrate the superficial mucosa, spread horizontally and cause the overyling mucosa to slough. The margins of the ulcers are raised as mucosal tags that project into the lumen (inflammatory pseudopolyps). Except in the most severe forms the muscle layers are spared. Occasionally the last few centimetres of the terminal ileum is ulcerated, i.e. the so-called condition of 'backwash' ileitis.

Complications These include toxic dilatation, haemorrhage, stricture and perforation. Carcinomas may occur, the overall incidence being around 2%. However, in patients who have had the disease for over 25 years this rises to 10%. Factors associated with higher risk include onset in childhood, a severe first attack, total colonic involvement, and continuous rather that intermittent symptoms. Extracolonic complications include seronegative arthritis (sacroilitis, ankylosing spondylitis), sclerosing cholangitis, cirrhosis, pericholangitis, iritis, uveitis, episcleritis, erythema nodsum, pyoderma gangrenosum, and apthous stomatitis. Rarely, systemic amyloidosis may occur.

Diverticular disease

Diverticulae are herniations of mucosa through the colonic wall. They occur at weak points where blood vessels pierce the bowel wall. They consist of mucosa and submucosa that have pierced the muscular coats. They are pulsion diverticula, being pushed out by increased intraluminal pressure. Although they may involve the whole of the colon, they are most common in the sigmoid colon. Diverticular disease is most common in Western society, where refined diets are more common than diets rich in fibre and hence the stool is less bulky. Patients with diverticular disease have shortened, thickened colonic muscle which reflects work hypertrophy from years of a low fibre diet and consequent small hard stools. High intraluminal pressures occur, pushing the diverticulae out through the wall. The propensity of diverticulae to form in the sigmoid colon is explained by Laplace's law which states that the pressure within a tube is inversely proportional to the radius.

Complications include inflammation (diverticulitis), and perforation; (i) into the local tissues, where it becomes walled off and leads to a paracolic abscess, (ii) into the general peritoneal cavity, giving rise to faecal peritonitis, or (iii) into an adjacent viscus, e.g. colovesical fistula (bladder), vaginocolic fistula (vagina) and ileocolic fistula (ileum). Bleeding, which can be profuse, may occur from erosion into an adjacent vessel. Repeated attacks of diverticulitis may result in fibrosis and narrowing of the bowel, leading to intestinal obstruction.

Volvulus

Volvulus is rotation of a segment of the intestine on an axis formed by its mesentery. It may cause partial or complete obstruction of the intestine and may result in strangulation of the bowel. Volvulus may occur around a fixed point: e.g. on the apex of a loop of bowel, e.g. fixation of the bowel to the back of the umbilicus via a Meckel's diverticulum or an adhesive band. A long sigmoid colon is a predisposing factor in sigmoid volvulus. Caecal volvulus may occur if the caecum is hypermobile owing to incomplete embryological fixation of the ascending colon. As the bowel twists on its mesentery, closed loop obstruction occurs when the rotation has reached 180°. At 360°, strangulation occurs which leads to gangrene and perforation.

Intussusception

An intussusception is the invagination of one segment of bowel into another in a 'telescoping' fashion. The segment of bowel invaginating is the intussusceptum, the adjacent or receiving segment is the intussuscipiens. The commonest form occurs when the terminal ileum is telescoped into the right side of the colon — an ileocolic intussusception. The apex of the intussusception may be a polyp, Meckel's diverticulum, intramural haematoma, or a hypertrophied Peyer's patch. The process of intussusception may result in gangrene of the intussusceptum.

Intestinal ischaemia

This may be due to occlusive or non-occlusive ischaemia. Occlusive ischaemia occurs as a result of thrombosis or embolism reducing flow or completely occluding a vessel. Non-occlusive ischaemia results from reduced flow in the vessel, with failure to sustain adequate flow to sustain mucosal integrity, e.g. hypotension, vasoconstriction, or abnormal blood viscosity. Total vascular occlusion results in intestinal infarction, the extent depending on the degree of collateral supply: e.g. with superior mesenteric artery occlusion, approximately 25 cm of jejunum will survive via flow from the coeliac axis via anastomosis between the superior and inferior pancreatico-duodenal arteries.

Acute ischaemia

This may result in mucosal infarction, mural infarction (not involving the muscularis propia), or transmural infarction. Mucosal infarction often results from systemic hypotension and may be followed by complete regeneration. Mural infarction is followed by fibrous stricture formation. Transmural infarction results in gangrene of the involved area, with subsequent perforation. Surgical treatment is required in the latter case.

Chronic ischaemia

Chronic mesenteric ischaemia describes a condition where there is inadequate blood flow to the small intestine because of partial occlusion of the superior mesenteric artery. The condition is sometimes described as mesenteric claudication or mesenteric angina. It occurs after a meal when the blood flow is inadequate to cope with the increased motility, secretion and absorption required. Cramping upper, or central abdominal pain occurs about 20 min after food. Patients become afraid to eat because of the pain, and lose weight.

In the large bowel, chronic ischaemia may lead to ischaemic colitis. This is usually a mural infarction and results in dark red bleeding initially from ulcerated ischaemic mucosa. It results usually at the 'watershed' area around the splenic flexure of the colon. The colon loses its normal outline and appears as a 'drain pipe' on barium enema. Strictures may occur.

Vascular abnormalities

Angiomas, arteriovenous malformation, and telangectasias may occur. Angiodysplasia may occur, usually in the elderly, and results in bleeding from the large bowel. Mesenteric angiography, often in the acute bleeding phase, is required to confirm the diagnosis.

Diseases of the anus and anal canal

Haemorrhoids

Haemorrhoids are vascular cushions occurring in the submucosa of the lower rectum and anal canal. There is an internal component covered by mucosa and an external component covered by skin.

Internal haemorrhoids are a plexus of superior haemorrhoidal veins above the mucocutaneous junction. They occur in three primary positions, i.e. at the 3 o'clock, 7 o'clock and 11 o'clock positions when the anal canal is viewed with the patient in the lithotomy position. External haemorrhoids occur below the mucocutaneous junction in the tissue beneath the epithelium of the anal canal and the skin of the perianal region. The two plexuses of internal and external haemorrhoids anastomose freely. The internal haemorrhoids drain via the superior haemorrhoidal veins and the portal vein, while the external haemorrhoids drain into the systemic circulation. Hence they are a site of portosystemic anatomosis.

Haemorrhoids may become symptomatic due to straining with chronic constipation, pregnancy, obesity, low fibre diet, or portal hypertension. Haemorrhoids are classified into three categories: (i) first degree, which manifest only by bleeding; (ii) second degree, which manifest by prolapsing on defaecation but return spontaneously; (iii) third degree, which prolapse and require manual reduction. Occasionally, haemorrhoids prolapse and become congested and oedematous and will not reduce. The venous return is obstructed by pressure from the anal sphincter, and thrombosis occurs. Infarction of the overlying skin and muscle may occur if surgical relief is not carried out. Rarely, septic emboli may occur from thrombosed piles and result in liver abscesses.

Anorectal abscesses

Infection occurs in an anal crypt and extends into one of

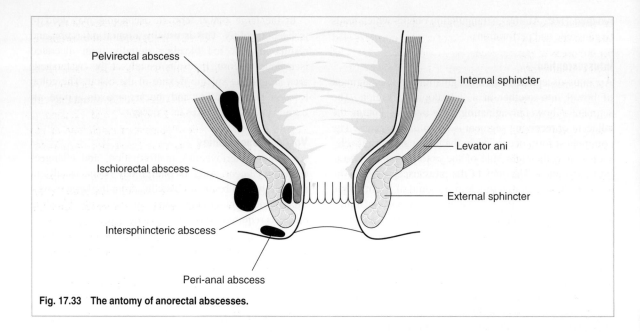

Fig. 17.33   The antomy of anorectal abscesses.

the pararectal spaces (Fig. 17.33), resulting in abscess formation. Infecting organisms include *E. coli, Proteus vulgaris,* faecal streptococci, bacteroides, and *Staph. aureus.* The infection is usually with mixed organisms. The incidence is higher in men. Abscesses may also result from: infection of hair follicles, sweat glands and sebaceous glands; following excoriation from scratching in pruritus ani; infection of a fissure-in-ano; infection of a perianal haematoma; infection of a thrombosed haemorrhoid; following injection of haemorrhoids; and in Crohn's disease.

Fissure-in-ano

A fissure represents a breach in the anal epithelium overlying the internal anal sphincter commencing just below the dentate line. They are painful because they occur in the area of somatic sensation below the dentate line. They are most common in the midline posteriorly because the anal mucosa is least well supported there, being in the 'V' shape where the two levator ani muscles join posteriorly, at the point of acute angulation between anal canal and rectum. A small number occur in the midline anteriorly. Chronic inflammation occurs in the fissure. Above the fissure there is usually a hypertrophied papilla adjacent to the anal crypt. Below the fissure there is usually a tag of oedematous fibrotic skin called a sentinel pile because it stands as a sentinel just below the fissure. Fissures often occur as a result of chronic constipation, passage of a hard stool tearing the anal mucosa. Other causes include Crohn's disease, tuberculosis, and carcinoma of

the anal canal, which must be carefully distinguished from a benign simple fissure-in-ano.

Fistula-in-ano

A fistula is an abnormal connection between two epithelial surfaces. By definition it must have at least two openings, as opposed to a sinus which is a blind-ended track with only one opening onto an epithelial surface. Most fistulae-in-ano originate in the anal crypts. An abscess is formed and, when it ruptures, a fistula occurs. Hence, perianal abscesses should be incised and drained promptly, but even then a fistula may result. Fistulae may result from perianal Crohn's disease, tuberculosis, or neoplasm.

Perianal haematoma

This is sometimes called a thrombosed external pile. It is characterised by a tense, painful, bluish rounded elevation beneath the skin at the anal verge. It may occur following a sudden increase in venous pressure, e.g. heavy lifting, straining, or paturition. There is usually no previous history of, or association with, internal haemorrhoids. Spontaneous resolution occurs, but evacuation of the thrombus is usually undertaken. Differentiation from a prolapsed internal haemorrhoid is important, as treatment is different.

Intestinal tumours

Polyps

Colorectal polyps are protuberant growths into the bowel lumen. They are a heterogeneous group of sessile or pedunculated, benign or malignant, mucosal, submucosal, or muscular lesions. Polyposis is a term reserved for hundreds of polyps occurring in the large bowel. The most common forms of polyps are listed in Table 17.1

Adenomas Most adenomas are tubular, tubulovillous, or villous. Adenomas may give rise to adenocarcinoma. The malignant potential of an adenoma depends on size, growth pattern, and degree of epithelial dysplasia. Malignant change is found in 1% of adenomas under 1 cm in diameter, 10% of adenomas 1–2 cm in diameter, and 40% larger than 2 cm. Malignant potential depends upon the type of adenomas: about 5% of tubuloadenomas, 20% of tubulovillous adenomas and 40% of villous adenomas become malignant. Sessile lesions are more likely to become malignant than pedunculated ones. Villous adenomas are usually sessile and may grow to a very large size. They may secrete copious amounts of potassium rich mucus, resulting in hypokalaemia.

Inflammatory polyps (pseudopolyps) These are associated with ulcerative colitis and result from mucosal ulceration.

Hamartomas These are rare. They may be solitary, e.g. juvenile polyps, or be present throughout the gastrointestinal tract as in Peutz–Jegher's syndrome.

Table 17.1 Large intestinal polyps	
Type	**Histology**
Neoplastic	Benign
	Adenoma
	Tubular
	Tubulovillous
	Villous
	Malignant
	Polypoid adenocarcinomas
	Carcinoid polyps
Inflammatory	Pseudopolyp (ulcerative colitis)
Hamartomatous	Peutz–Jegher's polyp
	Juvenile polyp
Unclassified	Metaplastic (hyperplastic)
Others	Mesenchymal in origin
	Benign
	Lipoma
	Fibroma
	Leiomyoma
	Haemangiomas
	Malignant
	Sarcomas
	Lymphomatous polyps

Metaplastic polyps These are not neoplastic and therefore do not become malignant. Their origin is unknown.

Malignant epithelial polyps The vast majority of adenocarcinomas arise within pre-existing adenomas. A very small number of polyps are carcinoid tumours with a low malignant potential. Complete local excision is usually curative. The development of carcinoma of the colon from polyps is discussed in the section on colorectal carcinoma.

Familial polyposis coli (familial adenomatous polyposis — FAP) This is a rare condition inherited as an autosomal dominant, with equal sex incidence. Hundreds of polyps of various sizes carpet the colon and rectum. Cancer develops before the age of 40 in almost all untreated patients. The gene responsible for FAP is on the long arm of chromosome 5.

Gardner's syndrome This is FAP-associated with desmoid tumours, osteomas of the mandible or skull, and sebaceous cysts.

Colorectal cancer

In Western countries, colorectal cancer ranks second to lung cancer in incidence and mortality rates. Adenomas are probably the precursors of most, if not all, colorectal cancers. Multiple synchronous colonic cancers, i.e. two or more carcinomas occurring simultaneously, are found in 5% of patients. Metachronous cancer is a new primary lesion in a patient who has had a previous resection for cancer. The risk of metachronous tumours reaches 25% after 20 years of follow-up. The incidence of colonic cancer appears to be rising, especially cancer of the right side of the colon and of the sigmoid colon.

Progression of adenoma to carcinoma

There is considerable evidence that most colorectal cancers develop from adenomas.

1. Colorectal cancer develops in familial adenomatous polyposis (FAP). FAP is an autosomal dominant carried by either parent. Adenomas develop in the colon during the second and third decades, undergoing malignant change with progression to cancer by the age of 40. The gene responsible for FAP is on the long arm of chromosome 5.
2. Adenomas and carcinomas frequently occur together in a resected specimen of bowel. Such patients have an increased risk of developing a metachronous cancer compared with those having carcinoma alone in the resected specimen.
3. There is a marked geographic variation in the prevalence of adenomas. There is a strong correlation

with the incidence of colorectal cancer in the same geographical areas.

Aetiology

The aetiology of colorectal cancer is unknown, but several theories have been put forward:

1. inherited genetic factors
   (a) familial adenomatous polyposis (see above)
   (b) autosomal dominant hereditary non-polyposis colorectal cancer (HNPCC). There are two types: cancer family syndrome (CFS: Lynch syndrome 2 with early onset — age 20–30 years) and associated with other adenocarcinomas, especially endometrial carcinoma; and hereditary site-specific colon cancer (HSSCC: Lynch syndrome 1) which shows the same characteristics except for extracolonic carcinomas. In the absence of the above syndromes, first degree relatives of patients with colorectal cancer have a 2–3 fold increased risk of the disease
2. environmental factors — there is a higher incidence in populations that are economically prosperous. Dietary factors may be important, i.e. low fibre, high fat diets. High fat leads to an increase in bile acid production, and bile acids are promoters of carcinogenesis. Dietary fibre contains plant lignans which are converted to human lignans by bacterial action in the colon. Lignans may protect against cancer. Low fibre diets also prolong intestinal transit time and therefore allow for a prolonged contact between any carcinogens and the bowel mucosa
3. inflammatory bowel disease — carcinoma may develop. There is a greater risk of ulcerative colitis than Crohn's disease
4. colorectal polyps — see above
5. schistosomal colitis
6. exposure to irradiation
7. the presence of a ureterocolostomy — this operation is rarely performed nowadays.

Molecular basis for development of colorectal carcinoma

The genetic basis for colorectal cancer is well established. Activation of oncogenes occurs. The oncogenes most frequently altered in colorectal carcinoma are c-Ki-*ras* and c-*myc*. Loss or mutations of tumour suppressor genes may occur. In FAP, mutations in tumour suppressor gene APC, localised on chromosome 5, occur. Defective gene of the DNA repair pathway may lead to genomic instability. Inhibitors of apoptosis, e.g. *bcl*-2 may be overexpressed. The cells then become more resistant to degrees of damage which would normally result in apoptosis and elimination of the cell. 'Abnormal' cells will therefore remain in the system. The P53 gene is also implicated in colorectal cancer. The P53 gene checks the integrity of the genome prior to mitosis. Defective cells are switched to apoptosis. The P53 gene product effects the G1 phase of the cell cycle, allowing time for successful DNA repair or diverting the cells towards apoptosis.

Distribution of colonic cancer

This is shown in Figure 17.34.

Methods of spread

Direct extension   The tumour may encircle the bowel lumen. Longitudinal submucosal spread occurs but rarely spreads more than 2 cm from the tumour edge unless there is concomitant lymphatic spread. The tumour eventually spreads to the bowel wall and into the neighbouring structures, e.g. liver, greater curve of the stomach, duodenum, small bowel, pancreas, kidneys, bladder, ureters, or vagina. Carcinoma of the rectum may invade the bladder, rectum, or sacrum.

Blood borne   The liver and lungs are most common.

Lymph nodes   Regional lymph nodes along the vessels are involved but not necessarily in a progressive and orderly fashion. Positive nodes may be found at some distance from the primary, intervening nodes being unaffected. Retrograde spread along lymphatics may occur,

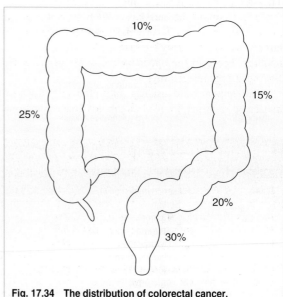

Fig. 17.34   The distribution of colorectal cancer.

with metastases in the lymph nodes at the porta hepatis resulting in obstructive jaundice.

Transcoelomic spread may occur, producing seedings on serosal surfaces, with resulting ascites. Rarely seedings on the ovaries may occur with development of Krukenberg-type tumours, but this is more common with carcinoma of the stomach.

Complications

These include obstruction, perforation (direct perforation of the tumour), perforation of the caecum in closed loop obstruction with a competent ileocecal valve, or perforation into an adjacent organ with development of a fistula, e.g. colovesical, and symptoms relating to direct extension.

Prognosis

This depends on the degree of differentiation of the tumour, the completeness of excision and the degree of spread. Examination of the resection margins (proximal, distal and circumferential) to assess completeness of excision is required. The extent of spread through the bowel wall and the presence of lymph node metastases are other major prognostic indicators. The extent of spread is given by the Duke's classification, which is also related to prognosis (Table 17.2).

Carcinoid tumours

These are apudomas that arise from the enterochromaffin cells throughout the gut. They may be associated with multiple endocrine neoplasia (MEN Type I and Type II). They are commonest in the midgut, the appendix being the most common site and the small intestine the second most common location. A small number occur in the large bowel. Mostly they are firm, yellowish, submucosal nodules. Those in the appendix are often an incidental finding at appendicectomy.

Small tumours are usually asymptomatic. Approximately 30% of small bowel carcinoids cause symptoms such as obstruction, pain or bleeding or the carcinoid syndrome.

Carcinoid syndrome

Extensive metastases from carcinoid, particularly the liver, result in a clinical syndrome, i.e. carcinoid syndrome, which consists of cutaneous flushing, diarrhoea, bronchoconstriction with wheezing, and right sided cardiac valvular disease (usually pulmonary stenosis) due to collagen deposition. Biologically active substances secreted by carcinoids are usually inactivated in the liver, but when hepatic metastases occur, these substances are released directly into the systemic circulation, where they produce the symptoms of carcinoid. The principal cause of the symptoms and signs of carcinoid syndrome is 5-hydroxy-tryptamine (5-HT). The 5-HT in the circulation is degraded to 5-hydroxy-indole-acetic acid (5-HIAA), which can be measured in the urine as a diagnostic marker of the disease.

Appendix

Appendicitis

Acute appendicitis is the commonest surgical emergency in Western countries but is rare in the third world. It may be related to the Western-style low fibre diets. Appendicitis is uncommon at the extremes of life, the lumen of the appendix being relatively large in infancy and the diet soft, while in old age the appendix tends to atrophy and the lumen becomes obliterated.

Factors predisposing to acute inflammation of the appendix include faecolith (hard pellets of faeces which reside in the appendiceal lumen), food residues, lymphoid hyperplasia (in childhood and occurring with some viral infections) and occasionally the presence of a carcinoid tumour.

The consequences of acute appendicitis include:

- resolution
- perforation with generalised peritonitis
- perforation within local adhesions, resulting in an appendix mass which may subsequently suppurate and form an appendix abscess.

Occasionally, the neck of the appendix may be obstructed either by a faecolith or tumour, leading to mucus retention within the lumen of the appendix and giving rise to a mucocele.

Other conditions of the appendix

Tuberculosis, actinomycosis and schistosomiasis of the appendix may occur. The appendix may also be involved in ulcerative colitis and Crohn's disease.

Table 17.2 Staging of colorectal carcinoma based on Duke's classification, with survival rates after surgery		
Duke's grade	Spread	5 year survival
A	Confined to the bowel wall	90%
B	Spread through the bowel wall	70%
C	Spread to lymph nodes	30%
Stage D was added to Duke's classification later, based on clinical rather than pathological evidence. Stage D implies distant metastases.		

Tumours of the anus and anal canal

Warts (condyloma acuminata)

Warts are the commonest benign tumour of the anal canal. They are usually associated with HPV infection and are usually sexually transmitted. There is an increased risk of anal carcinoma. Intraepithelial neoplasia (AIN) is associated with condylomas and HIV positivity. There is an increased incidence in homosexual males. Dysplastic changes or carcinoma in situ may be seen in the squamous epithelium and is graded AINI to AINIII. These changes are similar to cervical intraepithelial neoplasia (CIN) in females, which may coexist. AINIII may progress to invasive squamous cell carcinoma and is associated with HPV16. AIN may occur in the absence of pre-existing condylomata and HIV positivity.

Carcinoma

Anal margin   Bowen's disease (intraepithelial squamous cell carcinoma), Paget's disease, and squamous cell carcinoma may occur at the anal margin, the latter being the most common. It is distinguished from carcinoma of the anal canal. It is more common in elderly men and is usually a well-differentiated keratinising carcinoma. Lymphatic spread occurs to the inguinal nodes. The 5 year survival rate is 80% with appropriate treatment.

Carcinoma of the anal canal   There are three types of tumour relating to the different types of epithelium in the anal canal i.e. squamous cell carcinoma (arising below the dentate line), adenocarcinoma (arising above the dentate line), and basal cell carcinoma arising at the transitional zone. Squamous cell carcinomas grow upwards into the lower rectum and outwards to the sphincters. They spread to the inguinal nodes initially but, after crossing the dentate line, they may spread to the pelvic nodes. Adenocarcinomas spread to the pelvic nerves initially but may spread to the inguinal nodes if the tumour invades downwards beyond the dentate line. Squamous cell carcinomas and basal cell carcinomas are radiosensitive.

Malignant melanoma

This is rare, forming less than 1% of anal tumours. The prognosis is poor, lymph node metastases usually having occurred at the time of presentation. Blood borne spread occurs to the liver and lungs.

LIVER

Jaundice

Jaundice is defined as a yellowing of the skin, sclerae and mucous membranes because of the presence of bilirubin.

Jaundice is usually observed when the serum bilirubin concentration exceeds 40 mmol/L.

Classification of jaundice

Jaundice may be classified as prehepatic, hepatic or posthepatic. Posthepatic is often referred to as obstructive jaundice. This latter type is often amenable to surgical correction and has therefore also been referred to as surgical jaundice.

Prehepatic jaundice   The main cause is haemolysis, e.g. hereditary spherocytosis (congenital acholuric jaundice), autoimmune red cell destruction. Excessive production of bilirubin occurs as a result of breakdown of red cells. The bilirubin is unconjugated and therefore is not excreted in the urine (hence 'acholuric' jaundice). The bile may contain so much bilirubin that pure pigment stones are formed. Mismatched transfusions causing extensive haemolysis will result in acholuric jaundice, as will the absorption of large haematomas.

Hepatic jaundice   This may result from acute viral hepatitis, alcohol-induced hepatic damage, drug-induced liver injury, and decompensated cirrhosis.

Posthepatic jaundice   Obstruction of the extrahepatic bile ducts is an important cause of jaundice surgically. Urgent investigation and treatment is necessary to prevent liver damage. Important causes include: congenital biliary atresia; gall stone impaction in the common bile duct; strictures of the bile duct (e.g. following cholecystectomy); sclerosing cholangitis; carcinoma of the bile duct; extrinsic compression, e.g. carcinoma of the head of the pancreas; malignant nodes in the porta hepatis; damage to the bile duct at surgery. In this type of jaundice the bilirubin is conjugated and the urine is dark. As bile can not get into the intestine due to obstruction, the stools are pale.

The three categories of jaundice and their clinical and biochemical distinctions are shown in Table 17.3.

Acute liver injury

This may present with the acute onset of jaundice. It is necessary to be able to distinguish rapidly between 'medical' causes of jaundice and those which require surgery. The major causes of acute liver injury are viral infections, drug-induced reactions, alcohol and biliary obstruction, often due to gall stones. Jaundice occurs because of failure of the liver to secrete bilirubin at the rate at which it is formed in the body from the destruction of red cells. Accumulation of bile salts causes pruritis. Severe damage will lead to lack of clotting factors, with spontaneous bruising and haemorrhage. Ultimately, coma supervenes because of accumulation of toxic metabolites.

Table 17.3 The three types of jaundice and their biochemical and clinical differences

	Prehepatic (haemolytic)	Hepatic (hepatocellular)	Posthepatic (obstructive)
Jaundice	Usually mild	Variable	Variable Often deep
Colour of urine	Normal	Dark	Dark
Colour of faeces	Normal	Pale or normal	Pale
Serum bilirubin	Unconjugated	Unconjugated + conjugated	Conjugated
Serum transaminases	Normal	Grossly increased	Normal or mild increase
Serum alkaline phosphatase	Normal	Mild elevation	Grossly elevated

Liver cells contain many enzymes which are diagnostically important because they are released into the blood in liver disease. In acute liver injury, transaminases (AST and ALT) are elevated, as is the bilirubin. Liver damage results in impairment of bilirubin conjugation and also failure to excrete conjugated bilirubin and also any stercobilinogen absorbed from the gut. The urine is darkened by the presence of excessive bilirubin and urobilin that can not be excreted by the liver. As liver damage progresses, urobilinogen disappears from the urine because little or no bilirubin is being excreted by the liver. Acute liver injury may result in complete recovery, progression to chronic liver disease, or death from liver failure.

Liver tumours

Metastatic carcinoma is by far the most common hepatic tumour. Primary malignant tumours include hepatocellular carcinoma, cholangiocarcinoma, and more rarely angiosarcoma and hepatoblastoma. Benign tumours rarely cause clinical symptoms, although when large they may cause pain.

Benign tumours

Liver cell adenoma   This may arise spontaneously, but there is an increased incidence in patients taking anabolic, androgenic, or oestrogenic steroids. Adenomas may cause hepatomegaly or be clinically silent. Rupture may occur with haemoperitoneum.

Angioma   This is a benign vascular neoplasm. Angiomas are rarely of clinical significance. They rarely grow to more than a few centimetres in diameter.

Malignant tumours

These usually present with anorexia, weight loss, cachexia and jaundice. They are most often metastatic tumours.

Metastatic tumours   Common primary origins include the gastrointestinal tract, lung and breast. Deposits are normally multiple. When seen at surgery on the surface

of the liver they are usually white and umbilicated. Liver metastases may occur from malignant melanomas, in which case they are black or brown. Liver metastases need to be extensive before jaundice occurs.

Hepatocellular carcinoma   Aetiological factors include:

- cirrhosis — over 70% of hepatocellular carcinomas in the UK arise in cirrhotic livers
- geographical — common in Africa and the Far East
- hepatitis B
- aflatoxins — these are mycotoxins produced by *Aspergillus flavus.* The fungus contaminates food stored in hot, humid conditions and may be responsible for the geographical distribution
- anabolic steroids, androgenic steroids, and oral contraceptive agents have been implicated.

Spread of the tumour is by intrahepatic veins. Lymphatic spread occurs to lymph nodes at the porta hepatis, but distant metastases are uncommon. Hepatocellular carcinoma produces alpha-fetoprotein which is secreted into the blood stream, where it forms a useful diagnostic marker. The prognosis is poor, most patients being dead within 6 months of diagnosis.

Cholangiocarcinoma   This is an adenocarcinoma of bile duct epithelium. Aetiological factors include the liver fluke, *Clonorchis sinensis,* and primary sclerosing cholangitis (often in association with ulcerative colitis). Distinction of the tumour from metastatic adenocarcinoma can be difficult. The prognosis is poor, most patients being dead within a few months of presentation.

Liver cysts

These include simple cysts, hydatid cysts and choledochal cysts.

Simple cysts   These are usually small and multiple. They may be associated with congenital polycystic disease of the kidney, or von Hippel Lindau disase. Simple cysts of the liver have little clinical significance.

Hydatid cysts These are due to the parasite *Echinococcus granulosus.* They may reach over 20 cm in diameter. They have an outer fibrous, laminated capsule and contain numerous 'daughter' cysts. Cyst fluid is highly allergenic, and spillage at surgery may precipitate a Type I anaphylactic hypersensitivity reaction.

Choledochal cysts These are rare congenital cysts of the bile duct which may be intra- or extrahepatic. They may present with jaundice or cholangitis.

Portal hypertension

Cirrhosis is the commonest cause of portal hypertension in the UK. Worldwide, schistosomiasis the commonest cause. The causes of portal hypertension are shown in Box 17.2.

Portal venous pressure is normally in the range 7–10 mmHg. In portal hypertension, portal pressure exceeds 10 mmHg, averaging around 20–25 mmHg, and may rise as high as 50–60 mmHg. Portal hypertension leads to opening up of sites of portosystemic anastomosis.

Anatomy of portal hypertension

A portal vessel is one that has capillaries at each end. The portal venous system drains blood to the liver from the abdominal part of the alimentary canal (excluding the lower part of the anus), the spleen, the pancreas and the gall bladder. The portal vein is formed by the junction of the splenic vein and superior mesenteric vein behind the neck of the pancreas (Fig. 17.35). The inferior mesenteric vein ascends above the point of origin of its artery to enter the splenic vein behind the body of the pancreas. The portal vein ascends behind the first part of the duodenum entering the free edge of the lesser omentum in the anterior wall of the foramen of Winslow. At this point

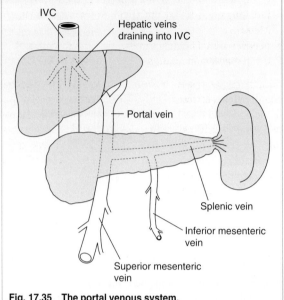

Fig. 17.35 The portal venous system.

the portal vein is immediately posterior to the bile duct and the hepatic artery. The portal vein then ascends to the porta hepatis, where it divides into the right and left branches and breaks up into the capillaries running between the lobules of the liver. These capillaries drain into radicles of the hepatic vein, eventually emptying into the inferior vena cava. There are no valves in the portal system, so that obstruction, e.g. due to cirrhosis of the liver, causes a rise in pressure throughout the system. In order for the blood to escape, the blood passes through any anastomosis between the portal and systemic system, and the anastomotic veins become dilated and may bleed. The site of collateral pathways between portal and systemic venous systems are as follows:

- between the oesophageal branch of the left gastric vein and the oesophageal tributaries of the azygos system; in the presence of portal hypertension, oesophageal varices will develop that may be the source of severe haematemesis
- between the superior rectal branch of the inferior mesenteric vein and the inferior rectal veins draining into the systemic system; this may give rise to dilated veins in the anal canal, which bleed
- between the portal tributaries in the mesentery and retroperitoneal veins, resulting in retroperitoneal varices
- between the portal veins in the liver, the veins of the abdominal wall via veins accompanying the ligamentum teres in the falciform ligament; this may

---

> **Box 17.2   Causes of portal hypertension**
>
> - prehepatic (obstruction of the portal vein)
>   - congenital atresia or stenosis
>   - portal vein thrombosis
>   - extrinsic compression, e.g. tumour
> - hepatic (obstruction to portal flow within the liver)
>   - cirrhosis
>   - hepatoportal sclerosis
>   - schistosomiasis
>   - sarcoidosis
> - posthepatic
>   - Budd–Chiari syndrome: idiopathic hepatic venous thrombosis e.g. polycythaemia, contraceptive pill, congenital obliteration, tumour invasion of hepatic veins
>   - constrictive pericarditis

result in the formation of a group of dilated veins radiating out from the umbilicus, known as a caput Medusae
- between portal branches in the liver and the veins of the diaphragm in relation to the bare area of the liver.

Surgery on patients with portal hypertension may be very complicated and very bloody. This is due to dilated veins in the abdominal wall, in the mesentery and in the retro-peritoneal area. Pressure in these veins may be extremely high, resulting in considerable portal venous bleeding.

Portal hypertension also results in the development of ascites and splenomegaly. The latter is probably due to passive congestion. Hypersplenism may result.

GALL BLADDER

Pathological conditions of the gall bladder are common surgical problems.

Gall stones (cholelithiasis)

In 80% of patients gall stones are composed predominantly of cholesterol with smaller amounts of calcium salts and bile pigments. They are referred to as mixed stones, are usually multiple with a faceted surface, and have a characteristic laminated surface on cross-section. Only about 10% of them contain sufficient calcium to be visible on a plain x-ray. Pure cholesterol stones form less than 10% of stones. They are usually solitary (the cholesterol 'solitaire'), up to 5 cm in diameter, and have a characteristic radial arrangement of crystals on cross-section. Cholesterol stones usually form in bile which is supersaturated with cholesterol. When bile contains more cholesterol than can be solublised in the bile-acid–lecithin micelles, crystals of cholesterol form in the bile. The greater the concentration of bile acids and lecithin in bile, the greater is the amount of cholesterol that can be contained in the mixed micelles. Lecithin is important because lecithin–cholesterol mixed micelles can solubilise more cholesterol than can micelles of bile acids alone. Following Crohn's disease of the terminal ileum or ileal resection the bile salt pool is reduced because of lack of absorption of bile salts, and the liver can not make good the losses. Such patients are prone to cholesterol stones.

Oestrogen increases the hepatic synthesis of cholesterol, and this may explain why females of child-bearing age have a higher incidence of cholesterol stones. A high animal fat, low fibre diet is also associated with cholesterol stones because of excretion in bile of the excess cholesterol absorbed from the gut. Clofibrate, a cholesterol-lowering agent, has been implicated in cholesterol stone formation, because it increases excretion of cholesterol in the bile. Decreased gall bladder motility probably plays a role in the aetiology of gall stones. Cholesterol and other substances which form the nuclei for gall stone formation must remain in the gall bladder long enough for crystal growth to occur. Stasis occurs during pregnancy due to the smooth-muscle-relaxing effect of progesterone. Motility of the gall bladder is also decreased during starvation and total parenteral nutrition, due to decreased stimulation of the gall bladder by CCK. Stones may also form after vagotomy, because of lack of vagal potentiation of CCK. Bile pigment stones account for about 10% of stones in the UK. The major constituent is the calcium salt of unconjugated bilirubin. They are associated with chronic haemolytic disease where there is breakdown of red cells with release of excessive bilirubin. Pure pigment stones occur in sickle cell disease, thalassaemia and hereditary spherocytosis. Pigment stones are found in the Far East, where they are associated with biliary tract infections with *E. coli* and *Bacteroides fragilis*. These organisms produce beta-glucuronidase which splits bilirubin diglucuronide and releases free bilirubin. The latter combines with calcium to form the relatively insoluble calcium bilirubinate.

Pathological consequences of gall stones

Consequences are:

- inflammation of the gall bladder; acute cholecystitis, chronic cholecystitis, acute-on-chronic cholecystitis
- obstructive jaundice due to impaction of a stone at the lower end of the common bile duct; secondary biliary cirrhosis may result
- ascending cholangitis
- empyema of the gall bladder
- mucocoele
- gall stone ileus — a fistula occurs between the gall bladder and duodenum, and a large stone enters the small bowel, causing obstruction, usually at the terminal ileum
- pancreatitis, usually associated with multiple small stones
- carcinoma of the bladder
- perforation of the gall bladder.

Cholecystitis Cholecystitis is inflammation of the gall bladder and is usually associated with stones. Occasionally it occurs without stones, i.e. acalculous cholecystitis. The latter may be due to infection with *E. coli*, *Clostridia*, or rarely *Salmonella typhi*. Acalculous cholecystitis may occur after prolonged starvation or total parenteral nutrition. Stasis is probably a contributing factor in the latter conditions.

The gall bladder becomes oedematous, with mucosal ulceration, and a fibrinopurulent exudate. Acute inflammatory cells infiltrate the wall. Even in the presence of thrombosis of the cystic artery, gangrene is rare, as the gall bladder gains a blood supply directly from the liver via the gall bladder bed. However, gangrene does occasionally occur with perforation of the gall bladder, resulting in generalised bile peritonitis or a localised abscess depending on whether the gall bladder has been walled off by adhesions or not. An empyema of the gall bladder may also result, suppuration occurring within the gall bladder and the gall bladder becoming distended with pus. Occasionally the gall bladder may fistulate into the duodenum.

Chronic cholecystitis Chronic cholecystitis is invariably associated with gall stones. It may develop after repeated episodes of acute cholecystitis but more often develops insidiously without any preceding clinically evident acute attacks. The gall bladder wall becomes thickened by fibrosis and relatively indistensible. The gall bladder wall is infiltrated with chronic inflammatory cells — lymphocytes, plasma cells and macrophages. Glandular outpouchings are formed by the lining of the mucosa and are known as Aschoff–Rokitansky sinuses. If obstructive jaundice occurs, it is due to a stone impacted in the common bile duct. The gall bladder does not usually distend, as the wall is relatively rigid due to fibrosis consequent on the associated chronic cholecystitis.

Mucocele This occurs when a stone impacts in the neck of the gall bladder in the absence of infection in the bile. The bile is absorbed from the gall bladder, and mucus is secreted into it from the mucus-secreting cells of the epithelium. The lack of inflammation in the wall allows the gall bladder to distend to several times its normal size. The gall bladder is usually palpable below the costal margin. The wall of a mucocele is usually very thin and is easily ruptured at surgery.

Cholesterolosis This is a condition where lipid-laden macrophages accumulate in the gall bladder mucosa to produce yellowish flecks in a reddish mucosa, appearing like the surface of a strawberry — hence the alternative name 'strawberry gall bladder'. This is often a symptomless condition but may accompany or predispose to cholesterol stones.

Tumours of the gall bladder

Benign tumours

An 'adenomyoma' is usually a fundal nodule composed of glandular structures mixed with hyperplastic smooth muscle fibres. It may be a hyperplastic condition rather than a true neoplasm. Adenomas of the gall bladder are rare and usually present as pedunculated polyps. Both are usually clinically silent but may show up on an ultrasound scan of the gall bladder and raise suspicion of a more sinister lesion.

Malignant tumours

Carcinoma of the gall bladder is the most common malignant tumour. It occurs in elderly people and is invariably associated with gall stones and chronic cholecystitis. About 0.5% of people with longstanding gall stones develop carcinoma of the gall bladder. The tumour is most often an adenocarcinoma, although in 10% of cases squamous cell carcinomas may occur. The tumour is usually advanced at presentation, having invaded directly into the liver or adjacent organs. Infiltration into the bile duct or metastases to the nodes of the porta hepatis will cause obstructive jaundice. Tumours are rarely resectable at presentation, and 5 year survival rates are less than 1%.

Conditions of the extrahepatic bile ducts

Congenital

These include extrahepatic biliary atresia and choledochal cysts. Biliary atresia presents as obstructive jaundice in the neonatal period. Choledochal cyst is a cystic dilatation of the common bile duct, the cyst reaching up to 5 cm in diameter. Complications include obstructive jaundice, cholangitis and stone formation. Malignant transformation may occur.

Sclerosing cholangitis

This is a rare condition of unknown aetiology, characterised by non-bacterial inflammatory narrowing of the bile ducts. There is a known association with chronic inflammatory bowel disease, particularly ulcerative colitis. Complications include chronic biliary obstruction with secondary biliary cirrhosis, episodes of ascending cholangitis, and malignant transformation to cholangiocarcinoma.

Carcinoma of the bile ducts

Ninety percent are adenocarcinomas. Ulcerative colitis is a common, associated condition. Chronic parasitic infection of the bile ducts is an aetiological factor in the Far East. Malignant transformation of choledochal cysts is also an aetiological factor. Most cases present with obstructive jaundice or ascending cholangitis if infection supervenes. Prognosis is poor, many patients surviving less than a year. The overall 5 year survival rate is less than 15%.

PANCREAS

Acute pancreatitis

Acute pancreatitis is an acute inflammatory process caused by the effects of enzymes released from the pancreatic acini. There are numerous aetiological factors (Box 17.3).

Pathogenesis

The pathogenesis of acute pancreatitis is obscure, but two main mechanisms may be involved:

1. duct obstruction — this may lead to reflux of bile into the pancreatic ducts causing injury. Alternatively, increased intraductal pressure may damage the pancreatic acini, leading to leakage of pancreatic enzymes which may further damage the pancreas
2. direct acinar damage — this may be caused by viruses, bacteria, drugs, or trauma.

The appearances of the pancreas in acute pancreatitis may be explained by release of pancreatic enzymes. Protease release causes widespread destruction of the pancreas and increases further enzyme release, with consequent further damage. Release of lipase causing fat necrosis resulting in characteristic yellowish-white flecks on the pancreas, mesentery and omentum, often with calcium deposition. Other enzymes, e.g. elastase, destroy blood vessels, leading to haemorrhage within the pancreas and a haemorrhagic exudate into the peritoneum. Haemorrhage may be extensive, leading to acute haemorrhagic pancreatitis.

Biochemical changes

1. Increased serum amylase. Amylase is released from the damaged acini and enters the blood stream. The serum amylase is released in the acute phase (24–48 h) but later falls to normal. Occasionally with acute haemorrhagic pancreatitis the destruction of pancreatic acini is so swift and complete that the serum amylase may not be raised by the time the patient reaches hospital.
2. Hypocalcaemia. This arises because of deposition of calcium in areas of fat necrosis.
3. Hyperglycaemia. This occurs because of associated damage to the pancreatic islets.
4. Abnormal liver function tests may occur, especially raised bilirubin and alkaline phosphatase due to mild obstruction of the bile ducts by oedema.

Complications

Complications include:

1. pancreatic pseudocyst — this is a localised collection of fluid in the lesser sac of peritoneum
2. pancreatic abscess
3. stress-induced gastric erosions with haematemesis or melaena
4. acute renal failure
5. toxic psychosis
6. multiple organ failure
7. chronic pancreatitis.

Prognosis

The overall mortality is between 10% and 20%. With severe haemorrhagic pancreatitis the mortality rate reaches 50%. The usual cause of mortality is multiple organ failure.

Chronic pancreatitis

Chronic pancreatitis is a relapsing disorder which may arise insidiously or following repeated attacks of acute pancreatitis. The commonest cause is chronic alcohol consumption. Other causes include cystic fibrosis, hypercalcaemia, hyperlipidaemia and a rare familial pancreatitis. Pathological changes include parenchymal destruction, fibrosis, loss of acini, calculi and duct stenosis with dilatation behind the stenosis. At operation the gland feels hard and irregular and may be mistaken for carcinoma. Calcification is often seen on plain abdominal x-ray. This is thought to be due to calcification of protein precipitates in the ducts.

Carcinoma of the pancreas

The incidence of carcinoma of the pancreas is increasing in many countries. The peak incidence is in the fifth and sixth decades. There is an association with diabetes mellitus, high fat diet and smoking. In two-thirds of cases the tumour is in the head of the pancreas. Most pancreatic

---

Box 17.3   Causes of acute pancreatitis

- gall stone disease
- chronic alcoholism
- infection, e.g. mumps, Coxsackie virus, typhoid
- hypercalcaemia, e.g. hyperparathyroidism
- trauma
- postoperative, e.g. after upper GI operations where pancreas is handled
- hyperlipidaemia
- drugs: corticosteroids, oestrogen-containing contraceptives, azathioprine, thiazide diuretics
- hypothermia
- vascular insufficiency, e.g. shock, polyarteritis nodosa
- scorpion bites
- iatrogenic, e.g. after ERCP

---

cancers are adenocarcinomas with a marked desmoplastic stromal reaction. Cancers in the head of the pancreas tend to present with obstructive jaundice due to compression of the common bile duct. Cancers elsewhere in the pancreas tend to remain silent until they are advanced, when the patient presents with dull back pain, nausea, weight loss and cachexia. Extensive tumours infiltrating the gland may present with diabetes mellitus.

Pancreatic carcinoma is characterised by early local spread to adjacent structures, lymph nodes and liver. Pulmonary and peritoneal metastases may occur later. Prognosis is poor because metastases or inoperable local extension are present at the time of diagnosis. Overall, 5 year survival of carcinoma of the head of the pancreas is less then 10%. Overall survival for tumours of the body and tail of the pancreas is even less.

Functioning endocrine tumours of the pancreas

Insulinoma
Insulinomas constitute 75% of endocrine tumours of the pancreas, and are most commonly found in the body and tail. They are derived from beta cells. The classic diagnostic criteria (Whipple's triad) are: (i) hypoglycaemic symptoms caused by fasting; (ii) a reduced blood glucose during symptomatic episodes; (iii) relief of symptoms by intravenous glucose. The majority are solitary non-metastasising lesions. 10% are malignant.

Gastrinoma
Although gastrin is usually produced by gastric antral G cells, tumours of the G cells, i.e. gastrinomas, most commonly originate in the pancreas. They are multiple in 50% of cases and malignant in 60%. Ten percent occur in extrapancreatic sites, e.g. duodenum. Excess gastrin production results in the Zollinger–Ellison syndrome, i.e. gastric hypersecretion, widespread peptic ulceration, and diarrhoea. Gastrinomas may occur as one of the MEN syndromes.

Vipomas
Vipomas are associated with the production of VIP and result in a syndrome of watery diarrhoea, hypokalaemia and achlorhydria.

Glucagonoma
This is much less common than insulinoma. It results in hypersecretion of glucagon, producing secondary diabetes. Other features include anaemia, weight loss, and characteristic rash known as a necrolytic migratory erythema. The tumour arises from the alpha cells of the pancreas. Twenty-five percent are benign and confined to the pancreas.

Somatostatinoma
This is rare and derived from the pancreatic delta cells. Clinically, diabetes mellitus, cholelithiasis, and steatorrhoea results.

18

Genitourinary system

Christopher Chapple

INTRODUCTION

The urinary system functions physiologically as a complex homeostatic mechanism for the regulation of acid–base balance, the excretion of waste products, and the control of water and electrolyte balance. Approximately one fifth of the cardiac output passes through the kidneys each minute, producing a renal blood flow of up to 400 mL/min per 100 g of kidney, which equates to approximately 650 mL/min per kidney. Under normal circumstances a total of 170–180 L of plasma per day are filtered by the glomeruli at an overall rate of 125 mL/min. Based on a normal fluid intake of approximately 2 L per day, between 1 and 1½ L is produced, which passes down the ureters to the bladder. Urine is produced within the kidneys at low pressure — not exceeding 15 cmH$_2$O, and is stored in the bladder at low pressure. The bladder is able to store urine at low pressure because of the particular property of smooth muscle known as tonus or receptive relaxation which permits the bladder to stretch and accommodate increasing volumes without any intrinsic rise in pressure until the functional capacity of the bladder is reached. In some situations structural limitation to distension of the bladder is imposed by an increased stiffness of the bladder wall as a consequence of fibrosis secondary to collagenous infiltration. This is most commonly associated with bladder outflow obstruction, although it can occur following radiotherapy and can also be due to failure of the bladder muscle to relax in association with neurological disorders. In these conditions filling of the bladder beyond 'anatomical' capacity will result in a linear rise in pressure and so-called 'low compliance'.

The bladder spends 99% of its time in a *storage phase*. The other function of the bladder, for which it is best recognised, is as a *voiding organ* — during which it contracts, expelling the contained urine within it, out via the urethra (with synchronous relaxation of the urethral sphincter mechanisms) and empties itself to completion.

The urinary tract is a complex system which subserves vital physiological functions resulting in the production of urine, its transfer from the kidneys via the ureters to the bladder, its low pressure storage and complete expulsion at a socially appropriate time. In order to understand the clinicopathological conditions affecting the urinary tract it is therefore important first to appreciate the anatomy (including structure, innervation and function), physiology and the techniques for structural and functional evaluation.

ANATOMY

KIDNEYS

Embryology
See Chapter 16.

Macroscopic anatomy
The kidneys have a characteristic shape and may retain a degree of fetal lobulation. Each kidney is approximately 11 cm long, 6 cm broad and 3 cm in thickness. Each kidney has the following features; two surfaces (anterior and posterior), two borders (medial and lateral), two poles (upper and lower) and a hilum which is situated at the middle of the medial border. The renal vein, renal artery and renal pelvis enter and leave the kidney at the level of the hilum and are situated anatomically in relation to each other in the order mentioned above, moving in an anteroposterior direction. The anatomy of the contents of the hilum can be variable: for instance the renal pelvis can be bifid, and the artery and vein may split into branches or receive tributaries, respectively, to a variable extent at the hilum — which can, on occasion, lead to confusion at the time of surgical dissection in this area.

The hilum of the kidney opens into a space called the renal sinus which is surrounded by the kidney parenchyma and contains branches of the renal artery, major tributaries of the renal vein, and both the major and minor

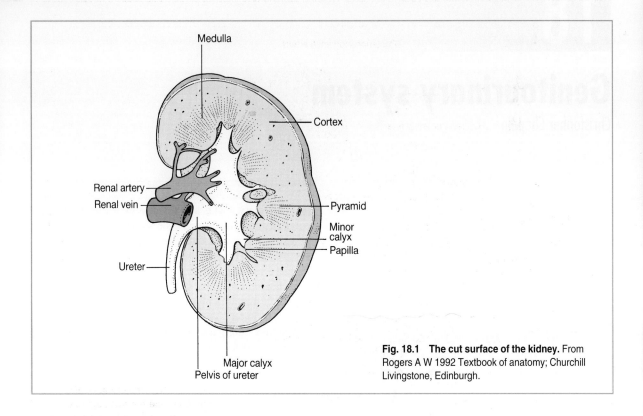

Medulla

Cortex

Renal artery

Renal vein

Pyramid

Minor calyx

Papilla

Ureter

Major calyx
Pelvis of ureter

Fig. 18.1   The cut surface of the kidney. From Rogers A W 1992 Textbook of anatomy; Churchill Livingstone, Edinburgh.

calyces (Fig. 18.1). All of the structures are surrounded and cushioned by fat.

There are two to three major calyces in each kidney, each of which comprises a number of minor calyces. An aid to visualising the anatomy is provided by the linguistic derivation of the term 'calyx' (latin for a wine glass). There are as many minor calyces as there are papillae, usually six to ten per kidney. The renal parenchyma comprises two zones (Fig. 18.1): (i) the medulla, which comprises six to ten pyramids of tissue, each with its base facing the outer capsule and its apex directed towards the hilum; (ii) the cortex, which lies between adjacent pyramids and separates the base of each pyramid from the outer capsule. The lobulation seen in fetal life represents each medullary pyramid with its associated rim of cortex. The cortex contains about one million glomeruli and their associated proximal and distal convoluted tubules. The medulla contains the loops of Henle, which sit up in the extracellular fluid, providing a gradient of increasing osmolarity (highest near the papillae). The collecting ducts run through this area and join together to form 30 to 40 papillary ducts with associated papillae. The microscopic structure and anatomy of the kidney is considered in more detail below when discussing physiological func-

tions of the kidney. The characteristic arrangement of vein, artery and pelvis (from before backwards) seen at the hilum is no longer present further into the renal parenchyma at the renal sinus. The nerves supplying the kidney are associated with the walls of blood vessels and comprise sympathetic and parasympathetic postganglionic fibres from the coeliac plexus. The renal arteries are direct branches from the aorta to each kidney, and in 30% of cases accessory renal arteries are present. The renal artery divides into three to five segmental arteries at the hilum, which divide within the sinus into six to ten lobar arteries — one for each each pyramid and associated cortex (Fig. 18.2). Each lobar artery divides into six interlobar arteries which are associated with papillae. The interlobar arteries give rise to arcuate arteries which run in a plane between cortex and medulla. The arterial supply to the cortex is derived from interlobular arteries which are branches of the arcuate arteries directed radially towards the kidney capsule, and each of these in turn gives off the afferent arterioles and supply glomeruli. The efferent arterioles that leave the glomeruli supply the capillary bed that surrounds the convoluted tubules. Arteries enter and leave each pyramid at its base and, as they penetrate deeper towards the papilla, they lose water

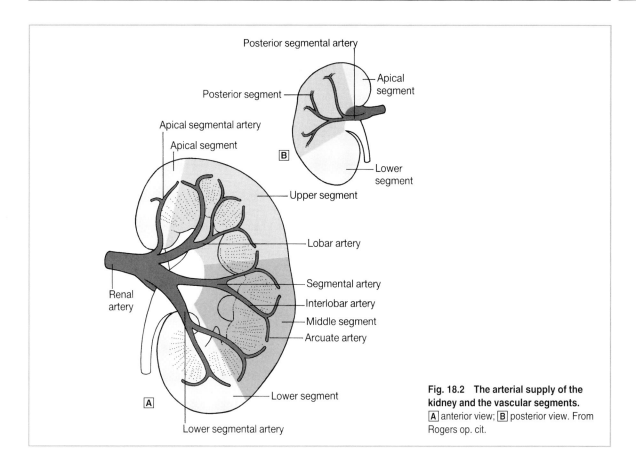

Posterior segmental artery

Apical segment

Posterior segment

Apical segmental artery

Apical segment

Lower segment

B

Upper segment

Lobar artery

Renal artery

Segmental artery

Interlobar artery

Middle segment

Arcuate artery

Lower segment

A

Lower segmental artery

Fig. 18.2 The arterial supply of the kidney and the vascular segments. A anterior view; B posterior view. From Rogers op. cit.

by osmosis and gain ions by diffusion — thereby reaching equilibrium with surrounding extracellular fluid. They then loop back towards the base of the pyramid, lose ions by diffusion and gain water by osmosis until they reach normal osmolarity at the base of the pyramid. These medullary vessels lie in bundles named vasa recta and are fed on the arterial side by efferent arterioles with adjacent glomeruli lying near the corticomedullary junction.

Venous drainage follows the arterial pattern closely. In the sinus of the kidney, interlobar veins unite into lobar veins then into segmental veins which join together to form the renal vein at the hilum of the kidney. The renal veins empty directly into the vena cava. Since the vena cava lies on the right side of the abdomen, the left renal vein is longer than the right and passes anterior to the aorta just caudal to the origin of the superior mesenteric artery. The left renal vein receives tributaries from the adrenal gland and gonad before entering the inferior vena cava. On the right side the adrenal vein usually drains directly into the inferior vena cava.

Each kidney lies within a cushioning bed of fat and tissue. The kidney itself is surrounded by renal fascia. There is a layer of perirenal fat which lies between the renal fascia and the true capsule of the kidney, which is continuous at the hilum with the fat and the renal sinus. In addition there is a layer of perirenal fat lying outside of the perirenal fascia (Gerota's fascia) which is particularly obvious posterior to the kidney (Fig. 18.3).

The adrenal glands lie within a separate compartment of the renal fascia. The surface markings of the kidney are shown in Figure 18.4. The hilum of both kidneys lie roughly at the level of L1 (the transpyloric plane).

In surgical practice it is very important to be aware of the anterior and posterior relationships of the kidneys — particularly in situations where normal tissue planes between the kidney and its adjacent structures are disordered due to either malignant or inflammatory disease processes, where it is important to be aware of which structures need to be mobilised (Figs 18.5 and 18.6). The relationship of the kidneys to surface markings is also important in planning the surgical approach to the patient during any procedure.

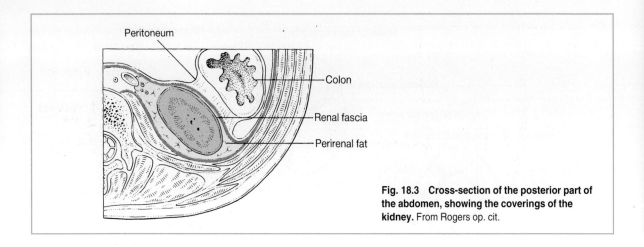

Fig. 18.3   Cross-section of the posterior part of the abdomen, showing the coverings of the kidney. From Rogers op. cit.

Peritoneum

Colon

Renal fascia

Perirenal fat

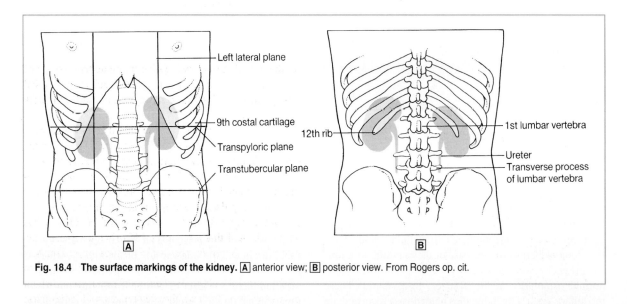

Left lateral plane

9th costal cartilage

Transpyloric plane

Transtubercular plane

12th rib

1st lumbar vertebra

Ureter

Transverse process of lumbar vertebra

Fig. 18.4   The surface markings of the kidney. A anterior view; B posterior view. From Rogers op. cit.

URETER

The ureters convey urine from the kidneys to the bladder. Each is 25 to 30 cm long and approximately 3 mm in diameter.

The ureter is a hollow muscular tube which commences at the renal pelvis and finishes at its entry into the bladder.

The wall of the ureter is composed of smooth muscle with a rich innervation comprising both sympathetic and parasympathetic fibres. The sympathetic fibres arise from spinal segments T11 to L1 and the parasympathetic fibres from sacral segments S2 to S4. Most of the nerves to the ureters are sensory. Stretching the wall, for instance, with the passage of a ureteric calculus produces acute pain. In view of the segmental innervation of the ureter this pain is usually referred to T11–L1. In addition the pain may radiate down the front of the thigh to the area supplied by L2. The ureter is lined by transitional epithelium continuous with that of the renal pelvis and calyces. The transitional cell lining of the urinary tract deserves some comment because this is a highly specialised epithelial layer designed to prevent diffusion of urine and other solids out of the urine and conversely passage of water into the urine by osmosis. Despite this it must be borne in mind that the urothelium is not purely an inert barrier, and there are a number of active transport mechanisms which are present, particularly within the

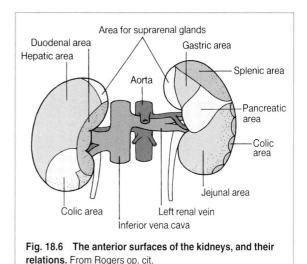

Fig. 18.6 The anterior surfaces of the kidneys, and their relations. From Rogers op. cit.

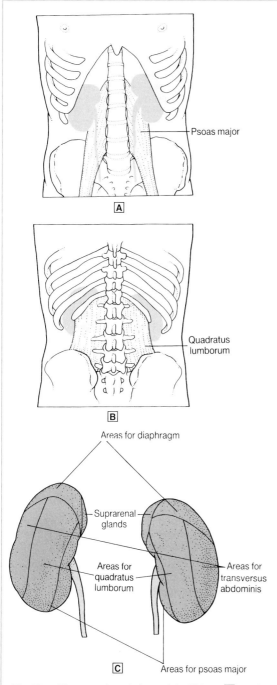

Fig. 18.5 The posterior relations of the kidney. A anterior view; B posterior view; C areas marked on the posterior surfaces of the kidneys. From Rogers op. cit.

urothelium of the bladder, which facilitate the passage of many substances, including drugs, through the urothelial lining and hence into surrounding tissues and ultimately the blood stream.

The entire ureter acts as a functional complex responsible for the transport of urine from the renal pelvis to the bladder. Whilst the mechanism is still a matter of some debate, it is very clear that there are one or more pacemakers situated in the renal pelvis which produce antegrade impulses which result in the propagation of a peristaltic wave down the ureter to the bladder. It has been estimated that a few drops of urine are transported down each ureter in peristaltic boluses approximately three to five times per minute. Each of these boluses of urine represents a high pressure localised segment which propagates rapidly down the ureter and which relies upon coaptation of the ureteric wall both proximal and distal to the 'bolus'. Any disruption of the normal ability of the ureter to form such 'boluses' results in severe pain and ureteric dysfunction as seen in the context of a diuretic challenge to a patient with pelviureteric junction obstruction and also commonly in a patient with a ureteric calculus undergoing an IVU, which may precipitate a further bout of renal colic.

In order to achieve its functional role the ureter must have a thick muscular coat, and indeed in its upper two-thirds it has an inner longitudinal and outer circular smooth muscle coat. In the distal third of the ureter, as it passes across the bony pelvis, the ureter acquires a third coat of longitudinal muscle which surrounds the other two. In its intramural portion, as it passes through into the bladder, the circular coat is lost but the remaining longitudinal muscle has an embryological relationship to the trigone of the bladder. The exact mechanism of action of the smooth muscle surrounding the ureter in its intramural portion remains the subject of some debate; it has been suggested that it has a sphincteric function to occlude the ureter at the time of detrusor muscle contraction to prevent vesico-ureteric reflux. A more important component of the sphincteric role of the lower ureter is likely to be its oblique position as it passes through the wall of the bladder, which results in the intramural portion of the ureter being closed off at the time of any rise in intravesical pressure to help prevent reflux — this remains the mainstay of most surgical procedures designed to correct vesico-ureteric reflux.

The ureters on either side run down the posterior abdominal wall overlying the transverse processes of L2 to L5 before crossing the pelvic brim overlying the bifurcation of the iliac vessels and running along the pelvic wall to the level of the ischial spine before turning medially and slightly upwards to enter the bladder at the level of the trigone.

The ureter can be considered to comprise three parts: (a) the pelvic ureter, (b) the abdominal part and (c) the part within the bony pelvis. The ureter receives a segmental innervation from both parasympathetic and sympathetic nerves. It is likely that the majority of the innervation is sensory in nature in view of the intrinsic peristaltic properties of the ureter. Each ureter receives a segmental blood supply from the following arteries:

- renal artery
- lateral branches directly off the abdominal aorta
- the gonadal vessels
- the common iliac arteries
- internal iliac arteries via the inferior vesical artery.

The venous drainage is by veins following similar lines to these arteries, and there is lymphatic drainage to periaortic and internal iliac groups of lymph nodes. There is a narrow area in each of the three segments of the ureter: namely at the pelviureteric junction, at the junction of the abdominal part and the part of the ureter passing into the pelvis as it crosses the bony pelvis/iliac vessels, and lastly as it passes through the wall of the bladder (the intramural portion). It is at these levels that a renal calculus is likely to become arrested on its descent into the bladder. Congenital abnormalities relating to the function of the muscle at the pelviureteric junction result in the condition known as pelviureteric junction obstruction, producing a functional outflow obstruction, which may require surgical resolution.

Surgical injuries to the ureter are most common in its lower third, owing to the close proximity of the ureter to the blood supply of the uterus, where the ureter is easily damaged during hysterectomy. It is important to appreciate the relations of the ureters and in particular the close proximity of the ureter to the gonadal vessels (Fig. 18.7), particularly the gonadal vein and its lower abdominal course through the bony pelvis, since in this area it is not unknown for the gonadal vein to be mistaken for the ureter and indeed mobilised instead of the ureter! The anterior relations of the ureter are easily dealt with in the majority of circumstances, providing its retroperitoneal position is borne in mind (Fig. 18.8).

BLADDER

Embryology
See Chapter 16.

Macroscopic anatomy and innervation
The bladder is a distensible reservoir with muscular walls. It lies in the true pelvis posterior to the symphysis pubis. The bladder does not rise above the pubis until it is very full, and when fully distended the adult bladder projects upwards from the pelvic cavity into the abdomen, lifting the peritoneum upwards from the abdominal wall as it distends.

The relations of the bladder are as follows:

- anteriorly — the pubic symphysis
- superiorly — the bladder is covered by peritoneum with coils of small intestine and the sigmoid colon resting on it. The relationship between the sigmoid colon and bladder is important in diverticular disease when a colovesical fistula may arise. In the female, the body of the uterus lies superior to the bladder
- posteriorly — in the male, the rectum and the seminal vesicles; in the female the vagina and supravaginal part of the cervix
- laterally — the bladder is separated from the levator ani and obturator internus muscles by loose connective tissue.

The relationship of the bladder to adjacent structures in both the male and female is best appreciated on a sagittal view (Fig. 18.9).

The bladder is a remarkable organ. As with the rest of the urinary tract it is lined by urothelium which acts as a watertight layer which nevertheless retains the ability to allow the active transport of a number of substances across its wall. The bladder should be considered to comprise two distinct functional and anatomical components.

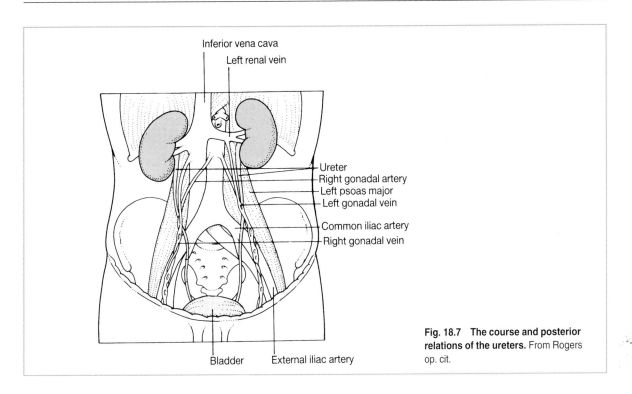

Inferior vena cava
Left renal vein

Ureter
Right gonadal artery
Left psoas major
Left gonadal vein

Common iliac artery
Right gonadal vein

Bladder   External iliac artery

Fig. 18.7   The course and posterior relations of the ureters. From Rogers op. cit.

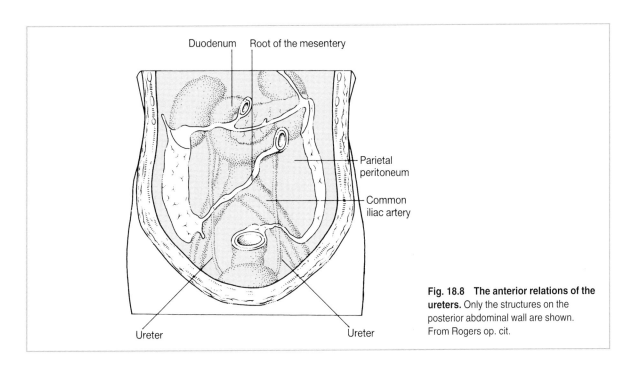

Duodenum   Root of the mesentery

Parietal peritoneum

Common iliac artery

Ureter   Ureter

Fig. 18.8   The anterior relations of the ureters. Only the structures on the posterior abdominal wall are shown. From Rogers op. cit.

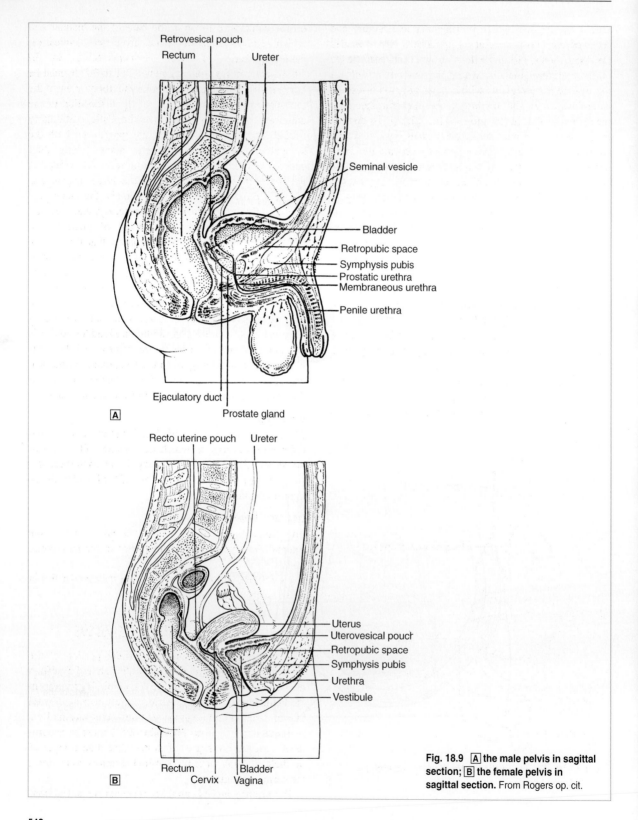

Fig. 18.9 A the male pelvis in sagittal section; B the female pelvis in sagittal section. From Rogers op. cit.

One is the trigone, which is triangular in structure and receives the two ureters at its uppermost lateral angles (Waldeyer's sheath) and extends down to its apex at the internal urethral meatus, where the smooth muscle of the trigone is contiguous with a ridge of smooth muscle extending down the urethra to the urethral sphincter mechanism. The innervation of the trigone is distinct from that of the remainder of the bladder muscle (detrusor muscle) in that it is predominantly adrenergic (sympathetic nervous system), relying upon the release of the neurotransmitter noradrenaline. The other component is the detrusor muscle, which constitutes the majority of the bladder and forms the cap on the base provided by the trigone. The word detrusor is derived from the term *detrudare* (= to drive out) and represents a complex admixture of muscle fibres, passing in different directions, which are predominantly under parasympathetic neural control acting via the release of the neurotransmitter acetylcholine acting on muscarinic receptors (the M_3 subtype is functionally predominant).

Despite the great deal of work that has been carried out looking at the innervation of the lower urinary tract, a number of aspects of the innervation of the bladder remain unclear. The extrinsic nerves innervating the bladder are demonstrated in Figure 18.10. The intrinsic nerves are derived from a perivesical plexus which lies on the connective tissue at the base of the bladder and which receives autonomic fibres from two sources: (a) parasympathetic fibres from segments S2 to S4, (b) sympathetic fibres from segments T11 to L2. It must be borne in mind that the contemporary textbook view of the innervation of the bladder and of the disposition of the autonomic nervous system is oversimplistic, particularly considering the fact that there are ganglia on both the sympathetic and parasympathetic nerves along their course from the spinal cord to the target organ with other ganglia both around and within the target organ, e.g. bladder, prostate, and that it is likely that there are interconnections between both the parasympathetic and sympathetic nervous systems at all of these levels. Furthermore it is now well recognised that there are a number of other sensory/motor neurotransmitters, additional to the classical neurotransmitters noradrenaline and acetylcholine, which may well be implicated in neural control pathways. There is considerable debate as to the sensory innervation of the bladder. No sensory end organs have yet been identified in the human bladder, and it is thought that sensory nerves are represented by non-myelinated fibres lying within the submucosa and proprioceptive receptors associated with the peritoneum and the adventitia overlying the detrusor muscle at its dome.

Blood supply

The arterial supply to the bladder is via the superior and inferior vesical arteries, which are branches of the anterior division of the internal iliac artery. In addition there is a rich venous plexus around the base of the bladder, draining into the internal iliac veins.

Lymphatic drainage

The lymphatics drain along the vesical vessels to the internal iliac lymph nodes and thence to the para-aortic nodes.

As with the rest of the urinary tract the bladder lies in an extraperitoneal position.

URETHRA AND URETHRAL SPHINCTER MECHANISMS

The urethra develops from the caudal portion of the urogenital sinus and associated Mullerian and Wolffian ducts. Whilst the urethra acts as a conduit for urine from the bladder to the outside world, it must be remembered that the urethra and its associated sphincter mechanisms play a vital role in terms of continence. It must be remembered that the urethra itself is no more than a layer of urothelium lying in a blood-filled arteriovenous sinus, the corpus spongiosum.

The urethra and its sphincter mechanisms act in con-

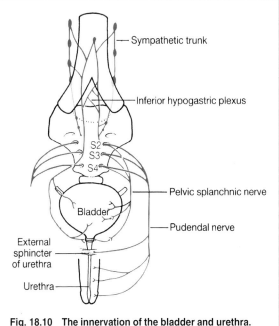

Fig. 18.10 The innervation of the bladder and urethra.
From Rogers op. cit.

Labels in figure:
- Sympathetic trunk
- Inferior hypogastric plexus
- S2
- S3
- S4
- Bladder
- Pelvic splanchnic nerve
- Pudendal nerve
- External sphincter of urethra
- Urethra

cert with the bladder for satisfactory voiding to occur; in other words when the bladder contracts the outlet must relax and vice versa during the storage phase. Whilst our level of knowledge relating to the cerebral control of micturition remains rudimentary, it is now recognised that there are important local spinal reflexes involved in micturition, with longer reflex tracts projecting to the pons acting under the influence of higher centres which impose voluntary control on the pons. In addition there is an important motor nucleus in the lower sacral region — the nucleus of Onufrowicz — which is important in the control of urethral sphincter muscle tone and is integral to the synchronisation of detrusor and sphincter function. It is very appropriate to consider the urethral sphincter mechanisms of the male and female separately and to bear in mind the similarities and differences which are present. In addition to the autonomic nervous system the striated urethral sphincter mechanism receives a somatic nerve supply which is both motor and sensory from the pudendal nerve.

Female urethra

The female urethra is approximately 4 cm long. It opens into the anterior wall of the vagina at the urethral meatus, situated in the vestibule between the anterior ends of the labia minora about 2.5 cm behind the clitoris. Like the rest of the urinary tract it is lined by transitional urothelium. There is an area at the internal urethral meatus on the trigone where the lining is comprised of squamous epithelium which appears to be under hormonal control and which changes its character at different phases during the menstrual cycle. In the female the principal sphincter mechanism is the urethral sphincter mechanism which extends down the length of the female urethra. There is an internal component composed of smooth muscle, the so-called lissosphincter, and an extrinsic component composed of striated muscle, the so-called rhabdosphincter. The sphincter is particularly well developed in the middle third of the urethra. In addition to this sphincter the submucosa of the urethra acts by producing a passive occlusive effect during urethral closure. This submucosa is under hormonal control and is very sensitive to changes in oestrogen levels. There is a very poorly developed bladder neck in the female which does not appear to have a significant functional role.

Male urethra

The male urethra (Fig. 18.11) is approximately 20 cm in length and comprises an anterior and posterior part. The posterior urethra, approximately 6 cm in length, is composed of that area which traverses the prostate, which

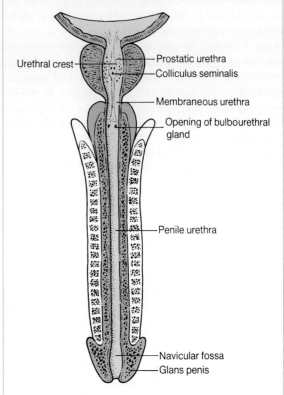

Urethral crest
Prostatic urethra
Colliculus seminalis
Membraneous urethra
Opening of bulbourethral gland
Penile urethra
Navicular fossa
Glans penis

Fig. 18.11   The posterior wall of the male urethra. From Rogers op. cit.

is approximately 3–4 cm in length, and that which lies within the confines of the distal sphincter mechanism, which is 2 cm in length. At the external border of the distal sphincter mechanism is the junction of the posterior urethra with the anterior urethra. The anterior urethra can be further subdivided into two areas which are divided on the basis of the areas anterior and posterior to the penoscrotal junction.

In the male there are two principal sphincteric mechanisms. The bladder neck mechanism lies at the outlet of the bladder around the internal urethral meatus and is composed principally of circularly oriented fibres, although there is a longitudinal component. This sphincter is sufficiently strong to maintain continence even if the distal sphincter mechanism is destroyed. Its principal role, however, is as a genital sphincter causing rapid closure of the bladder neck at the time of emission of semen into the prostatic urethra. The principal motor control of the bladder neck mechanism appears to be adrenergic via the release of noradrenaline from the sympathetic nerves.

Just distal to the bladder neck mechanism is the prostatic urethra, and it must be remembered that the human prostate comprises a significant smooth muscle component. At the apex of the prostate lies the distal sphincter mechanism, which is analogous to the urethral sphincter mechanism of the female and comprises both a lissosphincter and a rhabdosphincter as in the female urethra. Just as for the female sphincter mechanism there is a triple innervation from parasympathetic, sympathetic and somatic nerves (pudendal nerve).

In both the male and female urethra a number of glands open into the posterior urethra and can be the site of infection and source of confusion on occasion at the time of urethrography. There is slight dilatation of the urethra in the bulbar area where the urethra itself is surrounded by the bulbospongiosus muscle. There is a relative constriction of the urethra within the glans penis which helps focus the stream of urine as it comes through the dilatation present at the site of the navicular fossa; this is the narrowest part of the whole urethra.

The lining of the urethra varies in different portions. In the prostatic part it is transitional epithelium; in the membraneous and penile parts, pseudostratified and stratified columnar epithelium occur proximally, but, progressing more distally, islands of stratified squamous epithelium appear until in the distal part and the navicular fossa there is a complete sheet of stratified squamous epithelium.

REPRODUCTIVE SYSTEMS

Female reproductive organs consist of paired ovaries, paired fallopian tubes, a single midline uterus and a single midline vagina. Equivalent to the penis in the female is the clitoris, which is also composed of erectile tissue.

In the male there are paired testes where spermatozoa are produced. A pair of tubes, the vasa deferentia, carry sperm back from the testes into the pelvic cavity and into the urethra. There are paired seminal vesicles which produce materials, including sugars, needed for sperm to mature and which drain into the common termination of the vasa deferentia to form the paired common ejaculatory ducts opening into the prostatic urethra. The prostate gland produces much of the bulk of the semen. The penis is traversed by the urethra. In addition to the corpus spongiosum which surrounds the urethra, it comprises paired corpora cavernosa which represent the erectile tissue. It must be remembered that at the tip of the penis, the glans penis is contiguous with the corpus spongiosum and abuts against the corpus cavernosum (Fig. 18.12). Penile erection is essential to successful intercourse and is mediated by the nervi erigentes arising from the S2 to S4 nerve

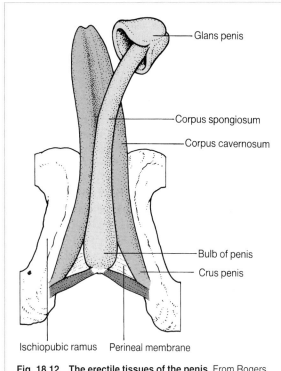

Fig. 18.12 The erectile tissues of the penis. From Rogers op. cit.

roots. Disorders of both penile and clitoral erection have been increasingly recognised in recent years to be a cause of significant concern within the population, and management of these disorders is an important mainstay of the subspecialty of andrology.

MALE AND FEMALE GERM CELLS

Both male and female germ cells present within either the testis or ovary respectively result from meiosis and contain 23 chromosomes. There are significant differences between male and female germ cells in terms of timing of production, the number of germ cells produced and their size and shape.

Cell division (mitosis) in the stem cells that result in germ cells ceases during embryonic life, and all the oogonia start their first meiotic division before birth. They remain in a resting phase until released from the ovary at ovulation, when the second meiotic division occurs rapidly after the ovum is penetrated by sperm. Meiosis can last up to 50 years. In contrast, mitosis in the male spermatogonia continues from puberty to old age and death. Cells are always entering meiosis, passing through the two divisions and maturing into sperm during a process that takes approximately 30 days. In the female, mitosis between oogonia in embryonic life produces a peak population of about 6 million cells two thirds of the way through intrauterinal life. There are approximately 2 million left at birth, which is followed by a dramatic loss of germ cells: by puberty there are only 150 000, and a thousand are left at the age of 50. In contrast, in the male, large numbers of germ cells persist through life, and in a healthy young man a single ejaculate contains 300 million sperm. The oocyte in the female is one of the largest cells in the body, measuring about 120 μm in diameter. It is spherical with a large active nucleus. In contrast the sperm comprises a head, which is the nucleus, containing tightly packed, condensed genetic material with a small cap. The acrosome and the body contain many mitochondria packed around a central cilium. The sperm relies upon energy reserves in the surrounding semen. It represents a motile cell packed with genetic material.

FEMALE REPRODUCTIVE TRACT

Ovary

The ovary is the size and shape of an almond and is attached to the posterior aspect of the broad ligament by the mesovarium (Fig. 18.13). At the superior (tubal) pole of the ovary is attached a prominent fold of peritoneum, the suspensory ligament of the ovary, which passes upwards over the pelvic brim and external iliac vessels to merge with the peritoneum over psoas major muscle. The ovarian artery gains access to the ovary through the mesovarium and suspensory ligament. A further ligament, the ovarian ligament, runs within the broad ligament to the cornu of the uterus.

Relations

These are extremely variable. The ovary lies in the shallow ovarian fossa. The upper margin of this fossa is formed by the external iliac vessels, whilst the posterior margin is formed by the ureter and internal iliac vessels. Fascia over the obturator internus muscle forms the floor of this fossa. The ovary is very variable in position and may be found prolapsed into the pouch of Douglas.

The relations of the ovary are of considerable importance clinically. They may be divided into:

- structures within the broad ligament
- structures on the lateral wall of the pelvis
- abdominal and pelvic viscera.

Blood supply

The arterial blood supply is from the ovarian artery, which is a branch of the aorta which comes off at the level of the renal arteries. The right ovarian vein drains into the inferior vena cava. On the left side, it drains into the left renal vein in a similar fashion to the testicular vein in the male.

Lymphatic drainage

Lymphatic drainage of the ovaries follows the ovarian arteries to the para-aortic lymph nodes.

Uterus

The uterus is a pear-shaped organ which is approximately 7 cm long, 5 cm from side to side at its widest point, and

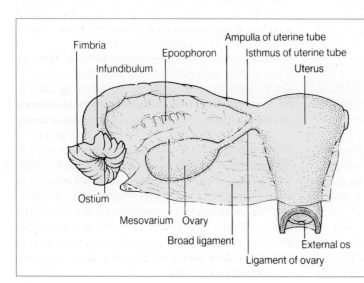

Fimbria
Infundibulum
Epoophoron
Ampulla of uterine tube
Isthmus of uterine tube
Uterus
Ostium
Mesovarium   Ovary
Broad ligament
Ligament of ovary
External os

Fig. 18.13   The uterus, broad ligament, and ovary — posterior view. From Rogers op. cit.

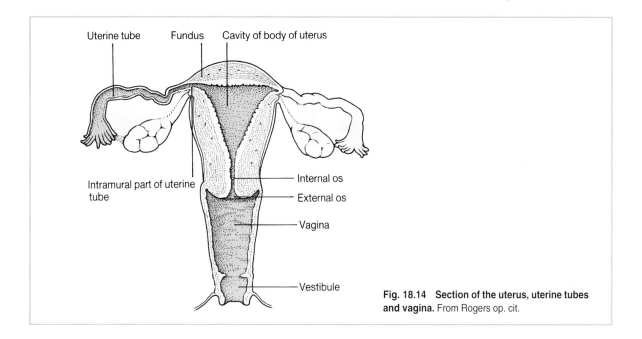

Uterine tube   Fundus   Cavity of body of uterus

Intramural part of uterine tube

Internal os

External os

Vagina

Vestibule

Fig. 18.14 Section of the uterus, uterine tubes and vagina. From Rogers op. cit.

3 cm anteroposteriorly. It is composed of a fundus, body and cervix. The fallopian tubes enter into each supra-lateral angle, above which lies the fundus. The features of the uterus, uterine tubes and vagina are shown in Figure 18.14.

Relations

- Anteriorly, the body of the uterus is related to the uterovesical pouch of peritoneum and lies either on the superior surface of the bladder or occasionally on coils of intestine. That part of the cervix lying outside the vagina is related directly to the bladder, whereas the infravaginal cervix has the anterior fornix as an immediate anterior relationship.
- Posteriorly lies the recto-uterine pouch (of Douglas), which is directly related to the coils of intestine lying in the pouch.
- Laterally lies the broad ligament; the ureter lies superior and lateral to the supravaginal cervix.

Blood supply

See Figure 18.15. The uterine artery, which is a branch of the internal iliac artery, runs in the base of the broad ligament, and about 2 cm lateral to the cervix it passes anterior and superior to the ureter, reaching the uterus at the level of the internal os. The artery then ascends in a tortuous manner, running up the lateral side of the body of the uterus before turning laterally and inferiorly to the uterine tube, where it terminates by anastomosing with

the terminal branches of the ovarian artery. The uterine artery also gives off a descending branch which supplies the cervix and the upper vagina. The uterine veins accompany the arteries, draining to the internal iliac vein.

Lymphatic drainage

Lymphatic vessels from the uterus drain in the following manner.

- The fundus drains along the ovarian vessels to the para-aortic nodes, although some drain with lymphatics which pass via the round ligament to the inguinal nodes. Metastases from the fundus of the uterus may therefore occur in the inguinal nodes.
- The body drains via lymphatics in the broad ligament to the iliac lymph nodes.
- The cervix drains laterally via the broad ligament to the external iliac nodes, posteriorly in the uterosacral fold to the sacral lymph nodes, and posterolaterally along the uterine vessels to the internal iliac nodes.

Fallopian tubes

The fallopian or uterine tubes are 10–12 cm long and run from the lateral side of the body of the uterus to the pelvic wall, where they end by opening near the ovary. The opening of the fallopian tube is called the ostium. The broad ligament of peritoneum is draped over the fallopian tube like a sheet over a washing line. Each tube comprises the following parts:

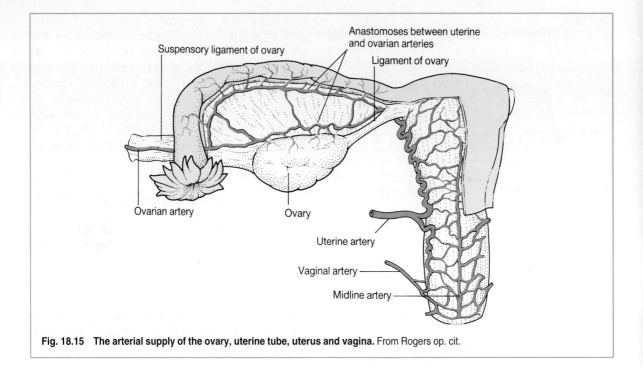

Fig. 18.15 The arterial supply of the ovary, uterine tube, uterus and vagina. From Rogers op. cit.

- the infundibulum — this is the trumpet shaped extremity which opens into the peritoneal cavity at the ostium. Its opening is fimbriated and overlies the ovary
- the ampulla, which is wide, thin walled and tortuous.
- the isthmus, which is narrow straight and thick walled.
- the intramural part — this pierces the uterine wall.

The fallopian tube is covered by peritoneum except for the intramural part. It contains a muscular coat of outer longitudinal and inner circular fibres, and the mucosa is formed of columnar-ciliated cells and lies in longitudinal ridges, each of which is thrown into numerous folds. The function of the tube is to propel ova along the lumen to the uterus. This is accomplished by muscular contraction, ciliary action and by the production of a lubricating fluid. A fertilised ovum may occasionally implant ectopically in the tube. This gives rise to an ectopic pregnancy which may cause rupture of the tube with consequent intraperitoneal haemorrhage. The distal end of the tube is open into the peritoneal cavity, providing direct communication between the peritoneum and the outside and therefore a potential pathway for infection.

Broad ligament

The broad ligament is a fold of peritoneum which connects the lateral margin of the uterus with the side wall of the pelvis. It drapes over the fallopian tube like a sheet on a washing line. The broad ligament contains or attaches to the following structures:

- the fallopian tube in its free edge
- the round ligament
- the ovarian ligament
- the uterine vessels and branches of the ovarian vessels
- the mesovarium attaching the ovary to its posterior aspect
- lymphatics.

In the base of the broad ligament the ureter passes forwards to the bladder lateral to and then immediately above the lateral fornix of the vagina.

Vagina

The vagina surrounds the cervix of the uterus and then passes downwards and forwards through the pelvic floor to open into the vestibule, which is the area enclosed by the labia minora and also contains the urethral orifice lying immediately behind the clitoris. The vagina is a muscular tube approximately 7 cm in length. The cervix opens into the anterior wall of the vagina superiorly bulging into the vaginal lumen. The vagina forms a ring around the cervix, and although this ring is continuous it is divided into anterior, posterior and lateral fornices.

Relations

- Anteriorly — the cervix enters the vagina above, and below this is the base of the bladder and the urethra which is embedded in the anterior vaginal wall.
- Posteriorly — the posterior fornix is covered by peritoneum in the recto-uterine pouch (of Douglas). Below this the anterior wall of the rectum is immediately posterior to the vagina, and below that the anal canal is separated from it by the perineal body.
- Superiorly — the ureter lies superior and lateral to the lateral fornix.
- Laterally — levator ani and the pelvic fascia.

Blood supply

The arterial blood supply is from several sources on each side:

- the vaginal artery
- the uterine artery
- the middle rectal artery
- the internal pudendal artery, supplying the lower third of the vagina.

Venous drainage is via a plexus of veins in the connective tissue around the vagina, draining into the internal iliac vein.

Lymphatic drainage

Those from the upper two thirds of the vagina drain into the internal and external iliac nodes. From the lower third, lymphatics pass to the superficial inguinal nodes.

MALE REPRODUCTIVE TRACT

Testis and epididymis

Each testis is ovoid, measuring 4 cm from upper to lower pole, 3 cm anterior to posterior and 2.5 cm from medial to lateral surface. The left testis lies at a lower level than the right within the scrotum. Each testis is contained by a white fibrous capsule, the tunica albuginea, and is covered by a double serous membrane into which it became invaginated in fetal life, the tunica vaginalis. Irregular septa arise from the tunica albuginea, dividing the testis into some 250 lobules, each lobule contains one to three tightly coiled tubules, seminiferous tubules, within which the sperm are produced.

The testes lie outside the body because spermatogenesis requires a temperature below that of the body, and if testes fail to descend properly this invariably leads to malfunction in spermatogenesis. At the hilum of the testis the seminiferous tubules drain into an irregular series of ducts called the rete testis from which efferent tubules arise, transporting the sperm into the head of the epididymis and subsequently down the epididymis through the vasa, joining with the seminal vesicles prior to forming the common ejaculatory ducts. The epididymis lies along the posterior border of the testis, somewhat to its lateral side. The epididymis is covered by the tunica vaginalis except at its posterior margin. The testis and epididymis each may bear at their upper extremities a small stalked body named respectively the appendix testis and the appendix epididymis. These may undergo torsion.

Blood supply

This is via the testicular artery, which arises from the aorta at the level of the renal arteries. The venous drainage is by the pampiniform plexus of veins, which becomes a single vessel, the testicular vein, at the deep inguinal ring. On the right this drains into the inferior vena cava and on the left into the renal vein.

Lymphatic drainage

Lymphatic vessels from the testis and epididymis accompany the testicular veins to drain into the para-aortic nodes.

Coverings of the testis

These coverings (Fig. 18.16) are important in a surgical approach to the testis through the scrotum. The following structures are encountered:

- scrotal skin
- dartos muscle
- external spermatic fascia
- cremaster muscle in cremasteric fascia
- internal spermatic fascia
- parietal layer of the tunica vaginalis.

Once the parietal layer of the tunica vaginalis has been divided, the visceral layer of the tunica vaginalis is seen covering the white tunica albuginea.

Vas deferens

The vas deferens (ductus deferens) commences at the inferior pole of the testis as the continuation of the epididymis. It is a thick muscular tube which transports sperm from the epididymis to the ejaculatory ducts within the prostate gland. It passes through the scrotum, inguinal canal and comes to lie on the side wall of the pelvis. Here it lies immediately below the peritoneum of the lateral wall of the pelvis. It then runs towards the tip of the ischial spine. It then turns medially to the base of the bladder. The vas ends by uniting with the ducts of the seminal vesicle to become the common ejaculatory duct. This occurs at the most superior and posterior aspect of the prostate gland.

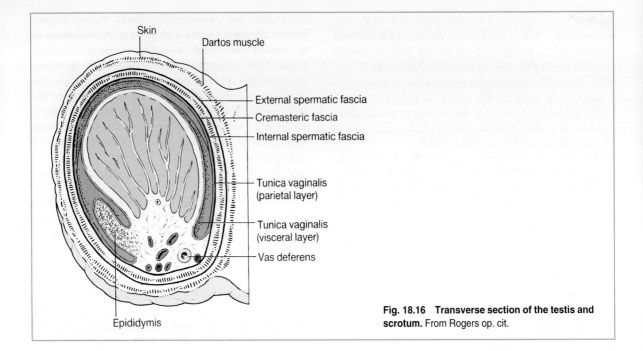

Skin
Dartos muscle
External spermatic fascia
Cremasteric fascia
Internal spermatic fascia
Tunica vaginalis (parietal layer)
Tunica vaginalis (visceral layer)
Vas deferens
Epididymis

Fig. 18.16   Transverse section of the testis and scrotum. From Rogers op. cit.

Prostate

The human prostate surrounds the prostatic urethra. There are two principal components to the prostate: the glandular component and a smooth muscle component. Approximately 25% of normal prostate is composed of smooth muscle, and with development of benign enlargement of the prostate, contrary to popular perception, although this is a glandular hyperplasia there is also a relative increase in the amount of smooth muscle such that smooth muscle in the hyperplastic prostate constitutes 40% of the gland. The majority of the prostate lies on the lateral and posterior aspects of the urethra, with little anterior prostatic tissue.

Relations
- Anteriorly — the pubic symphysis is separated by the extraperitoneal fat of the retropubic space.
- Posteriorly — the rectum is separated by the fascia of Denonvilliers.
- Superiorly — the prostate is continuous with the neck of the bladder.
- Inferiorly — the apex of the prostate rests on the external urethral sphincter within the deep perineal pouch.
- Laterally — levator ani.

Clinically the prostate gland is divided into lobes:

- The posterior lobe lies posterior to the urethra and inferior

to the plane defined by the course of the ejaculatory ducts.
- A median lobe lies between the ejaculatory ducts and posterior to the urethra.
- Two lateral lobes (or right and left lobes) are separated by a shallow posterior median groove which can be felt on rectal examination.
- Anterior to the urethra there is a narrow isthmus only, consisting mainly of fibromuscular tissue.

Blood supply
The arterial blood supply is derived from the inferior vesical artery, which is a branch of the internal iliac artery. The venous drainage is via the prostatic venous plexus, which drains into the internal iliac vein on each side. Some blood drains posteriorly around the rectum to the valveless vertebral veins of Batson. This is said to explain why prostatic carcinoma metastasises early to the bones of the lumbar spine and pelvis.

The prostatic urethra is the widest portion of the urethra, and on its posterior wall there is a prominent bulge known as the urethral crest, at the distal end of which lies the verumontanum, which has a midline opening on it leading to the prostatic utricle or uterus masculinus, which arises from the Mullerian ducts. Lying on either side of the opening of the utricle is the termination of the ejaculatory ducts, where seminal emission occurs.

The prostate has an important physiological role in producing secretions which are important to the survival and function of spermatozoa. It should not be forgotten that prostaglandins were so named having been first identified in the prostate.

Seminal vesicles

The seminal vesicles lie, one on each side, in the interval between the base of the bladder anteriorly and the rectum posteriorly. They lie lateral to the termination of the vasa. Each seminal vesicle has a common drainage with its neighbouring vas via the common ejaculatory duct (Fig. 18.17). The vesicles synthesise and secrete a sticky, yellowish fluid rich in fructose. The normal vesicles cannot be palpated on rectal examination. However, if they are enlarged by infection, e.g. tuberculosis, they become palpable.

PHYSIOLOGY

FLUID AND ELECTROLYTE BALANCE

The main physiological function of the urinary tract is the maintenance of fluid, acid–base and electrolyte balance and the excretion of waste products. A subsidiary but extremely important role is that of the production of certain hormones.

Approximately one fifth of the cardiac output passes through the kidneys each minute, resulting in a renal blood flow of up to 400 mL per 100 g of kidney per min (650 mL/min per kidney). The renal blood pressure remains extremely constant despite profound changes in systemic blood pressure, and the survival advantage of this mechanism is apparent on reflection. This phenomenon is described as autoregulation and is principally mediated via effects on preglomerular vascular resistance. Whilst the underlying mechanism is the subject of intensive study, it is thought to be related to intrinsic myogenic tone within blood vessels, independent of neural factors.

A total of 170–180 L of plasma per day are filtered through the glomeruli at an approximate rate of 125 mL/min. The glomerular membrane acts as a main filtration mechanism and is impermeable to molecules larger than 4 nm diameter, which relates to an average molecular weight of 70 000. The ultrafiltrate of plasma then passes down to the tubules.

The proximal tubule   This decreases the volume of glomerular filtrate by 75–80%, with active resorbtion of glucose, phosphate, bicarbonate, potassium and chloride. It is important to realise that glucose is resorbed entirely from the proximal tubules, unless the glucose load exceeds the capacity for absorption. The majority of filtered sodium and bicarbonate are reabsorbed from the proximal tubules, and sodium is actually pumped via hydrogen/potassium-linked pump mechanisms. The proximal tubular filtrate is iso-osmotic as a consequence of passive absorption of both water and urea. Sulphates, amino acids and low molecular weight proteins are reabsorbed, as is potassium.

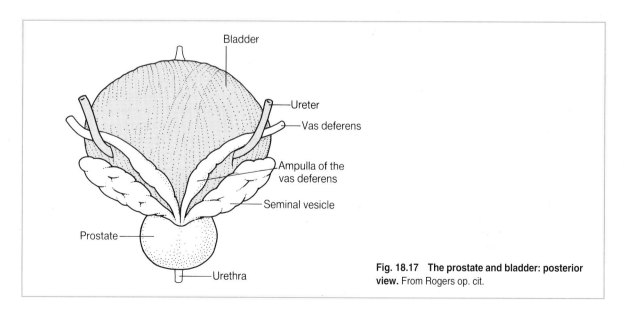

Fig. 18.17   The prostate and bladder: posterior view. From Rogers op. cit.

Loop of Henle Sodium chloride and water are resorbed passively. Water is resorbed from the more proximal part (descending limb) in combination with sodium, whilst the distal part (ascending limb) is impermeable to water, with active sodium resorbtion. This produces a concentration gradient in the renal medulla which is important in maintaining water balance. Loop diuretics, e.g. frusemide, inhibit chloride and sodium resorbtion from the descending limb.

Distal tubule and collecting duct The filtrate is hypotonic as it leaves the loop of Henle, entering the distal tubules where water resorbtion is under the control of ADH. Sodium is actively pumped out of the distal tubules, and resorbtion is modified by aldosterone secretion. The collecting tubules pass through the renal medulla, and water absorption is independent of sodium resorbtion and is regulated by ADH secretion. Sodium is actively pumped out of the collecting tubules against a concentration gradient to maintain the hypertonicity of the renal medulla, with associated passive resorbtion to a small degree. Large amounts of urea also are resorbed passively from the collecting tubules. A number of substances are secreted in the distal tubule, including potassium and hydrogen and drugs. Seventy-five percent of the potassium content of urine results at this level due to tubular secretion. Potassium secretion is linked with sodium and hydrogen concentrations and is modified by aldosterone secretion. Hydrogen secretion occurs in the distal tubules against a concentration gradient.

MAINTENANCE OF WATER BALANCE

The osmolality of urine varies between 50 mosm/L and 1200 mosm/L and depends upon the amount of water in the collecting tubule, which also is related to an appropriate corticomedullary osmotic gradient and the permeability of the collecting ducts under the control of ADH. Sodium and chloride are transported out of the ascending limb of the loop of Henle, and the sodium concentration falls progressively as the distal tubule is reached. The remainder of the loop of Henle is in osmotic equilibrium with the substance of the kidney. As the iso-osmolar filtrate reaches the bottom of the loop of Henle the contents of the descending limb become more concentrated as a result of being pushed towards the ascending limb. Further concentration occurs due to active sodium resorbtion in the ascending limb, resulting in an osmolar gradient in the renal medulla. Any increase in medullary blood flow results in dissipation of medullary osmolality, decreased water resorbtion and the production of large quantities of dilute urine. Dehydration results in release

of ADH, increasing permeability in the distal nephron and results in increased water resorbtion. ADH is released from the posterior lobe of the pituitary gland. The endogenous control of ADH release is under the regulation of osmoreceptors adjacent to the supraoptic nucleus, which is under the influence of sodium and chloride concentration in the plasma. There are also volume receptors in the atria and great veins which seem to be under the control of the vagus nerve.

MAINTENANCE OF ACID–BASE BALANCE

The kidney cannot excrete urine of pH < 4.5. Maintenance of acid–base balance relies upon a complex series of buffer mechanisms. In the proximal tubules the predominant buffer system is dependent on bicarbonate HCO_3^-/H_2CO_3, whilst in the distal tubules the predominant buffer is $HPO_4^{2-}/H_2PO_4^-$ and the weakest is the NH_4^+ system. The phosphate buffer system is the most important during normal renal function, but the NH_4^+ system has a particular advantage in that it allows excretion of acid without loss of metallic cations such as Na^+.

HORMONE PRODUCTION BY THE KIDNEY

A number of important hormones are produced within the kidney. The renin–angiotensin system is important, with renin being released from juxtaglomerular cells in response to sympathetic nerve stimulation via a decrease in afferent arteriolar pressure and hyponatraemia. Renin acts on circulating angiotensinogen to produce angiotensin I, which is converted by a circulating enzyme to angiotensin II. Angiotensin II stimulates the zona glomerulosa of the adrenal gland to produce aldosterone, which increases the sodium resorbtion by the kidneys and also produces vasoconstriction. These effects feed back in a negative fashion and switch off renin secretion and therefore maintain homeostasis. This is a gross oversimplification of an extremely complex system, but nevertheless it is evident that this homeostatic mechanism is essential to maintain a smooth blood pressure and compensate for changes in extracellular fluid volume and sodium excretion.

Other important hormones which are the subject of contemporary study include kallikrein (produced in the distal nephron) and other related agents. These substances are important vasodilators and also have been shown to have motor effects within the lower urinary tract and may be involved in sensorimotor mechanisms within the bladder.

The kidney is also involved in calcium metabolism and produces 1 α-hydroxylase in response to low circulating levels of calcium, which acts to convert 25-hydroxychole-calciferol into the active metabolite 1,25-dihydroxychole-calciferol, which then promotes calcium reabsorbtion and decreases urine excretion to maintain homeostasis.

Erythropoietin is produced by the kidney in response to hypoxia (either due to anaemia or respiratory causes), high circulating levels of the products of red cell destruction, and vasoconstriction. It is also produced in smaller amounts by the liver and spleen. Erythropoietin stimulates an increase in the number of nucleated red cells in the haemopoietic tissue, thereby raising red cell and reticulocyte counts in peripheral blood. Indeed synthesised erythropoietin is used in contemporary haematological practice, for these very purposes, especially in intractable anaemia associated with chronic renal failure.

The renal cortex and medulla synthesise a number of prostaglandins whose exact function remains obscure at present.

DISORDERS OF RENAL FUNCTION

Adverse effects of drugs on the kidney

As the kidneys act as the main detoxifying and filtration system within the body, it is not therefore a surprise that many drugs can affect the urinary tract either by a direct effect on the kidneys or bladder or indirectly by producing ureteric obstruction. Nephrotoxic drugs include heavy metals, organic solvents, radiological contrast media (the combination of radiological contrast plus metformin has recently been recognised as being toxic), antibiotics such as aminoglycosides, and some cephalosporins, chelating agents, paraquat and penicillamine. Ureteric obstruction can occur either as a direct result of drug action (predominantly of historical interest now), e.g. retroperineal fibrosis due to methysergide and practolol or as a consequence of blockage of the ureters due to renal papillary necrosis consequent upon analgesic abuse. Uric acid stones can result from the use of high dose aspirin, thiazide diuretics and frusemide. Increased symptoms can result from the effect of agents increasing urine production, e.g. diuretics, or acting directly on the bladder; and relative underactivity of the bladder possibly leading to retention can result from anticholinergics, particularly if there is an additional factor such as obstruction to the bladder outlet.

Acute renal failure

This is an abrupt decline in renal function with a loss of normal activity. A daily urine output of less than 500 mL is termed oliguria; the absence of urine formation is anuria. The underlying cause of acute renal failure is a persistent fall in renal blood flow to levels 30–40% of normal with a consequent reduction in glomerular filtration to less than 5 mL/min. The causes of acute renal failure can be divided broadly into prerenal, renal and postrenal. Prerenal acute renal failure usually results from dehydration or circulatory collapse producing hypovolaemia associated with conditions such as blood loss, septicaemia, or trauma. Renal causes can be broadly considered to be interstitial (drugs or infection), glomerular (autoimmune conditions, diabetes), tubular damage (antibiotics, drugs, toxic chemicals), or renal (vasculitis or thrombosis).

The diagnosis of acute renal failure is usually apparent from the history. Routine biochemical investigations which are useful in diagnosis of acute renal failure are summarised in Table 18.1.

An ultrasound scan is a particularly useful diagnostic investigation and is usually combined with a plain abdominal x-ray. The main aim of the treatment of patients with acute renal failure is to identify a cause and institute appropriate treatment. Fluid intake is restricted to 500 mL/24 h (equivalent to insensible loss). Fluids are usually given orally. Sodium intake is restricted to 20–30 mmol per day, and careful monitoring of metabolic and nutritional status is important. H_2 receptor antagonists and antacids are often used because of the associated incidence of upper gastrointestinal haemorrhage. Dialysis is indicated if conservative measures fail to control the situation, and usually in the acute situation it is instituted via haemodialysis. Indications for haemodialysis include:

- hyperkalaemia
- metabolic acidosis
- fluid overload with pulmonary oedema.

Table 18.1 Biochemical recognition of established acute renal failure		
	Physiological oliguria	Established ARF
Urine volume	Low (?high)	Low
Urine specific gravity	> 1020	1010
Urinary osmolality (mosm/kg H_2O)	> 500	250–300
Urinary sodium (mmol/L)	< 15	> 60
Urinary urea (mmol/L)	> 250	< 160
Urine/plasma osmolality	> 1.3	≤ 1.1
Urine/plasma urea	> 10	< 10
Response to fluid load	Always	Occasional

Reproduced from Bullock N, Sibley G, Whittaker R (eds) 1989 Essential urology; Churchill Livingstone, Edinburgh.

The clinical course of acute renal failure is highly variable depending upon the aetiology and can be considered to comprise oliguric, diuretic and postdiuretic phases. The oliguric phase usually starts early on but may be prolonged for up to 3 months or more. A diuresis can occur at any time and is often a sign that recovery is occurring. It is important to maintain vigilance particularly during this time because of the potential for loss of fluid and electrolytes. Renal function may continue to improve for up to a year, but distal tubular function is often permanently impaired, although this may be difficult to determine clinically. Acute renal failure is a condition with a high mortality, with the worst prognosis being associated with haemorrhage, trauma, peritonitis, advanced age and infection.

Chronic renal failure

A number of patients present each year in end stage renal failure, and it has been suggested that the incidence is approximately 50 to 60 patients per million of the UK population. Often no aetiological factor can be found as a cause for chronic renal failure, and it is important to try and differentiate the condition from acute renal failure, to determine its aetiology and the severity of the disease process. The commonest causes of chronic renal failure include chronic glomerulitis and pyelonephritis. Polycystic renal disease accounts for approximately 5% of cases and hypertension approximately 10%.

Patients with chronic renal failure usually have polyuria with loss of normal concentrating ability. Nocturia is often said to be an early sign and the urine contains protein with granular casts and white blood cells. Sodium is gradually retained in chronic renal failure, albeit the serum sodium level is a poor reflection of this. In end stage chronic renal failure potassium levels may rise and acidosis is inevitable due to decreased ammonium ion excretion and decreased excretion of buffer phosphate, the urine pH usually being less than 5. Since calcium levels may fall, secondary hyperparathyroidism is not uncommon and osteomalacia may occur which is sometimes vitamin D resistant. Magnesium levels may rise because of the inability to excrete a magnesium load. Characteristically the urea, uric acid and creatinine levels rise. Serum creatinine levels are a useful way of monitoring chronic renal failure. Anaemia occurs as a consequence of chronic renal failure, which is usually normochromic and normocytic and is likely to be due to marrow suppression with reduced red cell survival.

Appropriate investigation of patients with chronic renal failure in addition to biochemical investigations includes ultrasound scan of the upper tracts and a check on postvoiding residual urine. It must be remembered that up to a third of patients with chronic retention of urine present with chronic renal failure.

The aim of conservative treatment is to delay the progressive deterioration of renal function and its consequences. Fluid intake should be controlled to produce a urine output of approximately 1 L/24 h, blood pressure is controlled by the use of antihypertensive drugs, and cardiac failure is treated using standard measures. The anaemia of chronic renal failure responds well to the use of exogenous erythropoietin and may be treated by transfusion, although this is not usually used unless the patients are severely symptomatic. In some patients protein intake is restricted to 40 g/24 h in order to reduce the production of nitrogenous waste products.

When conservative measures fail, dialysis is instituted, and this is usually in patients in whom the serum creatinine has risen above 1000 mmol/L or if the creatinine clearance is less than 1 mL/min. The options for dialysis lie between haemodialysis and peritoneal dialysis.

A detailed discussion of dialysis lies outside the remit of this chapter. In brief, the principle of haemodialysis is to allow selective diffusion of molecules below a certain size from the peripheral blood into the dialysis fluid. Haemodialysis uses an artificial semipermeable membrane which is disposable. In contrast, peritoneal dialysis is less efficient and uses the peritoneum as a membrane, and is more commonly complicated by infective sequelae. However, it is particularly useful in the home situation and is cheaper than haemodialysis.

Wherever possible, renal transplantation is carried out, but this is limited by the availability of transplant organs, the suitability of those organs based on tissue typing, and the availability of appropriate resources.

INVESTIGATION OF UROLOGICAL SYMPTOMS

Urine analysis is best performed using a midstream urine. After cleansing the external urethral meatus the first 20 mL or so of urine is discarded before collecting the next part of the voided urine in a sterile container. It must be remembered that the commonly used dipsticks may detect an abnormality but this can be spurious, as they are subject to artefact and one cannot ascribe a positive stick test for blood to be equivalent to microscopic haematuria. Nevertheless stick tests are very useful and provide easy access to urine testing in a screening situation. The urine pH usually varies between 4.5 and 8, and a persistently alkaline urine is associated with infection with urea-splitting organisms such as *Proteus mirabilis*. The amount of protein in the urine is normally less than 100 mg/24 h, and glycosuria should always raise the suspicion of diabetes mellitus, which should be investigated further with a fasting blood glucose. Microscopy of the urine allows the presence of red cells, white cells and casts to be demonstrated. Early morning urines are classically collected to test for acid fast bacilli; usually three specimens are collected and cultured. Terminal stream urine specimens are characteristically recommended for examination of the urine for parasites and ova. Urine cytology should not be forgotten as a sensitive means of detecting carcinoma in situ of the urinary tract and the presence of high grade neoplasms. However, false positives and false negatives do exist, and urine cytology cannot be used to supplant conventional investigation.

Blood tests

Renal function is routinely assessed by measurement of the plasma urea and creatinine, but it must be remembered that significant renal dysfunction can occur (loss of two thirds of the renal reserve) before the urea and creatinine rise. The most accurate guide to renal function is creatinine clearance, normally 100–140 mL/min, which approximates to the glomerular filtration rates. This is calculated from measurement of urine volume (V), plasma creatinine (P_{creat}) and urine creatinine concentrations (U_{creat}). Creatinine clearance is calculated from the formula:

$$\frac{U_{creat} \times V}{P_{creat}} = Creatinine\ clearance$$

More sensitive measures for determining glomerular filtration rate involve the measurement of the plasmic clearance of compounds such as EDTA (ethylenediamine tetra-acetic acid). Haematology allows detection of anaemia and polycythaemia, and the ESR is characteristically elevated in cases of malignancy or retroperitoneal fibrosis. In patients who have urinary tract calculus disease, a serum calcium and uric acid are measured. A spot test of urine is sent for cystine analysis, and 24 h collection of urinary excretion of calcium and uric acid are estimated.

Diagnostic imaging

A plain abdominal x-ray is useful to detect soft tissue masses of the renal areas or pelvis and 90% of urinary tract calculi are radio-opaque. A plain abdominal x-ray is often called a KUB (kidney, ureter and bladder x-ray). The intravenous urogram, whilst it remains the gold standard investigation, is now less commonly used and has been supplanted in many areas by ultrasound scanning combined with a KUB x-ray. Nevertheless it remains the most sensitive investigation to pick up upper tract urothelial abnormalities. An ultrasound scan is often more useful in defining the presence of upper tract tumours. CT scanning is used to further refine the diagnosis following on from demonstration of an initial abnormality, and the spiral CT scan is being increasingly introduced as an alternative to intravenous urography particularly in the diagnosis and demonstration of upper tract calculous disease. Both ultrasound and CT scanning can be used to help guide biopsies of any abnormality seen. Arteriography now is uncommonly used but is particularly beneficial in the context of renal vascular disorders when associated with renal trauma. Venography is used in the context of therapeutic manoeuvres such as embolisation of varicoceles. Magnetic resonance imaging (MRI) scanning is used in conjunction with CT scanning but as yet has not replaced it.

Interventional radiology via the placement of nephrostomy tubes has revolutionised our management of urinary tract calculous disease and obstruction of the upper tracts. Such techniques allow the placement of a nephrostomy tube which decompresses the obstructed upper tract and allows the antegrade visualisation of the upper tract by the use of contrast media and can be used therapeutically for the placement of a stent in an antegrade fashion, which can be particularly useful in the context of malignancy causing obstruction to the ureter.

Radionuclide studies

Renography is an important aspect of the investigation of the upper urinary tract. When injected intravenously certain radio-isotope-labelled compounds are selectively taken up and excreted by the kidneys. The use of an externally placed counter allows important information on renal tract function and obstruction to be obtained.

Different isotopes can be used to study specific aspects of kidney function. Radiolabelled technetium (technetium-99) is the most commonly used isotope. The following compounds are used.

1. Dimercaptosuccinic acid (DMSA) is taken up by the renal tubules and allows assessment of size, position and function of the kidneys and some degree of anatomical definition with regard to scars, cysts, or tumours.
2. Diethylenetriamine penta-acetic acid (DTPA) is taken up and excreted in the urine. The initial uptake provides an assessment of blood flow to the kidney, the so-called vascular phase. The rate rises and slows as isotope is concentrated and passed into the collecting system of the kidney (the filtration phase). A peak is then reached as isotope passes down the ureter in

steady state with the amount arriving via the collecting system. As the amount arriving via the collecting system then drops off, the activity falls as isotope is transported down the ureter (excretion phase). Administration of this compound is often combined with that of a diuretic such as frusemide and allows some comment to be passed on the presence or absence of obstruction to the upper tract.

3. A technetium-labelled compound, MAG-3, is commonly used in patients with renal impairment, as this allows better definition of the kidney in these circumstances.

4. Technetium-labelled compounds are commonly used for bone scanning to check for metastases in association with prostatic carcinoma.

Lower urinary tract function

Urodynamic assessment of the urinary tract relates to the study of pressure and flow relationships within the urinary tract. Urodynamic tests should be considered to represent a hierarchy of investigations:

- fluid volume chart
- flow rate
- ultrasound residual
- urodynamic assessment
- video urodynamic assessment.

The simplest urodynamic technique is to assess the volume of fluid the patient takes in and the volume they pass out. By measuring the amount voided, one can assess the functional capacity of the bladder, and in addition the patient can record the number of incontinent episodes that they experience if incontinence is a problem. In the presence of symptoms suggesting bladder outflow obstruction then a flow rate produces objective documentation of the patient's flow. A flow rate by itself is not diagnostic of obstruction, since the reduced flow can occur either as a consequence of obstruction or in association with poor detrusor function. Poor detrusor function is usually associated with a large residual volume. In normal circumstances a patient should be able to void to completion. However, if the residual is 150 mL or more then increasingly one suspects poor detrusor function. Contrary to popular belief a large residual does not equate with bladder outflow obstruction. The most accurate way of defining lower urinary tract function is to measure the pressure within the bladder and synchronously the pressure within the rectum. The rectal pressure equates with the intra-abdominal pressure and is automatically subtracted from the total bladder pressure that is measured allowing calculation of the true detrusor

pressure. A number of computer programs exist to allow this calculation to be made simultaneously during any urodynamic study. A urodynamic study encompasses two components. The first is filling the patient's bladder and recording the volumes at which the patient experiences the first sensation of filling, discomfort and the final tolerated capacity. The pressure within the bladder can be measured at these various times, and in a patient with normal bladder function the pressure within the bladder should not rise above zero. Any rise in pressure whilst the patient is conscious and cooperative leads to the definition of detrusor instability. If bladder overactivity of this nature is defined and there is any history of relevant neurological disease, then by definition the patient has detrusor hyperreflexia. Any impairment of bladder filling in the absence of a pressure rise leads to the diagnosis of a hypersensitive bladder (provided that other pathology such as infective and neoplastic disorders has been excluded), a so called *sensory* disorder.

When a patient's tolerated bladder capacity is reached then the second phase of the urodynamic study is reached and they are asked to void; a normal bladder should accommodate 450–500 mL before capacity is reached. The patient then voids, in women with a pressure of 30–40 cmH$_2$O and in men of 40–50 cmH$_2$O with a flow rate of up to 30–40 mL/s in women and up to 25–30 mL/s in men. Combining a cystometrogram with the use of contrast media leads to the so-called videocystometrogram, which represents the gold standard investigation, as anatomical detail relating to the lower urinary tract can be seen in addition to the presence of reflux towards the upper tracts.

Approximately 15–20% of patients presenting with symptoms suggestive of bladder outflow obstruction require cystometrography, and indications for this include patients with equivocal symptoms, a neurological history, those who cannot carry out an adequate flow rate, where the postvoiding residual is high, or where there is a history of previous failed surgery. Cystourethrography, and in particular videocystometry, are particularly useful in the investigation of patients with a storage problem presenting with frequency and incontinence. Cystourethrography, by allowing anatomical definition of the lower urinary tract, allows assessment of the degree of prolapse of the bladder base and also can allow the confirmation of stress urinary leakage on asking the patient to cough.

Pressure flow urodynamics can be applied via a nephrostomy tube to the kidney, but this represents a specialist investigation which is now uncommonly used as it is often difficult to interpret. Other investigative techniques relating to the lower urinary tract, including electromyography and urethral pressure profile, are research tools and not in widespread clinical use. The assessment of Valsalva-induced leakage can be difficult to quantify and interpret and, although it is popular in certain centres, is an inaccurate technique and can not be recommended for general use.

PATHOLOGY

CONGENITAL ANOMALIES OF THE URINARY TRACT

See Chapter 16.

PRACTICAL PHARMACOLOGY OF THE URINARY TRACT

It must be remembered that the bladder spends most of its time as a storage organ, with less than 1% of its time contracting in the normal situation to empty its contents. The parasympathetic nervous system acts to expel urine from the bladder. The parasympathetic acts in synergy with the sympathetic nervous system, which opposes its action and therefore acts to store urine. Disease states affecting the lower urinary tract can be considered as:

- failure to store
- failure to empty.

Failure to store

This can result from overactivity of the bladder, underactivity of the sphincteric outlet mechanism, or lastly because of an oversensitivity of the lower urinary tract. In practical terms the principal pharmacotherapeutic agents used for bladder overactivity are anticholinergics. The smooth muscle relaxant Urispas (flavoxate) has not been shown to be effective in placebo-controlled trials and cannot therefore be recommended for use. An additional therapeutic avenue which can be utilised is to stop urine production, using an ADH analogue, which is used for patients with severe bladder overactivity and in particular, nocturia. A commonly used agent is DDAVP (an artificial analogue of ADH). This is available as either an intranasal preparation or in tablet formulation. It can be prescribed for patients as long as it is only used once per day and should be avoided in patients with a history of heart failure or renal impairment. Alpha$_1$ agonists have been advocated for use for sphincteric weakness but are very non-specific in their action, with too many side effects to be used clinically for stress incontinence.

Sensory disturbances of the bladder are as yet poorly understood, and whilst a number of agents are used for their treatment, including intravesical instillations for dimethyl sulphoxide and steroids, and oral agents such as cimetidine and pentosan polysulphate, no agents have been found to be universally successful, and the choice of treatment will depend upon careful evaluation of the patient and the targeted administration of appropriate therapy based on the experience of the treating clinician.

Failure to empty

This can be due to bladder underactivity or obstruction to the outlet.

Pharmacotherapy directed at bladder underactivity, including the use of muscarinic agonists, is not effective, has a number of side effects, and is not routinely used in contemporary urological practice. Conversely, alpha$_1$ antagonists which act to relax the muscle in the outlet to the bladder both of the prostate and the bladder neck are efficacious in the management of prostatic obstruction. Box 18.1 documents the commonly used agents.

A number of other agents are marketed for the management of these disorders but have not been found to be particularly efficacious.

All autonomically active agents do have side effects, and anticholinergics produce a dry mouth, heartburn and can cause visual disturbances. Conversely, alpha$_1$ antagonists can reduce the blood pressure and produce dizziness, drowsiness and other non-specific effects. Patients should be counselled regarding these side effects before therapy is commenced. As a general rule drugs are titrated against efficacy and side effects.

Box 18.1   Drug treatment of diseases affecting the lower urinary tract

Failure to store (detrusor instability)
- anticholinergics
  — oxybutynin
  — tolterodine
  — imipramine
  — propantheline
  — propiverine
- desmopressin

Failure to empty (bladder outflow obstruction)
- alpha I antagonists
  — prazosin
  — indoramin
  — terazosin
  — doxazosin
  — alfuzosin
  — tamsulosin

ERECTILE DYSFUNCTION

Erectile dysfunction affecting the penis in the male and the clitoris in the female is the subject of considerable interest at present. The innervation of these structures is provided by the nervi erigentes (S2 to S4). Nitric oxide has been identified as a relaxant agent within the erectile structures. Unfortunately nitric oxide agonists are too toxic for use in routine clinical practice, and this forms the basis of treatment with the new agent sildenafil (Viagra) which acts to prevent the breakdown of cyclic GMP, which is a substance produced via the nitric oxide pathway. Other pharmacotherapeutic agents used to treat erectile dysfunction act as smooth muscle relaxants and include agents such as papaverine or prostaglandins which can be injected into the corpora cavernosa. More recent studies have investigated the intra-urethral administration of such agents, and in addition some interest has been aroused by the use of oral alpha$_1$ antagonists which do have some efficacy in this area.

Failing efficacy with drug therapy then either a vacuum artificial erection device can be utilised or alternatively prostheses can be inserted into the penis.

URINARY TRACT INFECTION

Urinary tract infection is common, particularly in women. Whilst urinary tract infection may be asymptomatic it is usually associated with the classical symptoms of 'cystitis', including dysuria, frequency and an unpleasant odour to the urine. Whilst the commonest organisms associated with urinary infection are derived from the bowel, more chronic and serious infections which should always be considered in clinical practice include tuberculosis and parasitic infections, particularly schistosomiasis. These are uncommon in routine surgical practice in the Western world.

In the infant, urinary infection is slightly more common in boys than girls, and this is usually associated with congenital anomalies. In the adult, however, urinary infection occurring in women relates to anatomical factors and is not investigated in women unless it occurs in a persistent fashion, usually two or more infections. In contrast any urinary infection of the male should be investigated. The routine investigation of urinary infection includes culture of the urine, assessment of the upper tracts by ultrasound scan and KUB x-ray and cystoscopy, usually via the flexible cystoscope. In men in particular it is important to assess the bladder outflow tract by an ultrasound residual, and flow rate estimation. In a number of male patients no specific pathogen can be demon-

strated. These patients often have persistent features suggestive of urinary infection, with perineal discomfort, and often are ascribed the diagnosis of abacterial prostatitis or prostatodynia. This condition is of unknown causation but may often be associated with bladder outflow obstruction.

Persistent infection of the upper tract may be associated with reflux of urine, and this should always be suspected in the patient who complains of pain on voiding or where there are recurrent bouts of pyelonephritis. Chronic pyelonephritis usually is well established by the time adult life is reached, as a consequence of vesicoureteric reflux, but there is no evidence that surgical treatment of such reflux is beneficial. Infection of the upper tracts (pyelonephritis) results in loin pain and pyrexia with associated rigors and is an indication for hospital admission and intravenous antibiotic therapy.

Renal abscess formation is uncommon now that urinary infections are treated early with antibiotics but should always raise the possibility of complicating factors such as diabetes. An obstructed upper tract with features suggestive of infection is a surgical emergency requiring decompression of the upper tract, often by the placement of a nephrostomy tube. A chronically obstructed upper tract with poor function may present with insidious chronic symptoms of weight loss, lethargy and malaise. On examination, though few clinical signs may be evident, the patient may have a palpable kidney. Pyonephrosis presenting in this fashion can be difficult to diagnose and requires excision of the obstructed upper tract, although preliminary drainage is usually carried out to defunction the system and improve the patient's general state. The presence of such an infected upper tract, often with associated stone disease, may lead on to a pseudotumour known as xanthogranulomatous pyelonephritis, which can be difficult to remove surgically because of associated fibrosis.

Chronic infections of the urinary tract which deserve further consideration include tuberculosis and parasitic infections. The genitourinary tract is involved in 3–5% of cases of tuberculosis, usually as a consequence of *Mycobacterium tuberculosis*. The organism reaches the urinary tract via the blood stream from a primary focus elsewhere, usually in the lungs. It may also spread to the genital tract. Any patient with persistent sterile pyuria in the absence of a demonstrable abnormality should always be tested by early morning specimens of urine for acid fast bacilli. A number of parasites may infect the urinary tract, but all are rare in the United Kingdom. A diagnosis of parasitic infection must always be considered in patients originating from abroad, and the commonest parasitic infection is schistosomiasis. The organism

Schistosoma haematobium commonly affects the urinary tract. The chronic irritation resulting from egg laying in the bladder leads on to chronic irritation with squamous metaplasia, calcification of the bladder and, in untreated cases, squamous carcinoma. This is particularly common in certain countries where this disease is endemic.

HAEMATURIA

Haematuria is an important symptom and can be diagnosed on stick testing (chemical haematuria), microscopy (microscopic haematuria), or can be reported by the patient as macroscopic haematuria. The classical triad of loin pain, palpable mass and haematuria is uncommon as a presentation for renal tumour. Haematuria, particularly macroscopic haematuria, is a symptom which should always be investigated. Chemical haematuria should always be confirmed by microscopy. The standard investigation of patients with haematuria is screening of the upper tracts by ultrasound scan and KUB x-ray and cystoscopy. The persistence of haematuria in the absence of a structural abnormality defined by screening of the upper tracts and cystoscopy should alert one to the possibility of primary renal disease. Before drawing these conclusions, however, if an ultrasound scan is normal and haematuria persists then more specialised investigations such as urine cytology and intravenous urography of the upper tracts are indicated. Whilst much beloved of textbooks, spurious causes of haematuria are rare and one should always first consider whether the haematuria is occurring as a consequence of urinary tract calculi, infection, or renal tract neoplasia. Haematuria does occur in association with renal tract trauma, and this is considered in the next section.

In reviewing the aetiology of haematuria it is helpful to consider the kidneys, ureter, bladder, urethra and prostate as separate structural zones within the urinary tract, all of which should be investigated to exclude significant pathology. Causes of haematuria are shown in Box 18.2.

URINARY TRACT TRAUMA

Despite the number of people admitted to hospital each year as a consequence of trauma, only a small proportion have sustained genitourinary injuries. Indeed, urological injuries occur in 3–10% of patients who present following blunt or penetrating trauma. Of these about 10% involve the urethra. Nevertheless up to 10–15% of all patients with abdominal injuries have associated injuries to the urinary tract. Many of these are overshadowed by the injuries to other systems which take precedence, and

---

Box 18.2   Causes of haematuria

- kidney
  — glomerular diseases
  — polycystic kidneys
  — carcinoma
  — stone
  — trauma (including renal biopsy)
  — tuberculosis
  — embolism
  — renal vein thrombosis
  — vascular malformation

- ureter
  — stone
  — neoplasm

- bladder
  — carcinoma
  — stone
  — trauma
  — inflammatory/infective — cystitis, tuberculosis, bilharzia

- prostate
  — benign prostatic hypertrophy
  — neoplasm

- urethra
  — trauma
  — stone
  — urethritis
  — neoplasm

- general
  — anticoagulants
  — thrombocytopaenia
  — haemophilia
  — sickle cell disease
  — malaria

---

many of these injuries are appropriately managed conservatively. In the United Kingdom the majority of injuries are as a consequence of blunt trauma usually associated with road traffic accidents. In order to diagnose urinary tract trauma it is important to have a high index of suspicion with reference to the nature of the injury, and to carry out a clinical examination looking for injuries in the region of the loin, including to the lower ribs, deformities of the pelvis, superficial bruising of the abdomen, loins and perineum, and obvious swelling, deformity, or tissue loss in the genital region and the presence of blood at the urethral meatus. Rectal examination may be helpful in this context by demonstrating dislocation of the prostate or a boggy swelling in the area.

An important indicator of potential urinary tract trauma is the presence of blood in the urine, either macroscopic or microscopic in nature. Blood is present in over two thirds of patients with renal injury and in all patients with bladder or urethral injuries.

Renal injury

Two thirds of injuries to the kidney occur as a consequence of blunt trauma and result from a crush injury between the anterior ends of the lower ribs and the upper lumbar spine. There is often associated bony injury and bruising in the flank. After initial clinical assessment, whilst an ultrasound scan can be helpful it is recommended that a contrast study should be carried out. CT scanning is the gold standard, but intravenous urography is more readily available, particularly in the acute situation, and is important not only in demonstrating deformity of the collecting system and extravasation, but also whether there is significant filtration of contrast by the kidney.

The main aim of management is to preserve renal function and minimise blood loss. In the majority of instances renal trauma is managed by bed rest, appropriate analgesia and careful sequential review, usually by ultrasound scan. Antibiotics are given as a routine to prevent the development of associated infection, particularly if there is any evidence of extravasation. Such a conservative policy results in only a small proportion of patients coming to operation. If surgical exploration is required in the context of blunt trauma to the kidney then the majority of cases do result in either total or partial nephrectomy. Innovative work from the United States of America, where penetrating injuries are more common, has resulted in a much higher level of renal preservation. In such circumstances preoperative evaluation of the situation by arteriography is often carried out.

In the longer term following renal injury, hypertension can occur. This is usually renin-mediated and often transient in nature as a consequence of renal arterial damage. Long term follow-up of all patients with renal injuries is therefore essential with particular reference to their blood pressure. If there is any evidence of significant damage to the renal parenchyma or the vascular supply then other measures of renal function are routinely employed.

Ureteric injury

Injuries to the ureter are uncommon as a consequence of external trauma; they can occur in the context of penetrating injuries, but the commonest cause is iatrogenic during the course of intra-abdominal surgery, usually pelvic surgery. The majority of ureteric injuries occur in the lower third of the ureter, and it has been reported that ureteric injury complicates up to 0.5% of routine hysterectomies, with a much higher incidence for radical hysterectomies (up to 5%). The diagnosis of injury to the ureter is difficult in the immediate postoperative period unless the diagnosis is suspected. Any patient who develops loin discomfort or a persistent pyrexia, or indeed any evidence of per vaginam urinary leakage, should be investigated fully, initially by ultrasound scan, but if any doubt exists as to potential diagnosis then an intravenous urogram should be carried out even in the presence of an apparently normal ultrasound scan.

Bladder injury

The bladder is very flexible in being able to alter its shape and size radically to accommodate a large volume of urine. Rupture of the bladder tends to occur either in the context of patients who have undergone previous surgery to the bladder or more commonly in patients with an overdistended bladder, often related to excessive alcohol consumption. Two types of bladder rupture are recognised: intraperitoneal and extraperitoneal. Unless a diagnosis of bladder injury is suspected, it may be missed at an early stage due to other associated injury and should always be excluded in a patient who is either unable to void or on catheterisation where the urine is heavily blood stained. The diagnosis may be suspected on ultrasound scan and can be confirmed by the passage of contrast into the bladder, when extravasation will be seen. Intraperitoneal rupture usually occurs in the context of compression by an external force such as a seat belt with the consequence of a penetrating suprapubic injury piercing a full bladder. Iatrogenic intraperitoneal rupture can occur at the time of endoscopic surgery but is usually recognised at an early stage by the surgeon. Extraperitoneal rupture of the bladder is usually associated with fractures of the pelvis, with a reported occurrence in up to 10% of cases.

Intraperitoneal extravasation, if it is of significant degree, should be dealt with by open surgical repair and appropriate drainage. Extraperitoneal rupture will often settle with catheter drainage of the bladder.

It is important to diagnose bladder ruptures since, if untreated, major perforations are associated with a high mortality.

Injuries to the penis, scrotum and testes

Injuries to the genitalia are relatively uncommon. The commonest injury seen is the so called 'zipper' injury to the foreskin, which is managed conservatively in the accident and emergency department. A torn frenulum can occur as a consequence of intercourse and is usually managed conservatively in the first instance. Rupture of the penis is an uncommon cause of presentation to the accident and emergency department, where it is often difficult to get a clear history from the patient, though it is likely that this usually results from sexual excess. It should be managed by early surgical exploration and repair. Paraphimosis is not a true injury but usually results from a failure to replace the foreskin after intercourse and is managed by reduction of the paraphimosis in the majority of cases. Direct injuries of the scrotum and testes can occur as a consequence of any injury. Direct blows to the testicle, causing its rupture, are uncommon but may occasionally require orchidectomy. It is important to adequately investigate significant injuries to the testis and scrotum because of the consequent sequelae in terms of infection that may ensue otherwise. All scrotal injuries should be managed by appropriate debridement, with the use of antibiotics as appropriate, because of the risk of Fournier's gangrene ensuing.

Urethral injuries

Urethral injuries by themselves are never life threatening except as a consequence of their close association with pelvic fractures and multiple organ injuries. Because of this close relationship to trauma, it is of no surprise that the highest incidence of urethral injuries is in adults 15 to 25 years of age. There is also a significant number that occur iatrogenically. Urethral injuries can range from a mild contusion with preservation of epithelial continuity, to a partial tear of the urethral epithelium or a full urethral transection and disruption. They can also be classified by site into anterior urethral injuries and posterior urethral injuries — which is probably the best way to consider them, as both sites are exposed to different mechanisms of injury.

Anterior urethral injuries

Injuries to the anterior urethra occur with a frequency one third that of those to the posterior urethra (Box 18.3).

Posterior urethral strictures

Unfortunately, the term posterior urethral stricture is still widely used to include both simple sphincter strictures and subprostatic pelvic fracture urethral distraction defects (PFUDDs). This is confusing because they, and the principles of their surgical resolution, are entirely different. Logically, the term urethral stricture should be used to indicate a narrowing of urethral continuity, not a gap. Simple continuity strictures of the membraneous urethra are commonly the result of an internal urethral injury (prostatic surgery, instrumentation, indwelling catheters, or tumour invasion); they are best referred to as sphincter-strictures because this emphasises that, although the function is generally impaired to a variable extent, the distal urethral sphincter mechanism has not

---

Box 18.3 Aetiology of anterior urethral injuries

1. blunt trauma
   — fall astride
   — go-kart injuries
   — kicks in the perineum
   — skateboarding
2. penetrating trauma
   — gunshot
   — stab wounds
   — scissors
3. sexual excess
   — penile fractures
   — urethral stimulation
4. constriction bands
   — paraplegics
5. iatrogenic injuries
   — urethral catheters
   — endoscopic instrumentations
6. postcardiac surgery
   — usually as a consequence of ischaemia

---

been destroyed. The primary aim of the treatment of a sphincter stricture must be the preservation of the residual distal sphincteric function, just as the primary aim of the management of a pelvic fracture urethral distraction defect (PFUDD) is the preservation or functional reconstruction of the residual sphincter mechanism at the bladder neck only, because in all but the most minimal lesions the function of the intramural distal urethral sphincter is destroyed by the subprostatic urethral rupture through its mechanism.

The posterior urethra has a close relationship with the bony pelvis and is often associated with serious injury as a result of a severe external force to the pelvis and lower abdomen. Sixty-five percent of posterior urethral ruptures are complete. The aetiology of posterior urethral injuries is shown in Box 18.4.

Box 18.4 Aetiology of posterior urethral injuries

1. penetrating injuries
   — gunshot wounds
   — stab wounds

2. urethral injuries associated with pelvic fractures
   — road traffic accidents
   — falls from heights
   — industrial accidents

3. iatrogenic injuries
   — TURP complications

Diagnosis

Anterior urethral injuries can present with blood at the meatus, inability to pass water, or the rapid development of a perineal urinoma or haematoma forming down a sleeve of Buck's fascia. Extension of the penile bruising down beyond the shaft is due to rupture of Buck's fascia allowing the Colles fascia to act as the limiting tissue. This results in a characteristic butterfly pattern of bruising in the perineum.

The diagnosis of posterior urethral injuries requires a high index of suspicion and should be excluded before a urinary catheter is inserted, often by an experienced person in the emergency service. Urethral injury is to be suspected in any patient with a fracture of the pelvis. The likelihood of urethral injury increases with

- blood at the urethral meatus
- difficulties/inability to void
- palpable bladder from distension, failure to void, pelvic haematoma
- bruising of the perineum
- high riding prostate, although this might be difficult to appreciate in the presence of a pelvic haematoma
- fractures involving displacement of the pubic rami relative to the rest of the pelvis.

Although this classic triad of blood at the external urethral meatus, inability to pass urine and a distended bladder is fairly indicative of urethral injuries, it must be noted that a very high lesion above the external sphincter may not produce blood at the meatus and a distended bladder may be related to a sphincter spasm as a result of pain rather than a complete urethral rupture. Rectal examination helps to exclude a dislocated prostate, but swelling and oedema may mask the presence of a normally positioned prostate. Rectal examination is more important as a tool to screen for rectal injuries that can be associated with pelvic fractures. Blood on the examining finger is highly suggestive of such an injury.

URINARY TRACT CALCULI

Urinary calculi occur relatively commonly in the population, as evidenced by the large number of patients that present with ureteric colic. It is difficult to obtain accurate figures on the true prevalence of renal calculi, but it has been estimated that up to 2–3% of the UK population may have significant calculous disease. There are wide variations in the incidence of renal calculi, relating to geographical features, in particular environmental temperature. Over the last century there has been a significant change in the United Kingdom in the location of urinary tract calculi. Bladder calculi used to be relatively common, no doubt relating to untreated bladder outflow obstruction and also possibly dietary factors. These are now much less often seen than upper tract calculi.

Most patients with renal calculi present in early adult life, where the peak is around 28 years, but there is a second peak around the mid part of the fifth decade, principally as a consequence of infective stones in the female population. Nevertheless calculi are four to five times more common in men than in women. Precipitating factors in the development of urinary calculi include:

- diet
- dehydration
- stasis
- infection
- hyperparathyroidism
- idiopathic hypercalcuria
- milk-alkali syndrome
- hypervitaminosis D
- cystinuria
- inborn errors of purine metabolism
- gout
- chemotherapy (excess uric acid following treatment of leukaemia or polycythaemia).

Anatomical abnormalities can also predispose to stone formation, probably by producing stasis in the urinary tract.

Types of calculi

Calculi are often classified according to their composition. The types of calculi are as follows.

- Calcium oxalate (75%) are usually mulberry-shaped stones covered with sharp projections. They cause bleeding and are often black because of altered blood on their surface. Because of their sharp surface they often give symptoms when comparatively small. They usually occur in alkaline urine. Diets rich in rhubarb, spinach, tomatoes and strawberries may be contributory to the development of oxalate stones.
- Phosphate stones (15%) are usually composed of magnesium ammonium phosphate with calcium. They are smooth and dirty white in colour. They may enlarge rapidly and fill the calyces, taking on their shape: i.e. staghorn calculus. They occur in strongly alkaline urine and may be associated with urinary tract infections with bacteria such as *Proteus* which are able to break down urea to form ammonia.
- Urate stones (5%) arise in acid urine and are hard, smooth, faceted and light brown in colour.

- Cystine stones (2%) are usually multiple and arise in acid urine, being of metabolic origin due to decreased resorption of cystine from the renal tubules. They are white and often translucent.
- Xanthine and pyruvate stones are very rare and arise due to inborn errors of metabolism.

Ninety percent of calculi are radio-opaque. Usually only urates are radiolucent, cystine stones being faintly to moderately radio-opaque because of their sulphur content.

Calculi do occur elsewhere in the lower urinary tract, both in the urethra (usually consequent upon passage of a calculus from the ureter or bladder) and the prostate where they can be seen on x-ray in the prostatic parenchyma. Prostatic calculi are of no clinical significance.

TUMOURS OF THE URINARY TRACT

Renal tumours

Renal tumours can be either benign or malignant, but as a general rule any patient with a tumour identified within the kidney should be considered to have a malignant tumour unless proven otherwise. Benign renal tumours are rare. A benign developmental tumour of the kidney, known as an angiomyolipoma, has a characteristic CT scan appearance, due to the high fat content within the tumour, which can be used diagnostically, but in the absence of this appearance any solid lesion within the kidney should be considered as an indication for nephrectomy. Routine biopsy of solid masses within the kidney is not carried out, because the histology can be difficult to interpret and a benign appearance on biopsy does not exclude a malignant tumour. Certainly in the past it had been suggested that adenomas and adenocarcinomas were representative of a spectrum of disease and indeed a watershed size of 2.5 cm between the two conditions was once suggested as a cut-off point, although this has largely been abandoned.

Hypernephroma (renal adenocarcinoma)

The commonest renal tumour is the hypernephroma (renal adenocarcinoma, Grawitz tumour). The incidence of renal adenocarcinoma increases steadily above the age of 40, reaching a peak in the sixth and seventh decades of life. It is more common in men than women and may occur bilaterally.

Aetiological factors include:

- smokers
- coffee drinkers
- industrial exposure to cadmium, lead, asbestos, aromatic hydrocarbons

- development in renal cysts in end stage kidneys in dialysis patients
- von Hippel–Lindau disease (this suggests a genetic predisposition).

Common presenting clinical features include:

- haematuria
- loin pain
- a palpable mass.

Renal adenocarcinoma is also associated with a number of paraneoplastic syndromes:

- hypertension (due to renin secretion)
- polycythaemia (due to erythropoietin secretion)
- hypercalcaemia (due to ectopic parathyroid hormone production).

Additionally the patient may have a fever and develop anaemia, abnormal liver function tests, amyloidosis and neuromyopathy. Renal adenocarcinoma is being increasingly diagnosed in contemporary practice because of the more widespread use of ultrasound scans, and it is being picked up incidental to other conditions. Spread of hypernephroma occurs as follows:

- direct extension into perinephric tissues and adjacent organs; direct extension may occur into the renal vein and inferior vena cava
- lymphatic spread to the para-aortic nodes
- blood spread to liver, brain, bone and lung (cannon ball metastases).

Prognosis

In patients with no evidence of metastasis at presentation the 5 year survival may be as high as 70% but falls to 20% when the renal vein is involved or there is extension into the perinephric fat. Rarely metastases from renal adenocarcinoma can regress spontaneously after removal of the primary tumour, but this occurs in less than 1% of cases, with a limited duration for regression of those metastases in the majority of cases.

Wilms' tumour

This is the commonest intra-abdominal malignancy in children under the age of 10 years. The majority occur in the first 3 years of life. Less than 5% are bilateral. The most common presentation is with an abdominal mass, but haematuria, abdominal pain, hypertension and intestinal obstruction may occur. Metastases occur to the liver, lungs and regional nodes. Treatment is by surgical excision with aggressive chemotherapy and radiotherapy. There is an 80–90% chance of cure.

Carcinoma of the renal pelvis

These are relatively rare and are usually transitional cell tumours, although squamous cell carcinomas have been reported in areas of squamous metaplasia. Transitional cell carcinomas frequently infiltrate the wall of the pelvis and may involve the renal vein. With poorly differentiated tumours the prognosis is not good and multiple tumours may occur in the ureters and bladder. Aetiological factors include:

- analgesic abuse
- exposure to aniline dyes used in the dye, rubber, plastics and gas industries.

Squamous metaplasia of the urothelium may occur due to chronic irritation. This may be associated with calculi and chronic infection. Occasionally, squamous cell carcinomas arise de novo from transitional epithelium. Squamous cell carcinomas carry a poor prognosis.

Urothelial tumours

Urothelial tumours arise in the transitional epithelium, which extends from the tips of the renal papillae to the navicular fossa in men and half way down the urethra in women, and represent an important pathological entity within urological practice. Urothelial tumours may occur at any level within the urinary tract and are often multifocal. The majority, however, occur in the urinary bladder (90%), and renal pelvic transitional cell carcinomas (9%) and transitional cell carcinomas of the ureter (1%) are uncommon. In patients with bladder transitional cell carcinoma there is a higher prevalence of coincidental upper tract tumours.

Several thousand new cases of urothelial cancers present in the United Kingdom each year. Urothelial neoplasms were first recognised at the turn of the century to be associated with industrial carcinogens, but these now account for only approximately 10% of patients who present. Whilst in the majority of patients no specific aetiological causation is apparent, there is a widely held view that smoking is an important factor, and indeed it has been calculated that the risk of developing a bladder cancer as a consequence of smoking is doubled. The commonest presenting feature of transitional cell carcinoma of the bladder is painless macroscopic haematuria. A number of other lesions are identified on the basis of investigation of either sterile pyuria or microscopic haematuria.

The investigation of all patients with demonstrable haematuria, recurrent urinary infection, or symptoms of persistent cystitis, includes not only screening of the upper tracts but also cystoscopy, principally to exclude transitional cell carcinomas of the urinary tract. Urine cytology can be helpful if there is persistent microscopic haematuria and is particularly useful in alerting the clinician to the possible diagnosis of carcinoma in situ. Normal urine cytology does not exclude the presence of an early stage or well-differentiated tumour. With regard to screening of the upper tracts in all patients with a transitional cell carcinoma of the bladder then intravenous urography is recommended to check on the upper tracts. An abdominal CT scan is useful routinely in terms of staging of tumours if radical treatment is being considered. Clinical staging of transitional cell carcinoma of the bladder is notoriously inaccurate, and confirmation of tumour stage usually awaits histological examination of any resected tissue.

Transitional cell carcinomas of the bladder occur primarily on the posterior and lateral walls of the bladder in over two thirds of cases. One fifth of cases present with a tumour at the trigone or bladder neck and the remainder over the vault of the bladder. Whilst diverticula are a well-recognised predisposing factor for the development of tumours, less than 5% develop in a diverticulum. The prognosis for transitional cell carcinoma of the bladder is defined by its underlying histological grade, which reflects the predilection of the tumour to aggressive behaviour. Tumours are usually graded as well differentiated, moderately differentiated, or poorly differentiated. Carcinoma in situ, which elsewhere in the body is usually a premalignant and relatively benign condition, is quite the reverse in the bladder. Certainly it is premalignant, but such patients have a tendency, in at least 50% of cases, to develop a poorly differentiated aggressive tumour. Therefore, in the urinary tract, carcinoma in situ is treated in a very proactive fashion.

A patient's prognosis depends to a large extent upon the grade of tumour, and this is also reflected in the tumour stage in many cases. Poorly differentiated tumours, even if superficial, have a tendency to be rapidly progressive and are treated as such. At the very least, following resection of such a tumour then early endoscopic follow-up of the patient is essential.

The majority of superficial bladder tumours are dealt with endoscopically. In approximately 30% of patients after resection of the primary tumour no further recurrence is seen. In the remaining patients, however, recurrent tumours may occur within the bladder. Recent evidence supports the early use of intravesical chemotherapy following resection to reduce the incidence of recurrent disease as a consequence of tumour cell implantation.

Certainly muscle-invasive tumours and those with a

poorly differentiated appearance are an indication for aggressive intervention. Whilst the mainstay of treatment in the United Kingdom has tended, traditionally, to be radical radiotherapy, there is an increasing trend towards radical surgery at an early stage. Carcinoma in situ of the bladder, as mentioned above, is an indication for early intervention. Many of these patients will respond favourably to the use of intravesical BCG which acts as immunotherapy to promote the activation of T-cell-mediated killing of abnormal urothelial cells. If carcinoma in situ is widespread and does not respond to BCG, or is poorly differentiated, then most clinicians would proceed to radical treatment at an early stage.

Other tumours of the bladder include adenocarcinomas and squamous carcinomas. Adenocarcinomas in the United Kingdom are relatively uncommon and are usually associated with a urachal remnant on the anterior wall of the bladder, although the presence of adenocarcinoma on histology should always raise the possibility of the direct extension of an adenocarcinoma of the bowel. Squamous cell carcinoma is uncommon in the United Kingdom but is most commonly associated with situations where there has been chronic stasis or irritation within the bladder and in this context is seen in patients with a previous history of tuberculosis or paraplegics. In areas of the world where schistosomiasis is endemic, squamous cell carcinoma represents the commonest histological type and usually presents in patients from the second or third decade of life onwards. The tumour arises as a consequence of a chronic irritation within the bladder, leading on to squamous metaplasia and the subsequent development of a squamous carcinoma. This is precipitated by the parasite laying its eggs in a submucosal position.

Carcinoma of the prostate

Carcinoma of the prostate is one of the commonest malignant tumours in the male. The majority of cases present clinically in the sixth or seventh decade of life, but it must be recognised that, if a male lives long enough, there is a high chance of him developing carcinoma of the prostate, although it may not be manifest clinically. Indeed, postmortem series have reported a prevalence of carcinoma of the prostate in up to 80% of 80-year-old patients. Prostate carcinomas traditionally develop in the peripheral zone of the prostate and are adenocarcinomas. Unfortunately the majority of patients presenting with carcinoma of the prostate (two thirds) do so with either locally advanced disease or metastatic disease already present. Spread of prostatic carcinoma is as follows:

- direct — by local extension through the prostatic capsule to the urethra, bladder base, or seminal vesicle

- lymphatic — to the pelvic and para-aortic nodes
- blood borne — via the prostatic venous plexus to the vertebral venous plexus and to the bones of the lumbar spine and pelvis; and to the lungs and liver.

Clinical presentations include:

- urinary symptoms — features of bladder outflow obstruction
- routine rectal examination may reveal a hard craggy prostate
- bony metastases — bone pain, pathological fracture, anaemia due to extensive neoplastic infiltration of marrow-containing bones
- lymph node metastases.

The advent of testing for prostate specific antigen (PSA) has allowed the earlier diagnosis of many cases, although it must be recognised that the PSA test has a relatively low sensitivity and specificity and a normal PSA does not exclude the presence of a coexisting prostate carcinoma, although conversely a markedly raised PSA level makes the diagnosis very likely. Elevation of the PSA occurs following instrumentation of the prostate or can occur in association with a urinary tract infection. There is no evidence that digital rectal examination significantly raises the PSA.

The diagnosis of prostate carcinoma rests on the histological identification of prostatic adenocarcinoma on fine needle biopsy, which is usually carried out transrectally — either under digital guidance if there is a palpable abnormality or using ultrasound guidance. This technique should be carried out with full antibiotic cover because of the risk of bacteraemia, and the patients are also counselled preoperatively with regard to other complications such as haematuria and an incidence of retention of urine.

Following the diagnosis of prostate cancer, in addition to routine blood investigations, including a baseline serum PSA, a bone scan is carried out, and if the tumour is considered possibly to be localised then baseline imaging with a transrectal ultrasound scan and a CT scan are usually the preferred staging modalities. The radical treatment for prostate carcinoma involves either radical radiotherapy or radical prostatectomy. The latter has become increasingly popular in recent years. Radical prostatectomy should however be confined to patients where biologically a life span of at least 10 years is to be expected or where the tumour is locally confined; in support of this, results would suggest that PSA level in excess of 20 ng/mL is a relative contraindication.

In patients where the tumour is locally advanced or metastatic, then hormonal therapy is instituted. The mainstay of treatment is to remove testosterone production either by surgical orchidectomy or chemical measures designed to achieve the same aim (anti-androgens and LHRH analogues). There is no evidence that surgical orchidectomy is superior to chemical measures. The prognosis of patients with carcinoma of the prostate depends upon the stage of the tumour at presentation, and it is likely that in those where the tumour is detected at an early stage with a low tumour bulk, if a curative option such as radical surgery is carried out at an early stage then they can be cured. As a rule of thumb, patients presenting clinically with prostatic carcinoma before the sixth decade of life tend to have a more aggressive tumour which is reflected in a poorer prognosis.

Carcinoma of the testis

Tumours of the testis are relatively uncommon, accounting for 1–3% of malignant tumours in men; nevertheless they predominantly affect young men. There is a well-established link between undescended testes and testicular tumour, and it has been estimated that adults with maldescent of the testes have a 20 to 30 fold greater incidence of developing a testicular tumour then men with a normally descended testis. Testicular tumours may be derived from germ cells or non-germ cells. The majority (90%) are of germ cell origin. Germ cell tumours include seminomas and terratomas. Non-germ cell tumours include those arising from the Sertoli cells and Leydig cells. Testicular tumours may be classified as follows:

- seminoma
- teratoma
- combined germ cell tumours (seminoma and teratoma)
- malignant lymphoma
- interstitial (Leydig) cell tumour
- Sertoli cell tumour.

The two most common types of tumour are seminoma and teratoma. Metastatic tumours are rare and include bowel, bronchus and prostate.

Any patient presenting with a palpable mass in the testis should be considered to have a malignancy of the testis until proved otherwise.

Clinical features of testicular tumours include:

- unilateral painless enlargement of a testis
- secondary hydrocele
- retroperitoneal mass
- lymph node metastases (occasionally in the cervical nodes)
- symptoms from other metastases
- gynaecomastia from hormone-secreting interstitial tumours.

Ultrasound scanning is a non-invasive and very accurate way of defining primary testicular abnormalities. The treatment of choice is radical orchidectomy via an inguinal route, with preclamping of the inguinal cord prior to orchidectomy to prevent manipulation of the testis from disseminating tumour cells into the circulation. It is recommended that serological tumour markers such as αFP and β-HCG should be estimated prior to orchidectomy. It is now recognised that carcinoma in situ in the testis predisposes to the subsequent development of a tumour and may occur in a proportion of patients presenting with a primary testicular tumour in the contralateral testis. Whilst some workers have recommended biopsy of the contralateral testis in all patients presenting with a primary testicular neoplasm, the evidence in support of this is not yet available and this is not recommended in routine practice unless there are other predisposing features such as maldescent of the contralateral testicle, where the incidence of carcinoma in situ is much higher.

Staging of patients with a primary testicular tumour is principally carried out on the basis of the serological tests mentioned above and also CT scanning of the abdomen and pelvis to look for lymph node extension and retroperitoneal tumour mass. With a combination of radiotherapy and chemotherapy the cure rate for the majority of patients with testicular tumours approaches 100%.

Carcinoma of the scrotum

Carcinoma of the scrotum is rare. It is of historical interest, as in the 18th century it was one of the first tumours to be recognised to have a relationship to occupational exposure to carcinogens. The association occurred in chimney sweeps where the skin of the scrotum came into contact with carcinogens contained in soot. Later the lubricating mineral oils used to lubricate machinery in the cotton industry were discovered to be another responsible carcinogen. At the present time carcinoma of the scrotum is uncommon and is usually seen in elderly patients. It is of the squamous type and may spread to the inguinal lymph nodes. Treatment is by wide excision.

Carcinoma of the urethra

This is a rare tumour classically associated with chronic irritation within the urethra, often in association with a urethral stricture. Treatment involves radical excision.

Carcinoma of the penis

Carcinoma of the penis is rare. It occurs between 60 and 80 years and is almost unknown in circumcised males. Poor hygiene and accumulation of smegma may be aetiological factors. Histologically the tumour is a squamous cell carcinoma. It frequently starts in the sulcus between the glans and the foreskin. Spread is usually to the inguinal nodes. Intraepidermal carcinoma may occur on the glans penis, presenting as a red velvety lesion termed erythroplasia of Queyrat.

Benign disorders of the penis

Balanoposthitis

Balanitis is inflammation of the glans penis. Posthitis is inflammation of the foreskin. They usually occur together as balanoposthitis. It is often associated with phimosis. Smegma accumulates beneath the prepuce, which may become infected with staphylococci, coliforms, or gonococci. In patients with balanoposthitis the possibility of diabetes should always be excluded. In the case of diabetes, candida is the most likely infecting organism.

Phimosis

Phimosis is a tightness of the foreskin, which prevents it retracting back over the glans penis. The foreskin is adherent until the age of 3 years and then gradually separates by the age of 6 years. If the foreskin is not retractable by the age of 7 years and is causing problems then circumcision is justifiable. Phimosis occurring in the adult and causing interference with voiding or sexual activity is an indication for circumcision.

Paraphimosis

This occurs as a consequence of pulling a tight foreskin back over the glans penis and failing to reduce it. Venous return from the glans and prepuce is obstructed, and results in oedematous swelling of the glans and prepuce. Principles of treatment are to compress the oedematous foreskin to reduce the oedema and then attempt to reduce the foreskin. Appropriate analgesia, including a local anaesthetic block and occasionally injection of hyaluronidase into the oedematous tissue, may be helpful.

Balanitis xerotica obliterans

This is a condition of the foreskin characterised by loss of skin elasticity, and fibrosis, resulting in phimosis. The condition occurs mainly between 30 and 50 years of age. The aetiology is unknown and treatment is by circumcision.

Priapisim

Priapisim is rare and represents a persistent painful erection unassociated with sexual desire. Aetiological factors include:

- idiopathic
- leukaemia

- sickle-cell disease
- disseminated and pelvic malignancy
- neurological conditions, especially spinal cord injury
- patients on haemodialysis
- iatrogenic due to injection of vasoactive agents into the penis as treatment for impotence.

Therapy includes aspiration of the penis and injection of alpha-adrenergic agonists. In recalcitrant cases surgery can be used, but the success rate is limited. Priapisim associated with sickle-cell disease is often resistant to any of these measures, and many of the cases are managed conservatively.

Peyronie's disease

This is a fibrotic condition of the corpora cavernosa. It occurs between 40 and 60 years and the aetiology is unknown. Fibrotic plaques in the corpora cavernosa result in discomfort, pain and deformity on erection. The fibrous plaques are palpable along the shaft of the penis. They may become calcified. Spontaneous resolution may occasionally occur. The exact cause of the lesion is unclear. Some cases are associated with Dupuytren's contracture and others with retroperitoneal fibrosis.

Impotence

This is a common problem in the population, occurring with an increasing incidence with age. It is defined as the inability to initiate or sustain an erection sufficient to allow satisfactory sexual intercourse to occur. Whilst the precise neural mechanisms underlying erectile function are as yet not fully understood, it is clear that certain aetiological factors are of importance:

- psychogenic problems
- diabetes
- alcohol
- liver dysfunction (resulting in endocrine dysfunction)
- primary disorders of endocrine function
- atherosclerosis
- neurological disorders
- miscellaneous, e.g. Peyronies disease.

The principal causes therefore relate to inadequate libido / loss of confidence, reduced blood flow into the penis (occasionally, increased venous blood flow out of the penis) and disorders of the neural control of erection. Pathophysiological measures of innervation and penile blood flow and associated dynamics are useful research tools but are of limited use in routine clinical practice. Patients should be investigated to exclude any of the endocrine or metabolic abnormalities mentioned above.

Therapeutic options include counselling; vacuum devices

to produce an artificial erection; the use of vasoactive agents acting to relax the smooth muscle surrounding the intracavernosal vascular sinusoids by a direct smooth muscle relaxant effect (papaverine, prostaglandins); via the prolongation of endogenous nitric oxide effects (e.g. Viagra); or via blockade of alpha-adrenergic receptors. Failing these measures then surgical intervention using artificial prostheses inserted into the penis can be considered.

Scrotal swellings

The cardinal features of a scrotal swelling are the ability to get above it, whether it is solid or cystic in nature as defined by transillumination, and whether it is painful and/or associated with signs of inflammation or infection. Any patient presenting with a solid testicular swelling should be considered to have a tumour unless proven otherwise and should undergo an urgent ultrasound scan. Likewise any man presenting with a hydrocele, particularly a young adult or if there is an atypical history, should have further investigation of the testis to exclude tumour (e.g. drainage of the hydrocele and examination, or ultrasound scan).

The following are scrotal swellings encountered in surgical practice:

- indirect inguinal hernia
- hydrocele
- epididymal cyst
- epididymo-orchitis
- testicular tumour
- torsion of the testis
- varicocele
- hematocele
- sperm granuloma
- torsion of testicular appendage.

Indirect inguinal hernia and testicular tumour are dealt with elsewhere in this book.

Hydrocele

A hydrocele is a collection of fluid in the tunica vaginalis. A primary or idiopathic hydrocele develops slowly and becomes large and tense. It usually occurs in patients over the age of 40. A secondary hydrocele may be small and lax and occurs secondary to inflammation or tumour of the underlying testis. They tend to occur in a younger age group.

A congenital hydrocele is associated with a hernial sac and connects with the peritoneal cavity. A hydrocele of the cord lies along the cord anywhere from the deep inguinal ring to the upper part of the scrotum. It does not connect with either the peritoneal cavity or the tunica

vaginalis. A similar swelling may develop in the female and is known as a hydrocele of the canal of Nuck.

Epididymal cyst

These may be small, large, multiple, unilateral, or bilateral. Acquired cysts of the epididymis are usually caused by the obstruction of passage of sperm along the narrow lumen of the vas or obstruction of an epididymal tubule, resulting in a cystic dilatation of the duct system in the epididymis and efferent ductules of the testis. The majority of these contain clear straw-coloured fluid. However, if they contain opalescent milky fluid, containing sperm, which may be demonstrated on aspiration, they are known as spermatoceles. It is important to realise that surgical excision of an epididymal cyst may damage the epididymis on that side and may result in impairment of fertility.

Epididymo-orchitis

Acute inflammation of the body of the testis is known as orchitis. However, this most frequently develops in association with inflammation of the epididymis, and the combined condition is known as epididymo-orchitis. The commonest underlying cause is a urinary tract infection with coliform organisms. It may follow prostatitis or urethritis. The infection is thought to spread along the vas deferens or the lymphatics in the perivasal tissues. The condition may be unilateral or bilateral. It may be associated with a secondary hydrocele. Suppuration is unusual. Orchitis may occur as a complication of mumps.

Chronic epididymo-orchitis may develop as a result of tuberculous infection. The inflamed epididymis may become adherent to the scrotal skin, with the formation of sinuses. Tuberculous epididymo-orchitis is usually secondary to tuberculosis elsewhere in the urinary tract. Microscopy often shows 'sterile' pyuria with the presence of acid fast bacilli.

Torsion of the testis

In the majority of cases this should be termed torsion of the spermatic cord rather than torsion of the testis. Torsion of the spermatic cord involves twisting of the testis and epididymis together on their axis. In other cases the testis may twist on a long mesorchium. Torsion of the spermatic cord is often precipitated by exertion which causes contraction of the cremaster muscle. Torsion represents a surgical emergency and should be treated by surgical exploration as soon as possible whenever the diagnosis is suspected.

Anatomical abnormalities often predispose to testicular torsion. These include:

- an abnormally long spermatic cord

- the presence of a long mesorchium
- maldescent of the testis. This is often identified by the horizontal lie of the testis on clinical examination.

These conditions are often bilateral and, if torsion occurs on one side, once that has been dealt with, it is appropriate to fix the other testis in the scrotum so that it cannot undergo torsion. If treatment of torsion is delayed, infarction of the testis occurs, resulting subsequently in a small, shrunken, fibrotic testis and epididymis. Absorption of the products of dead spermatozoa may result in the development of antisperm antibodies, leading to sympathetic orchidopathia with consequent reduction in fertility.

Varicocele

A varicocele is a varicosity of the pampiniform plexus of veins in the spermatic cord. Varicoceles are extremely common in the population, with a reported incidence of up to 12%. The majority are left sided. Although they are widely considered to be associated with subfertility, a causal link between the two has not been clearly established. A primary varicocele is one that arises with no obvious underlying cause. A secondary varicocele is the result of venous obstruction. The commonest cause of this rare type of varicocele is obstruction of the renal vein due to carcinoma of the kidney growing down and obstructing the renal vein. As the testicular vein on the left side drains directly into the renal vein, back pressure may occur on the testicular vein, resulting in the development of a varicocele. Any patient over the age of 40 with rapid development of a varicocele on the left hand side should have an ultrasound scan of the kidney.

The main indication for treatment of varicoceles is if they are symptomatic. Contemporary management of a varicocele depends on local resources, but it may be very successfully managed in a minimally invasive fashion by percutaneous embolisation.

Haematocele

This is a result of testicular trauma either due to sports injuries or violence. Trauma results in bleeding into the layers of the tunica vaginalis resulting in a haematocele.

Sperm granuloma

This is an uncommon chronic inflammatory lesion resulting from extravasation of sperm from the tubules into the interstitium. The commonest cause of this is extravasated sperm, either from the site of transection of the vas, or within the epididymis, following vasectomy. A localised nodule forms which may require excision if it is symptomatic — often presenting as a painful lump.

Torsion of testicular appendage

There are several small testicular appendages, the most common of which is the appendix testis. This is attached to the front of the upper pole of the testis. Torsion results in sudden pain in the testis, with oedema and congestion of the cord, testis and epididymis. The condition is rare and usually mistaken for torsion of the testis. The diagnosis becomes apparent on exploration. Treatment is by excision of the appendix testis.

Acute scrotal pain

Acute scrotal pain is a urological emergency. Conditions include:

- torsion of the testis
- acute epididymo-orchitis
- torsion of testicular appendage
- Fournier's gangrene.

As a general rule any patient presenting with acute scrotal pain should be considered for urgent scrotal exploration because of the possibility that it may be due to testicular torsion. The availibility of colour Doppler ultrasound in the emergency situation may help confirm the diagnosis. However, even if the acute episode has resolved, where there is a history strongly supportive of torsion or findings suggestive of the diagnosis, e.g. a long mesorchium, or horizontal lie of the testes, then the patient should undergo orchidopexy on the next available elective list.

Fournier's gangrene which affects the scrotal skin is discussed in Chapter 7.

INCONTINENCE

Incontinence is defined as the involuntary loss of urine from the intact lower urinary tract that is socially or hygienically unacceptable. Incontinence may occur via the urethra or from an abnormal extra-urethral route such as, for example, via a fistula or a congenital ectopic ureteric opening. Incontinence can present as urge incontinence, stress incontinence, or total incontinence, or as a combination. Incontinence is extremely common in the female population, although its incidence increases with age in both sexes.

Postmicturition dribbling is a frequent symptom in men and, whilst it is associated with urethral stricture disease and bladder neck obstruction in younger men, most commonly it is a consequence of age-related weakness of the bulbospongiosus muscles. It is also common following urethral surgery in this area. Neurological conditions are commonly associated with incontinence. Depending on the underlying aetiology, associated urinary symptoms can range from urgency, frequency and nocturia to voiding difficulty and retention. A diagnosis is not possible on the basis of symptoms, and a full urodynamic analysis of the nature and cause of the urinary incontinence is mandatory.

Urinary incontinence is a disturbance of urine storage that comprises two major components: overactivity of the detrusor muscle or a weakness of urethral sphincter function, resulting in failure to store urine. It must not be forgotten that overflow incontinence can occur as a consequence of a failure of the bladder to empty, and it is important to exclude retention of urine with subsequent overflow incontinence.

A full history and physical examination is essential. This includes: the characterisation of the type, pattern and severity of the urinary incontinence; any precipitating factors and associated urinary symptoms such as frequency, nocturia, urgency, poor flow, hesitancy and terminal dribbling; its effect on activities of daily living, work, leisure and its impact on social and psychological wellbeing. Any previous surgery, medical problems, especially neurological ones, and medications are also important, especially in the elderly. In female patients an obstetric history and review of previous gynaecological surgery is helpful. Any predisposing factors for incontinence such as radical pelvic surgery, pelvic trauma, neuropathy and radical radiotherapy must be noted in detail. The prior state of the urinary tract before surgery and the operative notes made during the surgery should be reviewed with regards to the type and nature of surgery performed and the difficulties encountered.

Physical examination should start with a functional assessment of cognition, mobility and identification of other medical conditions. This includes a full abdominal examination to look for scars of previous operations, a distended bladder, palpable kidneys and a neurological examination of the lower extremities. A rectal examination allows assessment of perineal sensation, anal tone, impacted stools, and bulbocavernosal reflexes. Assessment of the presence of urinary leakage on coughing in the female patient and assessment of the degree of bladder base and urethral prolapse should be carried out.

A full assessment of urinary incontinence should include the recording of a voiding/incontinence diary by the patient for at least 3 days. Other initial investigations include serum urea, serum creatinine and electrolytes, urine analysis and cultures. If retention of urine is suspected, initial uroflowmetry is helpful together with a bladder ultrasound scan checking for postvoiding residual urine. If this is high, ultrasound assessment of the kidneys to exclude hydronephrosis should be performed.

Radiological studies are important to delineate anatomy where appropriate and are particularly useful when combined with pressure flow studies in video-urodynamics, particularly in the assessment of the degree of bladder base prolapse in the female patient or to assess sphincteric function following previous surgery. The urodynamic component of the study is essential to define detrusor over- or underactivity, and sensory abnormalities during bladder filling.

Detrusor overactivity is one of the commonest causes of urinary incontinence. It arises idiopathically in 10–15% of the normal population or secondarily in up to 80% of males with bladder outlet obstruction; the prevalence of bladder overactivity also increases with increasing age. It also occurs frequently in patients with central neurological lesions such as strokes, Parkinsonism, or multiple sclerosis and in spinal reflex bladders. Frequency, nocturia, urgency, and urge incontinence are the common symptoms encountered. These can occur on their own or more commonly in combination with the presenting symptoms of the underlying medical problem causing the incontinence. Detrusor overactivity is a urodynamic diagnosis. If it is secondary to an identifiable central neurological lesion, the term detrusor hyperreflexia is used. In cases where no upper motor neuron lesion is present, it is termed detrusor instability. The principal management of all incontinence is the provision of advice to the patient, the use of devices, catheters, pads, etc. In the context of detrusor overactivity, a combination of judicious fluid restriction to 1500 mL per day, bladder retraining and the use of anticholinergic agents is appropriate as first line management.

Detrusor underactivity is another cause of urinary incontinence. Many cases are idiopathic in origin, but neurological pathology must be excluded. In particular, it may result from a mechanical injury to the nerves supplying the bladder, such as in patients with prolapsed intervertebral discs or tumours involving the spine, or from pelvic plexus injury as a result of pelvic surgery, or autonomic neuropathy seen in diabetes, alcoholism, tabes dorsalis, Parkinsonism, or pernicious anemia. Alternatively, it can also result from the loss of detrusor muscle in patients with decompensated bladder outlet obstruction. Although the relationship between outlet obstruction and detrusor underactivity is accepted by many urologists, the fact that chronic outlet obstruction leads on to detrusor underactivity has still to be proven. This condition must always be considered in any elderly male presenting with incontinence. Many of these patients will be found to have a palpable bladder and a third will have significant renal impairment at the time of presentation.

Female patients may present with idiopathic urinary retention at two characteristic age groups: either young patients with a history of lifelong voiding dysfunction, who are subsequently found to have poorly relaxing urethral sphincters (of unknown aetiology), or in the fifth decade of life, where in some cases a long term history of infrequent voiding can be obtained.

The management of this group of conditions relies upon emptying the bladder; the most commonly used technique is to teach the patient intermittent self catheterisation. Urethral dilatation can be helpful in some patients, and following recovery of bladder function some male patients may benefit from prostatectomy.

Sphincteric causes of urinary incontinence are of particular importance in the female patient and result in the majority of cases from postobstetric sphincteric weakness. This is usually a combination of a weakness of the pelvic floor and denervation of the urethral sphincter mechanism as a consequence of damage to the somatic nerve supply mediated via the pudendal nerve. Therapy for this is based on initial treatment with pelvic floor exercises which will benefit up to 40% of patients. In the remaining patients surgery represents the mainstay of treatment and aims to correct prolapse and increase the bladder outflow resistance by resuspension or compression of the urethra. In the male patient sphincteric weakness can occur following lower urinary tract trauma but is usually iatrogenic in origin; the mainstay of treatment is the implantation of an artificial urinary sphincter.

Functional urinary incontinence refers to urinary incontinence that is not related to an objectively demonstrable lower urinary tract dysfunction but rather to loss of cognition, mobility, manual dexterity, motivation and the effect of enviromental demands. These factors are commonly involved in the development of urinary incontinence in the mentally handicapped and the elderly. However, functional incontinence is a diagnosis of exclusion, and one must not automatically assume that all urinary incontinence in the elderly or mentally handicapped is functional in nature, as a large number have urodynamic abnormalities that are amenable to treatment. These patients can be considerably improved by careful review of concomitant medication, attention to constipation, and the judicious use of the other measures mentioned above under the supervision of specialised nursing care.

Extra-urethral incontinence as a consequence of an ectopic ureter(s) presents early in life; fistulae are usually either as a consequence of obstetric mishaps (particularly in the developing world) or are iatrogenic in origin. These conditions will usually require surgical intervention.

PROSTATE OBSTRUCTION AND RETENTION OF URINE

Benign prostatic hyperplasia (BPH) is the most common disease to affect men of middle age and beyond; histological BPH is present in up to 50% of men above the age of 60 years and nearly 88% by age of 80. It is estimated that 25% of men in their sixth decade have urinary symptoms and objectively measureable bladder outflow obstruction.

Lower urinary tract symptoms (LUTS) are not disease specific since only 60–70% of patients with typical LUTS suggestive of BOO (bladder outflow obstruction) have proven obstruction on urodynamic studies.

Symptoms related to BPH can be divided into two groups: voiding and filling. Voiding symptoms are:

- hesitancy
- poor stream
- straining
- prolonged micturition
- feeling of incomplete emptying.

Filling/storage symptoms are:

- nocturia
- daytime frequency
- urgency
- urge incontinence
- overflow incontinence.

Baseline evaluation of a patient relies upon the three pillars of:

- a history including a symptom score and a voiding diary
- a physical examination that includes a digital rectal examination (DRE)
- diagnostic tests.

A voiding diary can be sent to the patient prior to his clinical visit and is particularly useful in the event of nocturia and daytime frequency which are affected by patterns of fluid intake.

Appropriate evaluation of the symptomatic patient relies upon a careful clinical history augmented by the use of a symptom score such as the International Prostate Symptom Score (IPSS), a physical examination including a digital rectal examination and the use of appropriate diagnostic tests such as routine biochemistry, an MSU and a serum PSA, and prostate biopsy possibly combined with a transrectal ultrasound scan in appropriate patients to exclude malignancy (see Box 18.5).

The only blood test that is considered standard is the urea and electrolytes; serum creatinine is routinely used

Box 18.5   Assessment of lower urinary tract symptoms

- *Symptoms.* Quality of life. Urinary symptoms: degree of bother (International Prostate Symptom Score). Enquire about the presence of haematuria, neurological disease, medication, polyuria and urinary tract infection.
- *Physical examination.* General examination. Abdominal examination and digital rectal examination is essential.
- *Uroflowmetry.* Determine maximum flow rate, flow pattern and volumes voided. Patients with BOO tend to produce a typical flow pattern with a delayed and reduced maximum flow rate. Generally, maximum flow rate <10 mL/s BOO is more than likely, while a flow rate of > 15 mL/s makes BOO unlikely. Flow rates vary; obtain at least two voids of preferably > 150 mL. A slow flow may be due to detrusor underactivity, especially when associated with increased postmicturition residual.
- *Post micturition residual volumes.* Obtained using transabdominal ultrasonography. Incomplete emptying essentially reduces functional bladder capacity, and this may account for the patient's symptoms or the propensity to develop complications. An increase in residual urine is a sign of bladder decompensation rather than obstruction per se.
- *Renal function.* Bladder outflow obstruction may contribute to renal failure.
- *PSA.* The use of this assay is controversial. Essentially, its use is recommended in patients where radical prostate surgery/radiotherapy would be an option should localised prostate cancer be diagnosed and to augment equivocal digital rectal findings.
- *Urinalysis.* Exclude urinary tract infection. Identify microscopic haematuria and pyuria.
- *Transrectal ultrasonography.* Used to aid in the diagnosis of prostate cancer and to guide prostate biopsy. It is also helpful in determining prostate size and morphology which may influence treatment options.
- *Prostate biopsy.* Required to make the histological diagnosis of prostate cancer.
- *Cystometry and videocystometrography.* Sensory and motor function of the bladder during filling may be observed. The relationship between voiding detrusor pressure and flow rate allows classification of patients into various degrees of obstruction. The presence of documented obstruction usually leads to a satisfactory outcome in 90% of patients. Surgery on unobstructed patients leads to less than optimal results. Cystometry is invasive and is restricted to selected patients: younger patients, predominately filling symptoms, underlying neurology, recurrent symptoms after previous prostate surgery and to determine the adequacy of detrusor function.
- *Cystoscopy.* Reserved for patients where underlying intravesical pathology is suspected and including patients with predominant filling symptoms, haematuria and repeated urinary tract infections.

in a serial fashion to follow an individual patient's clinical progress with regard to renal function. Other tests relevant to concomitant conditions may be included at this time, especially if surgery is likely. As many as 10% of patients with BOO may have renal insufficiency, and they have a risk of postoperative complications rising from 17% to 25% and a six-fold increased risk of death after surgical treatment of BPH. A raised serum creatinine should prompt the clinician to carry out further investigation. PSA is specific to the prostate but it is not disease specific. PSA is secreted by normal, hyperplastic and cancerous prostatic tissue and increased by urinary infections and any instrumentation of the prostate (although not significantly by a digital rectal examination). The reference ranges for PSA levels are agreed by general consent but are by no means absolute. Indeed, anywhere between 21% and 86% (depending on various studies) of men with BPH have a PSA above the upper limit of normal (for most assays > 4.0 ng/mL), making it a far from ideal screening test for carcinoma, as it is only moderately sensitive, not very specific, and gives many false positives which need to be excluded by other techniques.

The actual quantification of BOO relies on the judicious use of urodynamics incorporating flow rate, transabdominal ultrasound for postmicturition residual volumes, and pressure flow studies.

Complications

Acute retention of urine occurs in a small proportion of men presenting with a history of bladder outflow obstruction, the incidence of this complication having been estimated to be approximately 2.5% of this group of men per year. Acute retention of urine is characterised by painful inability to void, and the residual obtained is around 1 L. This is in contrast to chronic retention, which is of insidious onset, characteristically painless, associated with renal dysfunction in 30% of cases and where the residual obtained may well exceed 2 L; whilst it is presumed that chronic retention follows longstanding obstruction, it has been suggested that it may originate as a consequence of pathology other than chronic BOO. Other serious complications of symptomatic BPH are relatively uncommon in contemporary practice, but include bladder stone formation, stasis (residuals, diverticula) leading to urinary infection and recurrent haematuria.

DISORDERS OF THE FEMALE REPRODUCTIVE SYSTEM

The surgical trainee should know enough gynaecological pathology to diagnose gynaecological conditions that may present to the surgical clinic or as surgical emergencies.

Disorders of the uterus

Fibroleiomyoma (fibroid)

Fibroids are common tumours of smooth muscle origin. They grow during the reproductive years but regress after the menopause, but do not completely disappear. They are firm, white, whorled, well-circumscribed lesions which may be submucous, subserosal, or intramural. The subserosal variety may be pedunculated. Their aetiology is unknown. Clinically they may present as follows:

- abdominal mass
- abnormal uterine bleeding
- urinary problems due to pressure on the bladder
- pain due to complications, e.g. red degeneration, torsion of the pedicle of a pedunculated fibroid.

Complications include cystic degeneration, necrosis with haemorrhagic infarction (red degeneration) and dystrophic calcification (calcified fibroids may be seen on abdominal x-ray). Sarcomatous change is extremely rare.

Endometriosis

This is the presence of endometrial glands and stroma in sites other than the body of the uterus. The sites include:

- ovaries (80%)
- round ligaments
- fallopian tubes
- pelvic peritoneum
- intestinal wall
- umbilicus
- laparotomy scars
- lymph nodes (rare)
- lung and pleura (rare)
- synovium (rare).

The aetiology is unknown. In the peritoneal cavity retrograde menstruation may be important but this certainly cannot explain the spread to distant sites. The endometrial tissue retains its senstivities to hormones and bleeding occurs into the lesions at the time of menstruation. Fibrosis may occur at the site of the lesion. In the peritoneal cavity this may lead to adhesion formation.

Endometrial carcinoma

Two types are recognised. The first type occurs in young women with the polycystic ovary syndrome or in peri-menopausal women. It may complicate postmenopausal oestrogen replacement therapy. This type usually is associated with a good prognosis. The second type affects elderly postmenopausal women and does not appear to be oestrogen related. It is poorly differentiated with deep myometrial invasion and carries a poor prognosis.

Aetiological factors for endometrial carcinoma include obesity, hypertension, diabetes mellitus, nulliparity and long term tamoxifen therapy.

Spread occurs by direct extension into the pelvis and adjacent viscera as well as to the iliac and para-aortic nodes and via the blood stream to the liver and lungs.

Fallopian tubes

These may be the sites of inflammation, cysts, pregnancy, or neoplasia.

Inflammation (salpingitis)

This is usually due to ascending infection from the uterine cavity. It may be acute or chronic. Organisms involved include *Chlamydia*, *Bacteroides*, *E. coli* and *N. gonorrhoea*. Clinical presentation may resemble acute appendicitis. Suppuration may occur with development of a tubule abscess (pyosalpinx). Longstanding chronic inflammation may lead to distension of the tube, loss of mucosa, and accumulation of a watery fluid (hydrosalpinx). Inflammation may also lead to loss of tubal patency with the development of secondary infertility.

Cysts

Small benign fimbrial cysts are common. They cause abdominal pain by undergoing torsion.

Ectopic pregnancy

The fallopian tube is the commonest site for ectopic pregnancy. The incidence is 10 per 1000 pregnancies in the UK. The presenting symptoms are due to distension of the tube. The common presenting symptoms are:

- lower abdominal pain
- rupture with haemoperitoneum.

Ovary

Cysts

Both the normal follicle and corpus luteum are cystic. Retention cysts form quite frequently and by definition must be greater than 2 cm. Luteal cysts are lined by an inner layer of large luteinised granulosa cells and outer thecal cells. They may rupture with slight haemorrhage into the peritoneal cavity. Follicular cells have an inner layer of granulosa cells and contain clear fluid. They are often multiple. 'Chocolate' cysts of the ovary are a feature of endometriosis.

Tumours

Ovarian tumours may be divided into five main categories:

- epithelial
- germ cell
- sex-cord stromal
- metastatic
- miscellaneous.

Epithelial tumours

The majority of ovarian tumours are derived from the surface epithelium. There are several varieties which depend upon their embryonic differentiation. One group of these is the mucinous type, which may be benign or malignant. A benign mucinous cystadenoma may grow to a very large size, filling the peritoneal cavity, and may be mistaken for ascites. Benign tumours may rupture, releasing tumour cells which seed in the peritoneum and continue to produce mucus (pseudomyxoma peritonei). This condition carries a poor prognosis and is often complicated by intestinal obstruction. Some tumours are borderline between cystadenoma and cystadenocarcinoma. The commonest malignant ovarian tumour is the scrous carcinoma. They occur most frequently in women between 40 and 60 years. They may be largely cystic (25%) semisolid (65%), or entirely solid (10%).

Germ cell tumours

These may be either benign or malignant. The commonest is the benign or mature cystic teratoma (dermoid cyst). It may present at any age, although usually in younger patients, as a smooth-walled unilateral ovarian cyst. It characteristically contains hair, sebaceous material and teeth, the latter often being apparent on a plain abdominal x-ray. They may undergo torsion. Malignant transformation is rare.

Sex-cord stromal tumours

These form about 5% of all ovarian tumours, with fibromas comprising about half the cases. Ovarian fibromas are not associated with steroid hormone production as are other sex-cord stromal tumours, e.g. thecoma, granulosa cell tumour, Sertoli–Leydig tumours. Meig's syndrome occurs in approximately 1% of patients with ovarian fibromas and includes ascites and pleural effusions which disappear following removal of the ovarian fibroma.

Metastatic tumours

Large intestine, stomach and breast are the most common sites giving rise to metastatic tumours of the ovary. Krukenberg tumours of the ovaries relate specifically to secondary deposits of signet-ring mucus-secreting adenocarcinoma, usually of gastric origin.

Clinical presentations of ovarian tumours include:

- pain
- rupture or torsion of a cyst
- abdominal mass
- ascites — peritoneal seedlings, pseudomyxoma peritonei, Meig's syndrome
- excess hormone production — abnormal uterine bleeding with oestrogen production; virilisation due to androgen production
- pleural effusion — Meig's syndrome, lung secondaries
- symptoms of other distant metastases.

Index

Index

M

1. Finish Raftery

2. Anatomy diagrams.
3. Physiology — Respiratory
— Cardio
Endocrine

4. Bayley
Fluid balance
Abdomen
Genito urinary.

5. Important topics.

Mon 26/9/05
Tue 27/9/05
Wed 28/9/05
Thr 29/9/05   : Revise.
Fri 30/9/05   : Revise
Sat 1/10/05   : Revise
Sun 2/10/05   : Revise
Mon 3/10/05   : Revise.
Tue 4/10/05   : Travel & relax
Wed. 5/10/2005   : Exam date.

Sun 25/9/05
Sat 24/9/05
Fri 23/9/05
Thur 22/9/05

Important points

1. Types of joints.
2.